Radionuclide Imaging of Infection and Inflammation

Elena Lazzeri • Alberto Signore
Paola Anna Erba • Napoleone Prandini
Annibale Versari • Giovanni D´Errico
Giuliano Mariani
Editors

Radionuclide Imaging of Infection and Inflammation

A Pictorial Case-Based Atlas

Second Edition

Springer

Editors
Elena Lazzeri
Regional Center of Nuclear Medicine
University Hospital of Pisa
Pisa
Italy

Paola Anna Erba
Department of Translational Research and
Advanced Technologies in Medicine and Surgery,
Regional Center of Nuclear Medicine
University of Pisa
Pisa
Italy

Annibale Versari
Nuclear Medicine
Azienda Unità Sanitaria Locale-IRCCS di Reggio Emilia
Reggio Emilia
Italy

Giuliano Mariani
Department of Translational Research and
Advanced Technologies in Medicine and Surgery,
Regional Center of Nuclear Medicine
University of Pisa
Pisa
Italy

Alberto Signore
Department of Medical-Surgical Sciences
and of Translational Medicine
Sapienza University of Rome
Roma
Italy

Napoleone Prandini
Nuclear Medicine Department
Azienda Ospedaliero-Universitaria di Modena
Modena
Italy

Giovanni D´Errico
Nuclear Medicine Department
Private Hospital "PIO XI"
Roma
Italy

ISBN 978-3-030-62177-3 ISBN 978-3-030-62175-9 (eBook)
https://doi.org/10.1007/978-3-030-62175-9

This Springer imprint is published by the registered company Springer Nature Switzerland AG
The registered company address is: Gewerbestrasse 11, 6330 Cham, Switzerland

Foreword

Molecular imaging with positron emission tomography (PET) and single-photon computed tomography (SPECT) combined with computed tomography (CT) is increasingly being used in Nuclear Medicine to diagnose, characterize, and monitor disease activity in the setting of infections and inflammatory disorders. Hybrid PET/CT and SPECT/CT both produce images based on the biodistribution of radiopharmaceuticals able to localize the inflammatory changes and to describe their response to therapy. Although several textbooks have been published on this subject, the most successful so far has been *Radionuclide Imaging of Infection and Inflammation: A Pictorial Case-Based Atlas* (published by Springer in 2013) that presented and discussed a whole host of clinical cases and imaging examples illustrating the manifestations of the commonly encountered infectious and inflammatory conditions.

This new textbook is the second edition of the same Atlas, still edited by *Elena Lazzeri, Alberto Signore, Paola Anna Erba, Napoleone Prandini, Annibale Versari, Giovanni D'Errico, and Giuliano Mariani*. Until now the first edition has been considered an important and successful reference for medical students, residents in nuclear medicine and radiology, and for all physicians involved in the management of patients with infection and inflammation. The main added value of the Atlas was both the high level of its scientific contents and the original structure of its educational contents. Alongside the description of the most important inflammatory and infectious diseases, the authors presented in each chapter a series of illustrated teaching cases with images of the most frequent scintigraphic findings, as well the anatomic variants and technical pitfalls. Thus, the reader had the opportunity to understand the pathophysiologic basis of infections and inflammation and to learn how to correctly interpret the images obtained with these studies.

Several years have now elapsed since that first very lucky edition, which received the general appreciation of the clinical and scientific community. Over this period scientific knowledge of the molecular mechanisms and biology of the inflammatory response has changed. The same happened for infections, which today show different patterns versus those most frequently observed previously; in particular, the spectrum of pathogen agents, including viruses, has changed over time and new infections have emerged. New guidelines and recommendations have been developed by scientific societies, some of them with direct or indirect effects on the indications for some nuclear medicine imaging procedures. Furthermore, important technological advances have taken place in nuclear medicine concerning both imaging instrumentation and radiopharmaceuticals.

The above reasons stimulated the authors to implement, integrate, and enlarge the first edition of the Atlas to become this textbook. This second edition maintains the same excellent original structure based on accurate information on the diseases, technologies, and case reports with a high number of associated images, addressing the common questions and problems that arise in the daily practice. Furthermore, the number of chapters has been increased from 13 to 16, the new chapters being devoted to miscellaneous bone and joint conditions, to inflammatory vessels' disease (vasculitis and atherosclerosis), and to infections and inflammation in pediatrics. All the chapters have been modified and/or rewritten to address the latest advancements in the field. References have been carefully updated and new clinical cases have been included and discussed according to the most recent protocols and guidelines.

This new edition of the Atlas is still organized by clinical entity, and all issues are clearly presented, well illustrated, and referenced. Clinical cases at the end of each chapter offer a good teaching tool that refreshes and supports the concepts discussed in the main text. The illustrations are of very high quality, most of them being illustrated with hybrid imaging. The contents of the textbook cover all indications of nuclear medicine imaging in the current scenario of infections and inflammation. The book begins with the normal findings by using different radiopharmaceuticals and techniques, discussing variants and pitfalls. The following three chapters are devoted to imaging of soft tissue infections, bone and joint infections, and imaging of miscellaneous bone and joint conditions. Joint prosthesis infections and peripheral bone infections, vascular prosthesis infections, and nonorthopedic or cardiovascular implantable device infections are discussed in the following chapters. Other chapters are dedicated to some less known or less frequent conditions, such as inflammation of the head and neck region (including the central nervous system), infective endocarditis and cardiovascular implantable electronic devices, and fever of unknown origin. The textbook also presents abdominal infections and inflammations, diabetic foot infections, lung infections, chronic inflammatory diseases, inflammatory vascular diseases, vasculitis and atherosclerosis, and finally infections and inflammation in pediatrics.

In conclusion, this renewed Atlas continues to offer an excellent example of a modern and educational textbook, which is intended to disseminate worldwide the most up-to-date knowledge on the current role of nuclear medicine in the field. The authors, among the most experienced and distinguished professionals in this field, accomplished a great work to keep the contents of this text at the highest level, and through a multidisciplinary approach they have implemented an exceptional learning tool very useful for all physicians with interest in radionuclide imaging of infection and inflammation.

Bergamo, Italy
May 2020

Emilio Bombardieri

Preface

Why a second edition of *Radionuclide Imaging of Infection and Inflammation: A Pictorial Case-Based Atlas*? This is the question that most people looking at this textbook will wonder about. The answer is easy: being an atlas of images and interesting cases, there are always more cases and more educational images to add, in order to improve the understanding of the role of nuclear medicine imaging in the field of infection and inflammation. Furthermore, in the time elapsed since the first edition the role of [^{18}F]FDG PET/CT for imaging infection and/or inflammation has greatly expanded. At the same time, hybrid imaging with SPECT/CT has revived interest in single-photon imaging for infection, and new radiotracers are being developed for imaging of infection/inflammation.

It comes as a second consideration that this new edition is not intended to merely replace the first one, but rather to integrate it—so that the two editions will constitute a unicum, a full educational tool for all physicians with interest in radionuclide imaging of infection and inflammation.

As in the first edition of the book, we kept the same chapters, but raised the number from 13 to 16 in order to address the growing applications of radionuclide imaging for infection and inflammation, with particular emphasis on inflammatory vessels' conditions, such as vasculitis and atherosclerosis and on infection and inflammation in pediatrics.

Furthermore, the structure of each chapter has been modified to include learning objectives for each chapter and key learning points for each condition. This is an important modification that provides to the reader the possibility to quickly focus on the most relevant aspects for correct interpretation of images.

Finally, the most relevant feature of this second edition is that text and images have been prepared according to the multidisciplinary guidelines developed by the European Association of Nuclear Medicine (EANM) in conjunction with several other European societies of clinicians and radiologists; a list of the most relevant of such joint guidelines is reported in the next page. Therefore, this textbook is not the mere result of the experience of a group of Italian nuclear medicine physicians, but rather the summary of a wide international experience in the field. Indeed, some of the authors have been involved for several years in international task groups or committees of several world leading scientific societies.

This upgrade makes the book a modern and up-to-date reference manual for students and physicians who are approaching or already working in this field of nuclear medicine.

Rome, Italy — Alberto Signore
Rome, Italy — Giovanni D'Errico
Pisa, Italy — Paola Anna Erba
Pisa, Italy — Elena Lazzeri
Modena, Italy — Napoleone Prandini
Reggio Emilia, Italy — Annibale Versari
Pisa, Italy — Giuliano Mariani
April 2020

List of International Guidelines on Radionuclide Imaging of Infection/Inflammation Imaging (Most Recent Publications Listed First)

Dorbala S, Ando Y, Bokhari S, Dispenzieri A, Falk RH, Ferrari VA, et al. ASNC/AHA/ASE/EANM/HFSA/ISA/SCMR/SNMMI expert consensus recommendations for multimodality imaging in cardiac amyloidosis: part 2 of 2—diagnostic criteria and appropriate utilization. J Nucl Cardiol. 2020;27:659–73.

Dorbala S, Ando Y, Bokhari S, Dispenzieri A, Falk RH, Ferrari VA, et al. ASNC/AHA/ASE/EANM/HFSA/ISA/SCMR/SNMMI expert consensus recommendations for multimodality imaging in cardiac amyloidosis: part 1 of 2—evidence base and standardized methods of imaging. J Nucl Cardiol. 2019;26:2065–123.

Lazzeri E, Bozzao A, Cataldo MA, Petrosillo N, Manfrè L, Trampuz A, et al. Joint EANM/ESNR and ESCMID-endorsed consensus document for the diagnosis of spine infection (spondylodiscitis) in adults. Eur J Nucl Med Mol Imaging. 2019;46:2464–87.

Sconfienza LM, Signore A, Cassar-Pullicino V, Cataldo MA, Gheysens O, Borens O, et al. Diagnosis of peripheral bone and prosthetic joint infections: overview on the consensus documents by the EANM, EBJIS, and ESR (with ESCMID endorsement). Eur Radiol. 2019;29:6425-6438.

Signore A, Sconfienza LM, Borens O, Glaudemans AWJM, Cassar-Pullicino V, Trampuz A, et al. Consensus document for the diagnosis of prosthetic joint infections: a joint paper by the EANM, EBJIS, and ESR (with ESCMID endorsement). Eur J Nucl Med Mol Imaging. 2019;46:971–88.

Glaudemans AWJM, Jutte PC, Cataldo MA, Cassar-Pullicino V, Gheysens O, Borens O, et al. Consensus document for the diagnosis of peripheral bone infection in adults: a joint paper by the EANM, EBJIS, and ESR (with ESCMID endorsement). Eur J Nucl Med Mol Imaging. 2019;46:957–70.

Slart RHJA; Writing group; Reviewer group; Members of EANM Cardiovascular; Members of EANM Infection & Inflammation; Members of Committees, SNMMI Cardiovascular; Members of Council, PET Interest Group; Members of ASNC; EANM Committee Coordinator. FDG-PET/CT(A) imaging in large vessel vasculitis and polymyalgia rheumatica: joint procedural recommendation of the EANM, SNMMI, and the PET Interest Group (PIG), and endorsed by the ASNC. Eur J Nucl Med Mol Imaging. 2018;45:1250–69.

Signore A, Jamar F, Israel O, Buscombe J, Martin-Comin J, Lazzeri E. Clinical indications, image acquisition and data interpretation for white blood cells and anti-granulocyte monoclonal antibody scintigraphy: an EANM procedural guideline. Eur J Nucl Med Mol Imaging. 2018;45:1816–31.

Van den Wyngaert T, Strobel K, Kampen WU, Kuwert T, van der Bruggen W, Mohan HK, et al. The EANM practice guidelines for bone scintigraphy. Eur J Nucl Med Mol Imaging. 2016;43:1723–38.

Bucerius J, Hyafil F, Verberne HJ, Slart RH, Lindner O, Sciagrà R, et al. Position paper of the Cardiovascular Committee of the European Association of Nuclear Medicine (EANM) on PET imaging of atherosclerosis. Eur J Nucl Med Mol Imaging. 2016;43:780–92.

Habib G, Lancellotti P, Antunes MJ, Bongiorni MG, Casalta JP, Del Zotti F, et al. 2015 ESC guidelines for the management of infective endocarditis: the Task Force for the Management of Infective Endocarditis of the European Society of Cardiology (ESC). Endorsed by: European

Association for Cardio-Thoracic Surgery (EACTS), the European Association of Nuclear Medicine (EANM). Eur Heart J. 2015;36:3075–128.

Jamar F, Buscombe J, Chiti A, Christian PE, Delbeke D, Donohoe KJ, et al. EANM/SNMMI guideline for ^{18}F-FDG use in inflammation and infection. J Nucl Med. 2013;54:647–58.

Panes J, Bouhnik Y, Reinisch W, Stoker J, Taylor SA, Baumgart DC, et al. Imaging techniques for assessment of inflammatory bowel disease: joint ECCO and ESGAR evidence-based consensus guidelines. J Crohns Colitis. 2013;7:556–85.

de Vries EF, Roca M, Jamar F, Israel O, Signore A. Guidelines for the labelling of leucocytes with ^{99m}Tc-HMPAO. Inflammation/Infection Taskgroup of the European Association of Nuclear Medicine. Eur J Nucl Med Mol Imaging. 2010;37:842–8.

Roca M, de Vries EF, Jamar F, Israel O, Signore A. Guidelines for the labelling of leucocytes with ^{111}In-oxine. Inflammation/Infection Taskgroup of the European Association of Nuclear Medicine. Eur J Nucl Med Mol Imaging. 2010;37:835–41.

Contents

Contributors

Francesco Bandera Department of Biomedical Sciences for Health, University of Milan, Milan, Italy

Cardiology University Department, Heart Failure Unit, IRCCS Policlinico San Donato, San Donato Milanese, Milan, Italy

Francesco Bartoli Department of Translational Research and Advanced Technologies in Medicine and Surgery, Regional Center of Nuclear Medicine, University of Pisa, Pisa, Italy

Andrea Bedini Infectious Diseases Unit, Department of Medical and Surgical Sciences for Children and Adults, University Hospital "Policlinico di Modena", Modena, Italy

Florent L. Besson Department of Biophysics and Nuclear Medicine-Molecular Imaging, Hôpitaux Universitaires Paris-Saclay, Assistance Publique-Hôpitaux de Paris, CHU Bicêtre, Le Kremlin Bicêtre, France

Université Paris Saclay, CEA, CNRS, Inserm, BioMaps, Orsay, France

Jan Bucerius Department of Nuclear Medicine, University Medicine Göttingen, Georg-August-University Göttingen, Göttingen, Germany

Massimiliano Casali Nuclear Medicine, Azienda Unità Sanitaria Locale-IRCCS of Reggio Emilia, Reggio Emilia, Italy

Emanuele Casciani Department of Nuclear Medicine, Private Hospital "Pio XI", Rome, Italy

Giovanni D'Errico Department of Nuclear Medicine, Private Hospital "Pio XI", Rome, Italy

Paola Anna Erba Department of Translational Research and Advanced Technologies in Medicine and Surgery, Regional Center of Nuclear Medicine, University of Pisa, Pisa, Italy

Maria Carmen Garganese Nuclear Medicine Unit, Department of Imaging, "Bambino Gesù" Pediatric Hospital, Rome, Italy

Tiziana Lanzolla Nuclear Medicine Unit, AOU Sant'Andrea, Rome, Italy

Chiara Lauri Department of Medical-Surgical Sciences and of Translational Medicine, Sapienza University of Rome, Rome, Italy

Nuclear Medicine Unit, AOU Sant'Andrea, Rome, Italy

Elena Lazzeri Regional Center of Nuclear Medicine, University Hospital of Pisa, Pisa, Italy

Giuliano Mariani Department of Translational Research and Advanced Technologies in Medicine and Surgery, Regional Center of Nuclear Medicine, University of Pisa, Pisa, Italy

Napoleone Prandini Nuclear Medicine Department, Azienda Ospedaliero-Universitaria di Modena, Modena, Italy

Alberto Signore Department of Medical-Surgical Sciences and of Translational Medicine, Sapienza University of Rome, Roma, Italy

Nuclear Medicine Unit, AOU Sant'Andrea, Rome, Italy

Riemer H. J. A. Slart Medical Imaging Center, Department of Nuclear Medicine and Molecular Imaging, University of Groningen, University Medical Center Groningen, Groningen, The Netherlands

Department of Biomedical Photonic Imaging, Faculty of Science and Technology, University of Twente, Enschede, The Netherlands

Saadi Sollaku Department of Nuclear Medicine, Private Hospital "Pio XI", Rome, Italy

Martina Sollini Department of Biomedical Sciences, Humanitas University, Pieve Emanuele, Italy

Humanitas Clinical and Research Center - IRCCS, Rozzano, Italy

Annibale Versari Nuclear Medicine, Azienda Unità Sanitaria Locale-IRCCS di Reggio Emilia, Reggio Emilia, Italy

Maria Felicia Villani Nuclear Medicine Unit, Department of Imaging, "Bambino Gesù" Pediatric Hospital, Rome, Italy

Roberta Zanca Department of Translational Research and Advanced Technologies in Medicine and Surgery, Regional Center of Nuclear Medicine, University of Pisa, Pisa, Italy

Normal Findings with Different Radiopharmaceuticals, Techniques, Variants, and Pitfalls

1

Annibale Versari and Massimiliano Casali

Contents

A. Versari (✉) ·
Nuclear Medicine, Azienda Unità Sanitaria Locale-IRCCS di Reggio Emilia, Reggio Emilia, Italy
e-mail: annibale.versari@ausl.re.it

M. Casali
Nuclear Medicine, Azienda Unità Sanitaria Locale-IRCCS of Reggio Emilia, Reggio Emilia, Italy

E. Lazzeri et al. (eds.), *Radionuclide Imaging of Infection and Inflammation*, https://doi.org/10.1007/978-3-030-62175-9_1

Learning Objectives

- To acquire basic knowledge on the main nuclear medicine techniques applied to the diagnosis and monitoring of inflammatory and infectious processes
- To focus the attention on biodistribution, normal variants and the main diagnostic pitfalls of the "old" and the "newest" nuclear medicine agents, the latter including radiolabeled UBI-fragments, [^{18}F]FDG-labeled leukocytes, ^{68}Ga-citrate, and ^{124}I-Fiualuridine for PET imaging
- To shed light on the possibile use of radiolabeled antibiotics for the scintigraphic detection of infections

1.1 Introduction

The pharmacokinetic and/or pharmacodynamic patterns of radiopharmaceuticals in patients may be affected by several factors including a variety of drugs, disease states, and, in some cases, surgical procedure [1]. Among the factors that can change radiopharmaceutical biodistribution, co-administration of interfering drugs is the most commonly reported occurrence [2]. Drug–radiopharmaceutical interactions may arise as a result of the mode of drug action, of physico-chemical interactions between drugs and radiotracers, and of competition for common binding sites [2–4]. Table 1.1 lists drugs that can interfere with the biodistribution of ^{67}Ga-citrate, radiolabeled autologous leukocytes, and [^{18}F]FDG in patients [5].

Also faulty radiopharmaceutical preparation (including contamination during dispensing or administration and errors in the labeling procedure of autologous leukocytes with ^{111}In-oxine or ^{99m}Tc-HMPAO) may alter the subsequent biodistribution of radiopharmaceuticals, thus affecting the diagnostic quality of scintigraphic images [3, 6–12]. Although less commonly, radiopharmaceuticals may also interact with the syringe's or intravenous line's components [13, 14]. Also some lifestyle factors such as smoking, alcohol intake, and dietary habits (i.e., high-dose vitamins) have the potential of interacting with radiopharmaceuticals [15]. Furthermore, the use of monoclonal antibodies of murine origin may induce generation of human antimouse antibodies (HAMA), which can lead to allergic reactions and altered pharmacokinetics upon repeated injections [16].

Finally, technical pitfalls that may affect the results of imaging include equipment-related artifacts (i.e., inadequate quality-control procedures/calibration) as well as image processing-related artifacts (i.e., misregistration of the CT component with the SPECT or PET component), patient-related artifacts (i.e., patient motion) [6], and radiopharmaceutical extravasation during administration [6, 17, 18] (Fig. 1.1).

Tables 1.2 and 1.3 summarize the main pathophysiological characteristics and biodistribution of the radiopharmaceutical preparations discussed in this chapter [16].

Table 1.1 Drugs that can interfere with biodistribution of the radiopharmaceuticals/procedures most commonly employed for imaging inflammatory and infectious diseases (adapted from AIMN procedural Guide-Lines: http://www.aimn.it/pubblicazioni/LG/RP_AIMN_infezioni.pdf)

Radiopharmaceutical	Pharmaceutical class	Drug
^{67}Ga-citrate ^{68}Ga-citrate	Mineral supplements	Iron Calcium gluconate (parenteral)
	Chemotherapeutics	All
	Steroids	Prednisolone
Radiolabeled leukocytes	Beta lactam antibiotics	Cefalosporin
	Immunosuppressive	Azathioprine Cyclophosphamide
	Steroids	Prednisolone
	Calcium-antagonists	Nifedipine
	Anticoagulants	Heparin
	Sulfamide	Sulfasalazine
	Iron	Iron
[^{18}F]FDG	Steroids	Prednisolone
	Antiepileptics	Valproate Carbamazepine Phenytoin Phenobarbital
	Catecholamines	Catecholamines

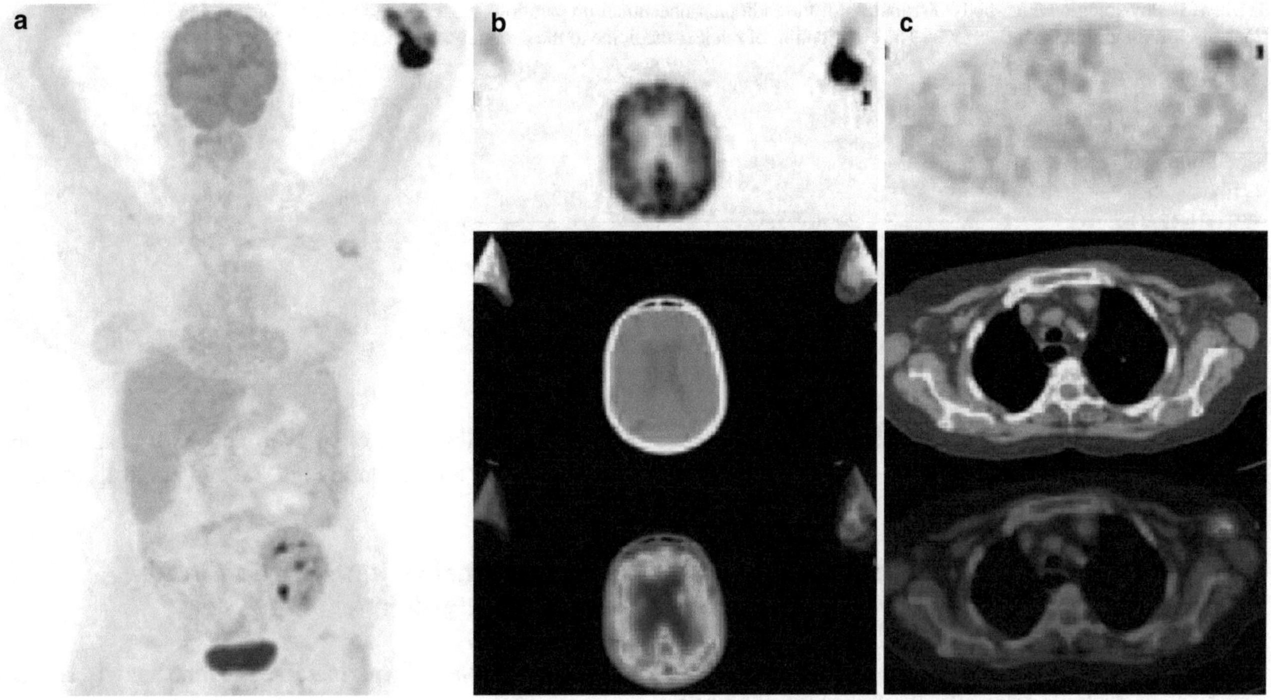

Fig. 1.1 MIP [^{18}F]FDG PET/CT image (**a**) shows intense radiopharmaceutical localization at injection site (left arm) as confirmed by transaxial views (**b**) associated with mild uptake in the left axilla (**c**) due to lymphatic drainage after [^{18}F]FDG extravasation during administration

Table 1.2 Targeting mechanisms of the radiopharmaceutical preparations most commonly employed for imaging inflammatory/infectious disease (modified from Laverman P et al. Current Radiopharmaceuticals. 2008)

Physiological characteristics	Targeting mechanism	Radiopharmaceutical
Enhanced vascular permeability	Transferrin and lactoferrin receptor binding	^{67}Ga-citrate ^{68}Ga-citrate
Enhanced vascular permeability and increased bone metabolism	Adsorption on hydroxyapatite crystals	^{99m}Tc-methylene diphosphonate (MDP)
Enhanced vascular permeability and endothelial activation	Uptake in activated endothelial cells	^{99m}Tc-sulfur colloid ^{99m}Tc-albumin nanocolloids
Enhanced vascular permeability and chemotactic activation	Chemotactic activation	Radiolabeled leukocytes (^{99m}Tc/[^{18}F]FDG)
Enhanced vascular permeability and cell binding	Antigen binding	^{99m}Tc-anti-NCA-95 IgG, BW 250/183, besilesomab (Scintimun®) ^{99m}Tc-anti-SSEA-1 IgM, falonesomab (Leu-Tech®, NutroSpec®) ^{99m}Tc-anti-NCA-90 Fab', Sulesomab (LeukoScan®)
Increased metabolic requirements	Enhanced glucose uptake in activated cells	[^{18}F]FDG
Incorporation into bacteria	Substrate of bacterial thymidine kinase	^{124}I-fialuridine
Electrostatic attraction to bacteria surface	Antimicrobial peptide (AMP) fragment	^{99m}Tc-ubiquicidin

Table 1.3 Physiologic whole-body distribution of the radiopharmaceutical preparations most commonly used for imaging inflammatory/infectious disease (modified from Becker W. The contribution of nuclear medicine to the patient with infection. Eur J Nucl Med. 1995)

Radiopharmaceutical	Liver	Spleen	Kidney	Bladder	Bowel	Bone cortical	Bone marrow	Blood
^{67}Ga/^{68}Ga-citrate	Yes	Yes	Yes	Yes	Yes	No	Yes	No
^{99m}Tc-MDP/HDP	No	No	Yes	Yes	No	Yes	No	No
^{99m}Tc-sulfur colloid and ^{99m}Tc-albumin nanocolloid	Yes	Yes	Yes	Yes	No	No	Yes	No
^{111}In-oxine-leukocytes	Yes	Yes	No	No	No	No	Yes	No
^{99m}Tc-HMPAO-leukocytes	Yes	Yes	Yes	Yes	Yes	No	Yes	No
^{99m}Tc-anti-granulocyte monoclonal antibodies	Yes	Yes	Yes	Yes	No	No	Yes	No
[^{18}F]FDG	Yes	Yes	Yes	Yes	No	No	No	No
Radiolabeled-UBI fragments	No	No	Yes	Yes	No	No	No	No
^{124}I-fialuridine	Yes	Yes	Yes	Yes	No	No	No	No

1.2 ^{67}Ga-Citrate Scintigraphy

1.2.1 Normal Biodistribution of ^{67}Ga-Citrate

About 10–25% of the injected activity is excreted through the kidneys during the first 24 h after administration, after which the principal route of excretion is the large bowel. By 48 h post injection, about 75% of the injected activity remaining in the body is equally distributed among the liver, bone/bone marrow, and soft tissues. ^{67}Ga-citrate localizes in bone marrow because it is incorporated as an iron analog into forming red blood cells; some (low degree) localization in bone is due to the $^{67}Ga^{++}$ ion weakly mimicking distribution of the calcium ions. Localization in the nasopharynx, lacrimal glands, salivary, thymus, breasts, spleen, and genitalia occurs with variable degrees [19–21]. Typical whole-body and spot images acquired at 24 h and 72 h post-injection of ^{67}Ga-citrate are shown in Figs. 1.2 and 1.3, respectively.

1.2.2 Normal Variants in ^{67}Ga-Citrate Scintigraphy

1. Below 2 years of age, increased thymic activity is common [22].
2. Hilar lymph node localization (usually low grade) can be seen in adult patients, particularly in smokers [23].
3. Increased breast activity, which is otherwise generally faint and symmetric, although it can be more intense in patients with hyperprolactinemia (associated physiologically with pregnancy and lactation, but possibly caused by numerous drugs, renal failure, in addition to prolactin-

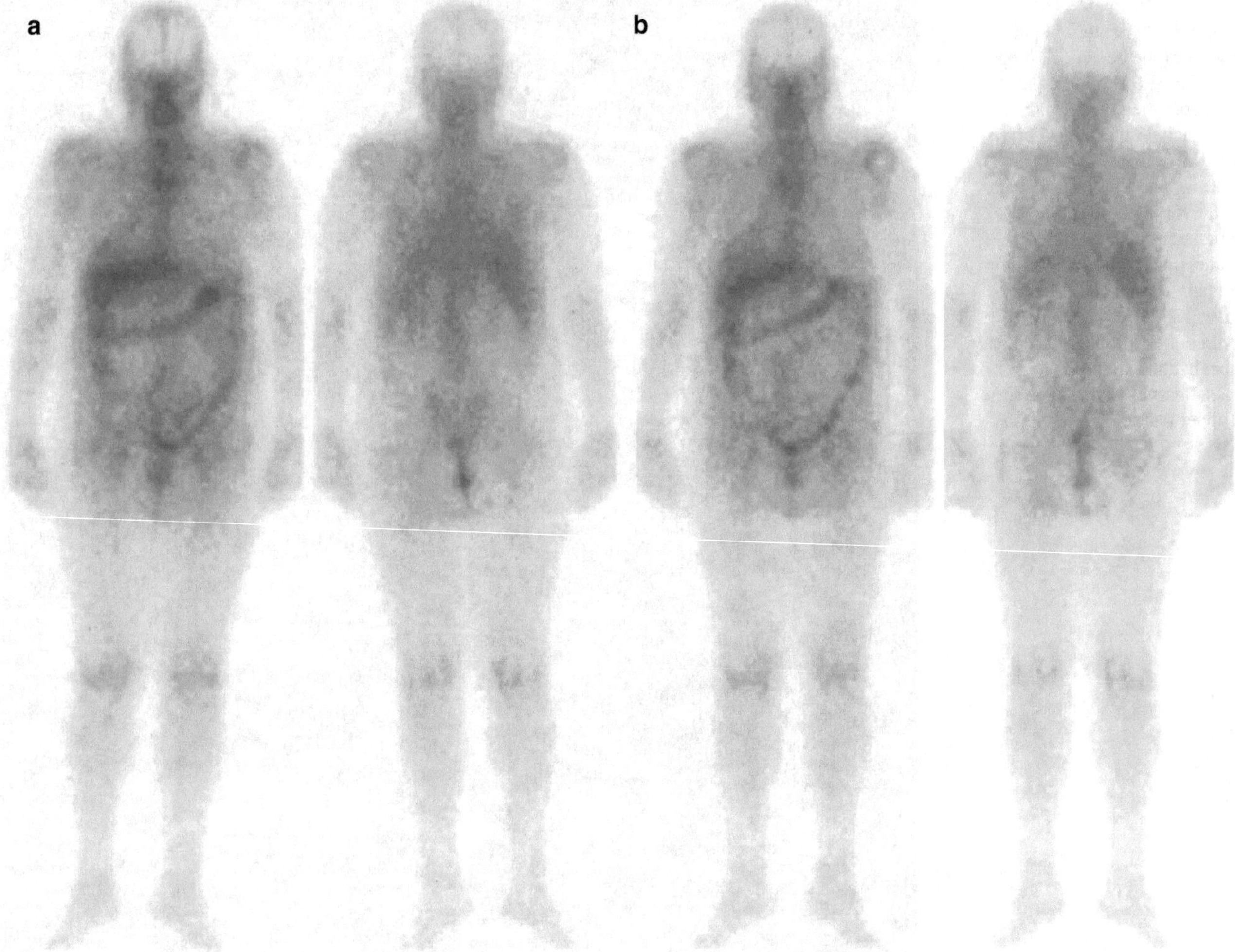

Fig. 1.2 ^{67}Ga-citrate scintigraphy: whole body images in anterior and posterior views obtained 48 h (**a**) and 72 h (**b**) after i.v. administration, showing physiologic biodistribution in the liver, bone and bone marrow, and soft tissues 48 h after injection. Similar pattern of distribution at 72 h. Both the images show radiopharmaceutical localization in the large bowel (major route of excretion from 24 h post-injection onward)

producing pituitary adenomas or to hypothalamic lesions which determine interruption of the hypothalamic–pituitary axis) [24, 25].

1.2.3 Pitfalls in ^{67}Ga-Citrate Scintigraphy

1. Residual bowel activity is probably the most common cause for both false-positive and false-negative interpretations [26], especially if planar images only are acquired rather than SPECT or preferably SPECT/CT images.
2. In children and teenagers, increased activity can be seen in case of thymic hyperplasia secondary to chemotherapy [27].
3. Gadolinium administered for MRI enhancement within 24 h before ^{67}Ga-citrate injection has been reported to decrease localization of the radiopharmaceutical at the sites of interest [28].
4. Saturation of iron-binding transferrin sites (i.e., hemolysis or multiple blood transfusions) causes altered ^{67}Ga distribution, thus resulting in increased renal, bladder, and bone activity and in reduced liver uptake and reduced accumulation in the colon [19].
5. ^{67}Ga uptake at sites of bone repair secondary to healing fractures (or prior orthopedic hardware sites, loose prostheses, or after successful treatment of osteomyelitis) may complicate interpretation in patients with suspected osteomyelitis [29].

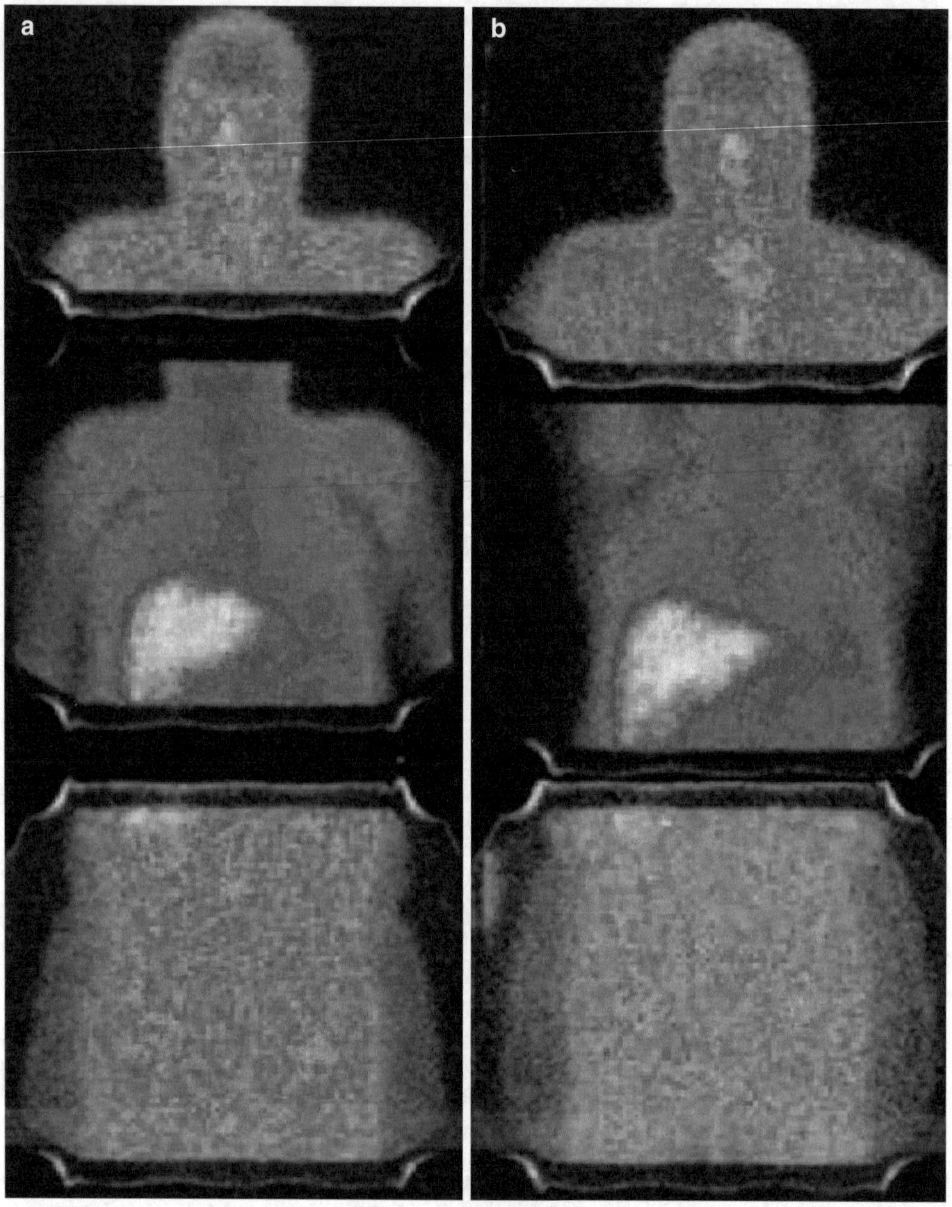

Fig. 1.3 Normal ^{67}Ga-citrate scintigraphy: anterior spot views of the head/neck (upper panels), chest (middle panels) and abdomen (lower panels) obtained 48 h (**a**) and 72 h (**b**) post-injection. Physiologic soft tissue visualization, with relatively intense tracer uptake in the liver (middle panels) and mild localization in pelvic bone and bone marrow (lower panels). Moderate radiopharmaceutical localization in the nasopharynx can also be seen (upper panels)

6. Recent chemotherapy and external beam radiation therapy [26].
7. Recent surgical wounds can induce increased radiopharmaceutical uptake, persisting up to 2 weeks after the event [29].
8. Uptake at cutaneous metal retention sutures, due to reaction at the site of insertion or other skin contact [29].
9. Desferoxamine therapy increases renal excretion of the tracer and enhances target-to-background ratios [30, 31].
10. Hilar, submandibular, and diffuse pulmonary localization in patients with lymphoma during therapy [20].
11. Radiation sialadenitis causes increased localization [32].
12. Possible uptake in a variety of tumors (i.e., lymphoma, lung cancer, mesothelioma, melanoma) [20, 33–37].
13. Physiologic liver uptake may be decreased in patients with AIDS or acute lymphocytic leukemia [26].
14. Diffusely increased pulmonary activity can occur in a variety of noninfectious disease as in cases of sarcoidosis, idiopathic pulmonary fibrosis, lymphoid interstitial pneumonitis, hypersensitivity pneumonitis, talc-induced granulomatosis, inhalational/occupational pulmonary diseases (asbestosis, berylliosis, coal worker pneumoconiosis, and silicosis), collagen vascular diseases (systemic lupus erythematosus and systemic sclerosis), eosinophilic pneumonia, multicentric reticulohistiocytosis, Wegener's granulomatosis, eosinophilic granuloma, drug toxicity (amiodarone, bleomycin, procarbazine, cyclophosphamide, nitrofurantoin, tocainide, busulfan), and reaction to iodinated contrast material (lipiodol) [38–62].

1.3 ^{99m}Tc-Diphosphonate (MDP/HDP) Scintigraphy

1.3.1 Normal Biodistribution of ^{99m}Tc-MDP/HDP

Excretion occurs primarily through the renal route, up to 70% of the injected activity being excreted within 6 h post-injection. Radiopharmaceutical uptake depends on local blood flow, osteoblastic activity, and extraction efficiency [6]. In a normal adult subject, the bone scan shows a higher concentration of activity in some parts of the skeleton, as in the spine (trabecular bone with large mineralizing bone surface), compared with the shafts of long bones (predominantly cortical bone) [63–68]. Renal and urinary bladder activities are normally present at the time of acquisition (about 3 h post-injection for a conventional bone scan) and minimal soft tissue activity is usually observed [6] (Fig. 1.4). This normal patten of distribution, however, is subject to considerable variation. In patients with significantly impaired renal function, the scans may be delayed to allow for better clearance of the extracellular fluid and vascular activity [67, 69].

1.3.2 Normal Variants in ^{99m}Tc-MDP/HDP Scintigraphy

1. Increased uptake at the confluence of sutures in the skull; this pattern can be more pronounced in patients with metabolic bone disease, such as renal osteodystrophy [65].
2. In elderly patients, increased uptake in the skull can be observed (especially in the frontal region and calvarium, due to hyperostosis frontalis interna) because of thickening of the frontal bones; such uptake can be more pronounced following chemotherapy in cancer patients, or in cases of metabolic bone disease [65].
3. Symmetrical or asymmetrical focal photopenia can be present in the parietal region, due to thinning of the parietal bone compared to the remaining portions of the skull [65].
4. Increased uptake at the manubriosternal junction [6].
5. A small photopenic defect (sternal foramina) surrounded by uniformly distributed radioactivity uptake can be observed in the inferior part of the sternum, due to the incomplete fusion of the cartilaginous bars in the distal sternum [65].
6. A vertical linear area of increased uptake can be seen distal to the sternum, due to benign tracer uptake in the xiphisternum [6].

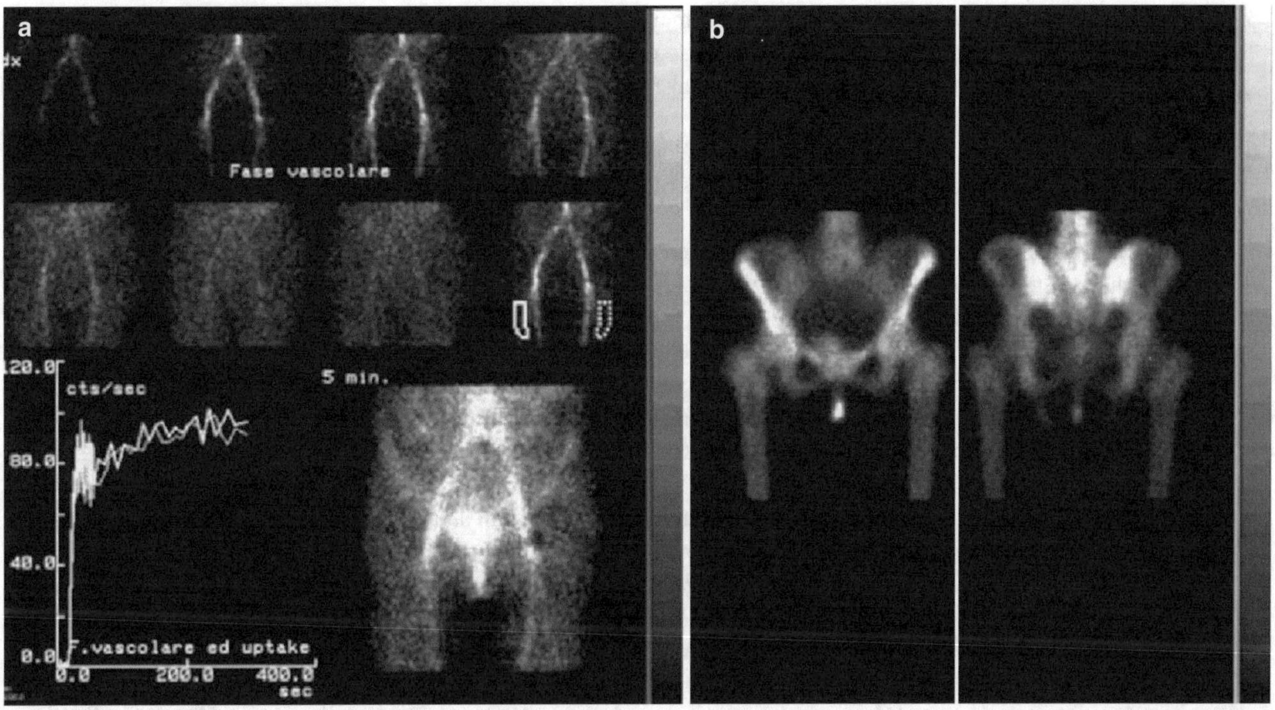

Fig. 1.4 ^{99m}Tc-MDP three-phase scintigraphy of the hip. (**a**) Arrival of the radiopharmaceutical in the region of interest; by drawing regions of interest (ROIs) on the suspected site of altered vascularization and on the corresponding contralateral, supposedly healthy site, it is possible to calculate time–activity curves. (**b**) Delayed scintigraphic acquisition (anterior and posterior images) obtained 3 h p.i., showing normal uptake of the pelvic bones

7. A focal area of increased uptake can be noted in the proximal/mid humeri at the site of insertion of skeletal muscles at the deltoid tuberosity [6].
8. Increased uptake in the pubic symphysis and possibly in the sacroiliac joints can be observed in women postpartum, as a consequence of increased stress reaction/pelvic diastases [65].
9. Diffuse breast uptake in women, especially if lactating [6].

1.3.3 Pitfalls in ^{99m}Tc-MDP/HDP Scintigraphy

1. Focally increased uptake in the mandible and/or maxillary bone is often due to underlying benign dental disorders [6].
2. Increased tracer uptake in the sinuses is frequently due to infection/inflammatory disease [6].
3. Hypertrophic pulmonary osteoarthropathy typically appears as symmetrically increased uptake of radiotracer in the cortices ("tram lines"), most often seen in the femora, tibiae, and wrists [6].
4. Decreased uptake in the presence of prosthesis (i.e., breast augmentation or orthopedic prosthesis) or metallic hardware (i.e., cardiac pacemaker), as well as at sites that have previously been included in an external beam radiation field [6].
5. Severe metabolic bone diseases may cause an abnormal radiopharmaceutical biodistribution (i.e., increased uptake at the confluence of head sutures, diffuse uptake in the calvarium) [65].
6. Symmetrical uptake in the acromioclavicular and/or sternoclavicular joint scan occur as consequence of degenerative disease [65].
7. Large vertical linear area of increased uptake in the sternum (sternal split) can be seen in patients who have undergone sternotomy [6].
8. A horizontal linear pattern of increased uptake in the vertebral body is typically observed in cases of vertebral fracture; however, it is difficult to distinguish fractures due to benign diseases, such as osteoporosis, from vertebral fractures due to a malignant condition [6].
9. Increased uptake in the patellae (hot patella sign), even if not be considered a real abnormal finding, can be seen in association with a wide variety of disorders, such as degenerative disease, Paget's disease, and osteomyelitis [65, 70].
10. In patients who have undergone recent surgery, such as knee or hip joint replacements, bone scintigraphy may result in false-positive findings [6].
11. Diffuse breast uptake in cases of gynecomastia induced by hormonal therapy in patients with prostate cancer. Focal breast uptake can be observed in other conditions, both benign and malignant [6].
12. Myocardial uptake can occur in case of myocardial necrosis/contusion, unstable angina, and ventricular aneurysm (focal pattern), or amyloidosis, hypercalemia, Adriamycin-induced cardiotoxicity, alcoholic cardiomyopathy, pericardial tumors, and pericarditis (diffuse pattern) [6].
13. Skeletal muscle uptake can be present in case of injury/trauma, renal failure, nontraumatic causes (i.e., alcoholic intoxication), scleroderma, polymyositis, carcinomatosis myopathy, muscular dystrophy, dermatomyositis, heterotopic bone formation/myositis ossificans (i.e., following direct trauma, complicated hip arthroplasty) [6].
14. Increased renal uptake can be observed after chemotherapy (vincristine, doxorubicin, cyclophosphamide) or in patients with nephrocalcinosis/hypercalcemia, iron overload, sickle cell disease, acute tubular necrosis (early stages), glomerulonephritis (diffuse pattern), and in the presence of obstructed collecting systems (focal pattern) [6].
15. Decreased renal uptake or non-visualization of the kidneys is generally observed as a consequence of nephrectomy, or in malignant/metabolic superscan. In cases of renal cyst, abscess, tumor, scarring as well as of partial nephrectomy, a focal area of reduced uptake can be observed [6].
16. Lung uptake can be observed in case of radiation pneumonitis, hyperparathyroidism, hypercalcemia, and, rarely, sarcoidosis [6].
17. Splenic uptake can be seen in case of Sickle cell disease, glucose-6-phosphtase deficiency, lymphoma, leukemia, and thalassemia [6].
18. Gastric uptake can be observed secondary to hypercalcemia with metastatic calcifications [6].
19. Bowel uptake can be observed in patients with surgical diversion, necrotizing enterocolitis, or ischemic bowel infarction [6].
20. Liver uptake can occur in the presence of amyloidosis and hepatic necrosis [6].
21. Soft tissue uptake can be observed in a variety of tumors (neuroblastoma, lung/liver tumors/metastases, breast tumors, sarcomas, malignant ascites/pleural effusion) [6].
22. Uptake in calcifications of the major arteries (i.e., femoral artery) [6].
23. Uptake in areas of cerebral infarct [6].

1.4 ^{99m}Tc-Sulfur Colloid and ^{99m}Tc-Albumin Nanocolloids

1.4.1 Normal Biodistribution of Radiocolloids

Following i.v. administration, the injected activity is rapidly cleared from the blood by the reticuloendothelial system (within approximately 2–4 h). About 55% of the

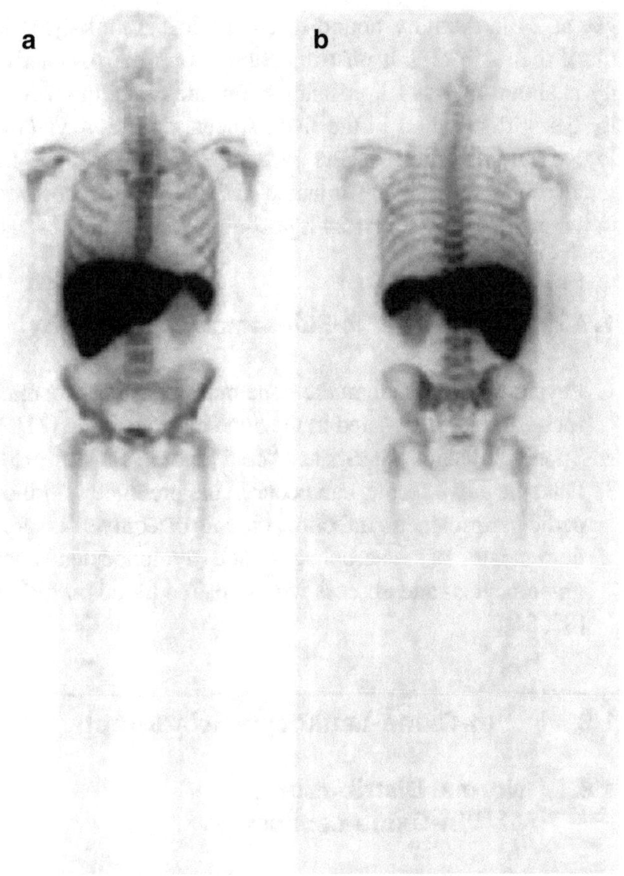

Fig. 1.5 Whole body scan following i.v. administration of 99mTc-albumin nanocolloids: anterior (**a**) and posterior (**b**) views show predominant uptake in the liver and spleen, with diffuse visualization of the hematopoietically active bone marrow

radiopharmaceutical is actively taken up by the reticuloendothelial system, to be degraded in the lysosomes of macrophages and excreted through the kidney within 24 h. An 80–90% of the injected particles is phagocytized by the Kupffer cells in the liver, 5–10% by macrophages in the spleen, and the remaining portion by macrophages in the bone marrow (see Fig. 1.5 for normal pattern of distribution as depicted in a whole body scan). However, uptake of the radiocolloid by the reticuloendothelial system is affected by both relative blood flow rates at the various sites and the functional capacity of the phagocytic cells, as well as by distribution of hematopoietically active marrow [21, 71].

1.4.2 Pitfalls in Radiocolloid Scintigraphy

1. Increased bone marrow uptake can be observed in case of aplastic anemia, myeloproliferative disease, and metastasis from solid tumors [72–74].

1.5 ^{99m}Tc-Besilesomab BW 250/183 (Scintimun®)

1.5.1 Normal Biodistribution of ^{99m}Tc-Besilesomab BW 250/183

About 10% of the injected activity is bound to neutrophils within 45 min post-administration, 20% of the radiopharmaceutical remaining free in the circulating blood. Up to 40% of the injected activity accumulates in the bone marrow [71, 75, 76] (see Fig. 1.6). Localization in the spleen, bowel, liver, bone marrow, thyroid, and kidney localizations is variable, occurring in up to 6%, to 4%, to 3%, and 2% of patients, respectively. Such normal distribution pattern is, however, subject to variation.

1.5.2 Pitfalls in ^{99m}Tc-Besilesomab BW 250/183 Scintigraphy

1. Physiological uptake in the bone marrow can mask small foci of infection located in the bone marrow space [71].
2. Spondylodiscitis and bone metastasis present as "cold" spots in the scan [75].
3. False-positive results can occur in case of myeloproliferative disease (i.e., multiple myeloma) [77].

1.6 ^{99m}Tc-Falonesomab (Leu-Tech®, NeutroSpec®)

1.6.1 Normal Biodistribution of ^{99m}Tc-Falonesomab

Following i.v. administration, activity is initially distributed in the circulating blood pool. The fraction bound to circulating neutrophils ranges between 11% and 51%, depending on neutrophil count. Bone marrow activity peaks shortly after administration (approximately 14% of injected activity at 2 h post-administration), with a longer washout time compared to background; the axial and appendicular bone marrow is well visualized. Spleen activity peaks at 5–12% of the injected amount 25–30 min post injection, declining to about half within 24 h. Similarly, rapid uptake is seen in the liver, with about 45–50% of the injected activity 35–65 min after administration, decreasing to 25–40% by 24 h. There is only minor retention of activity in the lungs [78]. Excretion occurs primarily through the renal route, radioactivity excreted in the urine being in the form of radiolabeled antibody fragments. Activity excreted through the gastrointestinal tract activity is variable [75, 79–82] (see Fig. 1.6).

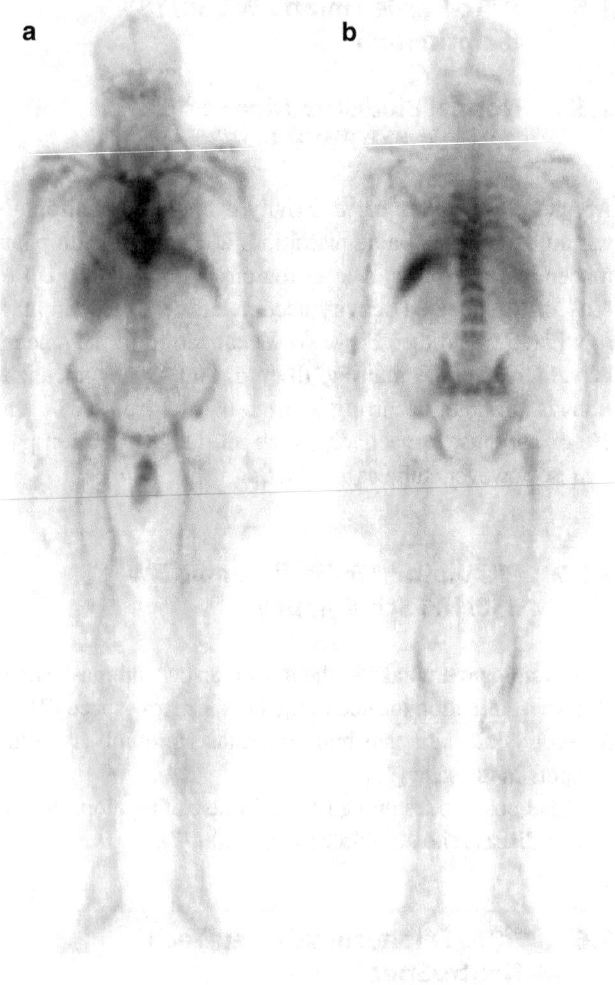

Fig. 1.6 Normal biodistribution of ^{99m}Tc-fanolesomab in the anterior and posterior views. Images obtained about 2 h after radiopharmaceutical administration (**a**) show activity within the cardiovascular system, genitourinary tract, liver, spleen, bone marrow, and soft tissues. By 24 h post injection of the radiolabeled antigranulocyte mAb, (**b**) blood pool activity has cleared and soft tissue activity has diminished, thus making bone marrow activity more prominent; diffuse colonic activity is also present. (Copyright permission from Love C et al. Imaging of infection and inflammation with ^{99m}Tc-fanolesomab. Q J Nucl Med Mol Imaging. 2006;50:113–20)

1.6.2 Pitfalls in ^{99m}Tc-Falonesomab Scintigraphy

1. Physiologic uptake in the bone marrow can mask small foci of infection located in the bone marrow space [71].

1.7 ^{99m}Tc-Sulesomab (LeukoScan®)

1.7.1 Normal Biodistribution of ^{99m}Tc-Sulesomab

About 25–34% of the injected activity circulates free in the blood 1 h after administration, declining to 17% at 4 h and 7% at 24 h. Activity bound to circulating granulocytes is more than 4% at 1 h post-injection. Bone marrow activity is about 43% at 1 h post-injection, the remaining activity being distributed in the liver, spleen, and kidneys (see Fig. 1.7). Excretion occurs virtually solely through the renal route, 41% of the injected activity being recovered in the urine over the first 24 h post-administration [81–84].

1.7.2 Pitfalls in ^{99m}Tc-Sulesomab Scintigraphy

1. Physiological uptake in the bone marrow can mask small foci of infection located in the bone marrow space [71].
2. Spondylodiscitis appears as a "cold" spot in the scan [75].
3. False-negative results can occur in the presence of orthopedic periprosthetic infection, chronic osteomyelitis (predominance of macrophages and lymphocytes over granulocytes) and abscess with impaired blood perfusion [85, 86].

1.8 ^{111}In-Oxine-Leukocyte Scintigraphy

1.8.1 Normal Distribution of ^{111}In-Oxine-Leukocytes

About 60% of the injected activity quickly localizes in the reticuloendothelial system of the liver, spleen, and bone marrow. There is only a transient migration of labeled cells in the lungs. The radiolabeled cells are cleared exponentially from the circulation, with a half-life between 5 and 10 h. Final distribution consists of about 20% of activity in the liver, 25% in the spleen, 30% in the bone marrow, and 25% in other organs. Images acquired up to 4 h post-injection may still show some pulmonary activity (Figs. 1.8 and 1.9). Clearance of activity from the liver and spleen is very slow. There is very low excretion of activity in both urine and feces, and no activity is normally observed in the bowel or bladder [87].

1.8.2 Normal Variants in ^{111}In-Oxine-Leukocyte Scintigraphy

1. Focal uptake can be seen in an accessory spleen [86].
2. Lymph node activity has been described in children—without however clinical significance [87–90].
3. Extramedullary hemopoiesis can result in lymph node activity [91].
4. Though usually solitary, multiple bilateral small round non-segmental lung foci of activity can occur, probably due to clumping of cells during the labeling process or during radiopharmaceutical injection; this occurrence may complicate interpretation of the images [85].

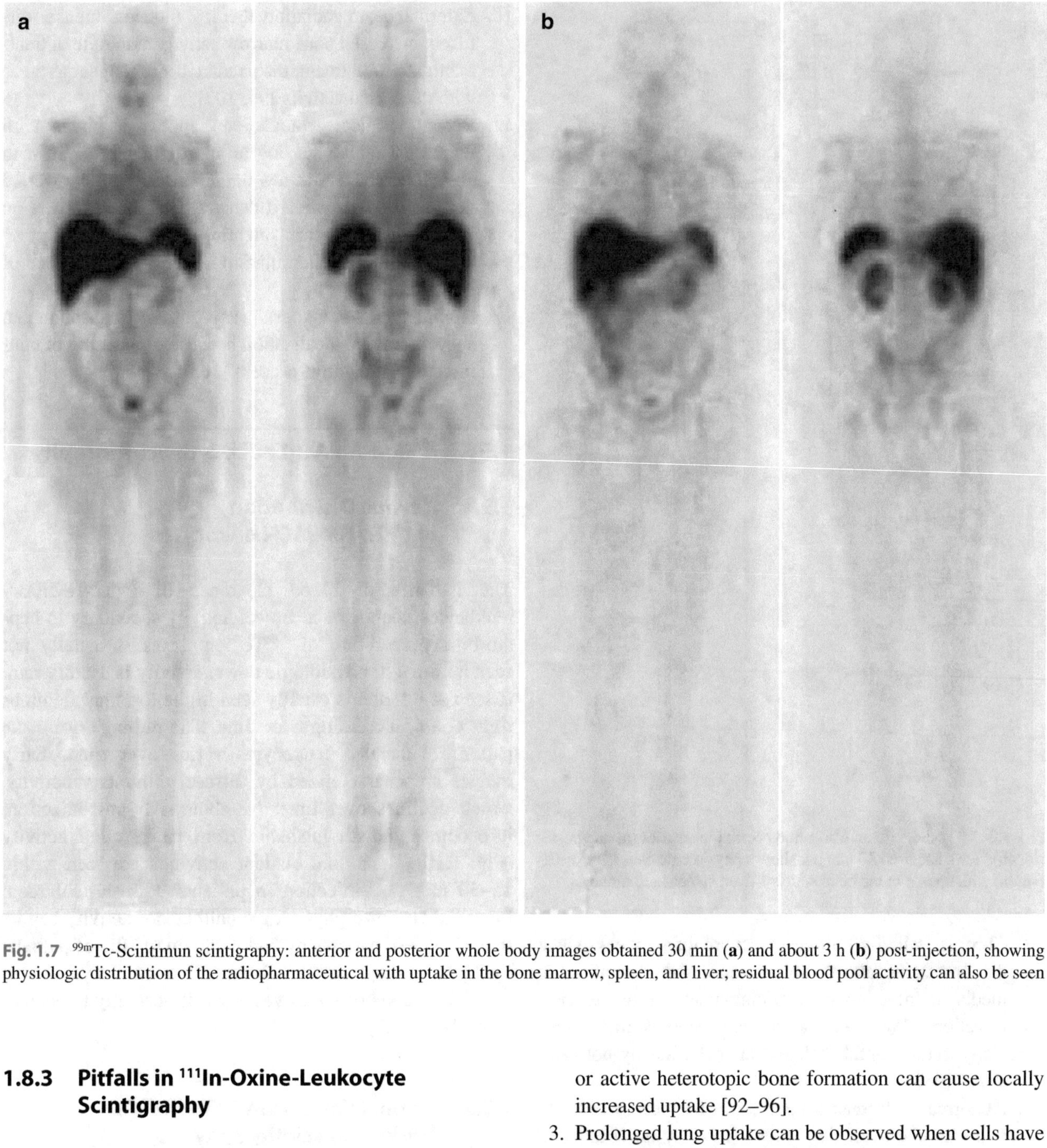

Fig. 1.7 ^{99m}Tc-Scintimun scintigraphy: anterior and posterior whole body images obtained 30 min (**a**) and about 3 h (**b**) post-injection, showing physiologic distribution of the radiopharmaceutical with uptake in the bone marrow, spleen, and liver; residual blood pool activity can also be seen

1.8.3 Pitfalls in ^{111}In-Oxine-Leukocyte Scintigraphy

1. In the presence of orthopedic hardware or prostheses, normal bone marrow is disrupted and displaced, making the interpretation of ^{111}In-oxine-leukocyte scintigraphy in these areas difficult [92].
2. Nonspecific bone/joint uptake can occur after bone marrow aspiration or at bone-graft donor sites and in the presence of traumatic/degenerative arthritis, gouty arthritis, acute fractures (less than 2 months), traumatic or neuropathic arthropathy, acute bone infarcts, or foreign body reaction. Although rarely, bone neoplasms (i.e., lymphoma with bone involvement) and metastasis, or active heterotopic bone formation can cause locally increased uptake [92–96].
3. Prolonged lung uptake can be observed when cells have been damaged during the labeling process.
4. Lung localization can be observed in cystic fibrosis and in patients with adult respiratory distress syndrome [85].
5. Focal uptake can be seen in cases of acute bleedings, hematomas, or recent myocardial/cerebral infarcts [21, 88].
6. Uptake can be observed in a variety of tumors (i.e., lymphoma, brain tumors) [92, 97].
7. Diffuse bowel uptake can occur in patients with noninfectious inflammatory bowel lesion(s) such as stomas, multiple enemas, gastrointestinal bleeding, or infarction [8].

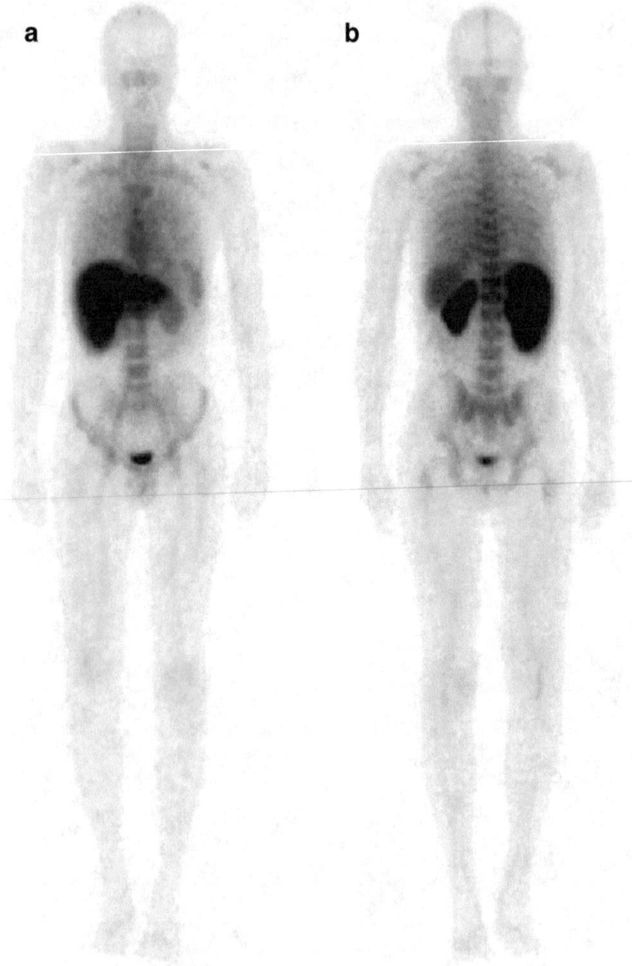

Fig. 1.8 ^{99m}Tc-Leukoscan whole body scan: the anterior (**a**) and posterior (**b**) views acquired 30 min p.i. show a physiologic pattern of distribution, with uptake in the bone marrow, liver, spleen, and kidneys

8. Chronic walled-off abscesses (more than 3 weeks since the onset), hepatic or splenic abscesses, lymphocytic mediated infection (i.e., granulomatous process, viral infection), low-grade or chronic osteomyelitis (especially in the central skeleton) are occasionally not visualized [98].
9. Abnormally decreased uptake can be seen in severely hypovascular/avascular sites (i.e., cysts, irradiated areas), implants (i.e., prostheses and cardiovascular implantable device), or spondylodiscitis (often appearing as focally decreased uptake compared with adjacent bone marrow) [21, 88, 99–101].
10. External beam radiation therapy induces intense, diffusely increased bone marrow activity at the site of treatment; after treatment, the irradiated sites appear as areas with decreased activity [99, 102].
11. Recent surgical wounds can appear as areas with increased uptake starting at approximately 72 h, with complete recovery in few days. When a surgical wound is not closed, or when it dehisces and is left to heal on its own by secondary intention, uptake persists as an area of intense accumulation—even in the absence of infection [21].
12. Noninfected vascular grafts and/or peritoneal shunts can show increased localization because of bleeding or noninfectious reparative process [103].

1.9 ^{99m}Tc-HMPAO-Leukocyte Scintigraphy

1.9.1 Normal Distribution of ^{99m}Tc-HMPAO-Leukocytes

The half-life of blood clearance of ^{99m}Tc-HMPAO-leukocytes is about 4 h. Bowel activity secondary to hepato-biliary secretion of ^{99m}Tc-complexes is usually not seen before 4 h; physiologic bowel activity is usually faint if seen at 4 h and is usually seen in the terminal ileum or right colon, increasing over time. The pulmonary uptake pattern of labeled leukocytes varies over time. Early images are characterized by diffuse pulmonary activity, which declines over time; by about 4 h post-injection, it becomes indistinguishable from background activity (Fig. 1.10). Renal and bladder activities are seen within 15–30 min post-injection in patients with normal renal function. Uniform physiologic gallbladder activity can be seen (in 4% of patients by 2–4 h and up to 10% of patients by 24 h). The spleen, liver, bone marrow, kidneys, bowel, bladder, and major blood vessels will normally be visualized [21, 71, 87].

1.9.2 Normal Variants in ^{99m}Tc-HMPAO-Leukocyte Scintigraphy

1. Bowel activity secondary to secretion of ^{99m}Tc-complexes can be detected in 20–30% of children as early as 1 h post-injection [102].

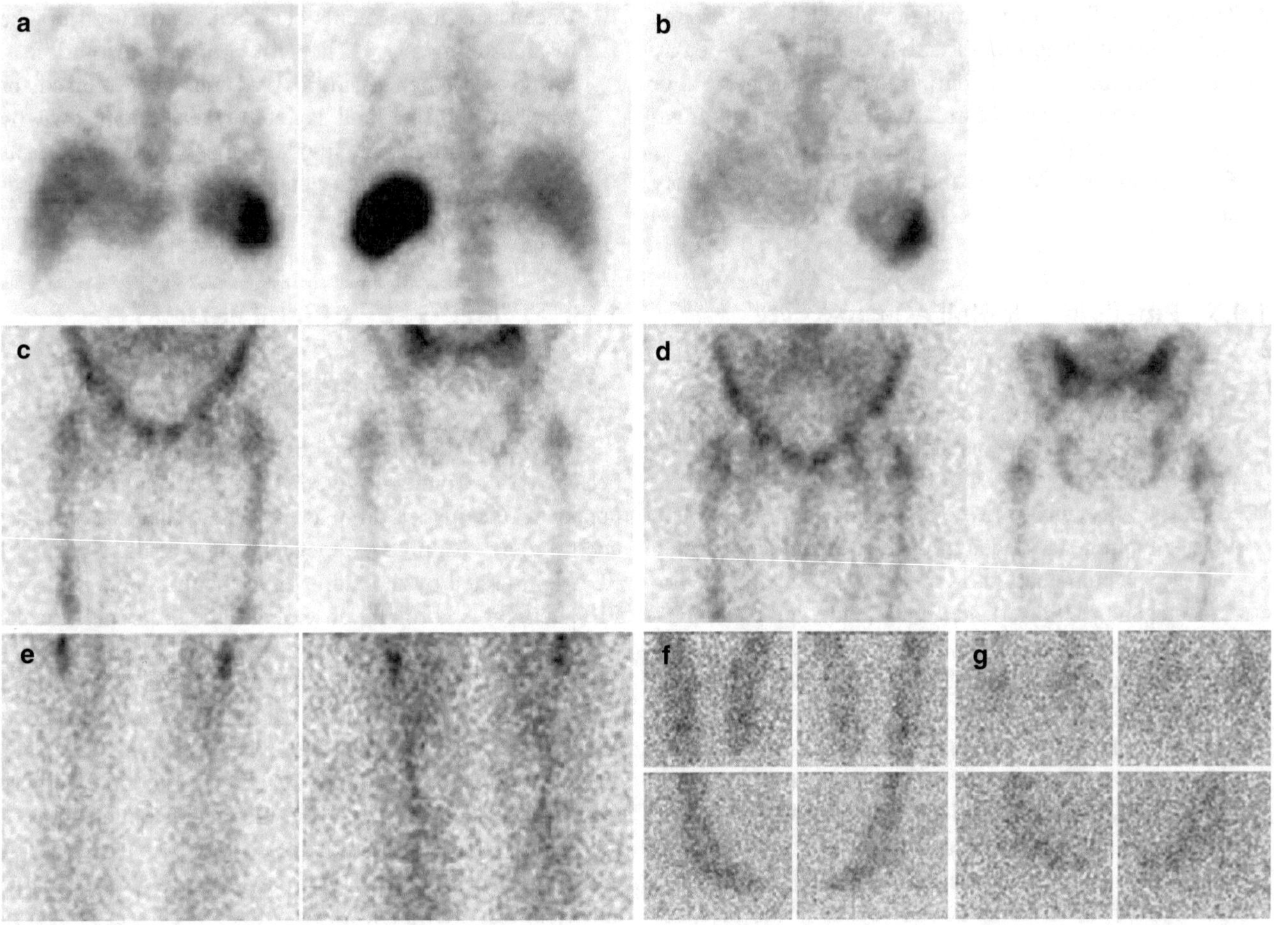

Fig. 1.9 ^{111}In-oxine-leukocyte scintigraphy. Planar spot views of the chest obtained 4 h (**a**) and 24 h (**b**) post injection. Early localization in the liver, spleen, and bone marrow (**a**), declining over time (**b**). Planar anterior and posterior spot views of the pelvis obtained 4 h (**c**) and 24 h (**d**) post injection show localization in the bone. Planar anterior and posterior views of the femora (**e**) obtained 24 h after administration show accumulation of the radiolabeled leukocytes in the bone marrow at the proximal portion of both femoral diaphyses. Planar spot views of the feet obtained 4 h (**f**) and 24 h (**g**) post injection obtained in anterior, posterior (upper panels) and lateral views (lower panels)

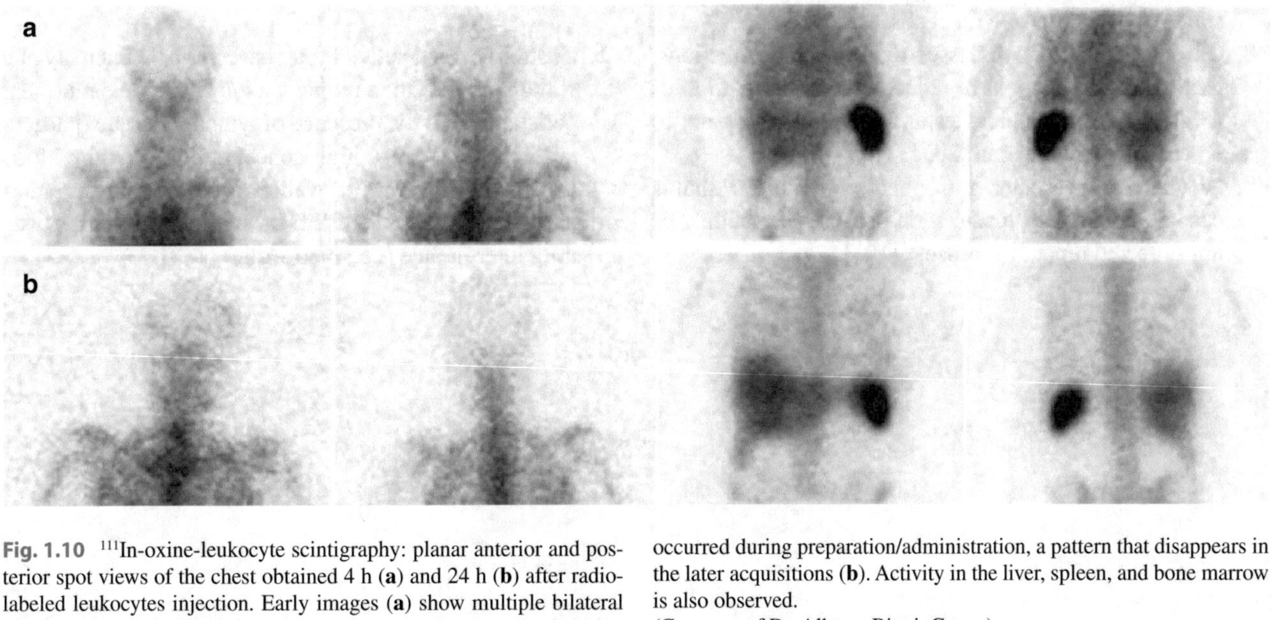

Fig. 1.10 ^{111}In-oxine-leukocyte scintigraphy: planar anterior and posterior spot views of the chest obtained 4 h (**a**) and 24 h (**b**) after radiolabeled leukocytes injection. Early images (**a**) show multiple bilateral small round non-segmental lung foci of activity due to cells clumping occurred during preparation/administration, a pattern that disappears in the later acquisitions (**b**). Activity in the liver, spleen, and bone marrow is also observed.
(Courtesy of Dr. Alberto Biggi, Cuneo)

2. Though usually solitary, multiple bilateral small round non-segmental lung foci of activity can occur, probably due to clumping of cells during the labeling process or during injection; this occurrence complicates interpretation of the scan [94].
3. Focal uptake can be seen in the presence of accessory spleen(s).

1.9.3 Pitfalls in ^{99m}Tc-HMPAO-Leukocyte Scintigraphy

1. Bone marrow expansion or hyperplasia can alter the normal scintigraphic patterns of bone marrow visualization [21, 100].
2. Lung activity can be present at 3 h post administration in case of pulmonary edema, diffuse inflammatory lung disease as pulmonary drug toxicity (bleomycin, methotrexate, and paclitaxel), atelectasis, radiation pneumonitis, heart or renal failure, sepsis, or adult respiratory distress syndrome, or due to cell damage during labeling [20, 87, 104–108].
3. Focal uptake can be seen in case of neoplasms (i.e., lymphoma, brain tumors) or hematomas [94, 109].
4. Spondylodiscitis may lead to either a spot of increased activity or more often a "cold" spot as compared with normal bone marrow localization [21, 110].
5. A "cold" spot in the spine may occur in the presence of compression fracture, neoplasm, post-irradiation changes, or postsurgical or anatomic deformities [94].
6. Bowel activity (prior to 4 h) can occur from intraluminal transit of labeled cells secondary to active gastrointestinal bleeding [21].
7. Normal renal activity can make it difficult to detect pyelonephritis and/or a renal abscess [104].
8. Chronic walled-off abscesses or low-grade infections, particularly in bone, have reduced the accumulation of ^{99m}Tc-HMPAO-granulocytes and are more likely not to be visualized in the scan [20, 111].
9. Non-infected vascular grafts and/or peritoneal shunts can show increased localization because of bleeding or non-infected reparative process [103].
10. Recent surgical wounds can induce increased uptake by approximately 72 h, with complete resolution in few days. When a surgical wound is not closed, or when it dehisces and is left to heal on its own by secondary intention, uptake persists and appears as areas of intense activity even in the absence of infection [21].

1.10 [^{18}F]FDG PET/CT (and PET/MR)

1.10.1 Normal Biodistribution of [^{18}F]FDG

[^{18}F]FDG uptake is physiologically most intense in the brain because of predominant glycolytic metabolism in neurons; uptake in the myocardium is variable, since the primary energy source for myocardiocytes is fatty acids. Since [^{18}F]FDG is excreted by the kidney into the urine, intense [^{18}F]FDG activity is normally observed in the intrarenal collecting systems, ureters, and bladder. Even 1 h after administration, the urinary excretion of [^{18}F]FDG continues in well-hydrated patients. Less intense and variable physiologic activity is present in the liver, spleen, bone marrow, and renal cortex. At 1 h post-injection, blood pool activity results in a moderate activity in the mediastinum against a low background lung activity (Fig. 1.11). Uptake in skeletal muscles is generally low if the patient has been allowed sufficient rest after physical activity before tracer injection. The larynx and vocal cords usually show either no uptake or mild symmetric uptake, which may have an inverted U shape [17, 111, 112].

1.10.2 Normal Variants in [^{18}F]FDG PET/CT

1. Gastrointestinal activity may have variable intensity and pattern related to multiple factors including muscular peristaltic activity, presence of lymphoid tissue (particularly in the cecum), high concentration of white blood cells in the bowel wall, swallowed secretions, intraluminal concentration of [^{18}F]FDG, colonic microbial uptake, drug interference (i.e., metformin) [113].

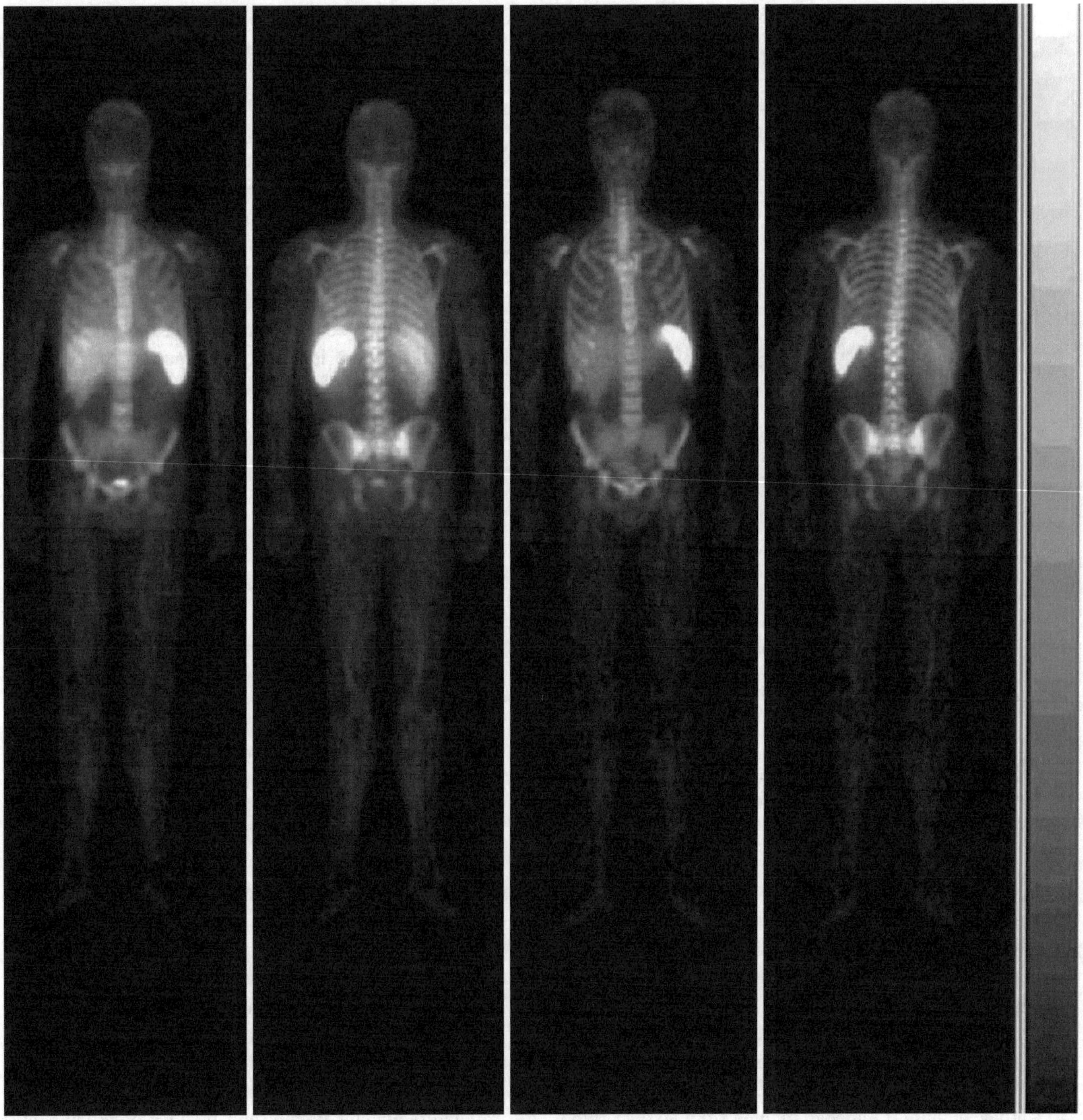

Fig. 1.11 ^{99m}Tc-HMPAO-leukocyte scintigraphy: anterior and posterior whole body images acquired 30 min p.i., showing physiologic uptake of labeled leukocytes in the spleen, liver, and bone marrow

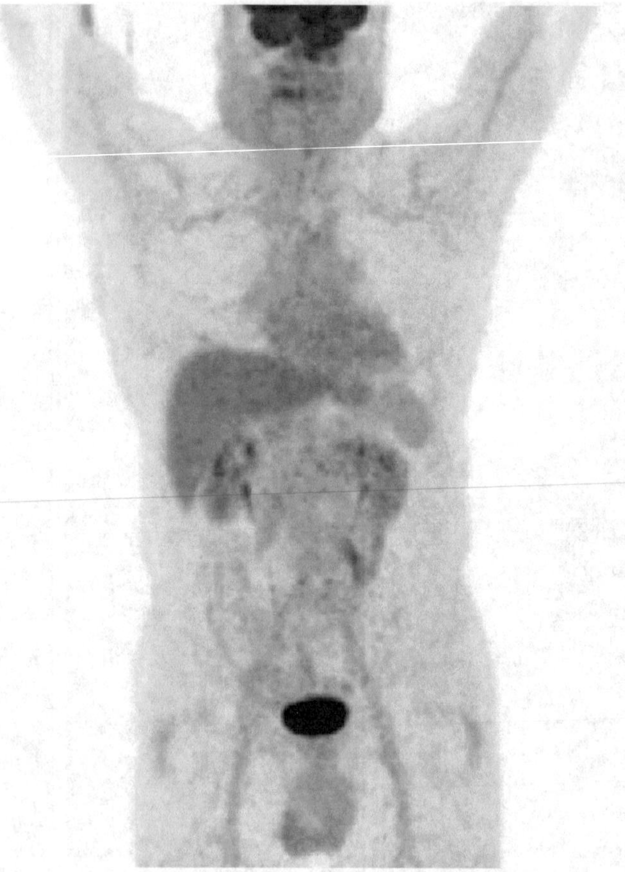

Fig. 1.12 PET/CT MIP image obtained 60 min after [^{18}F]FDG injection shows the physiologic pattern of biodistribution of this metabolic tracer

2. Intense uptake can be observed in the brown adipose tissue, commonly present symmetrically in the midaxillary line, posterior mediastinum, supra-clavicular, peri-hepatic, and para-spinal regions [114, 115] (Fig. 1.12).
3. Prominent activity in the laryngeal structures can occur in case of excessive talking while waiting after tracer injection, before the scan [112] (Fig. 1.12).
4. Cardiac activity is variable, ranging from no discernible activity above background blood pool activity to intense activity throughout the left ventricular myocardium, even in the fasting state [116]. Increased activity can present with a diffuse pattern (with/without heterogeneity), focally (i.e., papillary muscles), or regionally [116] (Fig. 1.13).
5. Physiologic thymic uptake can be observed in childhood, until puberty [117].
6. Mild to moderate uptake is usually seen in the adenoids, in the tonsils, and at the base of the tongue in children, due to the physiologic activity of lymphatic tissue in the Waldeyer ring [116]; this occurrence peaks around 6–8 years of age, declining then with increasing age.
7. Patients in the pediatric age range may have physiologic linear uptake in ephyses and apophyses, due to skeletal growth [110].
8. In children, uptake in the salivary glands is variable, but typically mild to moderate [115].
9. Endometrial uptake may increase during the ovulatory and menstrual phases in premenopausal women [17].
10. Moderate and diffuse uptake can be seen in the breasts, higher in adolescent girls with dense breasts or in lactating breasts (Fig. 1.14). Also the nipples normally demonstrate some activity uptake, better identified in the non-attenuation-corrected images [118].
11. Testicular uptake is usually symmetrical and diffuse, and it may decrease with age [119] (Fig. 1.15).
12. Increased uptake in skeletal muscles (generally symmetric) can occur due to excessive muscle activity during the uptake phase, or within a few days preceding the PET scan [112] (Fig. 1.16).

1.10.3 Pitfalls in [^{18}F]FDG PET/CT

1. Hyperinsulinemia may result in a “muscle scan” [120] (Fig. 1.17).
2. A well-defined focus of uptake in the lung on [^{18}F]FDG-PET without a detectable corresponding abnormality on the integrated CT (either above or below the diaphragm) can be observed as a consequence of microemboli secondary to paravenous injection. Since the blood clots are admixed with injected radiotracer, they may be very intense [120].
3. Increased bowel uptake can be seen in chronic inflammatory conditions, such as enterocolitis and inflammatory bowel disease [17].
4. Markedly increased uptake along the esophagus can occur in patients with esophagitis or after radiation therapy, or in patients with hiatal hernia and Barrett esophagus (in the distal esophagus) [112].
5. Focal pooling can be observed in renal calyces/pelvis, dilated/redundant ureters and bladder diverticula [17] (Fig. 1.18).
6. Diffuse myocardial uptake can occur in the presence of several myocardial diseases, including systemic and pulmonary hypertension, and valvular heart disease. Also myocarditis, both infective and radiation-induced, manifests as diffuse myocardial uptake. Increased activity localized in the atria is associated with atrial fibrillation. Myocardial and pericardial tumors and metastasis appear as focal [^{18}F]FDG uptake. The physiologic patterns of biodistribution of [^{18}F]FDG can mimic coronary ischemia. Left bundle-branch block is associated with a pattern of decreased [^{18}F]FDG septal activity. Radiation-induced pericarditis may result in a pattern of diffuse

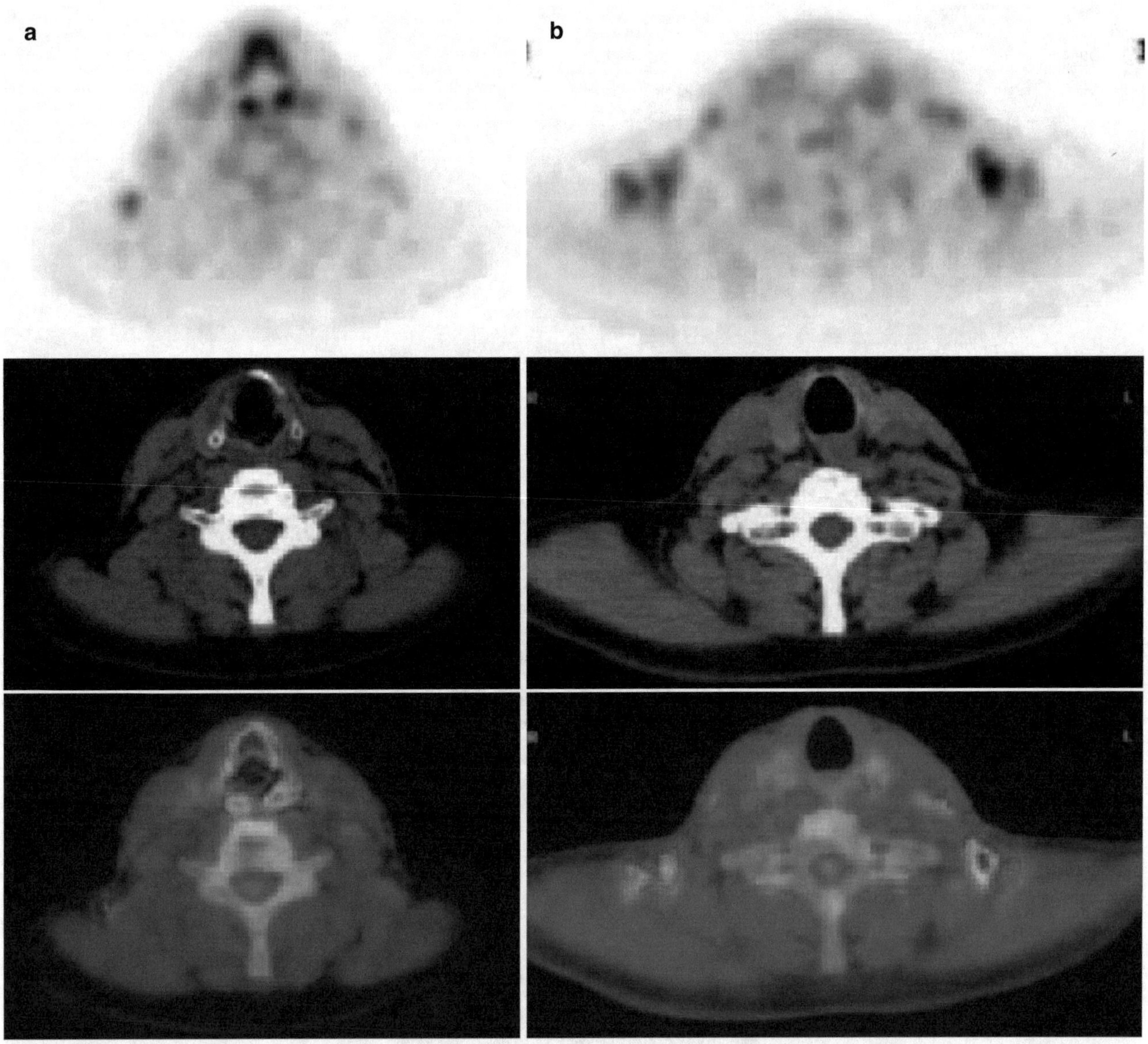

Fig. 1.13 [¹⁸F]FDG-PET/CT images (PET component in upper panels, CT component in middle panels, and fused PET/CT images in lower panels) showing two normal variants of [¹⁸F]FDG uptake in the same patient. (**a**) [¹⁸F]FDG uptake at the epiglottis and arytenoid muscles, due to excessive talking during waiting time between tracer injection and scan acquisition. (**b**) Increased uptake in the thermogenic brown fat of the sovraclavear regions (more prominent on the left side in this particular case)

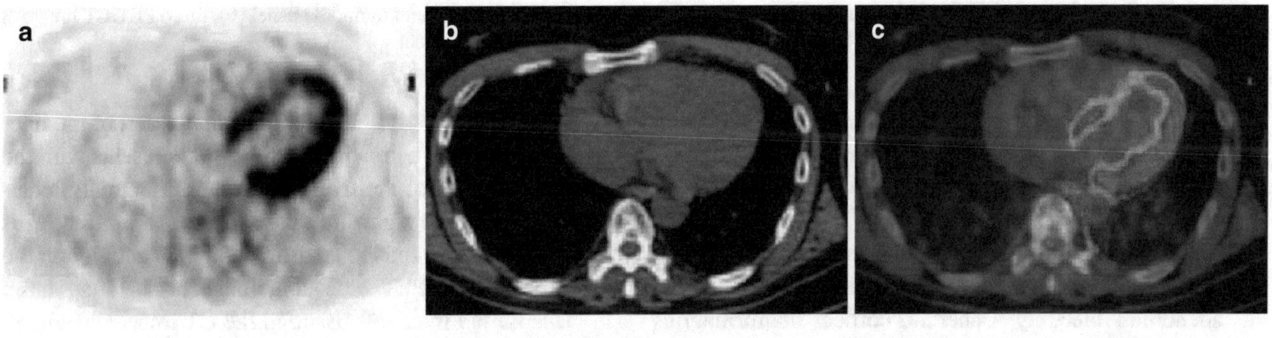

Fig. 1.14 Transaxial [¹⁸F]FDG PET/CT images [PET component in left panel (**a**), CT component in middle panel (**b**), fused PET/CT image in right panel (**c**)], showing intense myocardial [¹⁸F]FDG uptake, but with an area of reduced uptake in the septum in a patient with left bundle-branch block

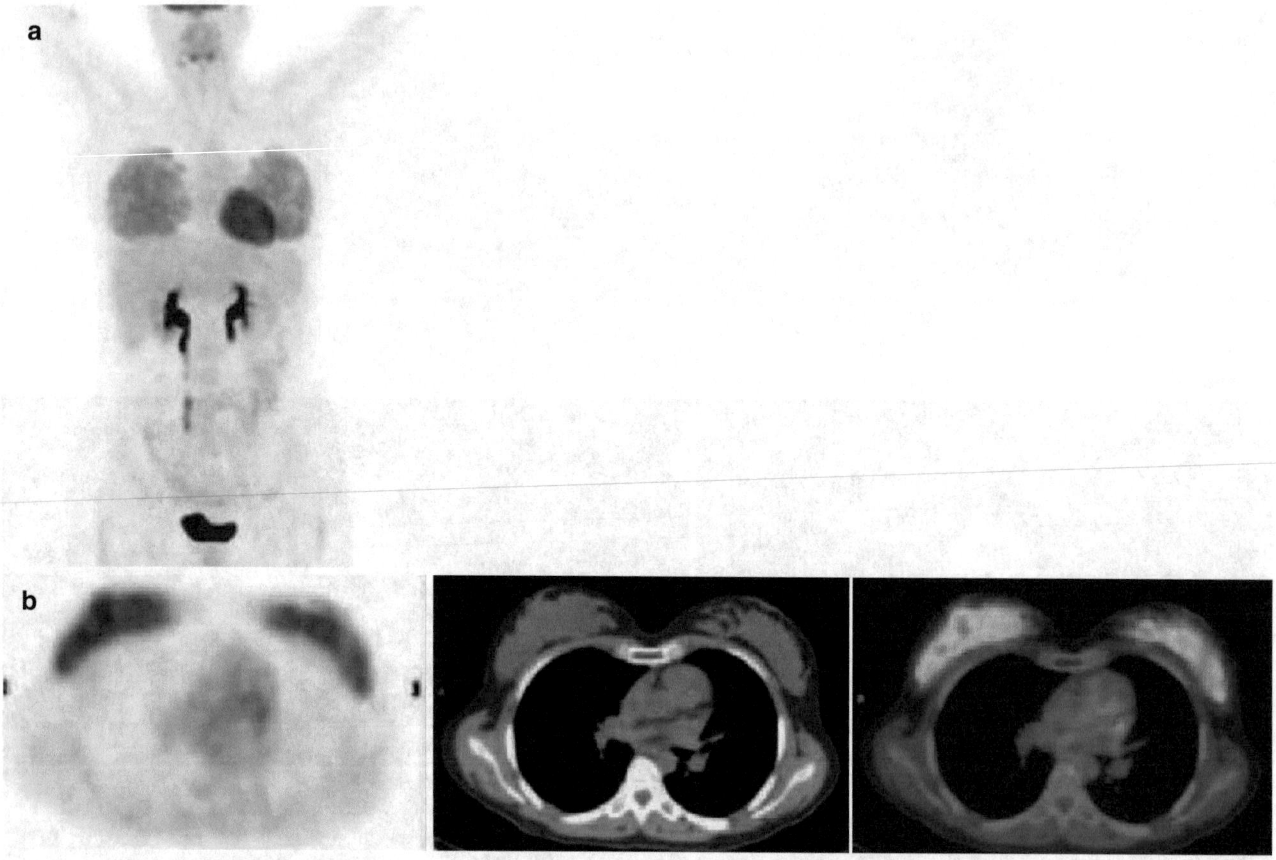

Fig. 1.15 Follow-up [18F]FDG PET/CT scan in a patient with Hodgkin's lymphoma (complete response lasting since 3 years) who has given birth to a child 2 months earlier. (**a**) MIP image showing intense [18F]FDG uptake in the myocardium as well as in the breasts, with radioactivity accumulation in the renal collecting systems, right ureter and bladder. (**b**) Transaxial [18F]FDG PET/CT section (PET component in left panel, CT component in middle panel, fused PET/CT image in right panel), showing intense [18F]FDG uptake at both lactating breasts (more prominent on the right side)

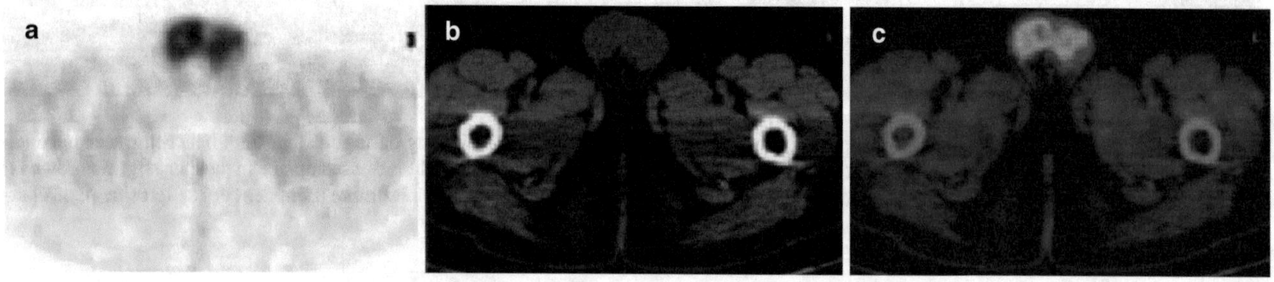

Fig. 1.16 Transaxial [18F]FDG-PET/CT sections [(PET component in left panel (**a**), CT component in middle panel (**b**), fused PET/CT image in right panel (**c**)], showing symmetric and diffuse [18F]FDG uptake at both testicles in an adult patient

[18F]FDG uptake rather than a nodular/focal pattern in the pericardium; the site of the increased [18F]FDG uptake corresponds anatomically to the radiation port [121, 122].

7. The pattern of physiologic brain uptake can vary in several conditions such as tumors, pituitary hyperplasia or adenomas, bleeding, ischemia, cortical malformations and epileptogenic foci, radiation-induced necrosis [123–128] (Fig. 1.19).
8. The base of the right lung and the upper part of the liver are affected by a breathing artifact that presents with the upper portion of the liver appearing artifactually localized within the right lung base in the CT images. This artifact corresponds to an artifactual high activity on the reconstructed PET emission image of the lung base, because the liver soft tissue in the CT images results in an overcorrection of photon attenuation of the lung tissue. The degree of respiratory artifacts may be more pro-

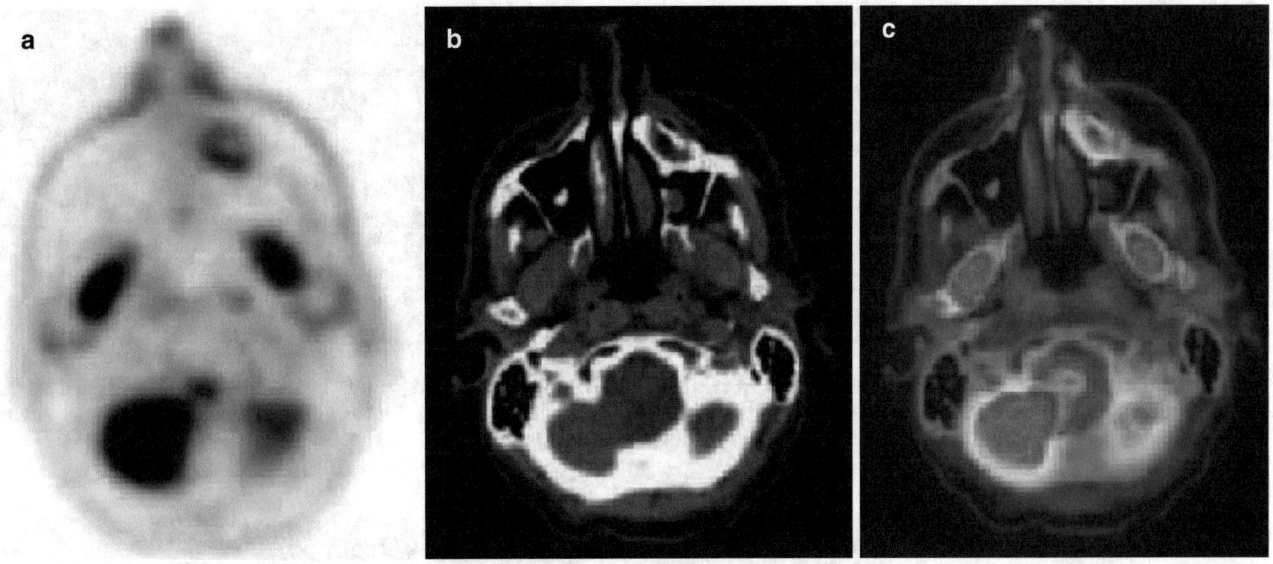

Fig. 1.17 Transaxial [^{18}F]FDG PET/CT images [(PET component in left panel (a), CT component in middle panel (b), fused PET/CT image in right panel (c)], showing intense bilateral symmetrical [^{18}F]FDG uptake in pterygoid muscles, due to chewing in the waiting time between tracer injection and acquisition of the scan

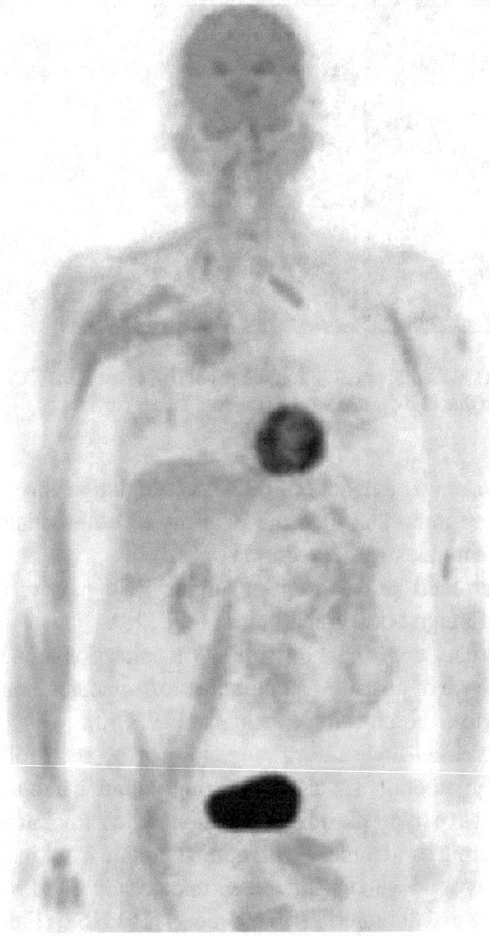

Fig. 1.18 MIP image of [^{18}F]FDG PET/CT in a diabetic patient who received insulin due to hyperglycemia 1 h before tracer injection. Diffuse and inhomogeneous tracer uptake in muscles and soft tissues (predominant on the right side) resulting in a high background with low brain, liver, and kidneys uptake. Intense radiopharmaceutical uptake is evident in the heart, and activity accumulation in the bladder

nounced, with increased respiratory mismatch between the CT and the PET images [17].

9. A moderate to high uptake in the chest wall muscles can occur in patients with chronic obstructive pulmonary disease. Furthermore, [^{18}F]FDG uptake in the diaphragmatic cruces may be increased in these patients because of enhanced abdominal breathing effort and increased anaerobic metabolism due to reduced oxygen delivery [129, 130].
10. Metallic objects (i.e., orthopedic hardware, dental implants) attenuate photons, with a degree of attenuation which is higher for the CT X-ray energy than for the annihilation gamma energy. Thus, CT-based correction overestimates the attenuation and results in artifactually increased [^{18}F]FDG activity in the CT attenuation-corrected PET images [131]. The intensity of uptake caused by this artifact depends on the size and shape of the metal hardware or prosthesis [131, 132].
11. Barium- or iodine-based oral contrast media may result in overestimation of photon attenuation and artifactually increased [^{18}F]FDG activity in the CT attenuation-corrected PET images [133, 134].
12. Systemic treatments such as chemotherapy and radioiodine therapy induce increased thymic uptake in both pediatric and adult patients [135–138] (Fig. 1.20).
13. Diffusely increased salivary gland uptake can be seen after chemotherapy or external beam radiation therapy [139] (Fig. 1.21).
14. Benign uterine/ovarian conditions including fibroids, endometriosis, dermoid/serous cyst, and inflammation can result in increased uptake [17, 140].

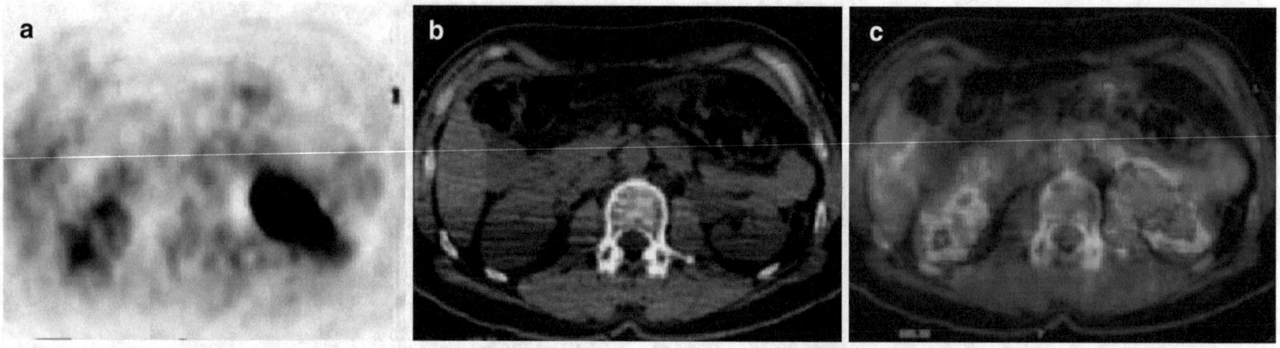

Fig. 1.19 Transaxial [18F]Transaxial [18F]FDG PET/CT images in a patient with left adrenal mass [(PET component in left panel (**a**), CT component in middle panel (**b**), fused PET/CT image in right panel (**c**)], showing increased [18F]FDG accumulation in the left renal pelvis; the CT image confirms dilation of the left renal pelvis, consistent with hydronephrosis

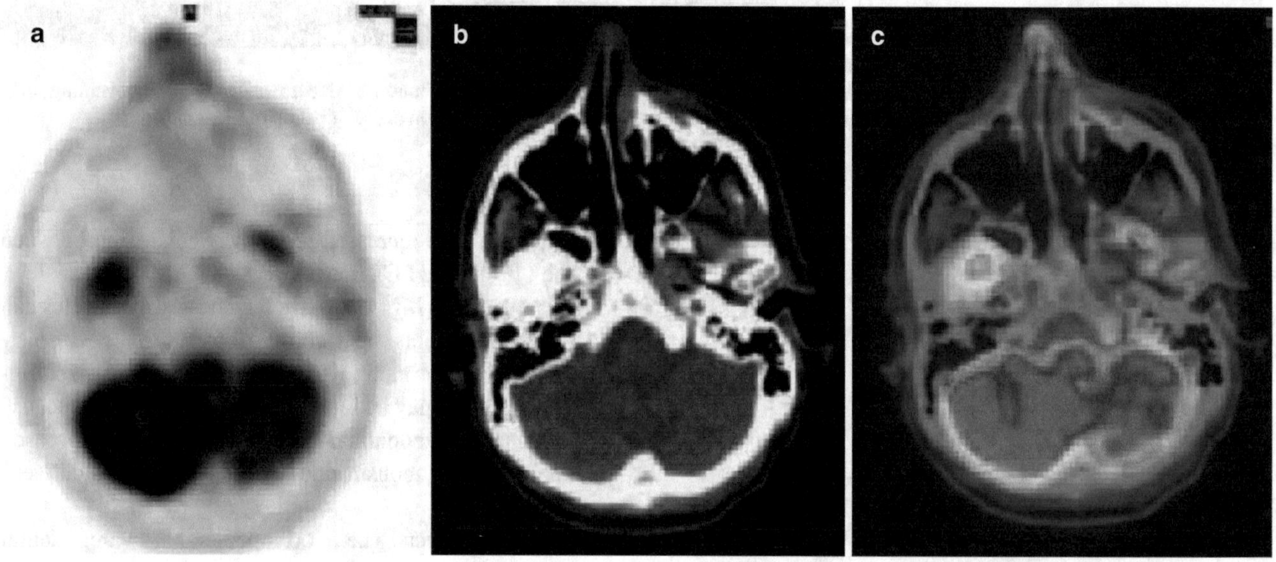

Fig. 1.20 Transaxial [18F]FDG PET/CT images [(PET component in left panel (**a**), CT component in middle panel (**b**), fused PET/CT image in right panel (**c**)], showing an area of reduced [18F]FDG uptake in the left cerebellum due to ischemic stroke occurred 1 year earlier

15. Increased uptake can be seen in adrenal adenomas and adrenal hyperplasia [17].
16. Increased uptake in malignancies (i.e., lymphoma and lung/liver/colon/gynecological tumors) can make it difficult to interpret a PET scan performed for localizing infection [17].
17. Radiation and chemotherapy may induce diffusely elevated [18F]FDG uptake [141].
18. Acute traumatic fracture causes significantly increased [18F]FDG uptake; moreover, hematoma and granulation tissue also account for [18F]FDG accumulation in the osseous callus [142–145]. Similarly, at the extremity of bone resection or amputation, focal-increased uptake is often noted for months [146].
19. Arthroplasty-related reactive increased uptake may persist for an extended period of time (many years) compared to surgical induced or traumatic fracture. Both the site and patterns of [18F]FDG accumulation appear to be more important than the intensity to differentiate reactive uptake from infection [144–147].
20. Increased uptake in a prior surgical field may correspond to foreign body granulomas [147, 148].
21. Surgery may induce [18F]FDG localization as a consequence of postsurgical inflammatory changes, persisting up to 6 months after treatment [149, 150].
22. Increased bone marrow uptake can be seen following chemotherapy (usually resolving within 1 month) or in cases of hyperplasia and hematopoietic stimulation from anemia or treatment with hematopoietic cytokines (possibly associated with spleen update, for up to 3 weeks after discontinuation of treatment) [151, 152] (Fig. 1.22).
23. Reduced bone marrow uptake can be noted several months after radiotherapy, due to replacement of bone marrow by fatty tissue [141, 153].

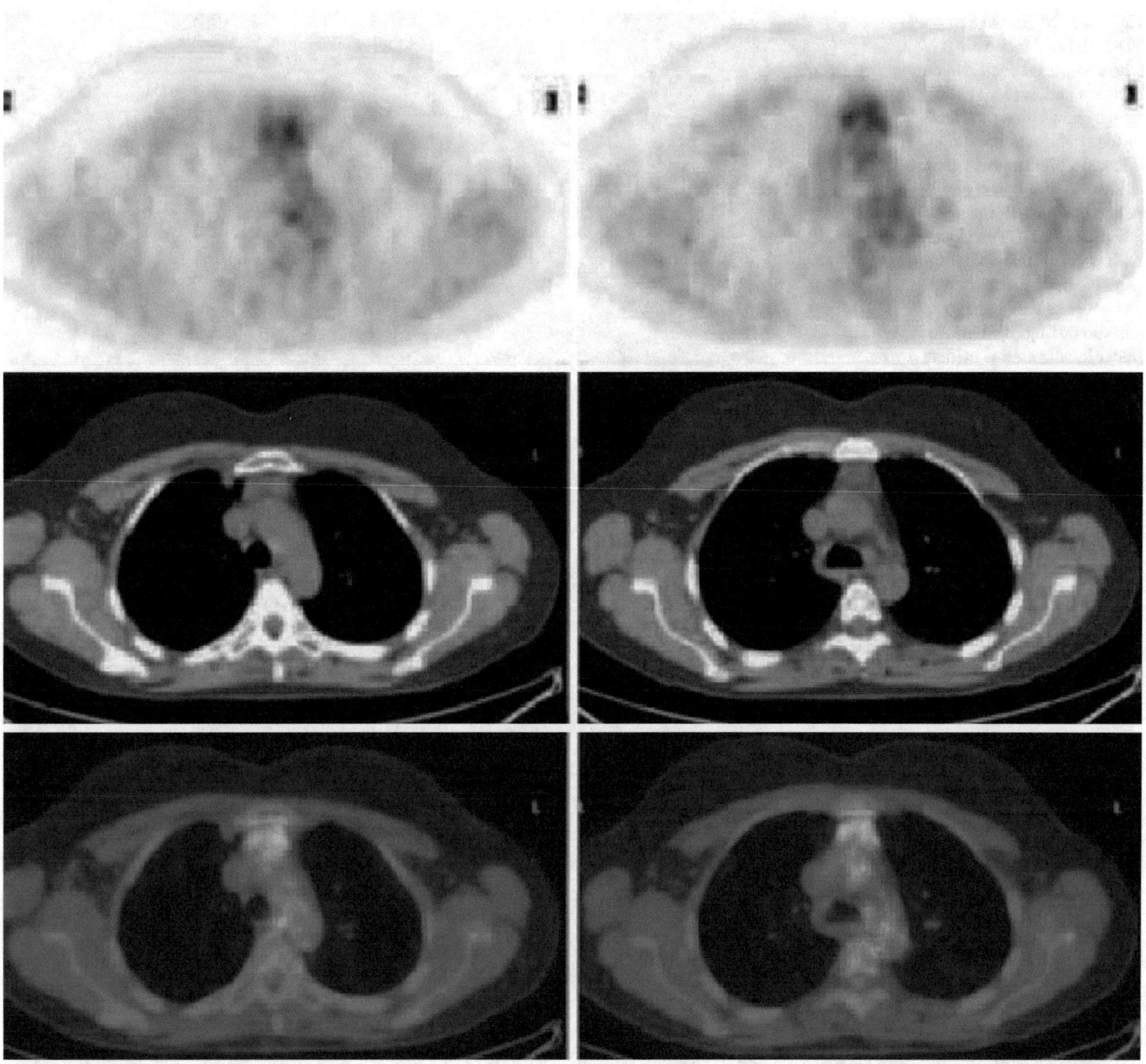

Fig. 1.21 Transaxial [^{18}F]FDG PET/CT views in a 46-year old woman, showing tracer uptake in the thymic lodge due to thymic hyperplasia induced by chemotherapy

24. The motion of patient during image acquisition can cause an artifact resulting in a different line-up between the [^{18}F]FDG localization and the corresponding anatomical structures in the fused PET/CT image (Fig. 1.23).

1.11 Novel Infection Imaging Agents

1.11.1 ^{99m}Tc-Ubiquicidin Fragments and ^{68}Ga-Ubiquicidin Fragments

Ubiquicidin (UBI) is a cationic, synthetic, antimicrobial peptide (AMP) fragment. These peptides are produced by several types of cells and constitute an important component of innate immune system against infection [154]. Electrostatic attraction is the basic mechanism of action of AMPs. The external surface of the bacterial cell membrane is charged negatively, thus attracting the AMPs which have positively charged domains. The UBI 29–41 fragment in particular has high sensitivity and specificity for the detection of bacterial and fungal infections in both human and animals, including immunocompromised animals [154–156]. Sepúlveda-Méndez et al. evaluated the role of ^{99m}Tc-UBI 29–41 scintigraphy in identifying foci of infection in patients with fever of unknown origin, reporting 97.52% sensitivity, 95.35% specificity, and 96.62% overall accuracy [157, 158]. The use of ^{99m}Tc-UBI 29–41 scintigraphy in diabetic foot infections reported perfect sensitivity,

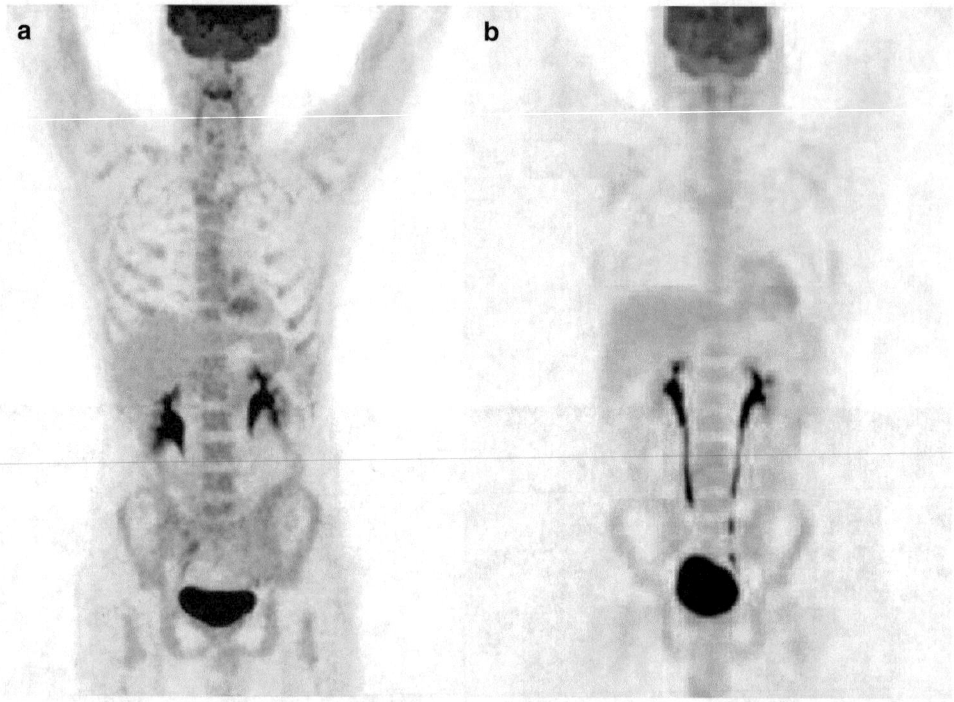

Fig. 1.22 MIP image of [^{18}F]FDG PET/CT in a patient who completed chemotherapy 1 month earlier (**a**). The image shows moderate and diffuse radiopharmaceutical uptake in bone marrow more evident in ribs, spine, and pelvic bones. MIP image of [^{18}F]FDG PET/CT in a patient with fever of unknown origin, negative bone marrow biopsy and severe anemia due to chronic oozing (**b**). Diffuse tracer localization is evident in blades, sternum, spine, and pelvic bones. In both the images, the genitourinary tract is visualized. These are two different examples of bone marrow activation induced by drug in the first case (**a**) and by physiological compensation in the second one (**b**)

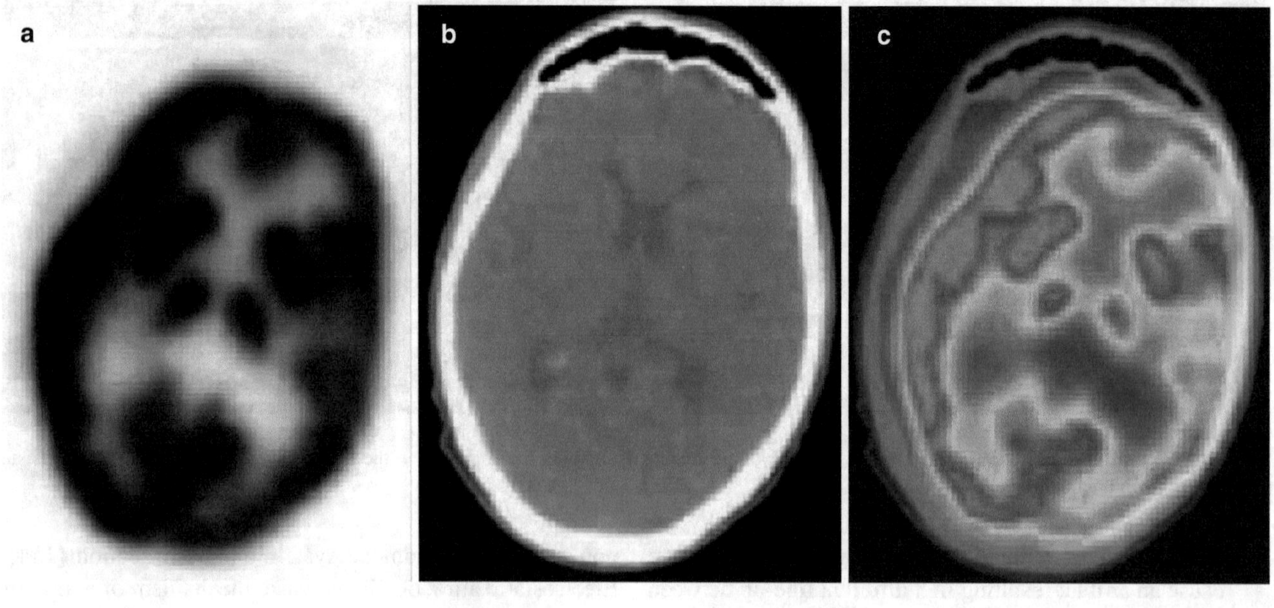

Fig. 1.23 Transaxial [^{18}F]FDG PET/CT images (PET component in the right panel-a, CT component in the middle panel-b, fused PET/CT image in the left panelc), showing technical pitfall due to patient motion. The patient-related artifact result in a discrepant line-up between the [^{18}F]FDG brain localization and the corresponding anatomic structures in the fused PET/CT image

specificity, and accuracy values of 100% [159]. SPECT/CT acquisition in addition to planar imaging could lead to an increased diagnostic performance and improved diagnostic confidence in differentiating soft tissue from bone infection, as well as a higher inter-observer agreement [159]. The optimum imaging time for distinguishing infection from inflammation is 60 min after intravenous administration of the radiotracer. The better resolution of the PET/CT camera and has led to interest in the use of ^{68}Ga-labeled UBI 29–41 for PET imaging of infection [160].

1.11.2 Radiolabeled Antibiotics

Radiolabeled antibiotics proposed for infection imaging mainly include fluoroquinolones, cephalosporins, inhibitors of nucleic acid synthesis, inhibitors of bacterial cell wall synthesis, and inhibitors of protein synthesis. Actually, a gold standard among radiolabeled antibiotics for bacterial infection imaging has not yet been defined, and none of the mentioned radiolabeled antibiotics is commercially available. Many factors contribute to this limited role: (1) minimal or very low specific activity for infection versus sterile inflammation; (2) selective specificity to one kind of bacteria only; (3) significant discrepancies in animal models, administered activity, time and type of scan acquisition; (4) extreme variability in the number of bacteria used for inducing the infection ranges; and (5) different clearance mechanism of the radiolabeled antibiotics [161].

1.11.3 [^{18}F]FDG-Labeled Leukocytes

Following the development of an in vitro procedure for labeling leukocytes (WBC) with [^{18}F]FDG (obtained simply by incubating the leukocyte population with the radiolabeled glucose analog), several studies have evaluated the diagnostic accuracy of this nuclear medicine imaging procedure in infections. However, the small number of enrolled patients has so far limited any kind of considerations on its diagnostic accuracy. In principle, [^{18}F]FDG-WBC PET/CT has two main advantages over [^{18}F]FDG PET/CT: (1) it represents a suitable imaging method in case of cerebral, cardiac, renal, and intra-abdominal diseases (where the use of [^{18}F]FDG is hampered by its physiological uptake/excretion); and (2) different types of inflammatory cells show [^{18}F]FDG uptake, while the sites of [^{18}F]FDG-WBC accumulation should be specific for granulocytes diapedesis, even if leukocyte accumulation is also seen at the site of sterile inflammation. On the other hand, the labeling efficiency of [^{18}F]FDG-WBC is variable and in general low. The short ^{18}F half-life does not allow late (24 h) acquisitions, when [^{18}F]FDG could also decay and detach from WBCs. Despite these limitations, a recent systematic review and a bivariate meta-analysis confirmed a good diagnostic performance in detecting infectious diseases, although the authors concluded that, because of the relative paucity of data available on [^{18}F]FDG-WBC PET/CT, this imaging method should not be considered as a standard clinical practice [162].

1.11.4 ^{124}I-Fialuridine

Fialuridine is a specific substrate of bacterial thymidine kinase. Since fialuridine is incorporated into bacteria rather than in the inflammatory cells, ^{124}I-fialuridine PET/CT is supposed to be a specific imaging method for infectious processes. Despite such theoretical advantages, the clinical use of ^{124}I-fialuridine PET/CT is limited by low image quality as a result of metal artifact and high background from non-specific muscle uptake. While in a pilot study by Luis et al. in eight patients with musculoskeletal infection, ^{124}I-fialuridine PET/CT demonstrated tracer uptake at the infection sites in all such patients, the results of subsequent investigations have been quite disappointing [163].

1.11.5 ^{68}Ga-Citrate

Nanni et al. reported the feasibility of ^{68}Ga-citrate PET/CT in patients with bone infections. The main advantages over the ^{67}Ga-citrate scan (with or without SPECT/CT) are the shorter half-life of ^{68}Ga (68 min versus 78.3 h for ^{67}Ga), the higher spatial-resolution of PET images versus single-photon imaging (especially because of the poor imaging properties of ^{67}Ga with standard gamma cameras), much shorter waiting time for recording diagnostic whole-body acquisition, and lower radiation dosimetry. Nevertheless, the ^{68}Ga-citrate PET/CT performance did not prove to be consistently really superior to that of a conventional imaging diagnostic flowchart. Nonetheless, ^{68}Ga-citrate PET/CT, as a new diagnostic tool, could be considered in the flowchart of patients with bone infection [164]. Tseng et al. investigated the use of ^{68}Ga-citrate PET/CT for detecting prosthetic joint infections and concluded that ^{68}Ga-citrate might have a complementary role to [^{18}F]FDG showing a higher specificity and the possibility to discriminate between an infectious condition and sterile inflammation [165]. Other larger-scale studies are required to validate the diagnostic performance of this novel infection imaging technique.

Key Learning Points

- The main nuclear medicine imaging procedures traditionally employed to evaluate inflammation and/or infection include scintigraphy with ^{99m}Tc-diphosphonate (MDP/HDP), with radiolabeled leukocytes (^{111}In-oxine- or ^{99m}Tc-HMPAO-labeling), with ^{67}Ga-citrate, or with ^{99m}Tc-albumin nanocolloids.
- Biodistribution of these imaging agents, the normal variants, and pitfalls related to many factors (e.g., drug interference, antibiotic therapy) must be kept in mind for correct interpretation of the scans.
- [^{18}F]FDG PET/CT constitutes a sensitive method of choice for characterization of inflammatory process (for either diagnosis or for assessing response to treatment).
- The use of PET/CT with [^{18}F]FDG-labeled leukocytes is currently limited by different shortcomings (e.g., labeling instability).

- A gold standard among the radiolabeled antibiotics for bacterial infection imaging has not yet been defined.
- Scintigraphy with ^{99m}Tc-ubiquicidine fragments is a promising technique, reported to exhibit high sensitivity and specificity for the detection of bacterial and fungal infections both in animal models and in humans.
- ^{124}I-fialuridine PET/CT is limited by low image quality as a result of metal artifacts and high background from nonspecific muscle uptake.

Acknowledgments All editors have contributed to the preparation of this chapter. We are particularly grateful to Dr. Elena Lazzeri (Pisa, Italy), Dr. Napoleone Prandini (Modena, Italy), and Martina Sollini (formerly in Pisa, and currently in Milan, Italy) for providing images that have been included in this chapter.

References

1. Hesselewood S, Leung E. Drug interaction with radiopharmaceuticals. Eur J Nucl Med. 1996;21:348–56.
2. Sampson CB. Drugs and chemicals which affect the purity, biodistribution and pharmacokinetics of radiopharmaceuticals. Aust J Biol Sci. 1990;1:381–400.
3. Santos-Oliveira R, Machado M. Pitfalls with radiopharmaceuticals. Am J Med Sci. 2011;342:50–3.
4. Spicer JA, Preston DF, Stephens R. Adverse allergic reaction to technetium-99m methylene disphosphonate. J Nucl Med. 1985;26:373–4.
5. Schmidt KG, Rasmussen JW, Frederiksen PB, et al. Indium-111-granulocyte scintigraphy in brain abscess diagnosis: limitations and pitfalls. J Nucl Med. 1990;31:1121–7.
6. Gnanasegaran G, Cook G, Adamson K, et al. Patterns, variants, artifacts, and pitfalls in conventional radionuclide bone imaging and SPECT/CT. Semin Nucl Med. 2009;39:380–95.
7. Al-Enizi E, Kazem N, Owunwanne A, et al. Dextrose solutions yield radiopharmaceutical impurities: the "sweet" scans. J Nucl Med Technol. 2003;31:33–6.
8. Saverymuttu SH, Peters AM, Danpure HJ, et al. Lung transit of ^{111}Indium-labelled granulocytes: relationship to labelling techniques. Scand J Haematol. 1983;30:151–60.
9. Love C, Tomas MB, Palestro CJ. Pulmonary activity on labelled leukocyte images: patterns of uptake and their significance. Nucl Med Commun. 2002;23:559–63.
10. Hung JC, Ponto JA, Hammes RJ. Radiopharmaceutical-related pitfalls and artifacts. Semin Nucl Med. 1996;26:208–55.
11. Roca M, de Vries EF, Jamar F. Guidelines for the labelling of leucocytes with In111-oxine. Eur J Nucl Med Mol Imaging. 2010;37:835–41.
12. De Vries EF, Roca M, Jamar F, et al. Guidelines for the labeling of leucocytes with Tc99m-HMPAO. Eur J Nucl Med Mol Imaging. 2010;37:842–8.
13. Cordova MA, Hladik WB, Rhodes BA. Validation and characterization of adverse reactions to radiopharmaceuticals. Noninv Med Imag. 1984;1:17–24.
14. Balan KK, Choudhary AK, Balan A, et al. Severe systemic reaction to ^{99m}Tc-methylene diphosphonate: a case report. J Nucl Med Technol. 2003;31:76–8.
15. Vidal MV, Gutfilen B, Barbosa-Da-Fonseca LM, et al. Influence of tobacco on the labelling of red blood cells and plasma proteins with technetium-99m. J Exp Clin Cancer Res. 1998;17:41–6.
16. Laverman P, Bleeker-Rovers CP, Corstens FHM, et al. Development of infection and inflammation targeting compounds. Curr Radiopharm. 2008;1:42–8.
17. Wang X, Koch S. Positron emission tomography/computed tomography potential pitfalls and artifacts. Curr Probl Diagn Radiol. 2009;38:156–69.
18. Dogan A, Rezai K. Incidental lymph node visualisation on bone scan due to subcutaneous infiltration of Tc99m MDP. Clin Nucl Med. 1993;18:208–9.
19. Palestro CJ. The current role of gallium imaging in infection. Semin Nucl Med. 1994;24:128–41.
20. Schuster DM, Alazraki N. Gallium and other agents in diseases of the lung. Semin Nucl Med. 2002;32:193–211.
21. Love C, Palestro CJ. Altered biodistribution and incidental findings on gallium and labeled leukocyte/bone marrow scans. Semin Nucl Med. 2010;40:271–82.
22. Connolly LP, Connolly SA. Thymic uptake of radiopharmaceuticals. Clin Nucl Med. 2003;28:648–51.
23. Ramsay SC, Yeates MG, Burke WM, et al. Quantitative pulmonary gallium scanning in interstitial lung disease. Eur J Nucl Med. 1992;19:80–5.
24. Desai AG, Intenzo C, Park C, et al. Drug-induced gallium uptake in the breasts. Clin Nucl Med. 1987;12:703–4.
25. Vazquez R, Oates E, Sarno RC, et al. Gallium-67 breast uptake in a patient with hypothalamic granuloma (sarcoid). J Nucl Med. 1988;29:118–21.
26. Society of Nuclear Medicine procedure guideline for gallium scintigraphy in inflammation. Version 3.0, approved 2 June 2004.
27. Rossleigh MA, Murray IP, Mackey DW, et al. Pediatric solid tumors: evaluation by gallium-67 SPECT studies. J Nucl Med. 1990;31:168–72.
28. Hattner RS, White DL. Gallium-67/stable gadolinium antagonism: MRI contrast agent markedly alters the normal biodistribution of gallium-67. J Nucl Med. 1985;31:1844–6.
29. Hoffer P. Gallium and infection. J Nucl Med. 1980;21:484–8.
30. Hoffer PB, Samuel A, Bushberg JT, et al. Desferoxamine mesylate (desferal): a contrast-enhancing agent for Ga-67 imaging. Radiology. 1979;131:775–9.
31. Lentle BC, Jackson FI, McGowan DG. Localization of gallium-67 citrate in salivary glands following radiation therapy. J Can Assoc Radiol. 1976;27:89–91.
32. Yoshida S, Fukumoto M, Motohara T, et al. Ga-67 tumor scan in malignant diffuse mesothelioma—comparison with CT and pathological findings. Ann Nucl Med. 1999;1:49–54.
33. Fink G, Krelbaum T, Yellin A, et al. Pulmonary carcinoid: presentation, diagnosis, and outcome in 142 cases in Israel and review of 640 cases from the literature. Chest. 2001;6:1647–51.
34. Shiojima K, Tamaki Y, Hashida I, et al. Gallium-67 scintigraphy in evaluation of malignant lymphoma of the thyroid gland. Radiat Med. 1996;14:31–4.
35. Yamamoto Y, Nishiyama Y, Kawasaki Y, et al. Evaluation of ^{99m}Tc-MIBI to predict chemotherapeutic response in patients with small cell lung carcinoma. Nippon Igaku Hoshasen Gakkai Zasshi. 1996;56:980–1.
36. Lee VW, Fuller JD, O'Brien MJ, et al. Pulmonary Kaposi sarcoma in patients with AIDS: scintigraphic diagnosis with sequential thallium and gallium scanning. Radiology. 1991;180:409–12.
37. Moinuddin M, Rockett J. Gallium scintigraphy in the detection of amiodarone lung toxicity. AJR Am J Roentgenol. 1986;147:607–9.

38. van Rooij WJ, van der Meer SC, van Royen EA, et al. Pulmonary gallium-67 uptake in amiodarone pneumonitis. J Nucl Med. 1984;25:211–3.
39. Richman SD, Levenson SM, Bunn PA, et al. ^{67}Ga accumulation in pulmonary lesions associated with bleomycin toxicity. Cancer. 1975;36:1966–72.
40. Garbes ID, Henderson ES, Gomez GA, et al. Procarbazine-induced interstitial pneumonitis with a normal chest x-ray: a case report. Med Pediatr Oncol. 1986;14:238–41.
41. MacMahon H, Bekerman C. The diagnostic significance of gallium uptake in patients with normal chest radiographs. Radiology. 1978;127:189–93.
42. Crook MJ, Kaplan PD, Adatepe MH. Gallium-67 scanning in nitrofurantoin-induced pulmonary reaction. J Nucl Med. 1982;23: 690–2.
43. Stein MG, DeMarco T, Gamsu G, et al. Computed tomography: pathologic correlation in lung disease due to tocainide. Am Rev Respir Dis. 1988;137:458–4.
44. Manning DM, Strirnlan CV, Turbiner EH. Early detection of busulfan lung: report of a case. Clin Nucl Med. 1980;5:412–4.
45. Lentle BC, Castor WR, Khaliq A, et al. The effect of contrast lymphangiography on localization of ^{67}Ga-citrate. J Nucl Med. 1975;16:374–6.
46. Kramer EL, Divgi CR. Pulmonary applications of nuclear medicine. Clin Chest Med. 1991;12:55–75.
47. Baughman RP, Fernandez M. Radionuclide imaging in interstitial lung disease. Curr Opin Pulm Med. 1996;2:376–9.
48. Schiff RG, Kabat L, Kamani N. Gallium scanning in lymphoid interstitial pneumonitis of children with AIDS. J Nucl Med. 1987;28:1915–9.
49. Nimkin K, Oates E. Gallium-67 lung uptake in extrinsic hypersensitivity pneumonitis. Clin Nucl Med. 1989;14:451–2.
50. Brown DG, Aguirre A, Weaver A. ^{67}Gallium scanning in talc-induced pulmonary granulomatosis. Chest. 1980;77:561–5.
51. Hayes AA, Thickbroom GW, Guelfi GR, et al. Computer quantitation of gallium 67 lung uptake in crocidolite (blue asbestos) workers of Western Australia. Eur J Nucl Med. 1990;16:855–8.
52. Deseran MW, Colletti PM, Ratto D, et al. Chronic berylliosis. Demonstration by gallium-67 imaging and magnetic resonance imaging. Clin Nucl Med. 1988;13:509–11.
53. Kanner RE, Barkman HW, Rom WN, et al. Gallium-67 citrate imaging in underground coal miners. Am J Ind Med. 1985;8: 49–55.
54. Siemsen JK, Grebe SF, Waxman AD. The use of gallium-67 in pulmonary disorders. Semin Nucl Med. 1978;8:235–49.
55. Lin RY. Severe spirometric defects in systemic lupus erythematosus. A possible role for bronchoalveolar lavage and gallium scanning. Clin Rheumatol. 1987;6:276–81.
56. Baron M, Feiglin D, Hyland R, et al. ^{67}Gallium scans in progressive systemic sclerosis. Arthritis Rheum. 1983;26:969–74.
57. Yeh SD, White DA, Stuver-Pepe DE, et al. Abnormal gallium scintigraphy in pulmonary alveolar proteinosis (PAP). Clin Nucl Med. 1987;12:294–7.
58. Morals J, Carrier L, Gariepy G, et al. Gallium-67 pulmonary uptake in eosinophilic pneumonia. Clin Nucl Med. 1988;13:41–3.
59. Widman D, Swayne LC, Rozan S. Multicentric reticulohistiocytosis: assessment of pulmonary disease by gallium-67 scintigraphy. J Rheumatol. 1988;15:132–5.
60. Alpert LI. Pulmonary uptake of gallium-67 in Wegener's granulomatosis. Clin Nucl Med. 1980;5:53–4.
61. Javaheri S, Levine BW, McKusick KA. Serial ^{67}Ga lung scanning in pulmonary eosinopbilic granuloma. Thorax. 1979;34:822–3.
62. Gnanasegaran G, Cook GJ, Fogelman I. Musculoskeletal system. In: Biersack HJ, Freeman LM, editors. Nuclear medicine concise. New York: Springer; 2007.
63. O'Connor MK, Brown ML, Hung JC, et al. The art of bone scintigraphy: technical aspects. J Nucl Med. 1991;32:2332–41.
64. Storey G, Murray IPC. Bone scintigraphy: the procedure and interpretation. In: Ell PJ, Gambhir SS Nuclear medicine in clinical diagnosis and treatment, Vol I. Churchill Livingstone, Elsevier, New York, 2004:593–622.
65. Cook GJ, Fogelman I. The role of nuclear medicine in monitoring treatment in skeletal malignancy. Semin Nucl Med. 2001;31:206–11.
66. Cook GJ, Fogelman I. Skeletal metastases from breast cancer: imaging with nuclear medicine. Semin Nucl Med. 1999;29:69–79.
67. O'Sullivan JM, Cook GJ. A review of the efficacy of bone scanning in prostate and breast cancer. Q J Nucl Med. 2002;46: 152–9.
68. Love C, Din AS, Tomas MB, et al. Radionuclide bone imaging: an illustrative review. Radiographics. 2003;23:341–58.
69. Fogelman I, McKillop JH, Gray HW. The "hot patella" sign: is it of any clinical significance? Concise communication. J Nucl Med. 1983;24:312–5.
70. Kipper MS, Alazraki NP, Feiglin DH. The "hot" patella. Clin Nucl Med. 1982;7:28–32.
71. Love C, Tronco GG, Palestro CJ. Imaging of infection and inflammation with ^{99m}Tc-Fanolesomab. Q J Nucl Med Mol Imaging. 2006;50:113–20.
72. Chu JY, Ho JE, Monteleone PL, O'Connor DM. Technetium colloid bone marrow imaging in Fanconi's anemia. Pediatrics. 1979;64:635–9.
73. Milner PF, Brown M. Bone marrow infarction in sickle cell anemia: correlation with hematologic profiles. Blood. 1982;60:1411–9.
74. Love C, Palestro CJ. Radionuclide imaging of infection. J Nucl Med Technol. 2004;32:47–57.
75. Gratz S, Braun HG, Behr TM, et al. Photopenia in chronic vertebral osteomyelitis with technetium-99m-antigranulocyte antibody (BW 250/183). J Nucl Med. 1997;38:211–6.
76. Becker W, Dölkemeyer U, Gramatzki M, et al. Use of immunoscintigraphy in the diagnosis of FUO. Eur J Nucl Med. 1993;20:1078–83.
77. Shanthly N, Aruva MR, Zhang K, et al. ^{99m}Tc-Falonesomab: affinity, pharmacokinetics and preliminary evaluation. Q J Nucl Med Mol Imaging. 2006;50:104–12.
78. Thakur ML, Marcus CS, Henneman P, et al. Imaging inflammatory disease with neutrophil-specific technetium-99m-labeled monoclonal antibody anti-SSEA-1. J Nucl Med. 1996;37:1789–95.
79. Mozley PD, Thakur ML, Alavi A, et al. Effects of a ^{99m}Tc-labeled murine immunoglobulin M antibody to CD15 antigens on human granulocyte membranes in healthy volunteers. J Nucl Med. 1999;40:2107–14.
80. Kumar V. Radiolabeled white blood cells and direct targeting of micro-organisms for infection imaging. Q J Nucl Med Mol Imaging. 2005;49:325–38.
81. Becker W, Repp R, Hansen HJ, et al. Binding characteristics and kinetics of a new Tc-99m-antigranulocyte Fab fragment (Leukoscan™). J Nucl Med. 1995;36:208P.
82. Quigley AM, Gnanasegaran G, Buscombe JR. Technetium-99m-labelled sulesomab (LeukoScan) in the evaluation of soft tissue infections. Med Princ Pract. 2008;17:447–52.
83. Gratz S, Schipper ML, Dorner J, et al. LeukoScan for imaging infection in different clinical settings: a retrospective evaluation and extended review of the literature. Clin Nucl Med. 2003;28: 267–76.
84. Becker W. The contribution of nuclear medicine to the patient with infection. Eur J Nucl Med. 1995;22:1195–211.
85. Love C, Opoku-Agyemang P, Tomas MB, et al. Pulmonary activity on labeled leukocyte images: physiologic, pathologic, and imaging correlation. Radiographics. 2002;22:1385–93.

86. Coleman RE, Welch D. Possible pitfalls with clinical imaging of indium-111 leukocytes: concise communication. J Nucl Med. 1980;21:122–5.
87. Oates E, Staudinger K, Gilbertson V. Significance of nodal uptake on indium 111 labeled leukocyte scans. Clin Nucl Med. 1989;14:282–5.
88. Williamson SL, Williamson MR, Seibert JJ, et al. Indium-111 leukocyte accumulation in submandibular gland saliva as a cause for false-positive gut uptake in children. Clin Nucl Med. 1987;12:867–8.
89. Palestro CJ, Finn C. Indium-111 leukocyte imaging in Gaucher's disease. J Nucl Med. 1993;34:818–20.
90. Cook PS, Datz FL, Disbro MA. Pulmonary uptake in indium-111 leukocyte imaging: clinical significance in patients with suspected occult infections. Radiology. 1984;150:557–61.
91. Palestro CJ, Love C, Bhargava KK. Labeled leukocyte imaging: current status and future directions. Q J Nucl Med Mol Imaging. 2009;53:105–23.
92. Propst-Proctor SL, Dillingham MF, McDougall IR, et al. The white blood cell scan in orthopedics. Clin Orthop. 1982;168:157–65.
93. Miron S, Minotti A, Crass J. Accumulation of In-111 tagged white blood cells in heterotopic new bone. Clin Nucl Med. 1992;17:972–3.
94. Kim EE, Pjura GA, Lowry PA, et al. Osteomyelitis complicating fracture: pitfalls of ^{111}In leukocyte scintigraphy. AJR Am J Roentgenol. 1987;148:927–30.
95. Sfakianakis GN, Mnaymneh W, Ghandur-Mnaymneh L. Positive indium-111 leukocytes scintigraphy in a skeletal metastasis. AJR Am J Roentgenol. 1982;139:601–3.
96. Bellotti C, Aragno MG, Medina M, et al. Differential diagnosis of CT-hypodense cranial lesions with indium-111-oxine-labeled leukocytes. J Neurosurg. 1986;64:750–3.
97. Mok YP, Carney WH, Fernandez-Ulloa M. Skeletal photopenic lesions in In-111 WBC imaging. J Nucl Med. 1984;25:1322–6.
98. Palestro CJ, Love C, Tronco GG, et al. Combined labeled leukocyte and technetium-99m sulfur colloid marrow imaging for diagnosing musculoskeletal infection: principles, technique, interpretation, indications and limitations. Radiographics. 2006;26:859–70.
99. Palestro CJ, Kim CK, Swyer AJ, et al. Radionuclide diagnosis of vertebral osteomyelitis: indium-111-leukocyte and technetium-99m-methylene diphosphonate bone scintigraphy. J Nucl Med. 1991;32:1861–5.
100. Palestro CJ, Kim CK, Vega A, et al. Acute effect of radiation therapy on indium-111 labeled leukocyte uptake in bone marrow. J Nucl Med. 1989;30:1889–91.
101. Palestro CJ, Love C, Tronco GG, et al. Role of radionuclide imaging in the diagnosis of postoperative infection. Radiographics. 2000;20:1649–60.
102. Society of Nuclear Medicine procedure guideline for ^{99m}Tc-exametazime (HMPAO)-labeled leukocyte scintigraphy for suspected infection/inflammation. Version 3.0, approved 2 June 2004.
103. McAfee JG, Samin A. In-111 labeled leukocytes: a review of problems in image interpretation. Radiology. 1985;155:221–9.
104. Palestro CJ, Padilla ML, Swyer AJ, et al. Diffuse pulmonary uptake of indium-111-labeled leukocytes in drug-induced pneumonitis. J Nucl Med. 1992;33:1175–7.
105. Marinelli WA, Walker Smith GJ, Ingbar DH. Inflammation and repair of the lung. In: Bone RC, editor. Pulmonary and critical care medicine. St Louis, Mo: Mosby; 1998. p. 1–6.
106. Girndt M, Kaul H, Leitnaker CK, et al. Selective sequestration of cytokine-producing monocytes during hemodialysis treatment. Am J Kidney Dis. 2001;37:954–63.
107. Palestro CJ, Goldsmith SJ. The role of gallium and labeled leukocyte scintigraphy in the AIDS patient. Q J Nucl Med. 1995;39:221–30.
108. Palestro CJ, Love C. Radionuclide imaging of musculoskeletal infection: conventional agents. Semin Musculoskelet Radiol. 2007;11:335–52.
109. Sonmezoglu K, Sonmezoglu M, Halac M. Usefulness of ^{99m}Tc-ciprofloxacin (infection) scan in diagnosis of chronic orthopedic infections: comparative study with ^{99m}Tc-HMPAO leukocyte scintigraphy. J Nucl Med. 2001;42:567–74.
110. Shammas A, Lim R, Charron M. Pediatric FDG PET/CT: physiologic uptake, normal variants, and benign conditions. Radiographics. 2009;29:1467–86.
111. Shreve PD, Anzai Y, Wahl RL. Pitfalls in oncologic diagnosis with FDG PET imaging: physiologic and benign variants. Radiographics. 1999;19:61–77.
112. Strauss GJ. Fluorine-18 deoxyglucose and false-positive results: a major problem in the diagnostics of oncological patients. Eur J Nucl Med. 1996;23:1409–15.
113. Abouzied MM, Crawford ES, Nabi HA. ^{18}F-FDG imaging: pitfalls and artifacts. J Nucl Med Technol. 2005;33:145–55.
114. Himms-Hagen J. Brown adipose tissue thermogenesis: interdisciplinary studies. FASEB J. 1990;4:2890–8.
115. Cook GJ, Wegner EA, Fogelman I. Pitfalls and artifacts in ^{18}FDG PET and PET/CT oncologic imaging. Semin Nucl Med. 2004;34:122–33.
116. Maurer AH, Burshteyn M, Adler LP, et al. How to differentiate benign versus malignant cardiac and paracardiac ^{18}F-FDG uptake at oncologic PET/CT. Radiographics. 2011;31:1287–305.
117. Patel PM, Alibazoglu H, Ali A, et al. Normal thymic uptake of FDG on PET imaging. Clin Nucl Med. 1996;21:772–5.
118. Hicks RJ, Binns D, Stabin MG. Pattern of uptake and excretion of ^{18}F-FDG in the lactating breast. J Nucl Med. 2001;42:1238–42.
119. Kitajima K, NakamotoY SM. Normal uptake of ^{18}F-FDG in the testis: an assessment by PET/CT. Ann Nucl Med. 2007;21:405–10.
120. Liu Y, Ghesani NV, Zuckier LS. Physiology and pathophysiology of incidental findings detected on FDG-PET scintigraphy. Semin Nucl Med. 2010;40:294–315.
121. Vilain D, Bochet J, Le Stanc E. Unsuspected hibernating myocardium detected by routine oncology ^{18}F-FDG PET/CT. Eur J Nucl Med Mol Imaging. 2010;37:409.
122. Zanco P, Desideri A, Mobilia G, et al. Effects of left bundle branch block on myocardial FDG PET in patients without significant coronary artery stenoses. J Nucl Med. 2000;41:973–7.
123. Zazulia AR, Videen TO, Powers WJ. Transient focal increase in perihematomal glucose metabolism after acute human intracerebral hemorrhage. Stroke. 2009;40:1638–43.
124. Akman CI, Ichise M, Olsavsky A, et al. Epilepsy duration impacts on brain glucose metabolism in temporal lobe epilepsy: results of voxel-based mapping. Epilepsy Behav. 2010;17:373–80.
125. Novak L, Emri M, Molnar P. Regional cerebral ^{18}FDG uptake during subarachnoid hemorrhage induced vasospasm. Neurol Res. 2006;28:864–70.
126. Weng JH, Lee JK, Wu MF, et al. Pituitary FDG uptake in a patient of lung cancer with bilateral adrenal metastases causing adrenal cortical insufficiency. Clin Nucl Med. 2011;36:731–2.
127. Poduri A, Golja A, Takeoka M, et al. Focal cortical malformations can show asymmetrically higher uptake on interictal fluorine-18 fluorodeoxyglucose positron emission tomography (PET). J Child Neurol. 2007;22:232–7.
128. Kostakoglu L, Hardoff R, Mirtcheva R, et al. PET-CT fusion imaging in differentiating physiologic from pathologic FDG uptake. Radiographics. 2004;24:1411–31.
129. Poole DC, Kindig CA, Behnke BJ. Effects of emphysema on diaphragm microvascular oxygen pressure. Am J Respir Crit Care Med. 2001;163:1081–6.
130. Alavi A, Gupta N, Alberini JL, et al. Positron emission tomography imaging in nonmalignant thoracic disorders. Semin Nucl Med. 2002;32:293–321.

131. Goerres GW, Ziegler SI, Burger C. Artifacts at PET and PET/CT caused by metallic hip prosthetic material. Radiology. 2003;226:577–84.
132. Bujenovic S, Mannting F, Chakrabarti R, et al. Artifactual 2-deoxy-2-^{18}F-fluoro-D-glucose localization surrounding metallic objects in a PET/CT scanner using CT-based attenuation correction. Mol Imaging Biol. 2003;5:20–2.
133. Cohade C, Wahl RL. Applications of positron emission tomography/computed tomography image fusion in clinical positron emission tomography—clinical use, interpretation methods, diagnostic improvements. Semin Nucl Med. 2003;33:228–37.
134. Wahl RL. Why nearly all PET of abdominal and pelvic cancers will be performed as PET/CT. J Nucl Med. 2004;45:82S–95S.
135. Kawano T, Suzuki A, Ishida A, et al. The clinical relevance of thymic fluorodeoxyglucose uptake in pediatric patients after chemotherapy. Eur J Nucl Med Mol Imaging. 2004;31:831–6.
136. Nakahara T, Fujii H, Ide M, et al. FDG uptake in the morphologically normal thymus: comparison of FDG positron emission tomography and CT. Br J Radiol. 2001;74:821–4.
137. Alibazoglu H, Alibazoglu B, Hollinger E, et al. Normal thymic uptake of 2-deoxy-2[F-18]fluoro-D-glucose. Clin Nucl Med. 1999;24:597–600.
138. Brink I, Reinhardt MJ, Hoegerle S, et al. Increased metabolic activity in the thymus gland studied with ^{18}F-FDG PET: age dependency and frequency after chemotherapy. J Nucl Med. 2001;42:591–5.
139. Burrell SC, Van den Abbeele AD. 2-Deoxy-2-[F-18] fluoro-D-glucose-positron emission tomography of the head and neck: an atlas of normal uptake and variants. Mol Imaging Biol. 2005;7:244–56.
140. Grab D, Flock F, Stöhr I, et al. Classification of asymptomatic adnexal masses by ultrasound, magnetic resonance imaging, and positron emission tomography. Gynecol Oncol. 2000;77:454–9.
141. Nakayama Y, Makino S, Fukuda Y, et al. Activation of lavage lymphocytes in lung injuries caused by radiotherapy for lung cancer. Int J Radiat Oncol Biol Phys. 1996;32:459–67.
142. De Winter F, Van de Wiele C, Vogelaers D. Fluorine-18 fluorodeoxyglucose positron emission tomography: a highly accurate imaging modality for the diagnosis of chronic musculoskeletal infections. J Bone Joint Surg Am. 2001;83:651–60.
143. Gorospe L, Raman S, Echeveste J, et al. Whole-body PET/CT: spectrum of physiological variants, artifacts and interpretative pitfalls in cancer patients. Nucl Med Commun. 2005;26:671–87.
144. Liu Y. Orthopedic surgery-related benign uptake on FDG-PET: case examples and pitfalls. Ann Nucl Med. 2009;23:701–8.
145. Zhuang H, Chacko TK, Hickeson M, et al. Persistent non-specific FDG uptake on PET imaging following hip arthroplasty. Eur J Nucl Med. 2002;29:1328–33.
146. Chacko TK, Zhuang H, Stevenson K, et al. The importance of the location of fluorodeoxyglucose uptake in periprosthetic infection in painful hip prostheses. Nucl Med Commun. 2002;23:851–5.
147. Nguyen BD, Ram PC, Roarke MC. Hip anthroplasty with mass-like pelvic granulomatous disease: PET imaging. Clin Nucl Med. 2006;31:30–2.
148. Lim JW, Tang CL, Keng GH. False positive F-18 fluorodeoxyglucose combined PET/CT scans from suture granuloma and chronic inflammation: report of two cases and review of literature. Ann Acad Med Singap. 2005;34:457–62.
149. Shon IH, O'Doherty MJ, Maisey MN. Positron emission tomography in lung cancer. Semin Nucl Med. 2002;32:240–71.
150. Henry G, Garner WL. Inflammatory mediators in wound healing. Surg Clin North Am. 2003;83:483–507.
151. Kazama T, Swanston N, Podoloff DA, et al. Effect of colony-stimulating factor and conventional- or high-dose chemotherapy on FDG uptake in bone marrow. Eur J Nucl Med Mol Imaging. 2005;32:1406–11.
152. Sugawara Y, Zasadny KR, Kison PV, et al. Splenic fluorodeoxyglucose uptake increased by granulocyte colony-stimulating factor therapy: PET imaging results. J Nucl Med. 1999;40:1456–62.
153. Kim EE, Chung SK, Haynie TP, et al. Differentiation of residual or recurrent tumors from post-treatment changes with F-18 FDG PET. Radiographics. 1992;12:269–79.
154. Esmailiejah AA, Abbasian M, Azarsina S, et al. Diagnostic efficacy of UBI scan in musculoskeletal infections. Arch Iran Med. 2015;18:371–5.
155. Meléndez-Alafort L, Rodrìguez-Cortés J, Ferro-Flores G, et al. Biokinetics of ^{99m}Tc-UBI in humans. Nucl Med Biol. 2004;31:373–9.
156. Jehangir M, Bashar M, Pervez S. Development of kits for ^{99m}Tc radiopharmaceuticals for infection imaging. Vienna: IAEA/IAEA-TECDOC-1414; 2004. p. 65–77.
157. Mikolajczak R, Korsak A, Gorska B, et al. Development of kits for ^{99m}Tc radiopharmaceuticals for infection imaging. Vienna: IAEA/IAEA-TECDOC-1414; 2004. p. 79–86.
158. Sepúlveda-Méndez J, de Murphy CA, Rojas-Bautista JC, et al. Specificity of ^{99m}Tc-UBI for detecting infection foci in patients with fever in study. Nucl Med Commun. 2010;31:889–95.
159. Saeed S, Zafar J, Khan B, et al. Utility of ^{99m}Tc-labelled antimicrobial peptide ubiquicidin (29-41) in the diagnosis of diabetic foot infection. Eur J Nucl Med Mol Imaging. 2013;40:737–43.
160. Sathekge M, Garcia-Perez O, Paez D, et al. Molecular imaging in musculoskeletal infections with ^{99m}Tc-UBI 29-41 SPECT/CT. Ann Nucl Med. 2018;32:54–9.
161. Auletta S, Galli F, Lauri C, et al. Imaging bacteria with radiolabelled quinolones, cephalosporins and siderophores for imaging infection: a systematic review. Clin Transl Imaging. 2016;4:229–52.
162. Meyer M, Testart N, Jreige M, et al. Diagnostic performance of PET or PET/CT using ^{18}F-FDG labeled white blood cells in infectious disease: a systematic review and a bivariate meta-analysis. Diagnostics. 2019;10(1). pii: E2. https://doi.org/10.3390/diagnostics10010002.
163. Zhang XM, Zhang H, McLeroth P, Berkowitz RD, et al. [124I] FIAU: human dosimetry and infection imaging in patients with suspected prosthetic joint infection. Nucl Med Biol. 2016;43:273–9.
164. Nanni C, Errani C, Boriani L, et al. ^{68}Ga-citrate PET/CT for evaluating patients with infections of the bone: preliminary results. J Nucl Med. 2016;51:1932–6.
165. Tseng JR, Chang YH, Wu CT, et al. Potential usefulness of ^{68}Ga-citrate PET/CT in detecting infected lower limb prostheses. EJNMMI Res. 2019;9(1):2. https://doi.org/10.1186/s13550-018-0468-3.

Nuclear Medicine Imaging of Soft Tissue Infections

2

Giovanni D'Errico, Emanuele Casciani, and Saadi Sollaku

Contents

Learning Objectives

- To become familiar with the different clinical presentations of soft tissue infections
- To provide a schematic classification of soft tissue infections into cellulitis, abscesses, necrotizing fasciitis, infectious bursitis, and infectious myositis
- To summarize a general imaging approach to soft tissue infection based on the use of ultrasound, plain X-ray, computed tomography, magnetic resonance imaging, and nuclear medicine imaging
- To emphasize, for each imaging technique, the advantages and drawbacks in order to direct the reader to the imaging procedure to use for rapid and accurate diagnosis of soft tissue infections

G. D'Errico (✉) · E. Casciani · S. Sollaku
Department of Nuclear Medicine, Private Hospital "Pio XI", Rome, Italy

2.1 Introduction

Soft tissues are defined all those tissues that do not have a density similar to that of bone. They therefore include, among others, the skin, muscles, abdominal wall, thoracic, or abdominal space. Infections of soft tissues constitute a group of frequently observed medical conditions (that are sometimes life-threatening), which may occur with different characteristics regarding site, location, clinical characteristics, and etiological agent. Their classification relies upon different criteria that can take into account anatomical site (depth of the plans involved, superficial and deep infections), patient's clinical status (possible comorbidity such as diabetes, AIDS, peripheral vascular diseases, sensory neuropathy, surgical or accidental trauma), and virulence of the causative microorganism. Soft tissue infections (acute or chronic) may arise by the hematogenous route, or "per continuitatem," or by inoculation, including surgical infection or spread from other areas. They can also be classified as follows: cellulitis, abscesses, necrotizing fasciitis, infectious bursitis, and infective myositis.

E. Lazzeri et al. (eds.), *Radionuclide Imaging of Infection and Inflammation*, https://doi.org/10.1007/978-3-030-62175-9_2

Cellulitis is usually diagnosed clinically, based on medical history and physical examination. Imaging may be helpful for characterizing purulent soft tissue infections and the associated osteomyelitis.

Necrotizing fasciitis, a medical emergency, is also diagnosed clinically, and imaging can reveal nonspecific or negative findings (particularly during the early phase of disease) [1]. Necrotizing fasciitis can mimic, in imaging investigations, non-necrotizing fasciitis, myositis, neoplasm, myonecrosis, and inflammatory myopathy.

Early and accurate diagnosis and identification of the anatomic boundaries of soft tissue infection/inflammation can be difficult, especially in some clinical situations, thus rendering complex the management of seriously ill patient.

If it is true that the gold standard method for diagnosing soft tissue infection is a positive culture from the affected tissue, it can often be problematic to obtain sufficient tissue for analysis for different reasons, among which the most frequent are the difficulty of anatomical access or the presence of contaminants on the surface. Moreover, the location and extent of the involvement largely influence management of these patients.

The most frequent questions that clinicians ask the imaging specialist (radiologist or nuclear medicine physician) to address are:

- Is there a focus of infection?
- What is the size and extent of the lesion?
- Can the patient stop antibiotic therapy?
- Is the infection/inflammation in the lesion over?

This chapter summarizes the soft tissue infection imaging approach performed with ultrasound (US), radiography, computed tomography, magnetic resonance imaging, and nuclear medicine. For each technique, the advantages and drawback are highlighted, directing the reader to the imaging procedure to be employed for rapid and accurate diagnosis of soft tissue infections.

Key Learning Points

- Soft tissue infections can occur with different characteristics in terms of site, location, clinical features, and causative agent.
- Soft tissue infections can be classified as cellulitis, abscesses, necrotizing fasciitis, infectious bursitis, and infective myositis.
- Early and accurate diagnosis of soft tissue infection/inflammation as well as identification of the anatomic boundaries can be difficult in some clinical conditions.
- The gold standard for reliable evaluation of soft tissue infection is a positive culture from the affected tissue, which can be problematic because of difficulties of anatomical access or the presence of contaminants on the surface.
- By providing a physiological evaluation, nuclear medical imaging tests are invaluable and sometimes represent the problem-solving diagnostic test, especially in those patients in whom other imaging tests provide equivocal/inconclusive results or are impossible to perform.

2.2 General Background on Imaging of Soft Tissue Infection

2.2.1 Ultrasound Imaging of Soft Tissue Infections

Although having low sensitivity, due to its low cost, availability, and portability, highlighting fluid collections and potential for real-time guidance of aspiration of fluids, ultrasound (US) can be particularly useful in soft tissue infections whose early diagnosis, together with clinical evaluation, represents the most immediate tool for adequate medical treatment and, possibly, also for surgical debridement [2].

Depending on internal composition, soft tissue abscesses may appear anechoic or may show a variable amount of internal echoes. Usually an abscess of the soft tissues presents in elliptical or spherical shape and is characterized by more or less irregular margins. This technique, however, is often unable to distinguish abscess from hematoma (which can be interpreted as a tumor). Furthermore, the US examination is heavily operator-dependent and, in the case of complex and deep lesions, may underestimate the extent of the lesion. Furthermore, the growing use of imaging such as magnetic resonance imaging (MRI) and computed tomography (CT) has significantly reduced the applications of ultrasound imaging.

2.2.2 Plain X-ray Imaging of Soft Tissue Infections

This relatively inexpensive and easy-to-perform procedure may identify soft tissue swelling, gas in soft tissue as in necrotizing fasciitis or bone involvement. However, it is actually considered as an ancillary imaging technique.

2.2.3 Computed Tomography (CT) Imaging of Soft Tissue Infections

By providing multi-planar images, CT (which is available also in any emergency department) can play an important role in the evaluation of soft tissue infection/inflammation. When administering intravenous contrast, rim enhancement helps to identify abscess collections.

The exact role of CT in the diagnosis of soft tissue infections has not yet been established. CT is certainly very useful in hybrid imaging studies (SPECT/CT) in which its role is enhanced in providing anatomical detail for exact anatomical characterization of the infection site. Martinez M et al. showed, in identifying soft tissues infection, sensitivity of 100%, specificity of 98%, positive predictive value of 76%, and negative predictive value of 100% [3].

2.2.4 Magnetic Resonance Imaging (MRI) of Soft Tissue Infections

MRI is the ideal technique to visualize the changes of the soft tissues produced by infectious processes; usually such changes consist of signal intensity changes that reflect the higher content of water of the soft tissues induced by inflammatory reactions. MRI provides more accurate information on local extent of the soft tissues and possible soft tissue abscess, particularly in patients with musculoskeletal infection. The main drawback of MRI is its long time of acquisition and higher costs versus other imaging modalities.

A multi-institutional comparative analysis [4] between MRI and radionuclide imaging (with SPECT/CT) showed sensitivity, specificity, positive predictive value, and negative predictive value of 86%, 88%, 60%, and 100% for MRI, whereas they were 93%, 97%, 90%, and 100%, respectively, for SPECT/CT.

2.2.5 Nuclear Medicine Imaging of Soft Tissue Infections

Scintigraphic procedures have gradually become an essential component of the diagnostic procedure. In order to address the questions asked by the clinician, the nuclear medicine specialist must be well aware of the pathophysiology of inflammation and infection. Knowing etiology and the mechanisms of infection/inflammation development is the starting point to carefully choose the most adequate nuclear medicine imaging method.

Inflammation is a nonspecific reaction of the body to any injury (which may be a simple trauma or an ischemia, or possibly also a tumor): if the tissue injury is not due to microorganisms, it will be inflammation without infection, otherwise it will be infection. The response is characterized by growth of local blood influx and increased vascular permeability in the affected area, enhanced transudation of plasma proteins, and increased influx of leukocytes. Leukocytes actively migrate from circulation into inflammatory tissues through sequential steps: adhesion to vascular endothelium, diapedesis crossing through the endothelium and the basal membrane, migration, and chemotaxis in the inflammatory site. In the acute phase, the site of infection and/or inflammation is infiltrated, largely, by granulocytes; in the chronic phase, the predominant cells are lymphocytes, monocytes, and macrophages.

Although many radionuclide imaging techniques that have been proposed over the years to classify the different inflammatory/infectious lesions, to date an ideal radiopharmaceutical has not yet been found. Wide availability, ease of preparation, low cost of both the drug and radionuclide, low toxicity, absence of immune response to the compound, and high specificity should induce nuclear physicians to evaluate, whenever possible, each individual case and choose the most suitable radiopharmaceutical for the patient's clinical situation.

Recent work has shown the advantages of using the high spatial resolution of PET/CT with [^{18}F]FDG, although further clinical trials are certainly required to better define the actual impact [^{18}F]FDG PET/CT, that targets the increased metabolic activity of infected areas. Limitations and pitfalls for the use of radiotracers in the assessment of infection and inflammation can be related to patient conditions (e.g., diabetes mellitus) or to biodistribution of a specific radiopharmaceutical [5].

To date, imaging with labeled white blood cells (WBC) is the procedure of choice, as a standard method for early assessment of functional damage due to an infectious process or for detecting and locating a hidden infection in soft tissues.

Labeling of leukocytes can be performed in vivo using antibodies or antibody fragments (a whole murine IgG anti-NCA-95 and a Fab' fragment anti-NCA-90) or in vitro using either ^{111}In-oxine or ^{99m}Tc-HMPAO.

^{99m}Tc-labeled antigranulocyte monoclonal antibody Fab' fragments can be used for imaging of acute infections of soft tissue. Finally they suffer from some limitations, with overall 76% sensitivity and 84% specificity for acute infections; moreover, false-negative results are likely in patients with chronic infections and are not widely available [6].

Despite the development of several new radiopharmaceuticals, imaging based on the use of in vitro labeled leukocytes remains the procedure of choice, the gold standard method for early assessment of functional impairment due to infectious process or to detect and localize an occult infection in soft tissues. Because of its more favorable radiation characteristics for imaging, labeling with ^{99m}Tc-HMPAO is more commonly used than labeling with ^{111}In-oxine [7].

Despite its high diagnostic accuracy, the in vitro labeled leukocyte procedure has significant limitations: it is not always available, is labor-intensive, and involves direct handling of blood products. The biological risk for healthcare professionals involved in the handling of blood products constitute additional disadvantages of the WBC labeling technique.

Furthermore, in patients with neutropenia, it is often difficult to obtain a sufficient amount of WBCs for labeling. In addition, the functional status of WBCs must be taken into account. Another concern involves patients receiving chemotherapy or other immune modulating agents that can affect WBC harvesting and/or function when injected back into the patient. Therefore, patients undergoing chemotherapy, receiving glucocorticoids, or infected with HIV may be difficult or impossible to image. The reported sensitivity and specificity for radiolabeled leukocytes ranges from 86 to 90%, with a slightly higher sensitivity for acute infections—most likely due to the increased granulocytic response.

A double-head γ-camera equipped with high-resolution collimators is used, with an acquisition matrix of 512 × 512. For an "in vitro quality control," the ^{99m}Tc-HMPAO-WBC images are acquired on lungs, liver, and spleen, to evaluate their in vivo biodistribution at 5 min and 60 min after administration. According to clinical indications, whole-body, planar and SPECT (preferably SPECT/CT) acquisitions should be recorded at 3–4 h (delayed images) and 20–24 h (late images) [8].

While SPECT imaging provides functional information and localization of all the foci of leukocyte accumulation, the CT images provide exact anatomical identification of the infection sites visualized by SPECT imaging. Thus, multimodality imaging with SPECT/CT identifies the morphological abnormalities that correspond to the areas of increased activity on the radionuclide images. Acquiring SPECT, more preferably SPECT/CT imaging improves the overall diagnostic accuracy [8, 9].

2.3 Conclusions

Wide availability, ease of preparation, low cost of both the drug and radionuclide, low toxicity, absence of immune response to the drug, and high specificity, particular characteristics necessary for an optimal imaging technique to detect an inflammatory/infectious soft tissue lesion, should induce the nuclear medicine specialist to evaluate, whenever possible, each individual case and choose the most suitable radiopharmaceutical for the patient's clinical situation.

Despite the development of several novel radiopharmaceuticals, imaging with in vitro labeled leukocytes is currently the approach of choice, the gold standard method for early assessment of functional impairment due to infectious process or to detect and localize an occult infection in soft tissues.

Key Learning Points

- Because of its wide availability and overall low cost, ultrasound imaging is generally employed as a preliminary investigation in patients with suspected soft tissue infection.
- However, it has generally low sensitivity, although it can be especially useful for real-time guidance for aspiration of fluids and subsequent microbiology.
- Plain X-ray imaging may identify soft tissue swelling or gas in soft tissues (as in necrotizing fasciitis); it is currently considered an ancillary imaging technique.
- CT imaging with contrast enhancement can identify the edge of abscess collections in patients with soft tissue infections.
- Rather than a separate imaging investigation per se, CT imaging has an important role when employed for hybrid PET/CT or SPECT/CT imaging in patients with soft tissue infections.
- MR imaging provides accurate information on local extent of soft tissue infections, particularly in case of musculoskeletal infections.
- Radionuclide imaging of soft tissue infections relies on two main modalities, PET/CT with [^{18}F]FDG and SPECT/CT with infection imaging agents, respectively.
- Leukocyte scintigraphy can be based on in vitro labeling (i.e., ^{111}In-oxine-WBC or preferably ^{99m}Tc-HMPAO-WBC) or on administration of radiolabeled anti-granulocyte antibodies.
- For single-photon imaging, scintigraphy with ^{99m}Tc-HMPAO-WBC remains the preferred imaging modality in patients with soft tissue infections, especially if including SPECT/CT acquisition.

Acknowledgments The authors express their gratitude to Drs. Alessandro Carbonara and Dario Di Luzio (Department of Radiology of the Private Hospital "Pio XI," Rome, Italy) for their precious contribution.

Clinical Cases

Case 2.1

Background

A 76-year-old woman submitted 3 years earlier to total arthroplasty of her right hip. The patient complained of persistent pain in right hip, with progressive worsening, and limited movement. A cutaneous fistula discharging pus-like fluid appeared on the anterior aspect of right thigh; besides the fistula, physical examination revealed the classical triad of infection/inflammation: "rubor," "calor," and "dolor" on the external aspect of the right thigh. Blood biochemistry revealed markedly increased values of the acute infection/inflammation markers (ESR 76 mm/h; C-reactive protein 30.1 mg/dL), while the leukocyte count was 7900/mm^3. Clinical diagnosis of possible infection was established, and the patient was referred for leukocyte scintigraphy to ascertain the presence of infection and to assess its extent.

Scintigraphy with ^{99m}Tc-HMPAO-WBC and especially SPECT/CT imaging (Fig. 2.1) visualized abnormal accumulation of labeled leukocytes to constitute an oval-shaped collection with cranio-caudal course, located deeply and externally to the right femoral head, parallel to the prosthesis stem (fused SPECT/CT images: coronal in upper left panel, sagittal in upper right panel, transaxial in lower left panel). An additional focus of labeled leukocyte accumulation was observed on the right pubic branch, continuing with a fistulous tract reaching the skin surface (fused coronal SPECT/CT image in lower right panel).

Suspected Site of Disease

Right hip prosthesis and adjacent soft tissues.

Radiopharmaceutical Activity

^{99m}Tc-HMPAO-WBC, 555 MBq.

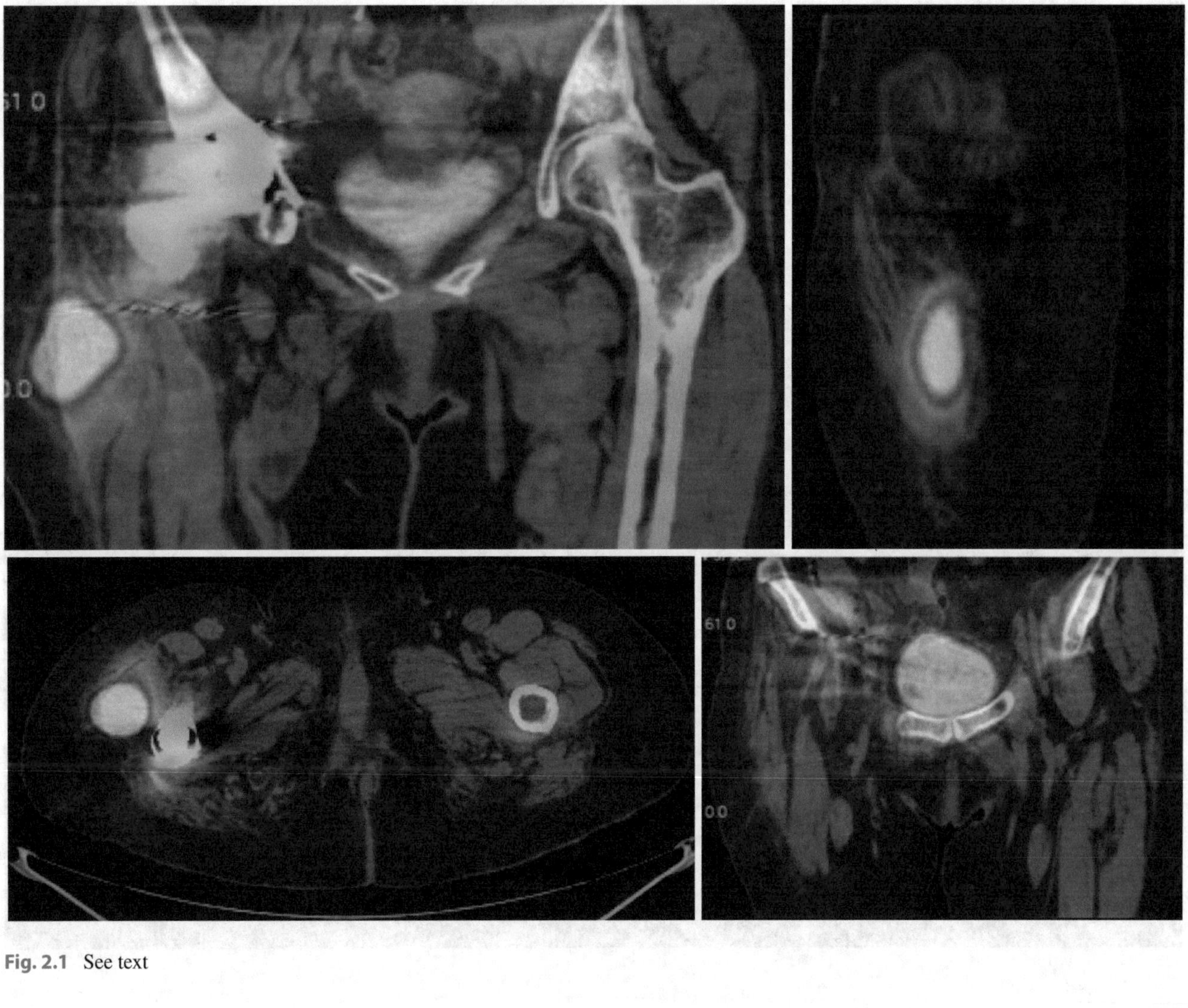

Fig. 2.1 See text

Imaging
Planar acquisitions at 1 h, 4 h, and 20 h after administration of the radiolabeled leukocytes. SPECT/CT imaging acquired immediately after acquisition of the 4-h planar image and also at the delayed 20 h time point.

Conclusion/Teaching Point
Although the 4-h planar imaging alone correctly visualized the focal accumulation of labeled leukocytes at the right thigh (thus confirming the presence of infection), it was SPECT/CT imaging that identified full extension of infection from the femoral head (parallel to the prosthesis stem) up to the skin (fistula). This information was crucial for decision-making when selecting the most adequate treatment of this infectious condition.

Case 2.2

Background
A 69-year-old diabetic man whose medical history included amputation of left leg (at the mid-diaphyseal portion of left tibia). Recent onset (about 1 month before being referred for labeled leukocyte scintigraphy) of severe pain at the left leg stump, with appearance of an abscess treated with antibiotic therapy and ice cube cryotherapy. Later on, onset of fistula with leak of sero-hematic fluid, treated with laser therapy and magnetic therapy leading to apparent healing. This was followed by recurrence and worsening of the abscess; the patient also suffered from hamstring syndrome of left lower limb. MRI of left tibia visualized sclerosis at the end of the tibial stump, hypotrophy of adjacent muscles, and fluid collection on the distal portion of the left tibial stump. Ultrasound showed diffusely increased echogenicity of the skin and subcutaneous tissue involved (Fig. 2.2).

Scintigraphy with ^{99m}Tc-HMPAO-WBC was performed to confirm the infectious nature of the lesion (versus simple inflammation) and to assess the actual extent of infection, i.e., to ascertain whether the infection was limited to soft tissues only or involving bone as well (concomitant osteomyelitis?). Planar imaging, but especially a SPECT/CT acquisition of the left lower limb (Fig. 2.3), visualized abnormal accumulation of labeled leukocytes in the soft tissues of the outer end of the left tibial stump (corresponding to the clinically detectable abscess) with extension up to the skin (fistula). Radiolabeled leukocytes accumulated in a wide area on the rear portion of left knee, corresponding to the hamstring muscles. Concomitant osteomyelitis was not detected.

Suspected Site of Disease
Left tibial stump and adjacent soft tissues.

Radiopharmaceutical Activity
^{99m}Tc-HMPAO-WBC, 555 MBq.

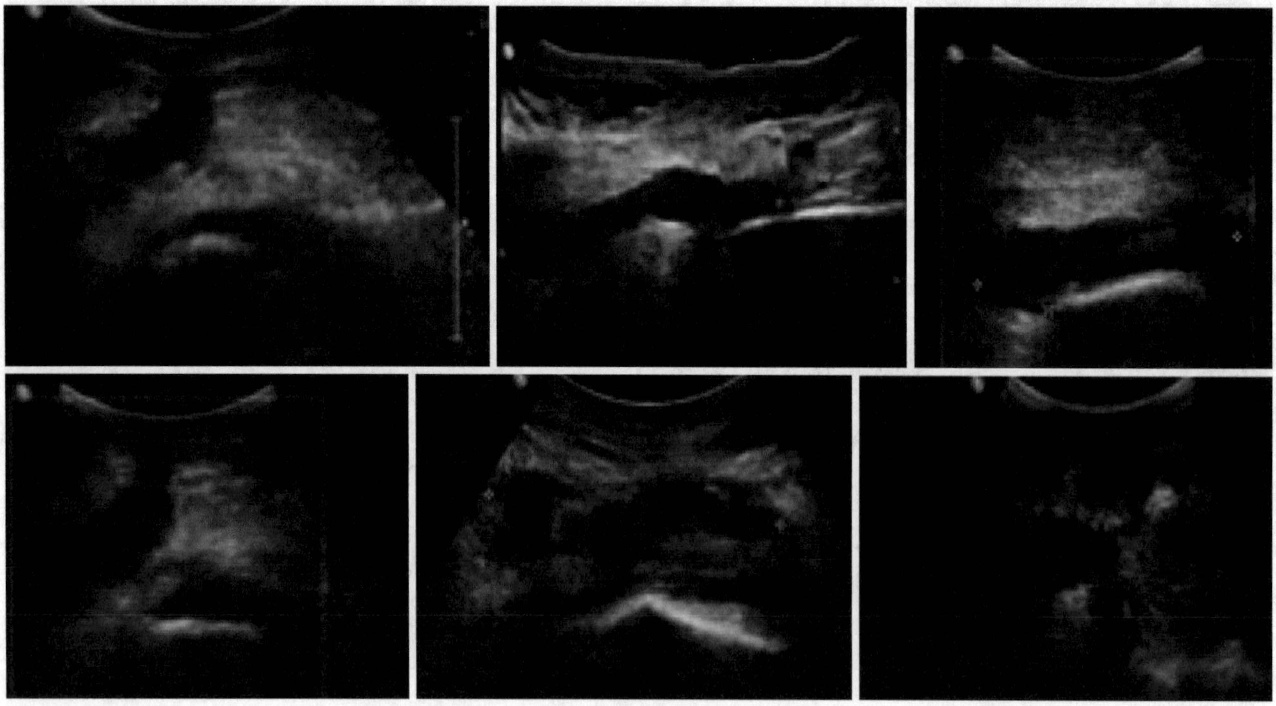

Fig. 2.2 See text

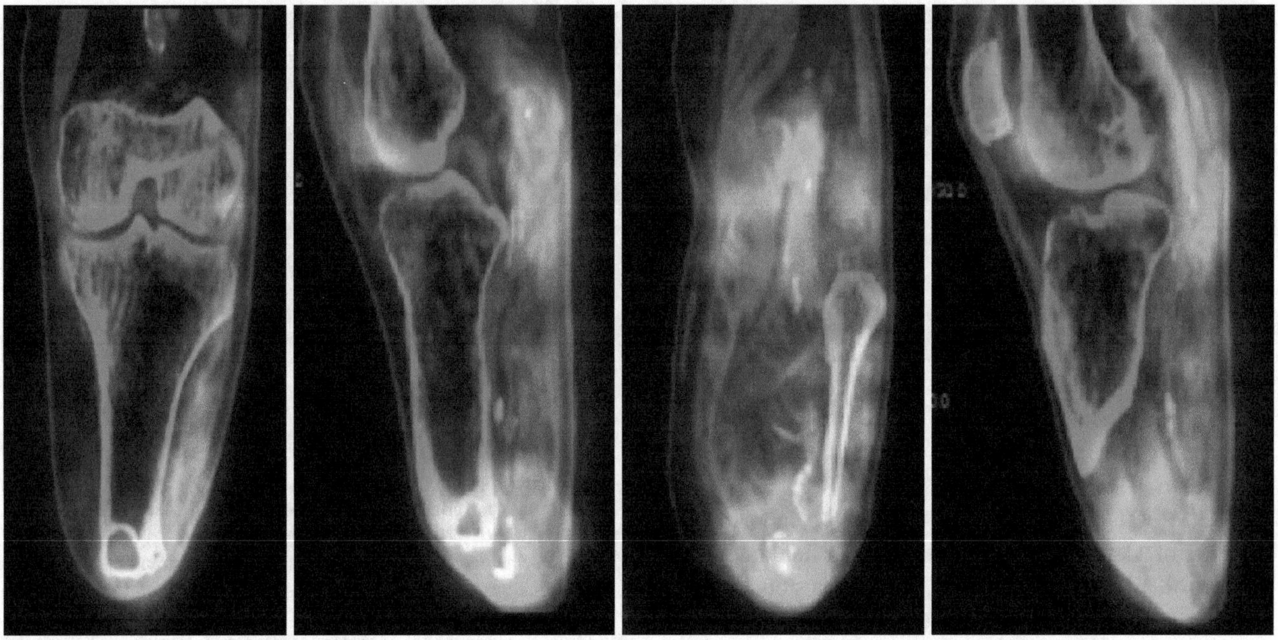

Fig. 2.3 See text

Imaging

Planar acquisitions at 1 h, 4 h, and 20 h after administration of the radiolabeled leukocytes. SPECT/CT imaging acquired immediately after acquisition of the 4-h planar image and also at the delayed 20 h time point.

Conclusion/Teaching Point

Hybrid SPECT/CT acquired during ^{99m}Tc-HMPAO-WBC scintigraphy excluded the presence of osteomyelitis. The presence of an abscess on the outer end of the left tibial stump with extension up to the cutaneous fistula was confirmed, despite the fact that the abscess site appeared as healed on visual inspection; furthermore, SPECT/CT imaging visualized the presence of infection at the hamstring muscles.

Case 2.3

A 70-year-old man submitted to total replacement of right hip prosthesis because of femoral trauma. Four months after hip prosthesis replacement surgery, onset of painful swelling in right thigh, fever, and reduced motion range of the right hip. A CT scan showed significant accumulation of fluid close to the trochanteric region and to the proximal third of the right femoral shaft. Medical history revealed a recent infection from *Klebsiella pneumoniae*. Ultrasonography of the right hip confirmed a significant periprosthetic abscess (>10 cm in size) extending into the subcutaneous levels of the anterolateral thigh and continuing superficially with a linear image interpreted as scarring or fistula.

Physical examination revealed the classical triad of infection/inflammation: “rubor,” “calor,” and “dolor” on the surgical scar of the right thigh. Two fistulas at the lower edge of the scar, with discharge of purulent material, were noticed. Blood biochemistry revealed markedly increased values of the acute infection/inflammation markers (ESR 58 mm/h; C-reactive protein 37 mg/dL), while the leukocyte count was 8600/mm^3 (neutrophils representing 69.9% of total leukocytes).

Scintigraphy with ^{99m}Tc-HMPAO-WBC was performed to confirm the presence of infection and to assess its actual extent. The planar views at 1 and 3 h (as well as SPECT/CT imaging at 3 h) visualized a photon-deficient area surrounded by a halo of increased radioactivity accumulation at the right hip; late SPECT/CT imaging at 22 h (Fig. 2.4) revealed complete filling with radiolabeled leukocytes of the area that was photon-deficient at the earlier acquisitions, with some residual inhomogeneity.

Suspected Site of Disease

Right hip.

Radiopharmaceutical Activity

^{99m}Tc-HMPAO-WBC, 600 MBq.

Imaging

Planar acquisitions at 1, 3, and 22 h after administration of the radiolabeled leukocytes. SPECT/CT imaging acquired immediately after acquisition of the 4-h planar image and also at the delayed 22 h time point.

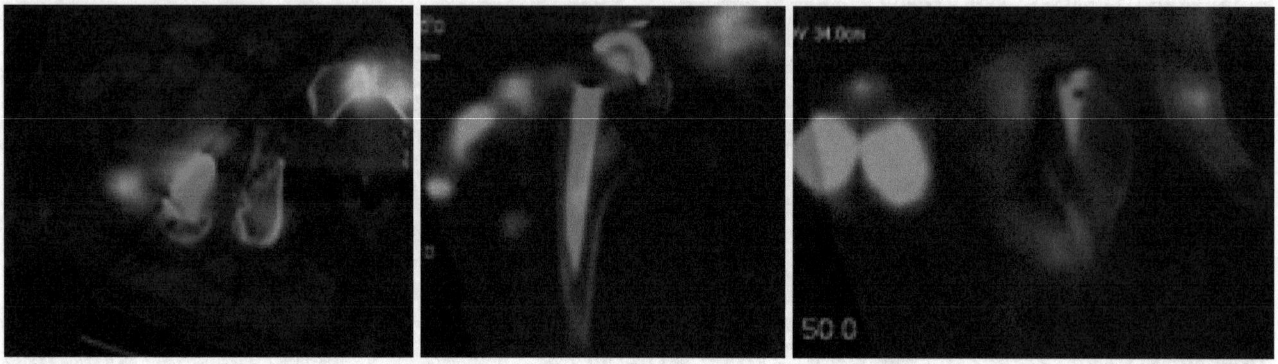

Fig. 2.4 See text

Conclusion/Teaching Point

Hybrid SPECT/CT imaging was crucial to demonstrate the presence of a large collection of corpuscular fluid in the right peri-prosthetic area (an abscess), with extension up to the skin surfaces (fistulas). The most informative SPECT/CT images were obtained at 22 h post injection.

References

1. Chaudhry AA, Baker KS, Gould ES, Gupta R. Necrotizing fasciitis and its mimics: what radiologists need to know. AJR Am J Roentgenol. 2015;204:128–39.
2. Altmayer S, Verma N, Dicks EA, Oliveira A. Imaging musculoskeletal soft tissue infections. Semin Ultrasound CT MR. 2020;41:85–98.
3. Martinez M, Peponis T, Hage A, Yeh DD, Kaafarani HMA, Fagenholz PJ, et al. The role of computed tomography in the diagnosis of necrotizing soft tissue infections. World J Surg. 2018;42:82–7.
4. Backer HC, Steurer-Dober I, Beck M, Agten CA, Decking J, Herzog RF, et al. Magnetic resonance imaging (MRI) versus single photon emission computed tomography (SPECT/CT) in painful total hip arthroplasty: a comparative multi-institutional analysis. Br J Radiol. 2020;93(1105):20190738.
5. Arnon-Sheleg E, Israel O, Keidar Z. PET/CT imaging in soft tissue infection and inflammation—an update. Semin Nucl Med. 2020;50:35–49.
6. Gratz S, Schipper ML, Dorner J, Höffken H, Becker W, Kaiser JW, et al. LeukoScan for imaging infection in different clinical settings: a retrospective evaluation and extended review of the literature. Clin Nucl Med. 2003;28:267–76.
7. Petruzzi N, Schipper ML, Thakur M. Recent trends in soft tissue infection imaging. Semin Nucl Med. 2009;39:115–23.
8. Signore A, Jamar F, Israel O, Buscombe J, Martin-Comin J, Lazzeri E. Clinical indications, image acquisition and data interpretation for white blood cells and anti-granulocyte monoclonal antibody scintigraphy: an EANM procedural guideline. Eur J Nucl Med Mol Imaging. 2018;45:1816–31.
9. Erba PA, Glaudemans AW, Veltman NC, Sollini M, Pacilio M, Galli F, et al. Image acquisition and interpretation criteria for ^{99m}Tc-HMPAO-labelled white blood cell scintigraphy: results of a multicentre study. Eur J Nucl Med Mol Imaging. 2014;41:615–23.

Nuclear Medicine Imaging of Bone and Joint Infection

3

Elena Lazzeri

Contents

Learning Objectives

- To understand that different radiopharmaceuticals used to image infection have different mechanisms of accumulation at the sites of infection
- To learn how PET/CT with [^{18}F]FDG can be employed to detect both infection and sterile inflammatory reaction
- To learn how scintigraphy with radiolabeled autologous leukocytes can discriminate between infection and inflammation
- To understand the rationale of using either three-phase bone scintigraphy or [^{18}F]FDG PET/CT to rule out disease in patients with low probability of infection
- To understand the rationale of using scintigraphy with ^{99m}Tc-HMPAO-leukocytes in patients with high probability of infection
- To learn that the optimal radionuclide imaging technique in patients with suspected spine infection is currently PET/CT with [^{18}F]FDG

Bone infection (osteitis and osteomyelitis) can be divided into infection of the peripheral bones, infection of the spine, and joint infection. Bone infection can be acute (being so defined within the first 8 weeks since onset) or chronic (when lasting than 8 weeks). Acute and chronic osteomyelitis are caused by different microorganisms and can occur in any age range. The origin of bone infection is most frequently exogenous, following trauma or surgery, or by contiguous spread from adjacent tissues; it is more rarely hematogenous [1]. The rate of peripheral bone infection in the developed countries is less than 2% per year [2], but it can increase after surgical procedures of an open or closed fracture in the acute setting (2–19%) [3–5].

E. Lazzeri (✉)
Regional Center of Nuclear Medicine, University Hospital of Pisa, Pisa, Italy
e-mail: e.lazzeri@ao-pisa.toscana.it

E. Lazzeri et al. (eds.), *Radionuclide Imaging of Infection and Inflammation*, https://doi.org/10.1007/978-3-030-62175-9_3

Table 3.1 Main indications for the clinical use of radionuclide imaging according to pretest probability of bone infection

Clinical suspicion	Nuclear medicine imaging
Infection of peripheral bone (low probability)	Three-phase ^{99m}Tc-diphosphonate bone scan
Infection of peripheral bone (high probability)	Labeled autologous leukocytes
Infection of axial skeleton (low probability)	^{99m}Tc-diphosphonate bone scan
Infection of axial skeleton (high probability)	[^{18}F]FDG PET/TC ^{99m}Tc-diphosphonate bone scan + ^{67}Ga-citrate
Infection of joint (low probability)	^{99m}Tc-diphosphonate bone scan
Infection of joint (high probability)	Labeled autologous leukocytes

The diagnosis of bone infection is based on clinical data (physical examination, high levels of ESR, RCP, leukocyte count, and positive blood and bone cultures) and on imaging findings obtained with radiologic and/or and nuclear medicine procedures. Although for diagnostic imaging the radiological approach represents almost always the first-line choice, recently published guidelines for bone infection diagnosis [6–8] state that nuclear medicine procedures such as labeled leukocyte scintigraphy (WBC), [^{18}F]fluorodeoxyglucose positron emission tomography ([^{18}F]FDG PET/CT), and combination of the ^{99m}Tc-diphosphonate (bone scan) and ^{67}Ga-citrate scan (^{67}Ga-scan) are complementary and sometimes can replace other imaging procedures such as ultrasound (US), computed tomography (CT), and magnetic resonance (MR). Nuclear medicine and radiological imaging is mandatory to confirm the presence of bone infection as well as to evaluate response to therapy.

Table 3.1 summarizes the main clinical indications and usefulness of radionuclide imaging procedures in patients with bone infection.

3.1 Infection of Peripheral Bones

The diagnosis of peripheral bone infection can be based on clinical parameters (physical examination, high levels of ESR, RCP, leukocyte count, and positive blood and bone cultures) and on imaging findings obtained with radiologic and/or and nuclear medicine procedures. The diagnosis requires the presence of at least two of the following four criteria: (a) purulent material draining from the site of osteomyelitis, (b) positive findings at bone tissue or blood culture, (c) localized classical physical findings of bone tenderness and edema, and (d) positive imaging findings. A positive bone culture obtained by fine needle aspiration or bone biopsy (when the bone is exposed) is considered the "gold standard" method to diagnose acute osteitis or osteomyelitis.

Radiological imaging includes plain X-ray [9, 10], US [11, 12], CT, and MR [13]. Bone destruction with deep soft tissue swelling, the typical X-ray signs of infection, may appear only 15 days after the onset of infection and are not specific for infection; in fact, fractures, surgical procedures, and/or reabsorption outcome can show some similar changes in bone structure.

Ultrasound (US) may be used especially for the evaluation of fluid collections and/or for guiding the biopsy; nevertheless, its usefulness is limited in the deep tissues evaluation and bone marrow infections.

A CT scan is often used to evaluate acute bone infection with soft tissues involvement. Medullary low-attenuation areas or trabecular enlargement, cortical erosions, periosteal reaction, and extramedullary fat-fluid level and overlying soft-tissue swelling are the typical CT features of bacterial osteomyelitis. CT is considered superior to MR imaging in the setting of chronic osteomyelitis for the demonstration of cortical destruction and gas. However, CT suffers from a certain time gap (14–21 days after the onset of infection) in the detection of structural bone changes [5].

MR imaging has good spatial resolution for defining the anatomical extent of osteomyelitis, but it is less accurate in chronic bone infection. Furthermore, MR imaging cannot easily distinguish latent infection from simple bone remodeling, even with intravenous administration of contrast media [14]. Moreover, pathologic changes in bone structure caused by chronic infection can persist for years in MR imaging.

The main limitation of radiological imaging is the inability to distinguish an acute from a chronic osteomyelitis, whereas nuclear medicine imaging procedures have made important advances in this regard, especially in the case of post-surgical infection.

The radiopharmaceuticals available for the diagnosis of peripheral bone infection are ^{99m}Tc-diphosphonate, ^{99m}Tc-HMPAO-, or ^{111}In-oxine-labeled autologous white blood cells (^{99m}Tc-HMPAO-WBC and ^{111}In-oxine-WBC, respectively), ^{99m}Tc-labeled anti-granulocyte antibodies (^{99m}Tc-anti-G mAb), [^{18}F]FDG, ^{67}Ga-citrate, and ^{68}Ga-citrate [15].

A negative ^{99m}Tc-diphosphonate three-phase bone scintigraphy or negative [^{18}F]FDG PET/CT is sufficient to rule out the presence of inflammation and infection. Therefore, in patients with low probability of bone infection, a three-phase bone scan is suggested for first-line imaging. When either the three-phase bone scan or [^{18}F]FDG PET/CT is positive, a second study with labeled WBC or anti-G mAb is suggested to distinguish bone infection from sterile inflammation.

Labeled WBC scintigraphy with SPECT/CT mode acquisition [16, 17] is the gold standard technique for diagnosing neutrophil-mediated infectious processes. Proper imaging acquisition and interpretation criteria for labeled leukocyte scintigraphy [16] allow the diagnosis of inflammation and/or infection in most cases. In some patients, however, labeled leukocyte scintigraphy combined with bone marrow radiocolloid scintigraphy can be helpful for the diagnosis of bone infection [18]. In particular, both labeled leukocytes and radiocolloids accumulate in the healthy bone marrow, while labeled leukocytes accumulate in infection and radiocolloids do not [19]. Labeled anti-G mAb [20] can also be used, particularly for the diagnosis of chronic osteomyelitis [18].

PET/CT with [^{18}F]FDG and/or ^{18}F-fluoride has been used in patients with suspected peripheral bone infection, although neither of them can be considered infection-specific [18, 21]. Autologous leukocytes can also be labeled in vitro with [^{18}F]FDG [22]; however, the short physical half-life of this preparation does not allow to reproduce the pathophysiology of leukocyte migration at delayed time-point after administration. ^{67}Ga-citrate scintigraphy can be helpful for the diagnosis of peripheral bone infections when leukocyte scintigraphy and [^{18}F]FDG PET/CT are not available. The high radiation burden and the long time required for acquisition of ^{67}Ga-scintigraphy represent the major limitations of this technique—especially considering the suboptimal imaging properties of ^{67}Ga with standard gamma cameras [23, 24].

3.2 Infection of the Axial Skeleton

Infection of the spine can involve the vertebral body (spondylitis), the intervertebral disk (discitis), or both (spondylodiscitis). The origin of spine infection can be primary (hematogenous) or secondary (post-surgical). Primary spine infections can be correctly diagnosed using MR or CT.

MR suffers from some limitations in secondary spondylodiscitis, often associated with metal implants fixation, particularly in the immediate post-surgical period. The associated tissues reactions can persist for many years [25, 26], and fat suppression sequences cannot be employed in these patients [27].

CT-guided biopsy has high specificity, associated however with variable sensitivity for the characterization of the microorganism; it is not routinely performed in most centers [28–32].

The radiopharmaceuticals used for the diagnosis of spine infection are ^{99m}Tc-Diphosphonate, [^{18}F]FDG, ^{67}Ga- or ^{68}Ga-citrate, or the combination of ^{99m}Tc-diphosphonate bone scintigraphy with ^{67}Ga-citrate scintigraphy [33]. Radiolabeled leukocytes may fail in the detection of vertebral infection, due to the frequent appearance as a "cold spot" in the scan [34].

A negative ^{99m}Tc-diphosphonate bone scan or a negative [^{18}F]FDG PET/CT rules out the presence of spine infection. Post-surgical infection, or some cases of primary spondylodiscitis with equivocal/inconclusive MRI findings, can be diagnosed using [^{18}F]FDG PET/CT or the combination of ^{99m}Tc-diphosphonate scintigraphy with ^{67}Ga-citrate scintigraphy [35–37].

Radionuclide imaging is strongly recommended to evaluate disease activity during follow-up after medical treatment [7]. Since the specificity of the radiopharmaceuticals currently available is suboptimal, alternative radiopharmaceuticals such as radiolabeled antibiotics [38] and radiolabeled vitamins [39, 40] are being developed and tested; although the preliminary data obtained so far showed highly encouraging results, there is the need for further large-scale validation studies.

3.3 Joint Infection

Diagnosis of joint infection (JI) should be made as early as possible to prevent or limit bone destruction. Nonspecific signs such as heat, redness, swelling, pain and/or fever, and movement limitations can be present in case of JI.

Although plain X-ray is often non-diagnostic, it is invariably performed as first-line imaging. Soft tissue swelling and bone lucency can be the radiographic signs of JI, but become detectable only when the loss of the bone mass is almost 30%; thus, 50% of radiographs remain normal despite the presence of infection [41]. Bone erosions are a sign of infection and can be easily detected by CT, which is the most sensitive imaging modality because of its high resolution [42]. The main limitation of CT is represented by a relatively high radiation burden to patients, especially in case of sequential evaluations during the follow-up. Ultrasound imaging has high accuracy for the evaluation of fluid collection during JI and can guide fluid aspiration for the bacterial culture analysis. Nevertheless, a negative bacteriological culture of fluid aspiration cannot rule out the presence of infection [43].

MR has shown high accuracy for the diagnosis of JI [44, 45]. Both bone and soft tissues can be evaluated by MR imaging, which can exclude an infection with a 100% negative predictive value if the bone marrow is normal on all pulse sequences. Intravenous contrast is useful to differentiate synovial thickening from fluid and to identify soft tissue abscesses and sinus tracts [46].

Nuclear medicine imaging procedures are very useful in patients with suspected JI; in particular, scintigraphy with ^{99m}Tc-HMPAO-WBC, especially if acquired with SPECT/CT, can distinguish infectious from inflammatory joint disease and can be employed to monitor response to treatment [16]. Bone scintigraphy with ^{99m}Tc-diphosponate can easily evaluate the extent of disease, by identifying the number of joints involved.

Key Learning Points

- Bone scintigraphy with ^{99m}Tc-diphosphonates is not specific for infection, as it only visualizes sites with increased osteoblastic activity that can be associated with a host of conditions including, among many others, infection, inflammation, trauma, and primary and metastatic tumor.
- Three-phase bone scintigraphy with ^{99m}Tc-diphosphonates is very sensitive for the detection of focal changes in blood perfusion and capillary permeability due to infection/inflammation.
- Because of such exquisite sensitivity, a negative three-phase bone scintigraphy with ^{99m}Tc-diphosphonates rules out the presence of infection/inflammation and can therefore be employed as the first-line radionuclide imaging approach in patients with low probability of bone/joint infection.
- Similar considerations hold true also for PET/CT with [^{18}F]FDG PET/CT (or PET/MR).
- While [^{18}F]FDG-PET/CT allows identification of the sites of bone and joints infection and/or inflammation, in general it does not enable to distinguish infection from inflammation.
- Except in the spine, scintigraphy with labeled autologous leukocytes (^{99m}Tc-HMPAO- or ^{111}In-oxine-WBC) detects sites of bone and joint infection and can be employed to distinguish infection from sterile inflammation.
- Scintigraphy with ^{99m}Tc-HMPAO-WBC or ^{111}In-oxine-WBC should be performed as the first-line radionuclide imaging approach in patients with high probability of infection.
- PET/CT with [^{18}F]FDG is the preferred radionuclide imaging modality in patients with suspected spine infection.
- Radionuclide imaging of infection provides important information also when assessing response to treatment in patients with bone and joint infection.

Acknowledgments All editors have contributed to the preparation of this chapter.

3.4 Examples of Imaging in Patients with Bone and Joint Infection

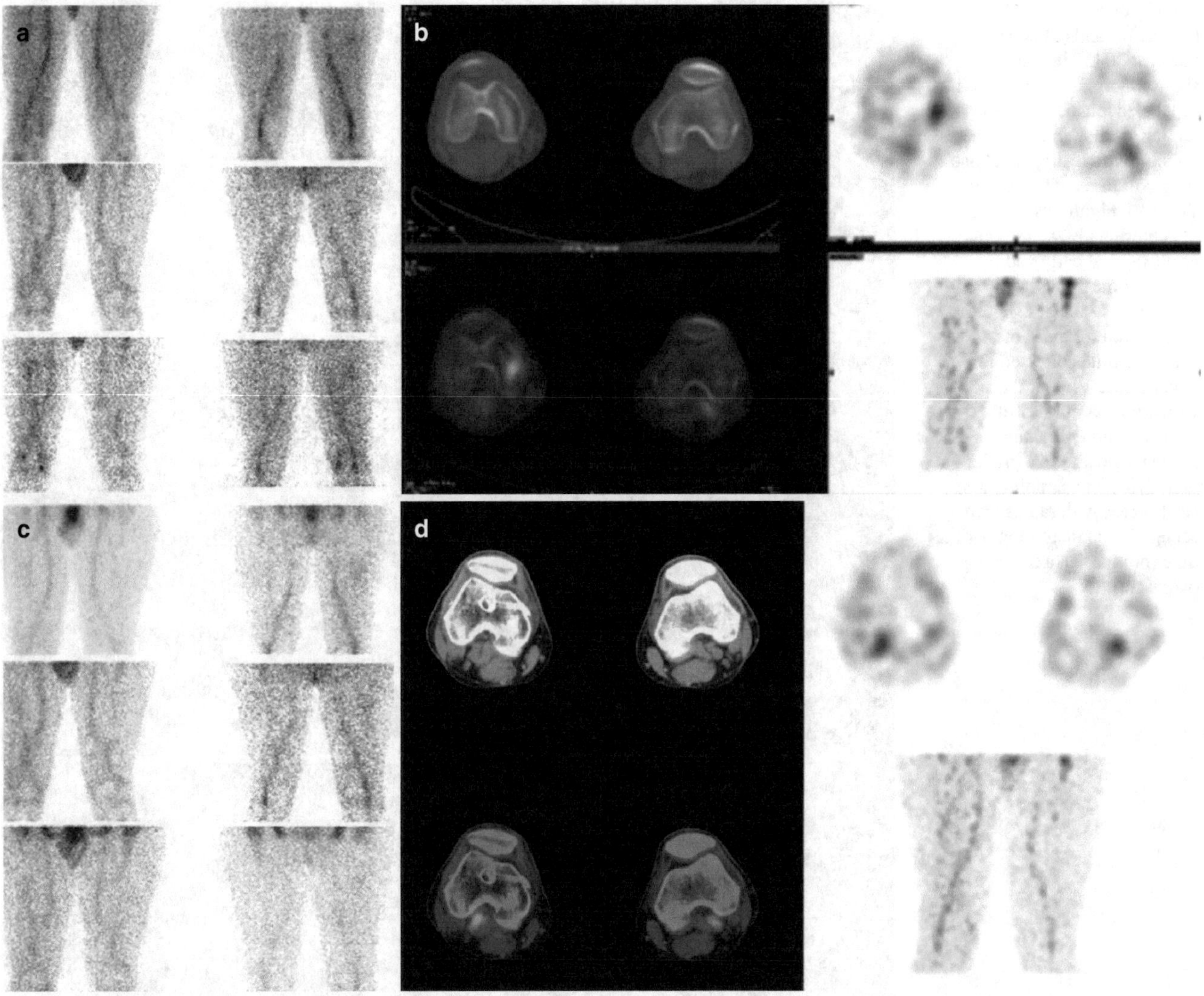

Fig. 3.1 Baseline ^{99m}Tc-HMPAO-WBC scintigraphy. Upper panel: (**a**) Planar images (anterior and posterior views, *left* and *right*) at 30 min (*upper*), 4 h (*middle*), and 20 h (*lower*) p.i. show mildly increased focal accumulation of labeled leukocytes in the rotula and in the medial condyle of right femur. (**b**) The transaxial CT (*upper left*), SPECT (*upper right*), fused (*lower left*) SPECT/CT images more precisely localize the site (medial condyle) of leukocyte accumulation. Lower panels: follow-up ^{99m}Tc-HMPAO-WBC scintigraphy performed after antibiotic treatment. (**c**) Planar images (anterior and posterior, *left* and *right*) at 30 min (*upper*), 4 h (*middle*), and 20 h (*lower*) p.i. show complete disappearance of the focus of leukocyte accumulation at the medial condyle of right femur, as also confirmed by the transaxial CT (*upper left*), SPECT (*upper right*), fused (*lower left*) SPECT/CT images (**d**)

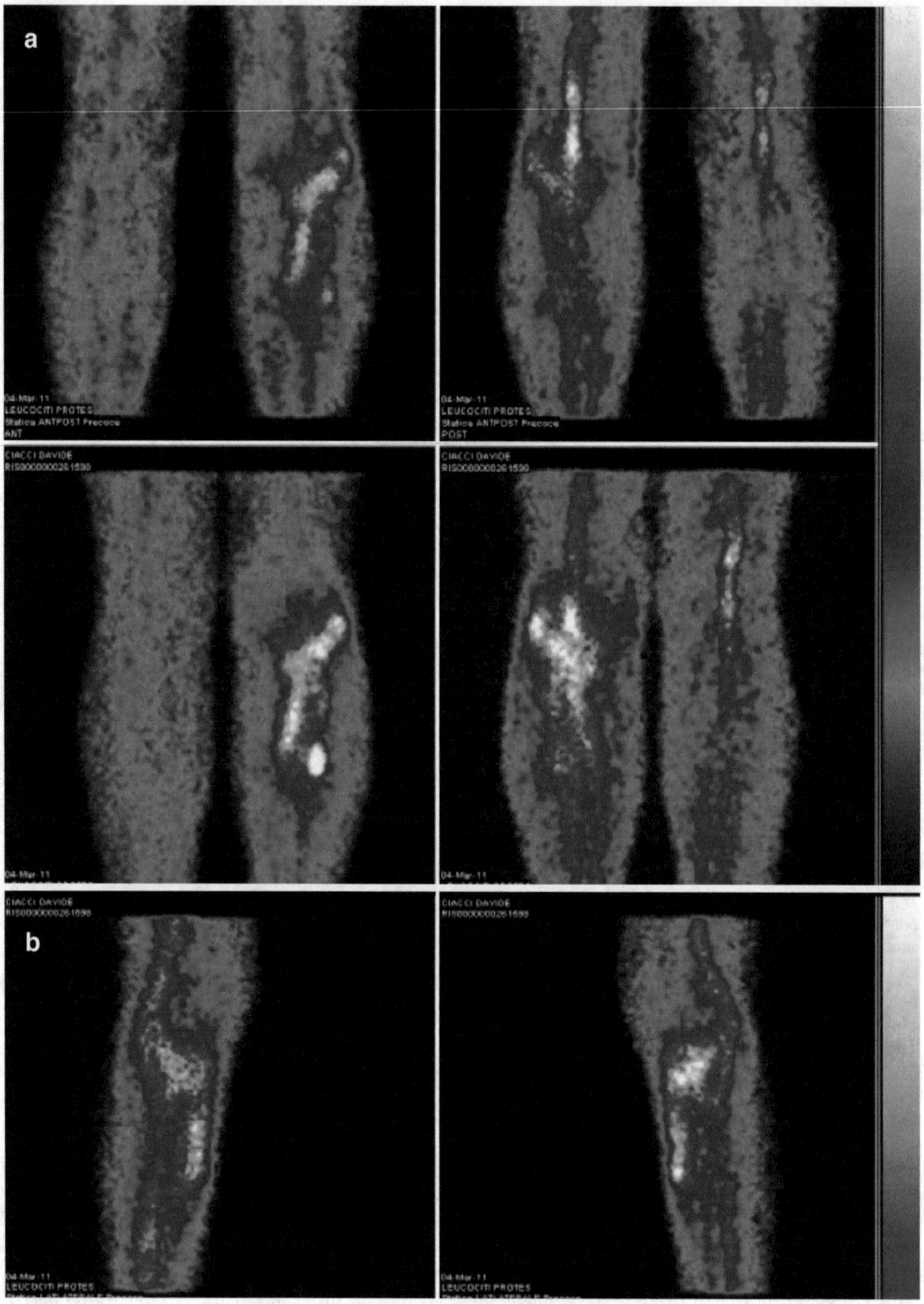

Fig. 3.2 ^{99m}Tc-HMPAO-WBC scintigraphy. (**a**) Spot planar images of the legs in anterior and posterior views 4 h p.i. (upper) and 20 h p.i. (lower) (**a**) and (**b**) lateral views at 20 h. The images show abnormal accumulation of labeled leukocytes at the left leg, without however the possibility to distinguish bone from soft tissue involvement. This case highlights the need of acquiring always the same projections at early and delayed time points. Furthermore, images should be acquired for the same period of time corrected for isotope decay, rather than with a pre-set number of counts, in order to compare all images with same grading of activity, thus defining more easily areas with radioactive accumulation increasing over time (or vice versa declining over time)

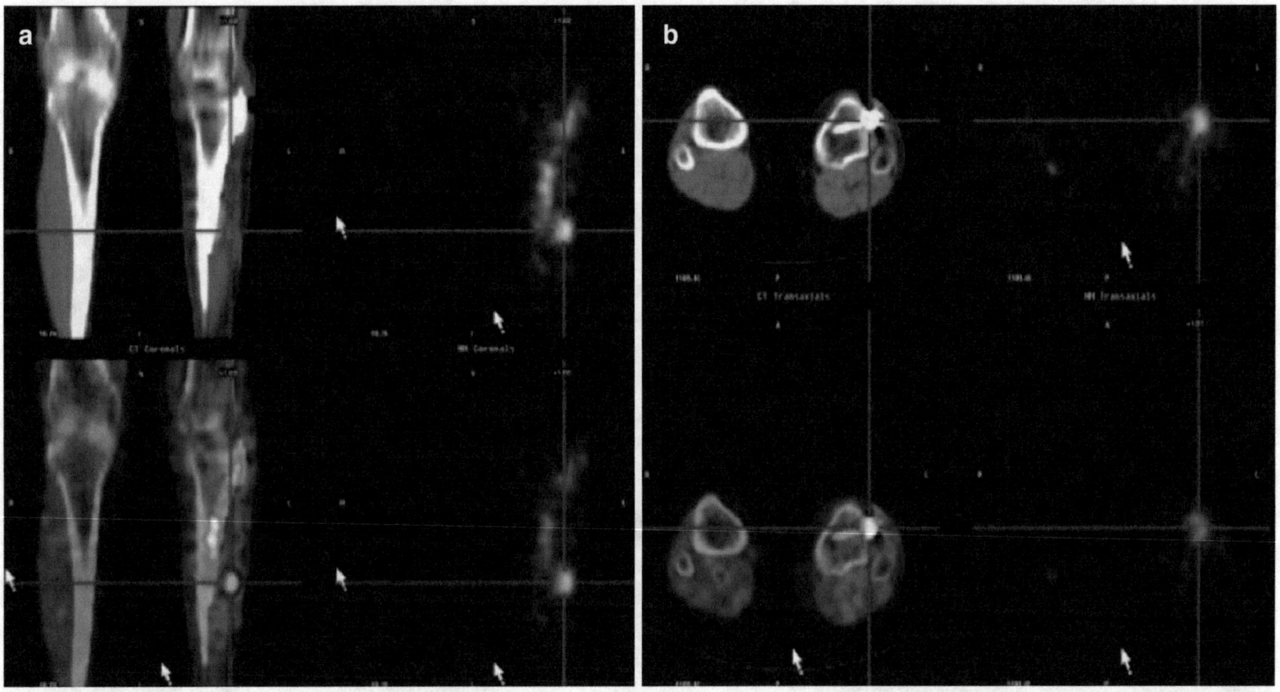

Fig. 3.3 ^{99m}Tc-HMPAO-WBC scintigraphy. The coronal (**a**) and transaxial (**b**) SPECT/CT sections demonstrate labeled leukocyte accumulation in cortical bone near the metallic implants and soft tissues

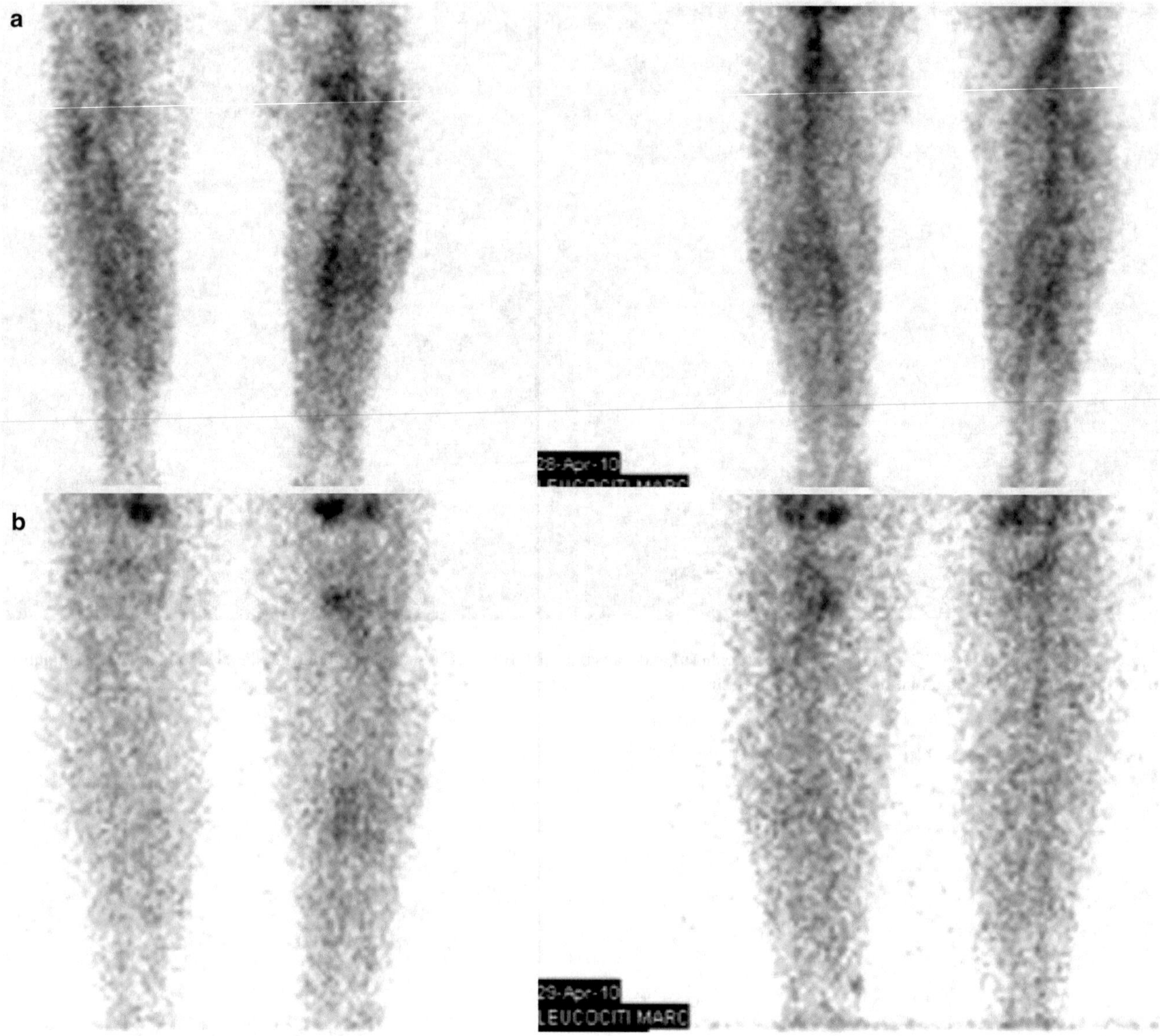

Fig. 3.4 ^{99m}Tc-HMPAO-WBC scintigraphy. Planar spot images (anterior and posterior views *left* and *right*, respectively) 4 h p.i. (**a**) and 24 h p.i. (**b**). The images show increased accumulation, stable overtime, of labeled leukocytes in the proximal and middle diaphyseal portion of left tibia, suggesting inflammation without infection

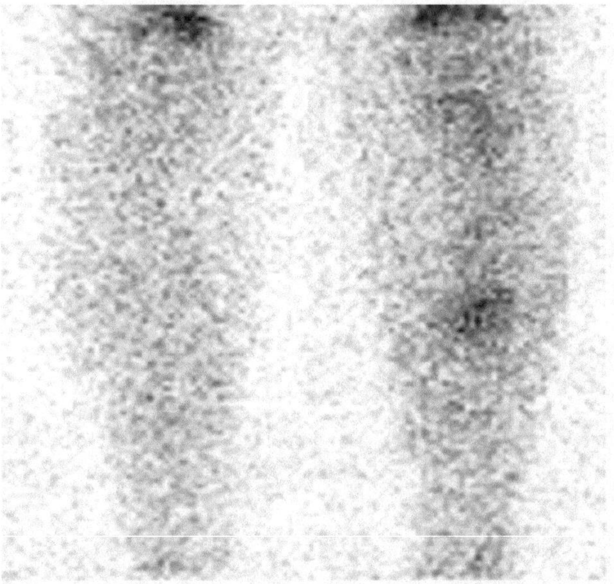

Fig. 3.5 ^{99m}Tc-colloid scintigraphy. Planar spot anterior view acquired 30 min p.i., showing tracer uptake in the same site as the labeled leukocytes in the prior scintigraphy. This finding confirms the presence of bone marrow at the site of interest, thus ruling out of the presence of acute infection

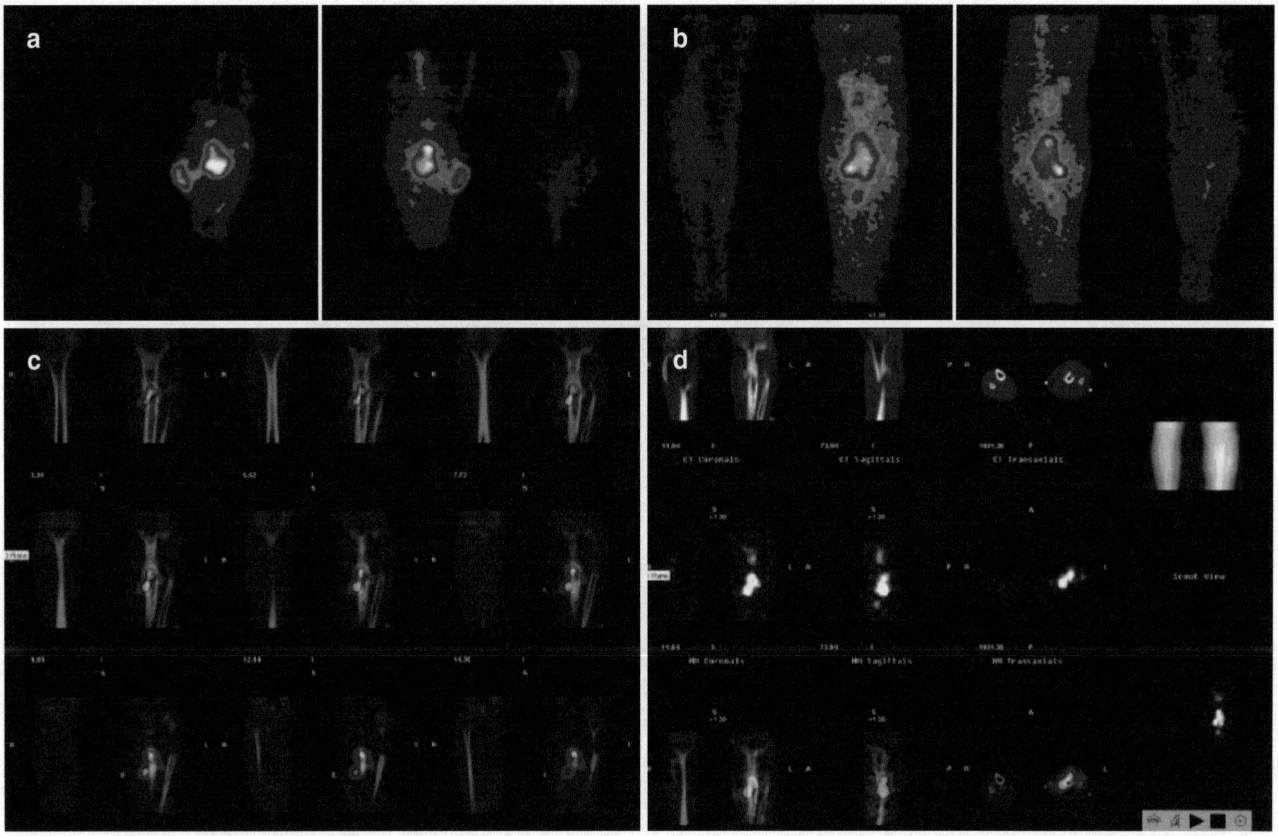

Fig. 3.6 ^{99m}Tc-HMPAO-WBC scintigraphy performed to evaluate the extent of infection. The planar spot views (anterior and posterior, *left* and *right*) at 4 h (**a**) and 24 h (**b**) p.i. show increased accumulation of labeled leukocytes in the diaphysis of left tibia. The coronal (**c**), sagittal and transaxial (**d**) SPECT/CT images allow precise assessment of the extent of infection in the affected bone and the adjacent soft tissues

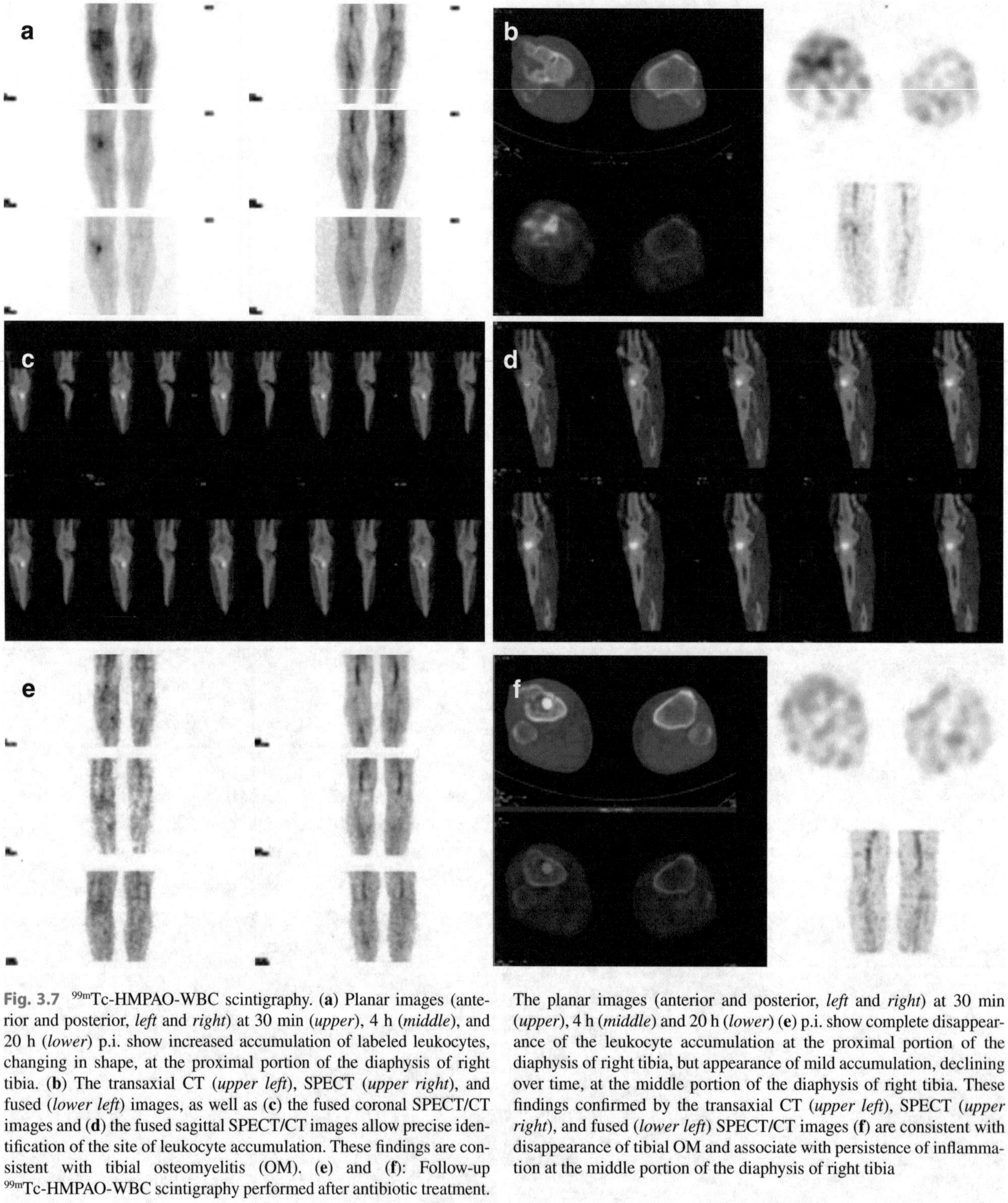

Fig. 3.7 ^{99m}Tc-HMPAO-WBC scintigraphy. (**a**) Planar images (anterior and posterior, *left* and *right*) at 30 min (*upper*), 4 h (*middle*), and 20 h (*lower*) p.i. show increased accumulation of labeled leukocytes, changing in shape, at the proximal portion of the diaphysis of right tibia. (**b**) The transaxial CT (*upper left*), SPECT (*upper right*), and fused (*lower left*) images, as well as (**c**) the fused coronal SPECT/CT images and (**d**) the fused sagittal SPECT/CT images allow precise identification of the site of leukocyte accumulation. These findings are consistent with tibial osteomyelitis (OM). (**e**) and (**f**): Follow-up ^{99m}Tc-HMPAO-WBC scintigraphy performed after antibiotic treatment. The planar images (anterior and posterior, *left* and *right*) at 30 min (*upper*), 4 h (*middle*) and 20 h (*lower*) (**e**) p.i. show complete disappearance of the leukocyte accumulation at the proximal portion of the diaphysis of right tibia, but appearance of mild accumulation, declining over time, at the middle portion of the diaphysis of right tibia. These findings confirmed by the transaxial CT (*upper left*), SPECT (*upper right*), and fused (*lower left*) SPECT/CT images (**f**) are consistent with disappearance of tibial OM and associate with persistence of inflammation at the middle portion of the diaphysis of right tibia

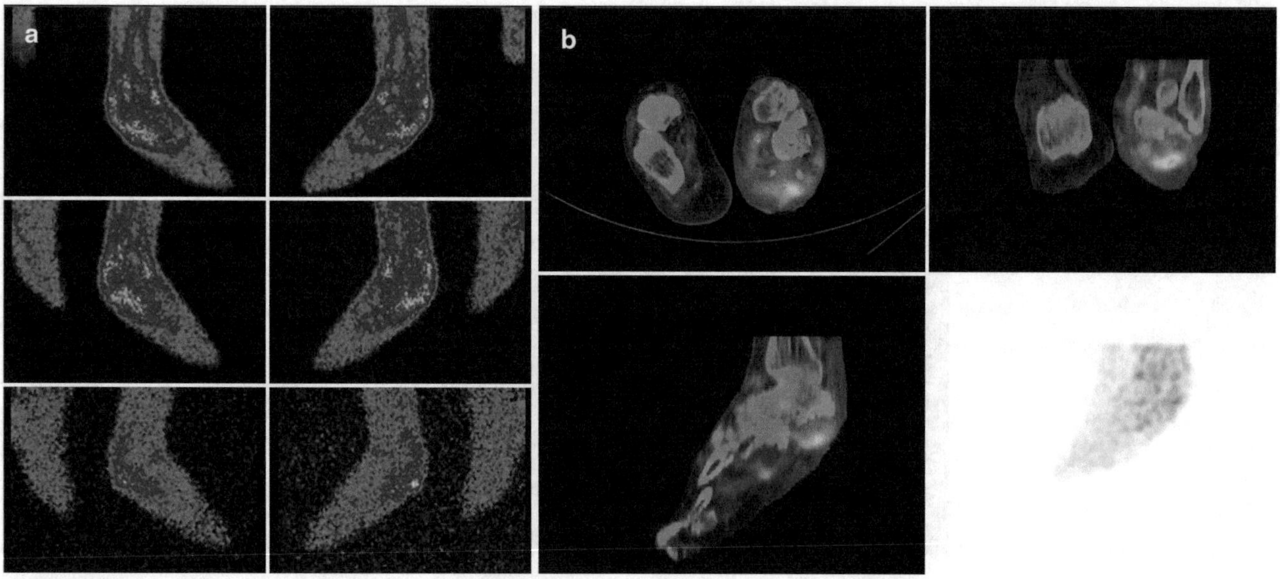

Fig. 3.8 ^{99m}Tc-HMPAO-WBC scintigraphy. (**a**) Planar images (anterior and posterior, *left* and *right*) at 30 min (*upper*), 4 h (*middle*), and 20 h (*lower*) p.i. show accumulation of labeled leukocytes at the forefoot, changing in shape. (**b**) The fused transaxial, coronal, and sagittal SPECT/CT images allow precise identification of the site of leukocyte accumulation, which in soft tissues under the heel without bone involvement

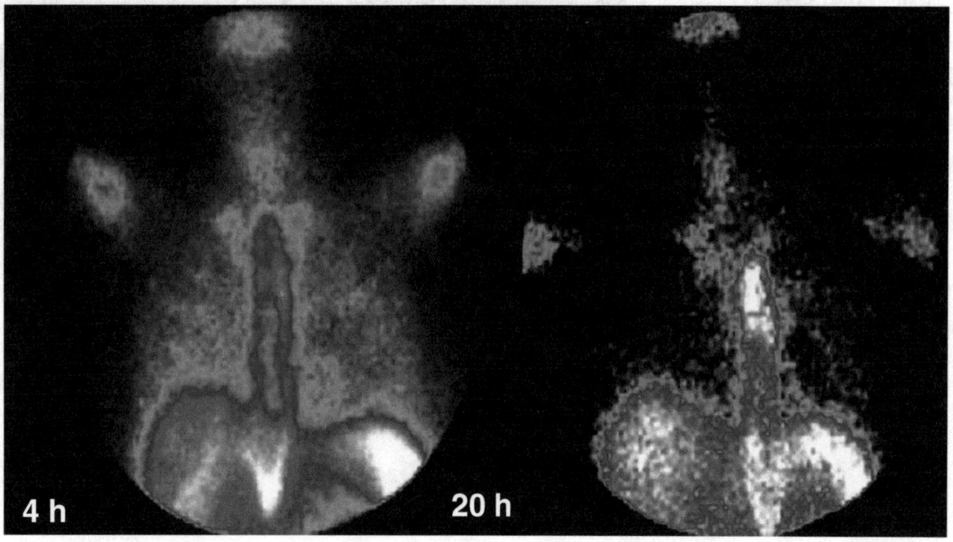

Fig. 3.9 Patient with deep sternal wound infection: planar images (anterior view) at 4 h (*left*) and 20 h (*right*) p.i. of ^{99m}Tc-HMPAO-WBC. The images show the increased leukocyte accumulation at the sternum increasing from the 4 h to the 24 h acquisition. The diffuse and intense sternal uptake at 20 h is greater than liver activity

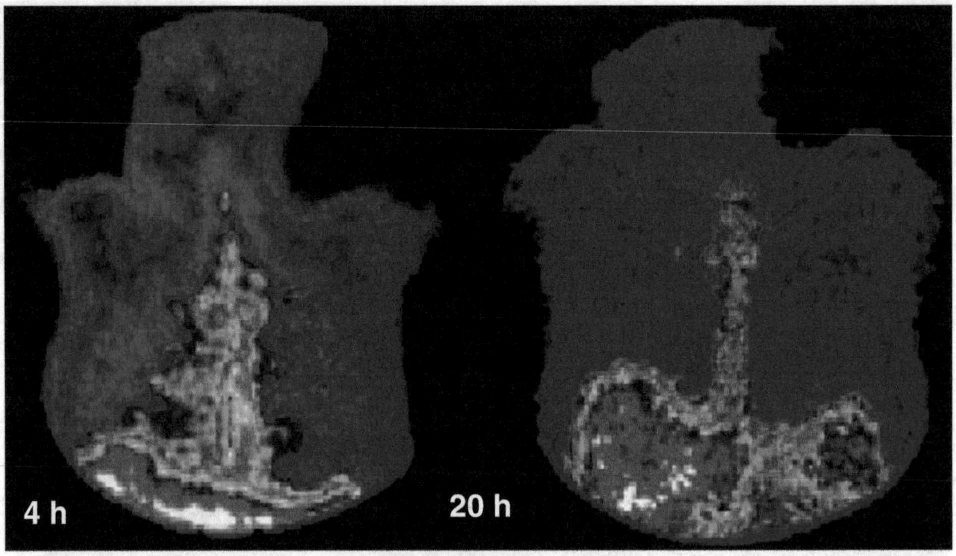

Fig. 3.10 Patient with superficial sternal wound infection. Planar images (anterior view) at 4 h (*left*) and 20 h (*right*) p.i. of ^{99m}Tc-HMPAO-WBC. The images show mildly increased activity with time and irregular sternal uptake in the 4 h image

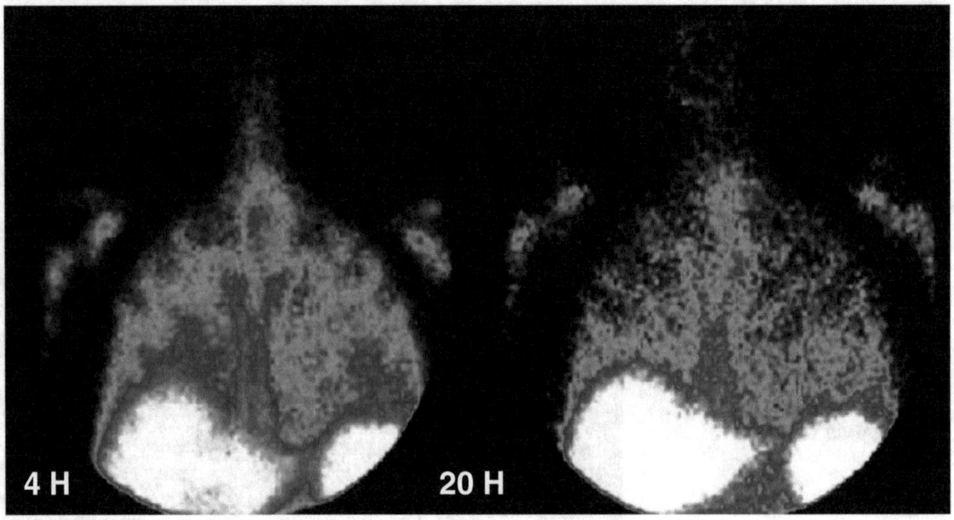

Fig. 3.11 Patient without sternal wound infection. Planar images (anterior view) at 4 h (*left*) and 20 h (*right*) p.i. of ^{99m}Tc-HMPAO-WBC. The images show mild and uniform sternal distribution (comparable to other bones of the ribcage), with a midline longitudinal defect due to surgical scar. Sternal activity does not increase with time

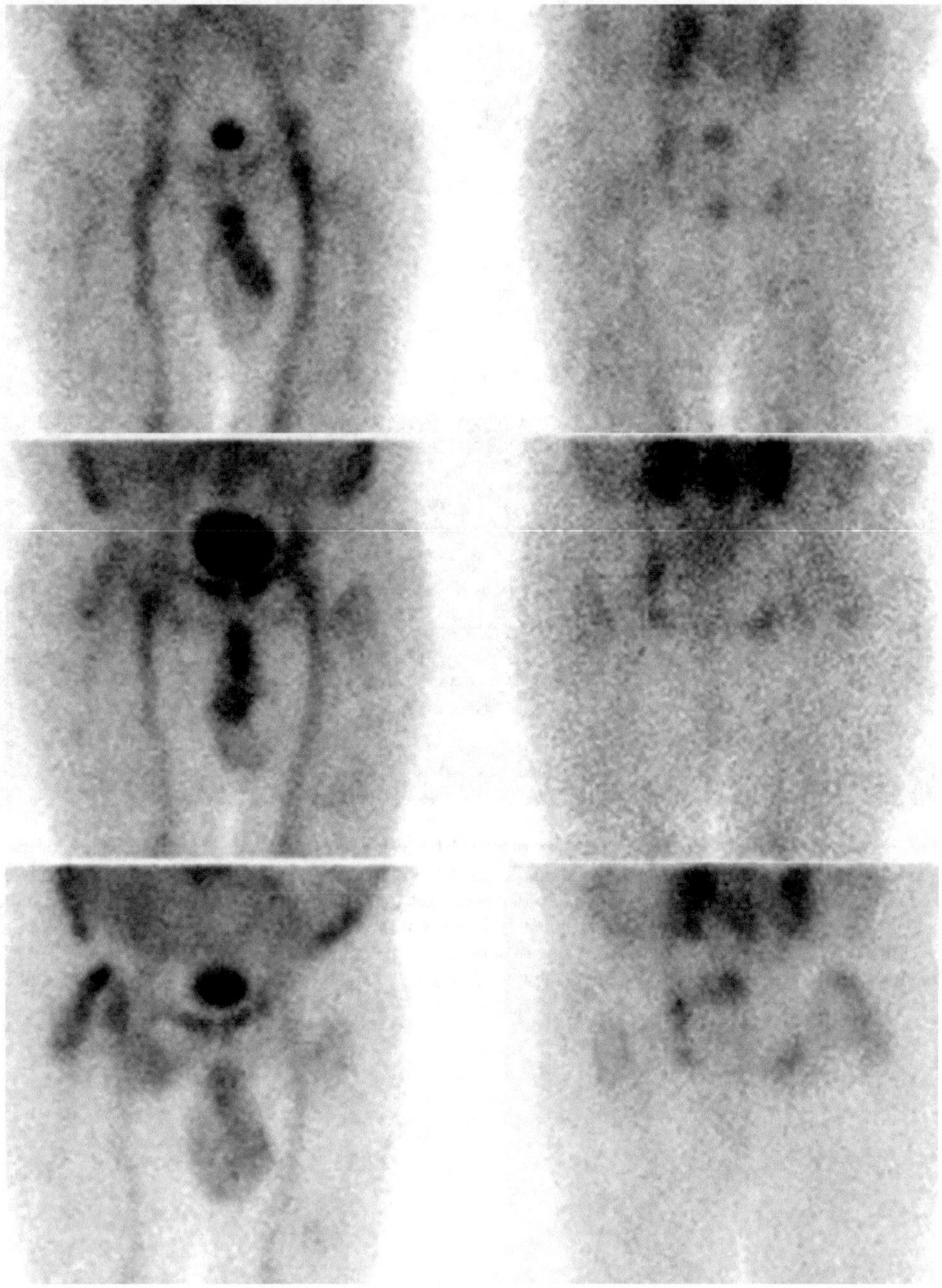

Fig. 3.12 ^{99m}Tc-HMPAO-WBC scintigraphy. Planar images (anterior and posterior, *left* and *right*) at 30 min (*upper*), 4 h (*middle*), and 20 h (*lower*) p.i. show accumulation of labeled leukocytes, increasing overtime and changing in shape, at right femur (head and neck). These findings are consistent with osteomyelitis involving also the adjacent anterior soft tissues, as later confirmed by microbiological culture of biopsy

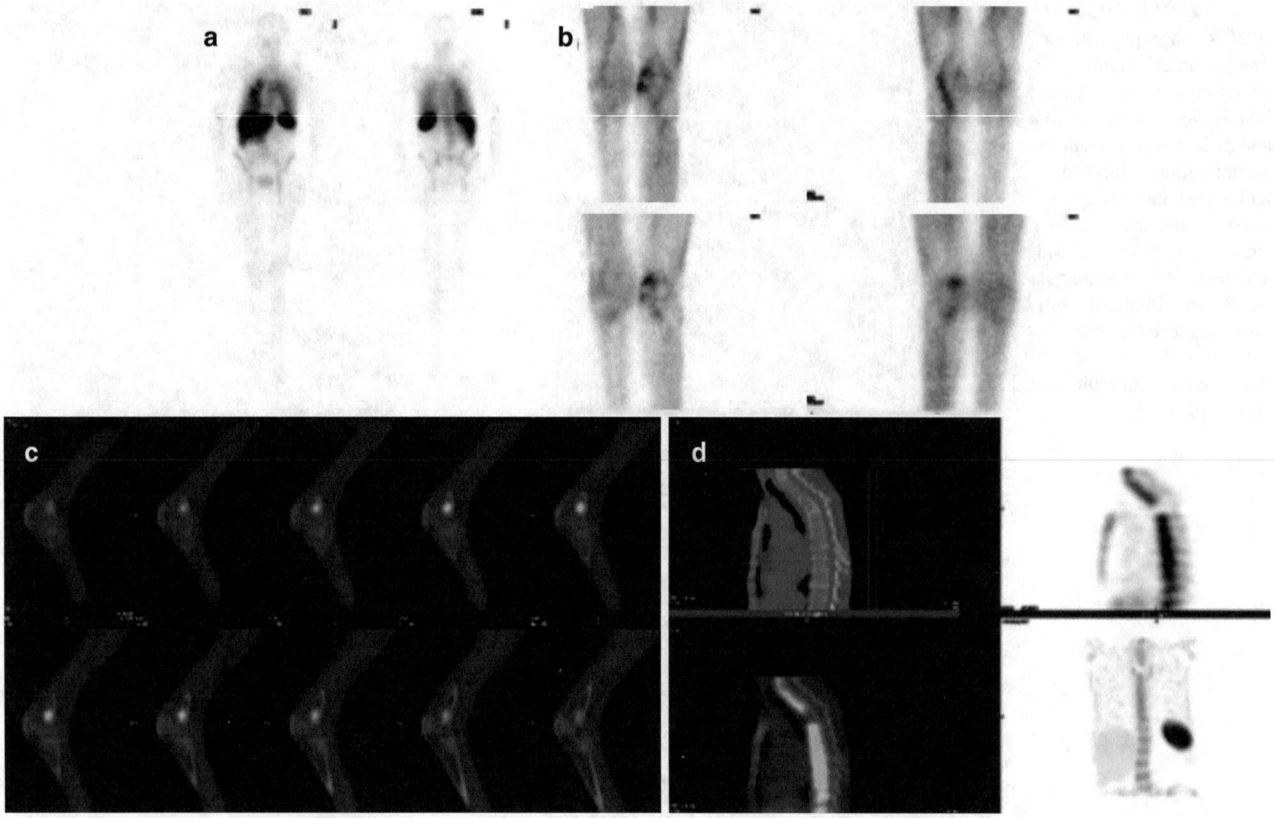

Fig. 3.13 ^{99m}Tc-HMPAO-WBC scintigraphy. (**a**) Total body images (anterior and posterior, *left* and *right*) at 30 min p.i. (**a**) showing focally reduced accumulation in thoracic skeleton. (**b**) Planar images (anterior and posterior, *left* and *right*) at 4 h (*upper*) and 20 h (*lower*) p.i. show an accumulation of labeled leukocytes, increasing over time and changing in shape, at left femur and tibia. (**c**) Fused sagittal SPECT/CT images allow precise identification of the site of leukocyte accumulation in the femur (above the medial condyle) and tibia (below the medial plate). (**d**) The lack of uptake in a thoracic vertebral body was confirmed in the transaxial CT (*upper left*), SPECT (*upper right*), and fused (*lower left*) SPECT/CT images at 4 h. These findings are consistent with femural and tibial OM with suspected infection of the thoracic spine

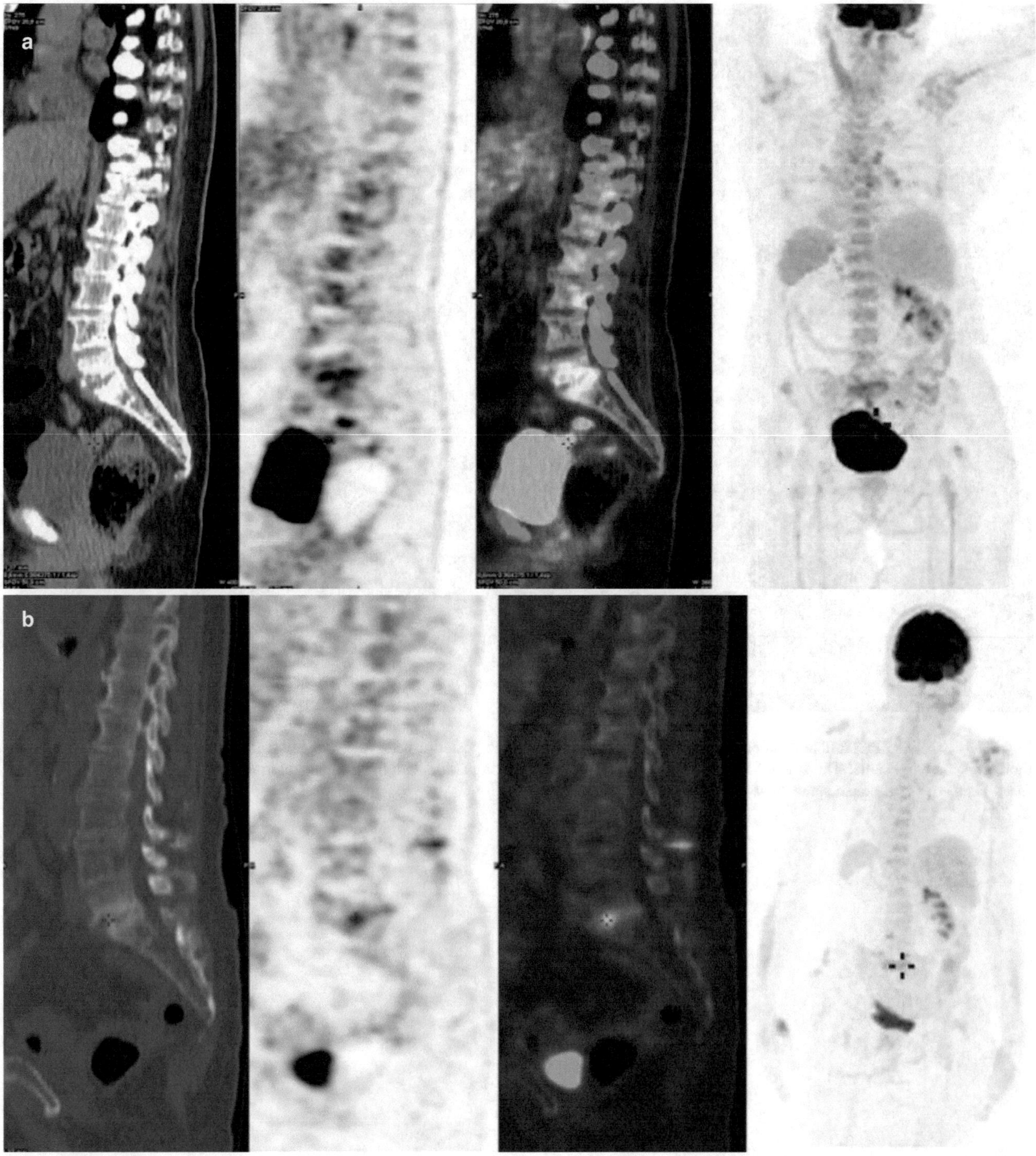

Fig. 3.14 [^{18}F]FDG PET/CT. (**a**) The baseline sagittal images (CT *left*; PET *middle*; fused *right*) of the lumbosacral skeleton show increased [^{18}F]FDG uptake at L5–S1 region (lower region of L5, disk space L5–S1, and upper region of S1). (**b**) Four months later, the follow-up sagittal images (CT *left*; PET *middle*; fused *right*) performed during antibiotic treatment show a significant reduction of [^{18}F]FDG uptake at the L5–S1 region, thus demonstrating good response to therapy

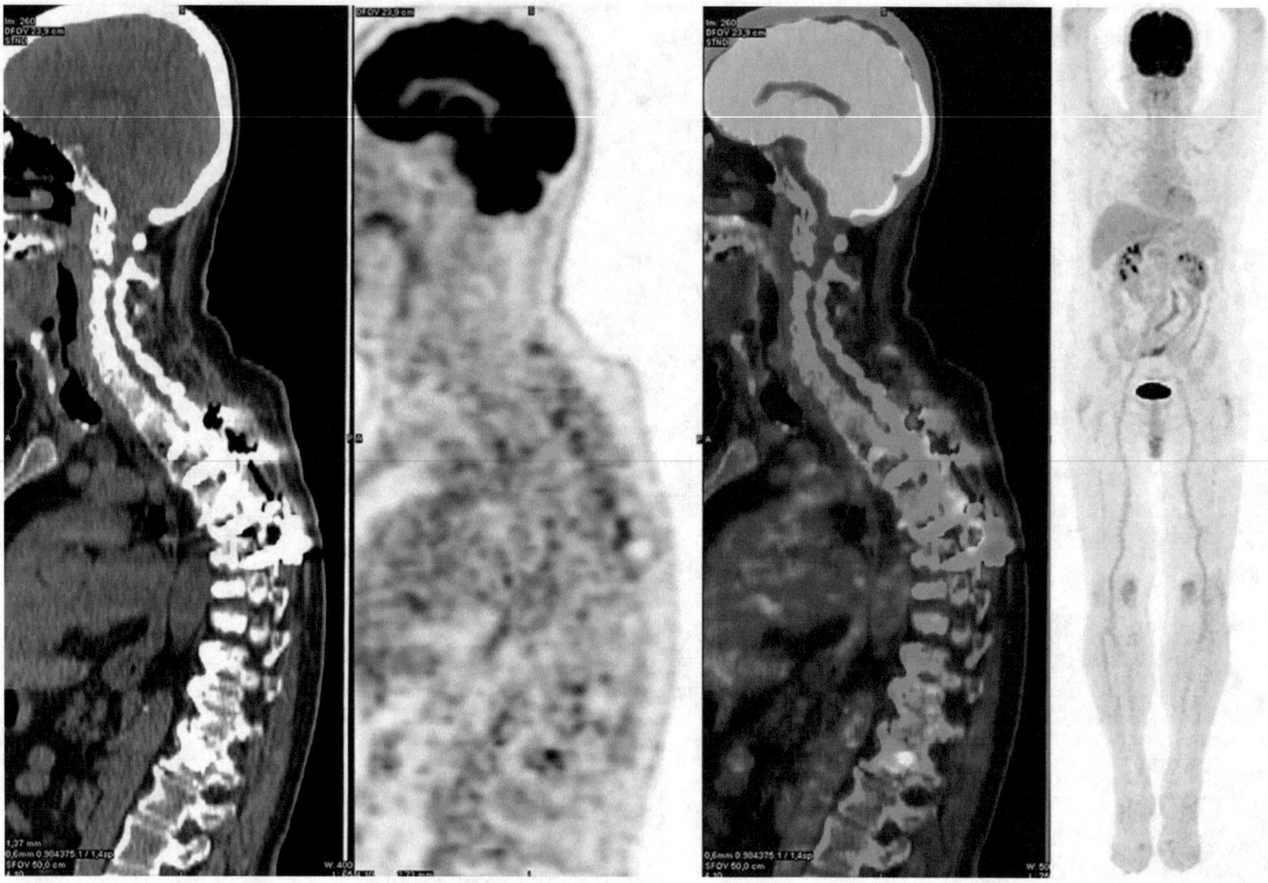

Fig. 3.15 [18F]FDG PET/CT in a patient with suspected post-surgical thoracic spondylodiscitis. The sagittal images (CT *left*; PET *middle*; fused *right*) of the thoracic spine show increased [18F]FDG uptake in the posterior para-vertebral and para-hardware soft tissues. The scan is compatible with the presence of infection

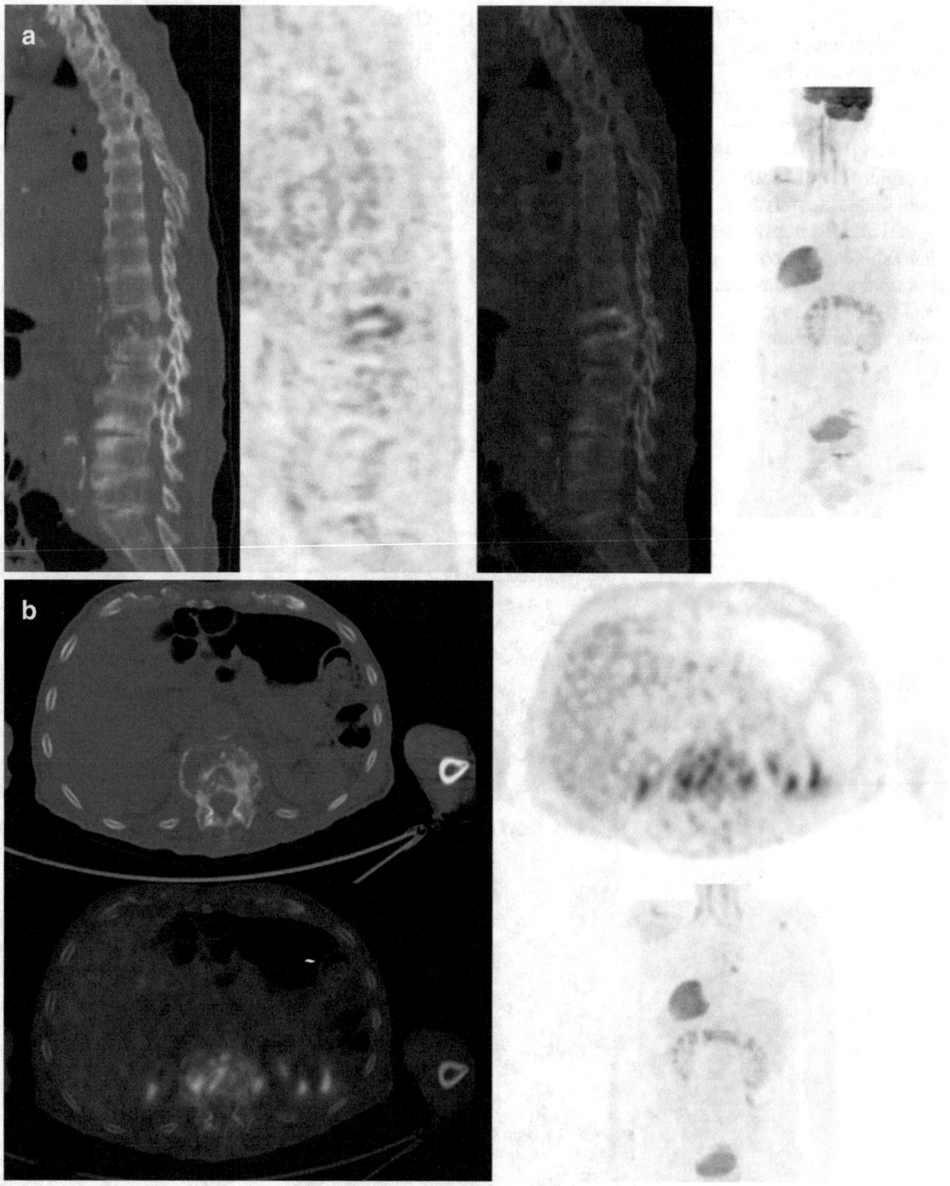

Fig. 3.16 [^{18}F]FDG PET/CT in a patient with dorsolumbar spondylodiscitis. (**a**) The sagittal images (CT *left*; PET *middle*; fused *right*) show increased [^{18}F]FDG uptake in the T12–L1 region (lower region of T12 and upper region of L1). (**b**) The transaxial images (CT *left*; PET *middle*; fused *right*) of T12 confirmed increased [^{18}F]FDG uptake, consistent with infection

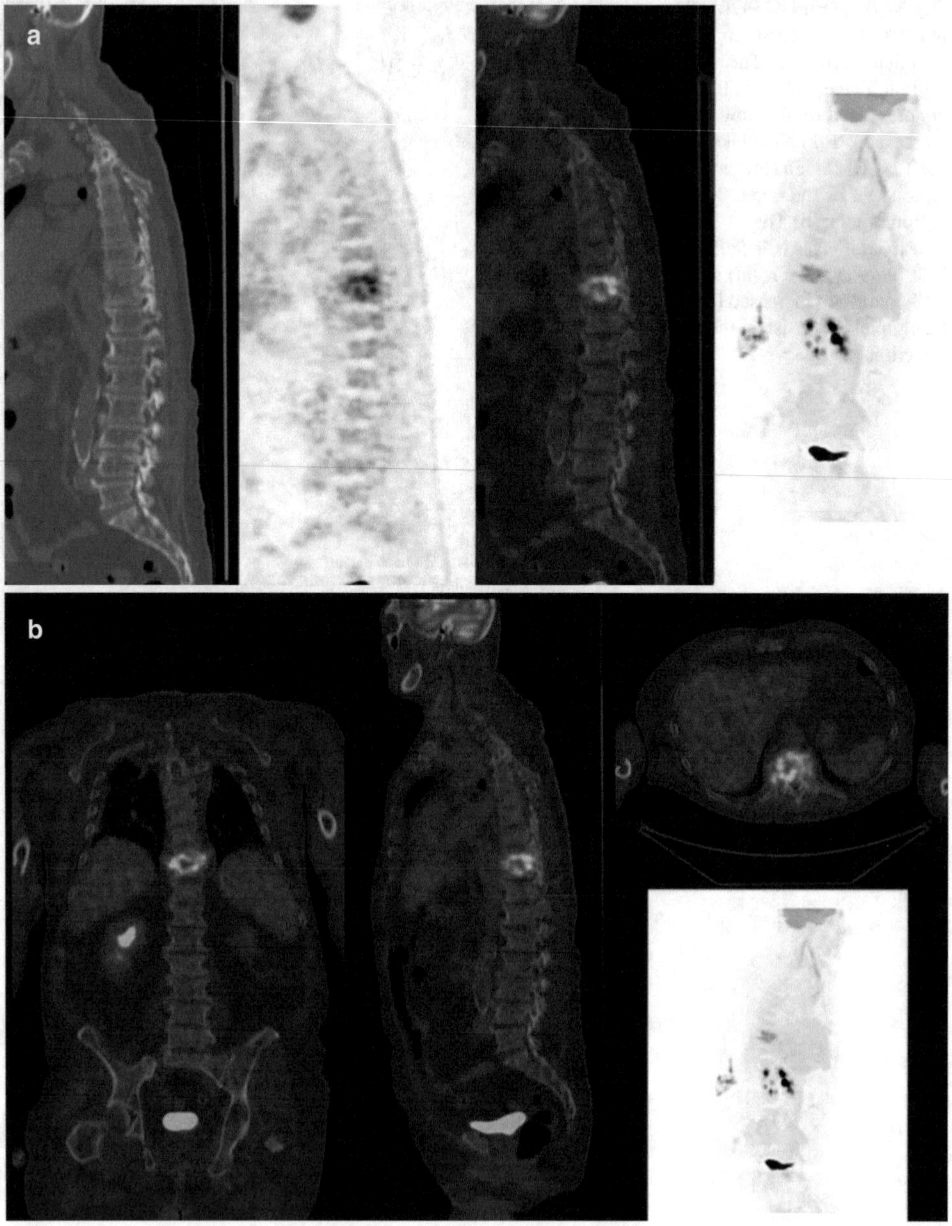

Fig. 3.17 [^{18}F]FDG PET/CT in a patient with thoracic spondylodiscitis. (**a**) The sagittal images (CT *left*; PET *middle*; fused *right*) show increased [^{18}F]FDG uptake in the region T10–T11. (**b**) The fused images (coronal *left*; sagittal *middle*; transaxial *right*) show the extension of abnormal [^{18}F]FDG uptake in the T10–T11 region, confirming infection

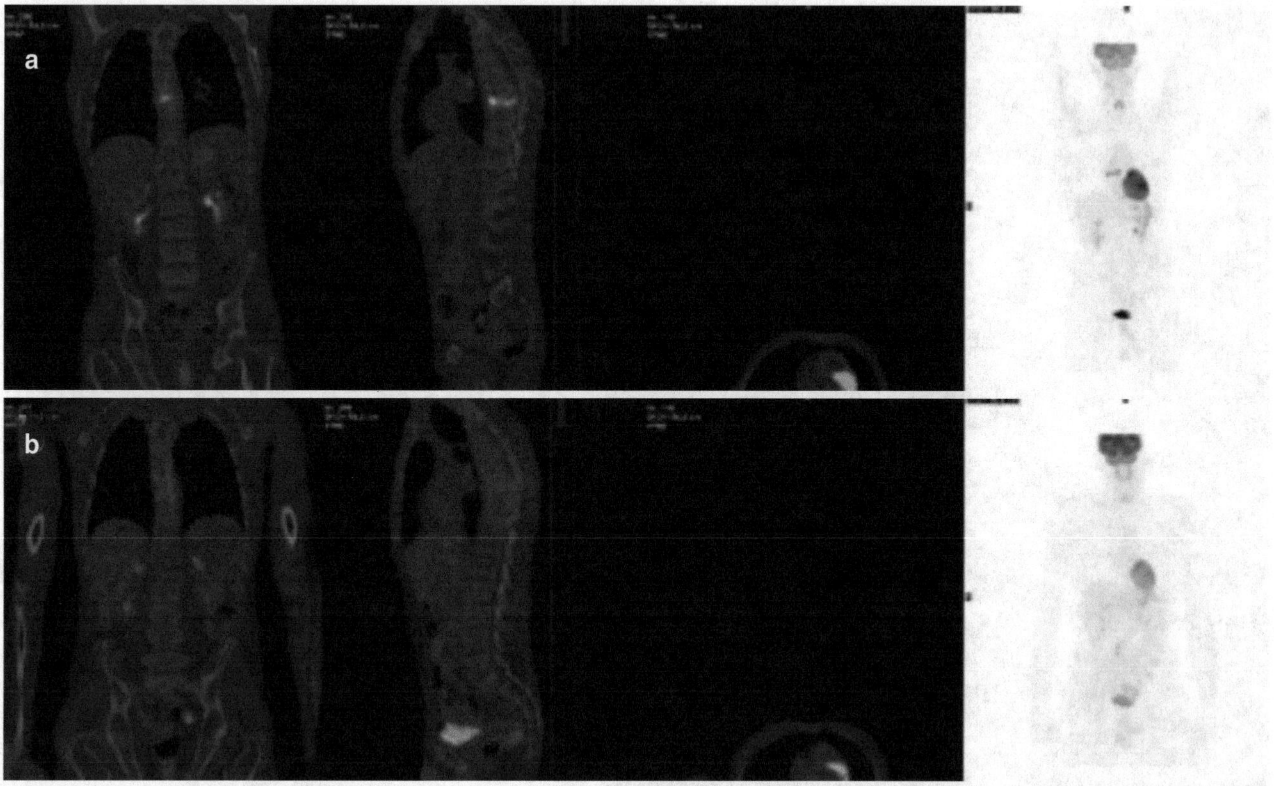

Fig. 3.18 [^{18}F]FDG PET/CT in a patient with thoracic spondylodiscitis. (**a**) The baseline fused images (coronal *left*; sagittal *middle*; transaxial *right*) show increased [^{18}F]FDG uptake in the T8–T9 region. (**b**) The follow-up fused images (coronal *left*; sagittal *middle*; transaxial *right*) performed after 6 months of antibiotic treatment show the disappearance of detectable [^{18}F]FDG uptake in the T8–T9 region

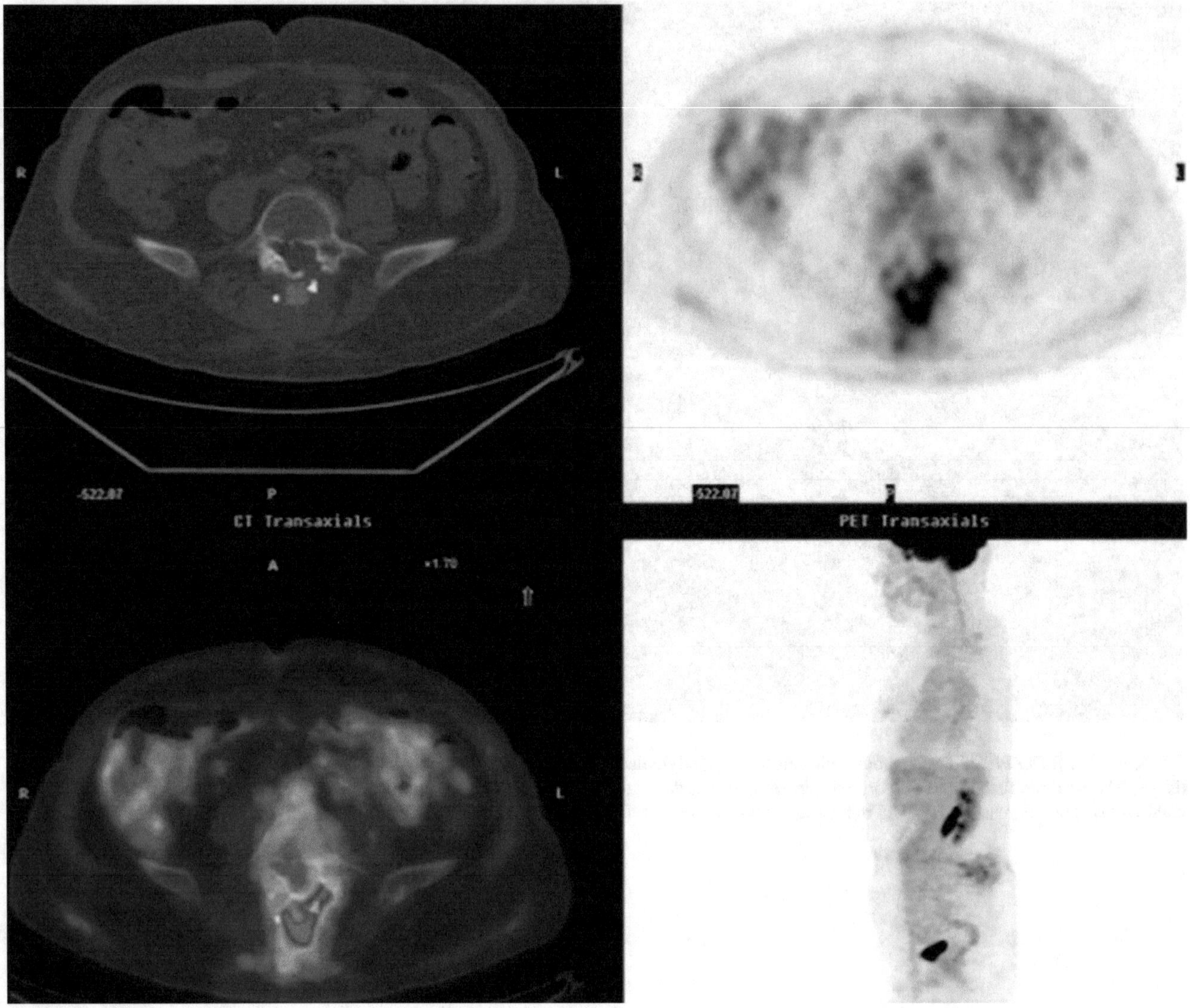

Fig. 3.19 [^{18}F]FDG-PET/CT in a patient with suspected lumbar spondylodiscitis. The transaxial images (CT *upper left*; PET *upper right*; fused *lower left*) of the lumbar spine show increased [^{18}F]FDG uptake in the posterior para-vertebral soft tissues in the L4–L5 region, with partial bone involvement (spinous process of L5). The scan allows correct evaluation of disease extent

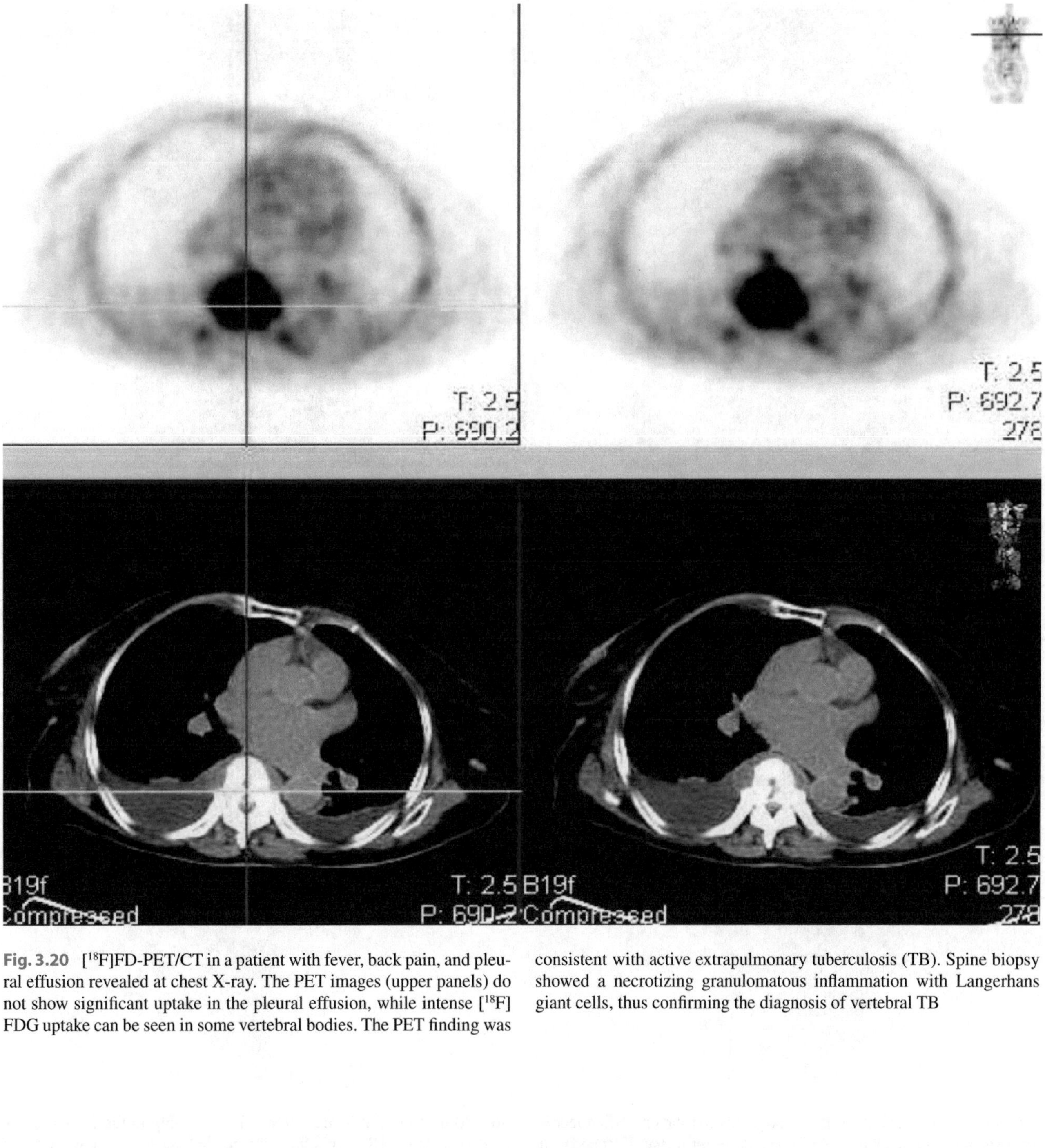

Fig. 3.20 [^{18}F]FD-PET/CT in a patient with fever, back pain, and pleural effusion revealed at chest X-ray. The PET images (upper panels) do not show significant uptake in the pleural effusion, while intense [^{18}F]FDG uptake can be seen in some vertebral bodies. The PET finding was consistent with active extrapulmonary tuberculosis (TB). Spine biopsy showed a necrotizing granulomatous inflammation with Langerhans giant cells, thus confirming the diagnosis of vertebral TB

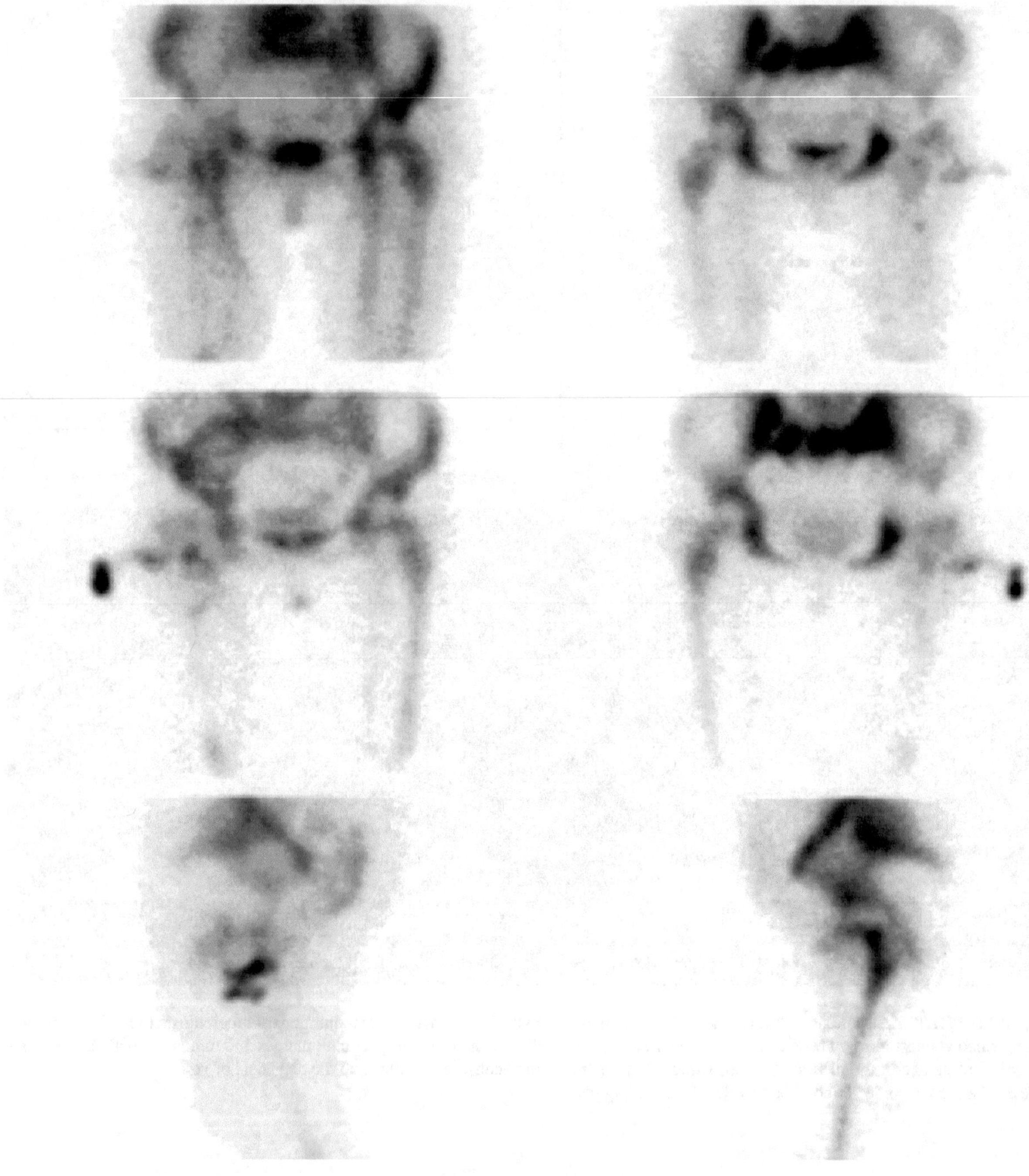

Fig. 3.21 ^{99m}Tc-HMPAO-WBC scintigraphy in a patient with infective arthritis of right hip. Planar anterior and posterior images (left and right images, respectively) at 4 h and 24 h p.i. of labeled leukocytes clearly show accumulation of activity increasing with time in the right hip joint, with appearance of a fistula at 24 h, associated soft tissue infection. Almost invariably, fistulae can be seen only in the 24 h scan. In case of a superficial infection, the wound must be medicated and cleaned before each image acquisition, in order to avoid false positivity due to accumulation of radioactive pus in the bandage

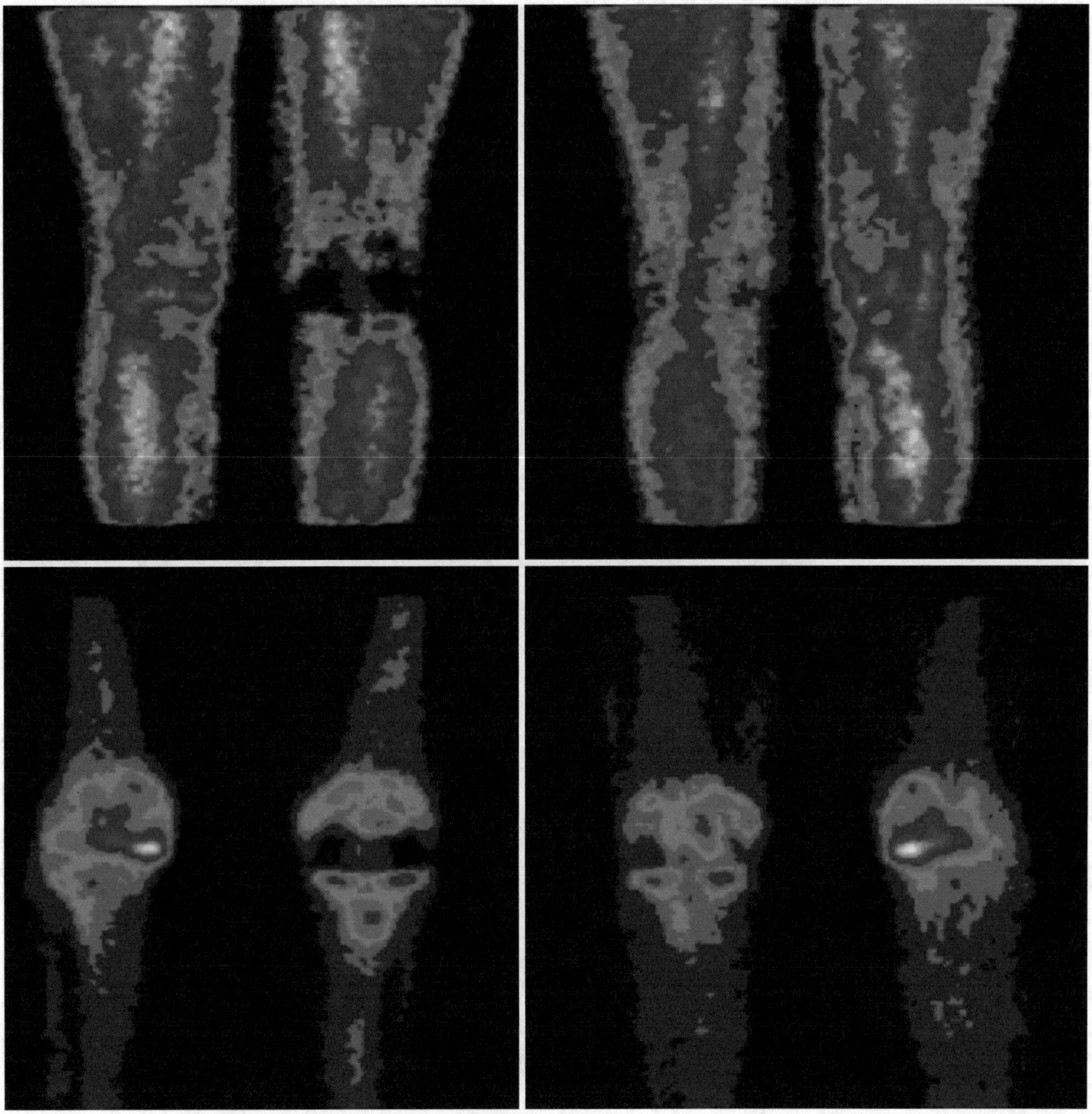

Fig. 3.22 ^{99m}Tc-HMPAO-WBC scintigraphy in a patient with suspected right knee arthritis. Planar anterior (*left*) and posterior (*right*) images at 1 h (*upper*) and 6 h (*lower*) p.i. show abnormal accumulation of labeled leukocytes, increasing with time, in the medial region of the right knee joint, indicating the presence of infected arthritis

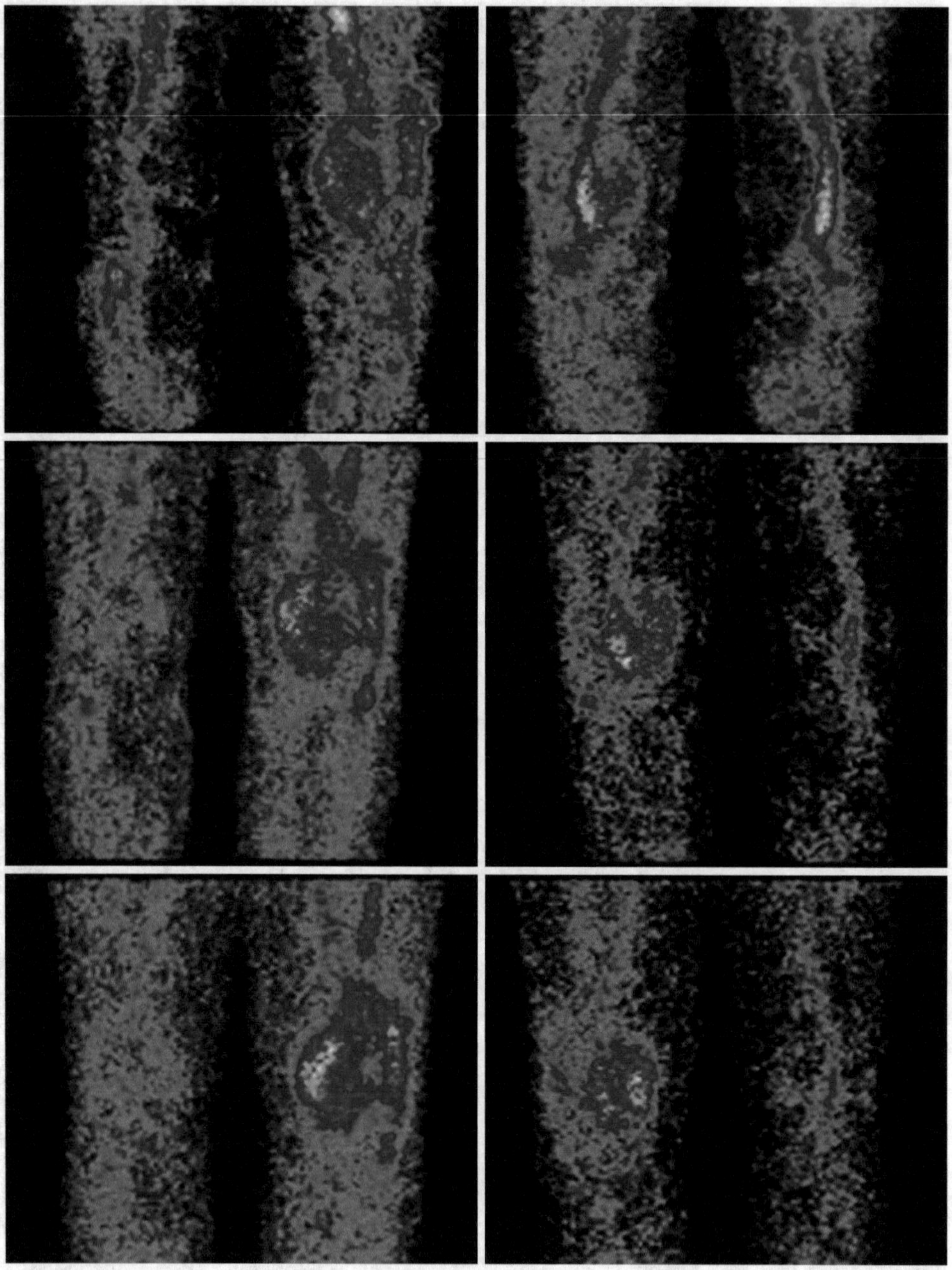

Fig. 3.23 ^{99m}Tc-HMPAO-WBC scintigraphy in a patient with suspected left knee arthritis. Planar anterior (*left*) and posterior (*right*) images at 30 min (*upper*), 4 h (middle), and 20 h (*lower*) p.i. show abnormal accumulation of labeled leukocytes, increasing with time, in the medial and lateral region of the left knee, indicating the presence of infected arthritis

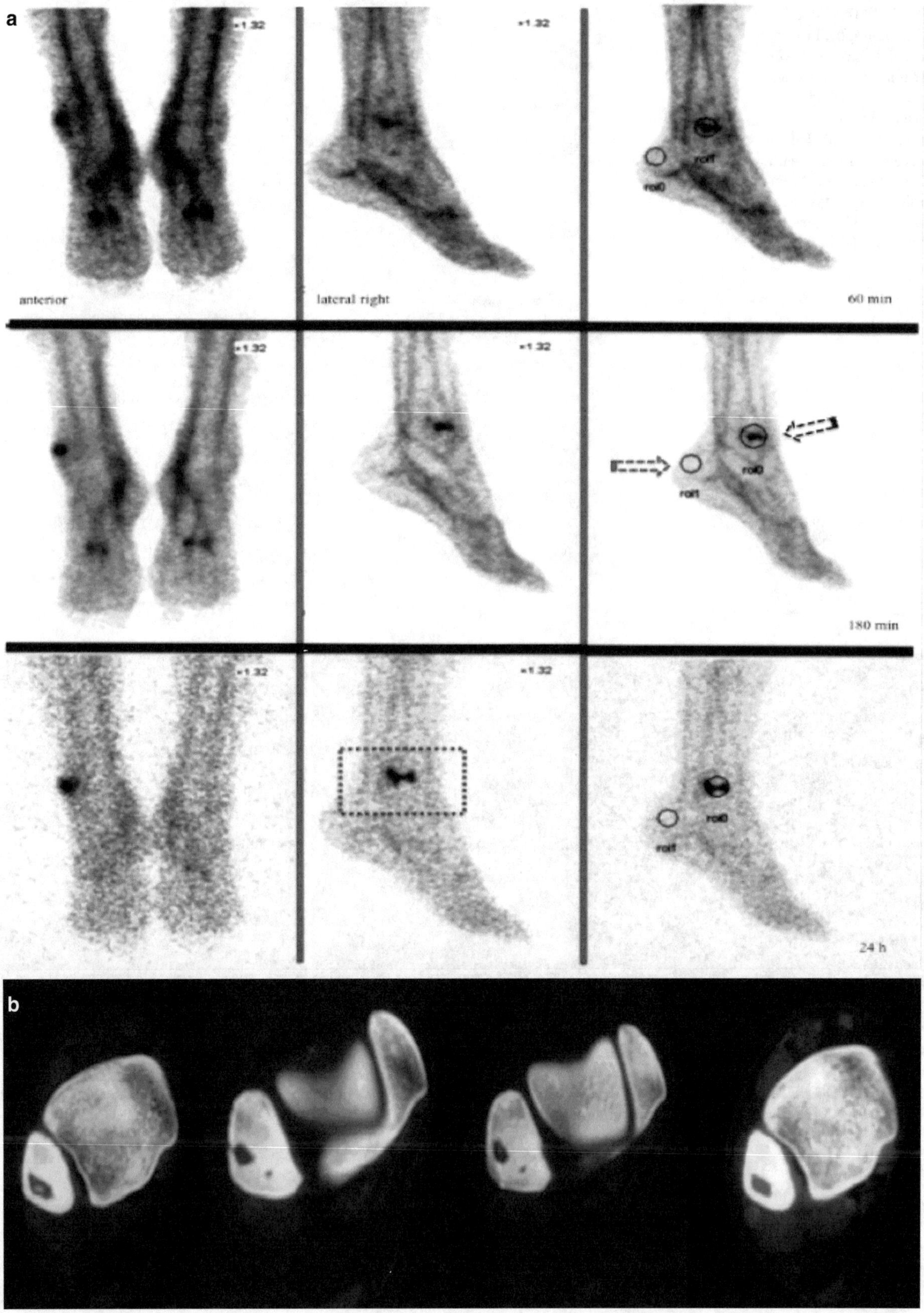

Fig. 3.24 ^{99m}Tc-HMPAO-WBC scintigraphy. (**a**) Planar anterior (*left*) and posterior (*right*) images at 1 h (*upper*), 3 h (middle), and 20 h (*lower*) p.i. show abnormal accumulation of labeled leukocytes, increasing with time, at right fibular malleolus. These findings are consistent with infectious disease. (**b**) MRI of right ankle showed abnormal MR signals, probably due to reactive sclerosis, edema, and inflammatory disease of cancellous bone, with extension to soft tissues around the right fibular malleolus. The ^{99m}Tc-HMPAO-WBC scan and MRI findings are consistent with the presence of a Brodie abs cess

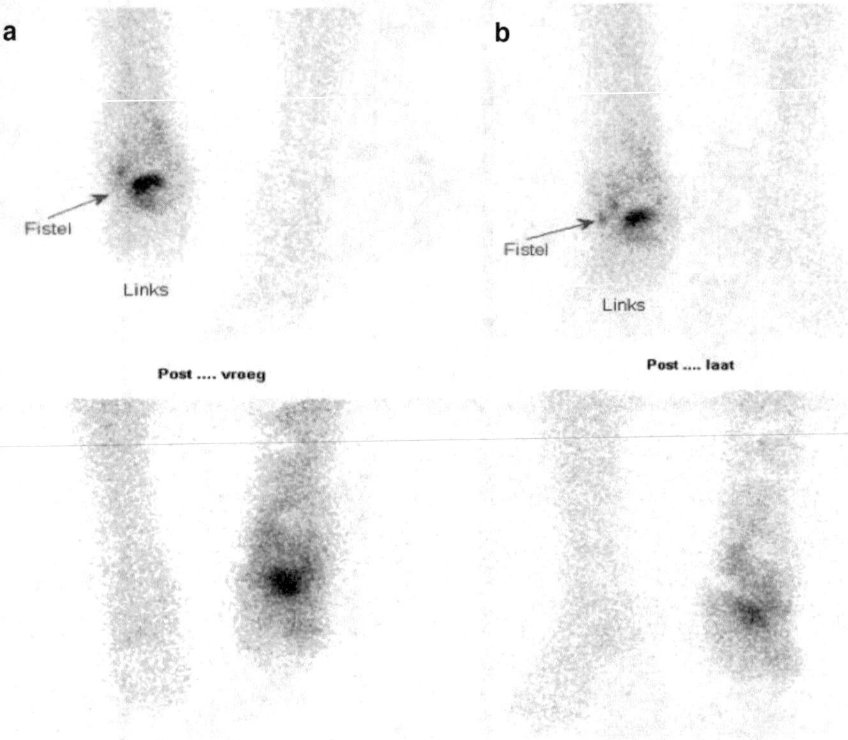

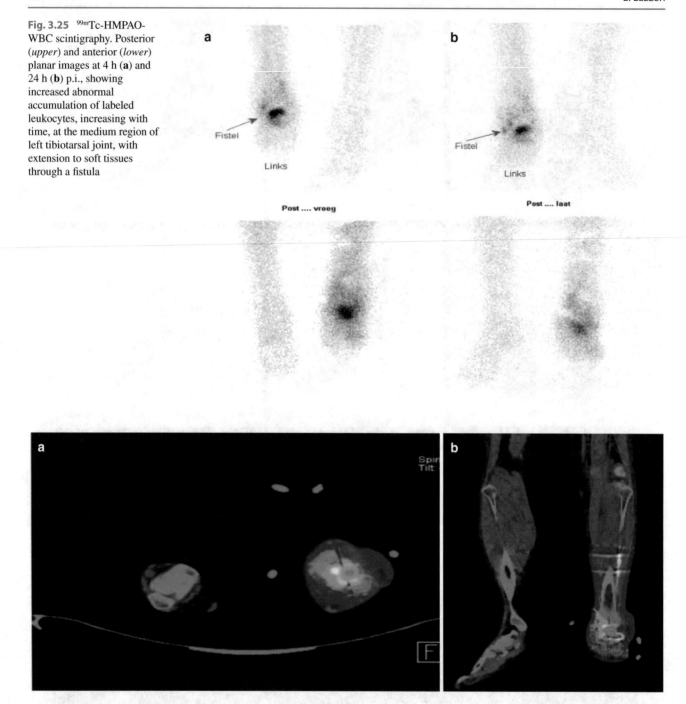

Fig. 3.25 ^{99m}Tc-HMPAO-WBC scintigraphy. Posterior (*upper*) and anterior (*lower*) planar images at 4 h (**a**) and 24 h (**b**) p.i., showing increased abnormal accumulation of labeled leukocytes, increasing with time, at the medium region of left tibiotarsal joint, with extension to soft tissues through a fistula

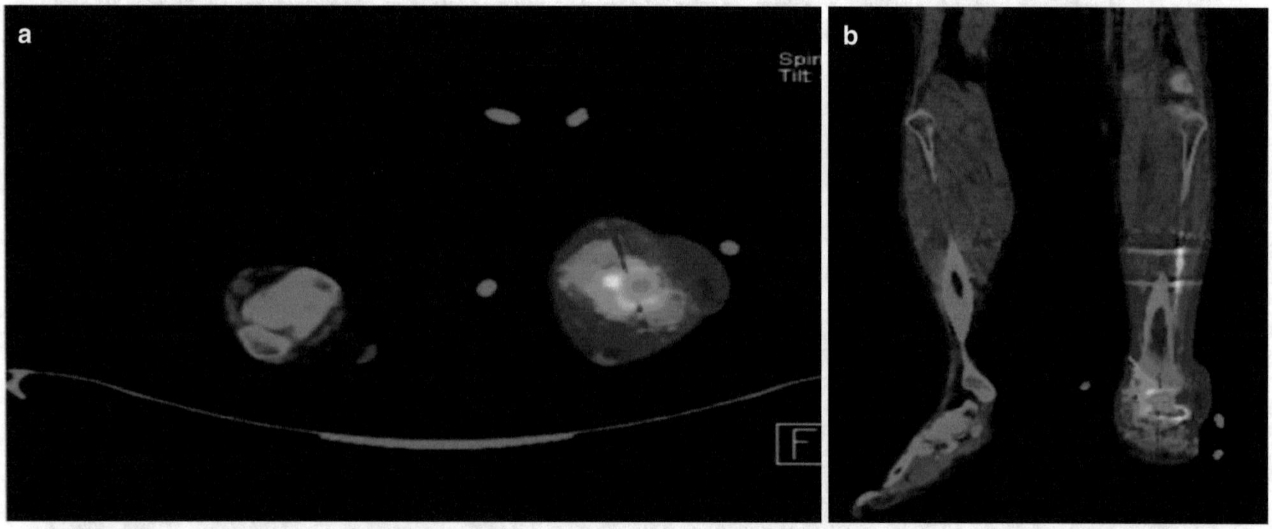

Fig. 3.26 [^{18}F]FDG PET/CT. (**a**) Transaxial and (**b**) coronal sections of fused PET/CT showing increased [^{18}F]FDG uptake along the middle portion of diaphysis of left tibia and all along the left tibiotarsal joint

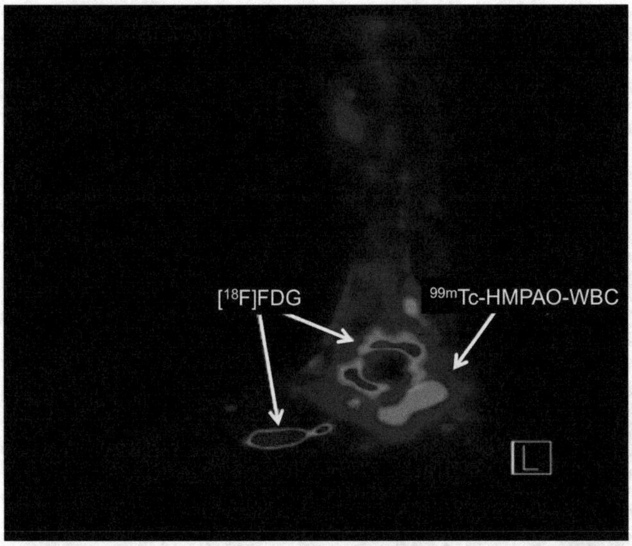

Fig. 3.27 [^{18}F]FDG PET/CT and ^{99m}Tc-HMPAO-WBC fused image (post-acquisition processing). In this sagittal section, it is possible to distinguish accumulation of the two different radiopharmaceuticals: ^{99m}Tc-HMPAO-WBC are localized in the inferolateral region of the calcaneous, whereas [^{18}F]FDG is localized in the upper region of the joint and in the plantar region of the foot. The two different radiopharmaceuticals localize at different sites because they target different biological events, therefore different specificities. In this case, [^{18}F]FDG concentrates in healing tissues and inflammatory reaction, while ^{99m}Tc-HMPAO-WBC accumulate in the infected portion of the joint

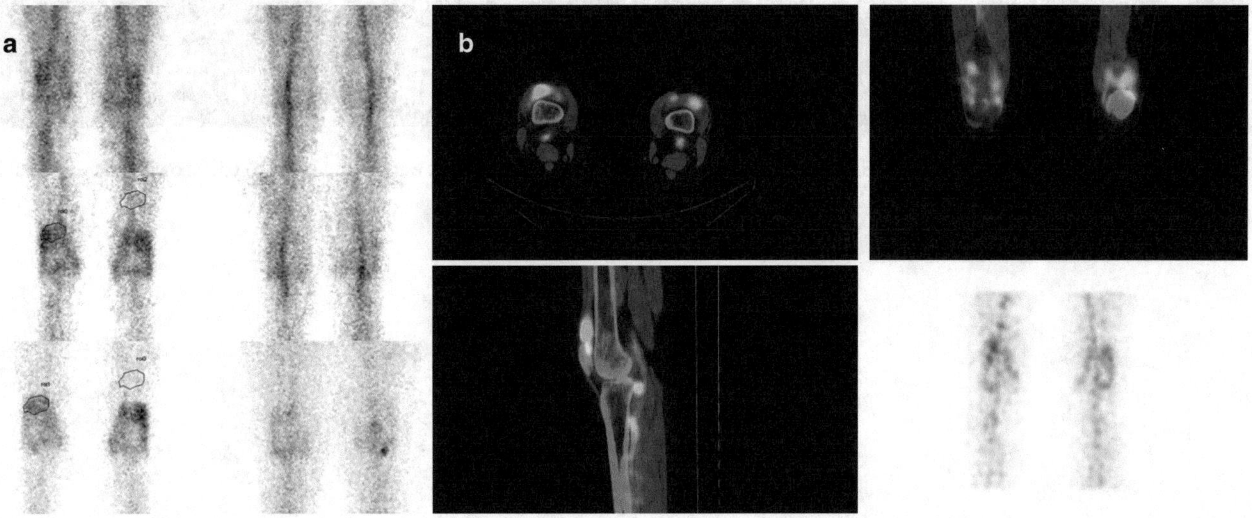

Fig. 3.28 ^{99m}Tc-HMPAO-WBC scintigraphy in a patient with infectious arthritis of left knee and inflammatory arthritis of right knee. (**a**) Planar anterior (*left*) and posterior (*right*) views at 30 min (*upper*), 4 h (*middle*), and 20 h (*lower*) p.i., clearly showing an increase of activity with time in the left joint and an apparent decline in accumulation of labeled leukocytes in the right knee. (**b**) Fused SPECT/CT transaxial (*upper left*), coronal (*upper right*), and sagittal (*lower left*) images, identifying the anatomical sites of leukocytes accumulation

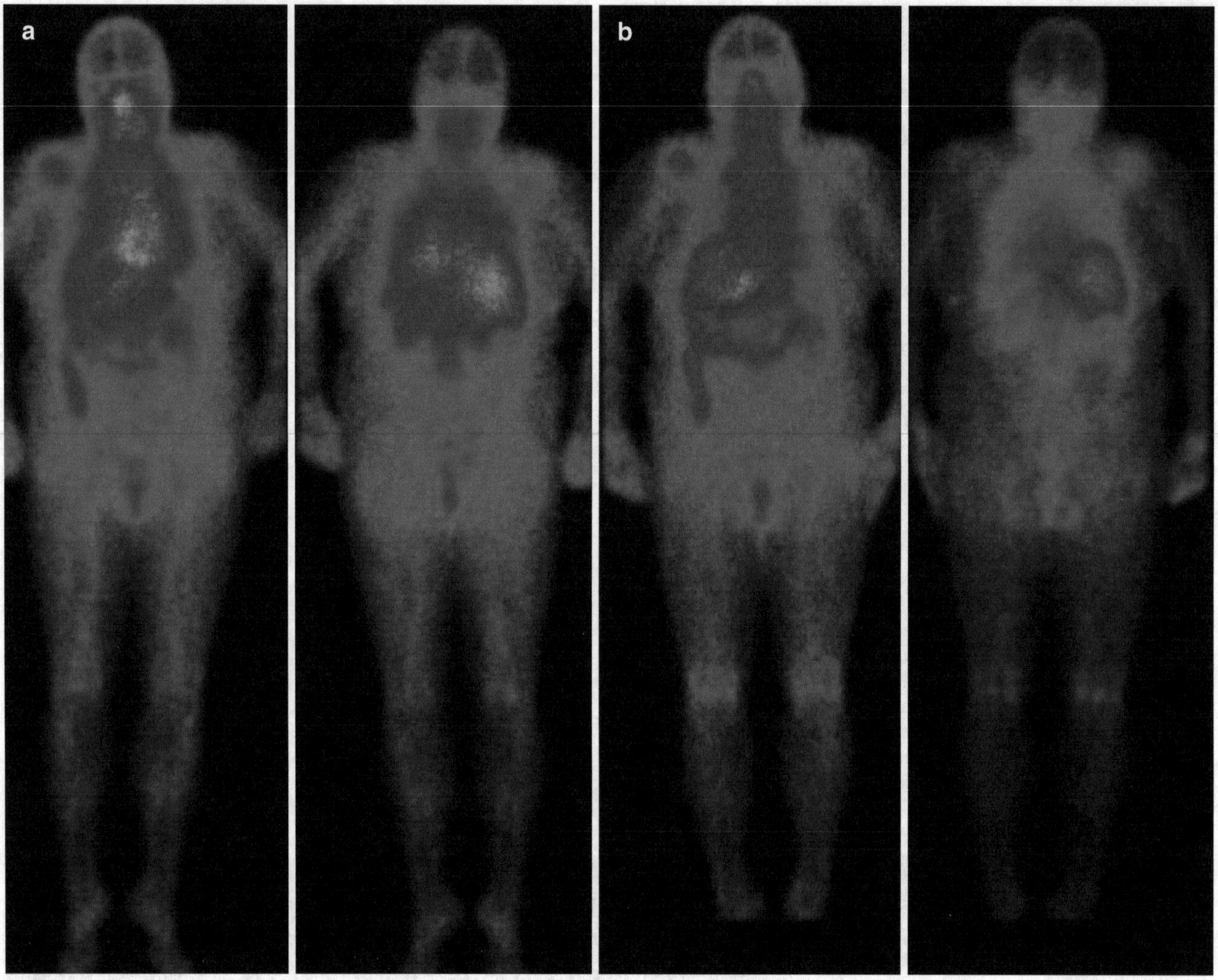

Fig. 3.29 ^{67}Ga-citrate scintigraphy: whole-body images (anterior, *left* and posterior, *right*) at 6 h (**a**) and 24 h (**b**) p.i., showing increased radiotracer uptake in right shoulder

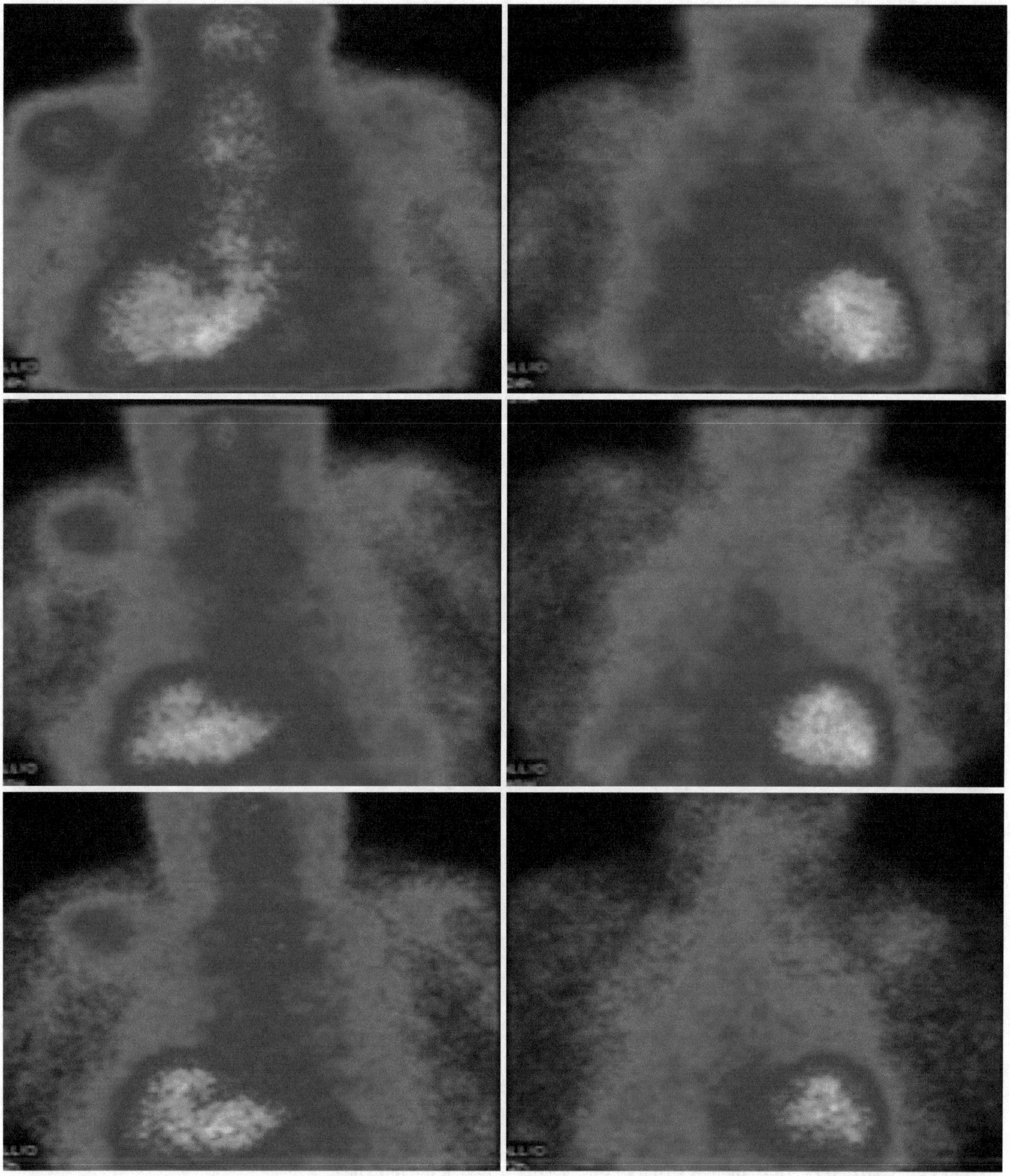

Fig. 3.30 ^{67}Ga-citrate scintigraphy. Spot images of the chest in anterior (*right*) and posterior (*left*) views obtained at 24 h (*upper*), 48 h (*middle*), and 72 h (*lower*) p.i., showing markedly increased tracer uptake in right shoulder

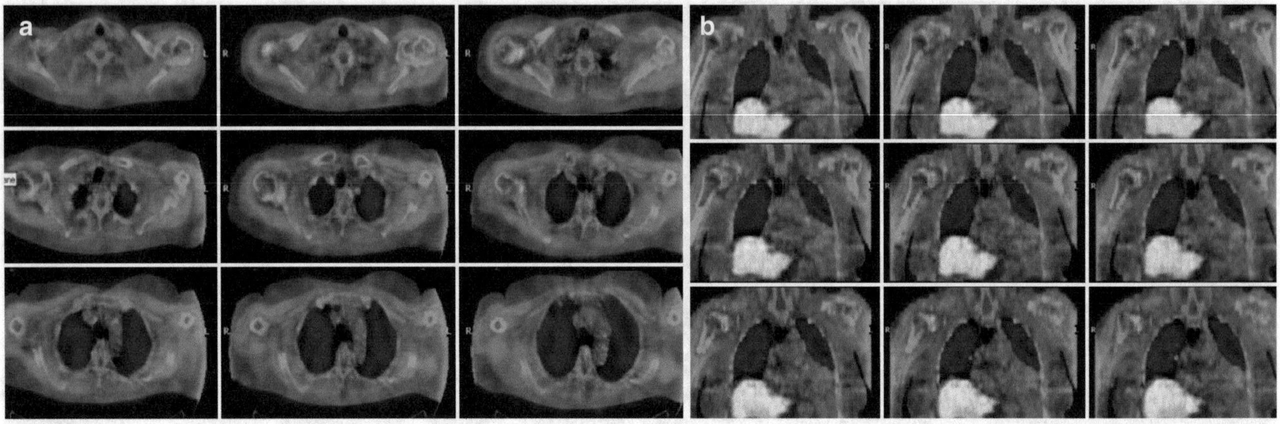

Fig. 3.31 ^{67}Ga-citrate scintigraphy, with SPECT/CT acquisition at 48 h p.i. Fused transaxial (**a**) and coronal (**b**) images showing intense tracer uptake in the right shoulder, suggesting infectious arthritis. Due to the low specificity of ^{67}Ga-citrate scintigraphy, fine-needle aspiration biopsy for microbiology culture is mandatory for final diagnosis. In this case, the scan indicates that there are no other sites of suspected infection in the body. In addition, ^{67}Ga-citrate scintigraphy may also serve for post-therapy follow-up

3.5 Clinical Cases

Case 3.1

Elena Lazzeri

Background

A 55-year-old man with fever, chronic pain at both knees, and long-lasting increase of inflammation indexes for rheumatoid arthritis; positive blood culture for *Staphylococcus aureus*. Transthoracic and trans-esophageal echocardiograms showed mitral valvular regurgitation. For the suspicion of infective endocarditis, [^{18}F]FDG PET/CT was performed, after a low carbohydrate/high fat diet for 24 h. No [^{18}F]FDG uptake was detectable at heart valves, whereas a focal area of increased tracer uptake was observed in the upper lobe of left lung (MIP image in lower right panel of Fig. 3.32a). In addition, increased [^{18}F]FDG uptake was found at bilateral knee joints (transaxial CT, PET, and fused PET images). These findings were consistent with lung infection and suspected for septic involvement of chronic arthritis.

^{99m}Tc-HMPAO-WBC scintigraphy was therefore performed for the differential diagnosis between septic and inflamed knee arthritis (planar images at 30 min, 4 h, and 20 h in Fig. 3.32b; SPECT/CT images at 4 h in Fig. 3.32c). The scan showed accumulation of labeled leukocytes at both knee joints, increasing over time especially in the right knee.

Suspected Site of Infection

Infected knees arthritis.

Radiopharmaceutical Activity

[^{18}F]FDG, 276 MBq.

^{99m}Tc-HMPAO-WBC, 740 MBq.

Imaging

[^{18}F]FDG PET/CT acquired 60 min post-injection, including CT scout view (120 kV, 10 mA), whole-body CT scan (140 kV, 80 mA), and PET (3 min/FOV). Images were reconstructed with and without attenuation correction using the low-dose transmission CT scan.

^{99m}Tc-HMPAO-WBC scintigraphy: acquisition of planar images at 30 min, 4 h, and 20 h; SPECT/CT acquisition at 4 h.

Conclusion/Teaching Point

[^{18}F]FDG PET/CT identified the sites of infection/inflammation, without however the possibility to discriminate between infection and inflammation. ^{99m}Tc-HMPAO-WBC scintigraphy identified septic arthritis at the right knee and inflammation at the left knee.

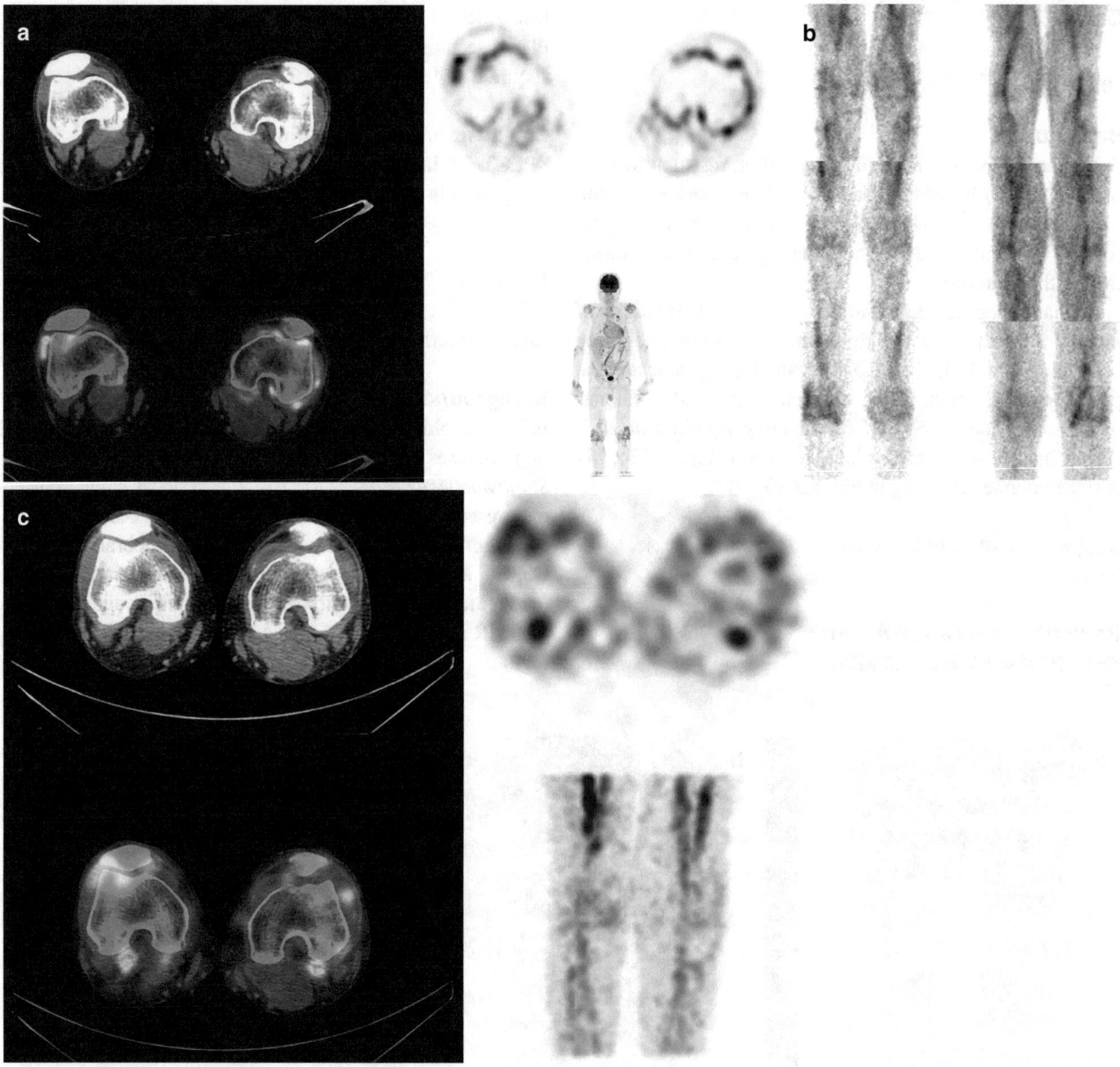

Fig. 3.32 [^{18}F]FDG-PET/CT (**a**). The transaxial CT (*upper left*), PET (*upper right*), fused (*lower left*) show high uptake of [^{18}F]FDG at left lung (superior lobe) and a diffuse and high uptake of [^{18}F]FDG at main joints particularly evident at knees (left higher than right). These findings are consistent with the presence of inflammatory and/or infective disease. ^{99m}Tc-HMPAO scintigraphy was performed 3 days later, to differentiate inflammatory and/or infective knees joint disease. Planar anterior (*left*) and posterior (*right*) images 30 min (*upper*) 4 h (*middle*) and 20 h (*lower*) p.i. (**b**) clearly showing an increase of activity over time in the right joint and a seeming stable accumulation of labeled leukocytes at the left knee. Semiquantitative evaluation, drawing regions of interest in the target and background regions, confirms the decrease of activity at the left knee. Fused SPECT/CT images (CT *upper left*; SPECT *upper right*; fused *lower left*) (**c**) show the anatomical regions of leucocytes accumulation. These findings are consistent with infective arthritis of right knee and inflammatory disease of left knee

Case 3.2

Napoleone Prandini

Background

A 67-year-old man with pain in right foot, resistant to various therapy with nonsteroidal anti-inflammatory drugs (no obvious fever). ^{99m}Tc-HMPAO-WBC scintigraphy was performed which allows to diagnose the presence of bone infection of the right foot.

Planar imaging demonstrated clear accumulation of labeled leukocytes at the right foot, persisting over time between 1 and 20 h (Fig. 3.32a). This finding indicates the presence of infection, which was better localized as talonavicular infection by SPECT/CT imaging acquired at 20 h (fused images in different planes shown in Fig. 3.32b; 3D surface volume rendering in Fig. 3.32c).

Suspected Site of Infection

Right foot.

Radiopharmaceutical Activity

^{99m}Tc-HMPAO-WBC, 740 MBq.

Imaging

Planar scan of lower limbs at 1 h, 4 h, and 24 h; SPECT/CT acquired at 4 h (Figs. 3.33, 3.34, and 3.35).

Conclusion/Teaching Point

SPECT/CT imaging during ^{99m}Tc-HMPAO-WBC scintigraphy precisely identifies the site of infection.

Case 3.3

Elena Lazzeri

Background

A 79-year-old woman with neck pain, increase of inflammation indexes and positive blood culture positive for *Staphylococcus aureus*. MRI of the cervical spine showed the presence of an anterior epidural abscess collection with concomitant cortical alterations of the vertebral bodies of C5, C6, and C7 consistent with spondylodiscitis (Fig. 3.36: (**a**) sagittal T1 image with low signal intensity and (**b**) sagittal STIR image with high signal intensity in the C5–C7 spine region).

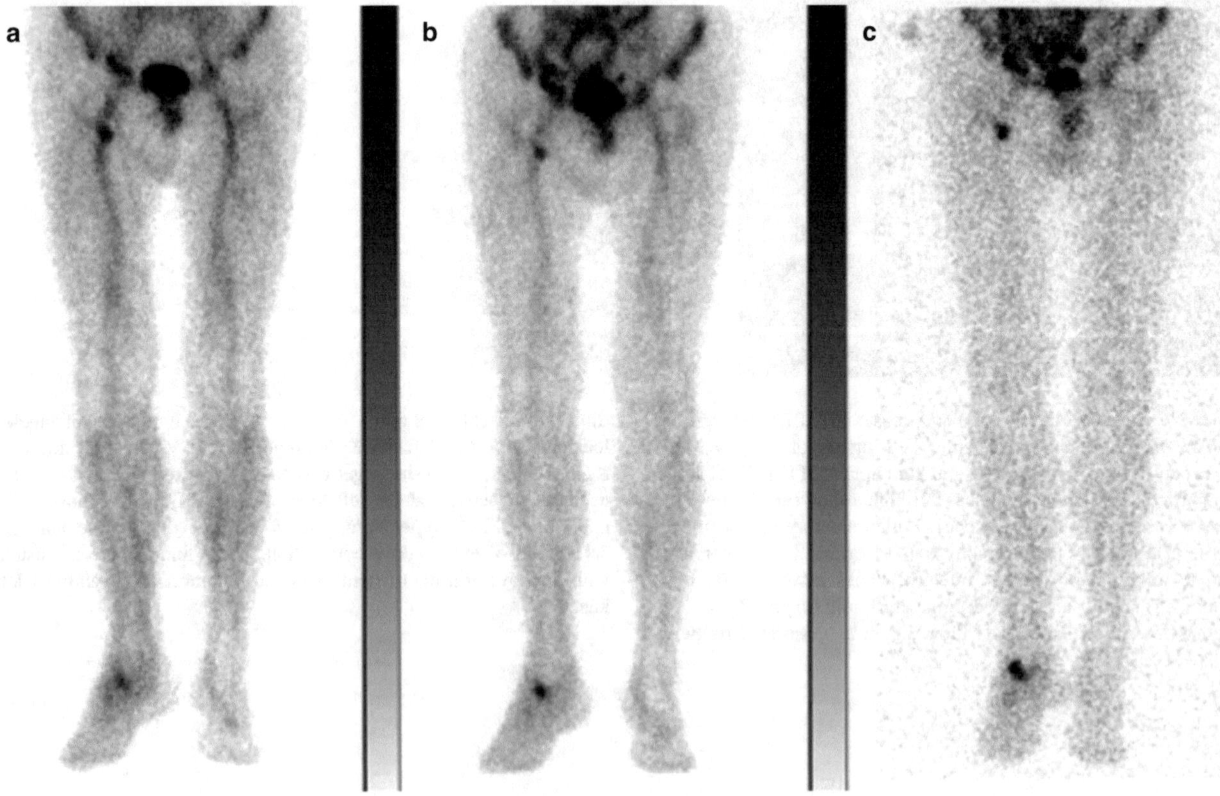

Fig. 3.33 ^{99m}Tc-HMPAO scintigraphy. Anterior scan images of lower limbs 1 h (**a**), 4 h (**b**), and 24 h (**c**) p.i. The images show accumulation of labeled leukocytes in right tarsus increasing over time, indicating infection. Increased activity in ipsilateral inguinal lymph nodes confirms this diagnosis

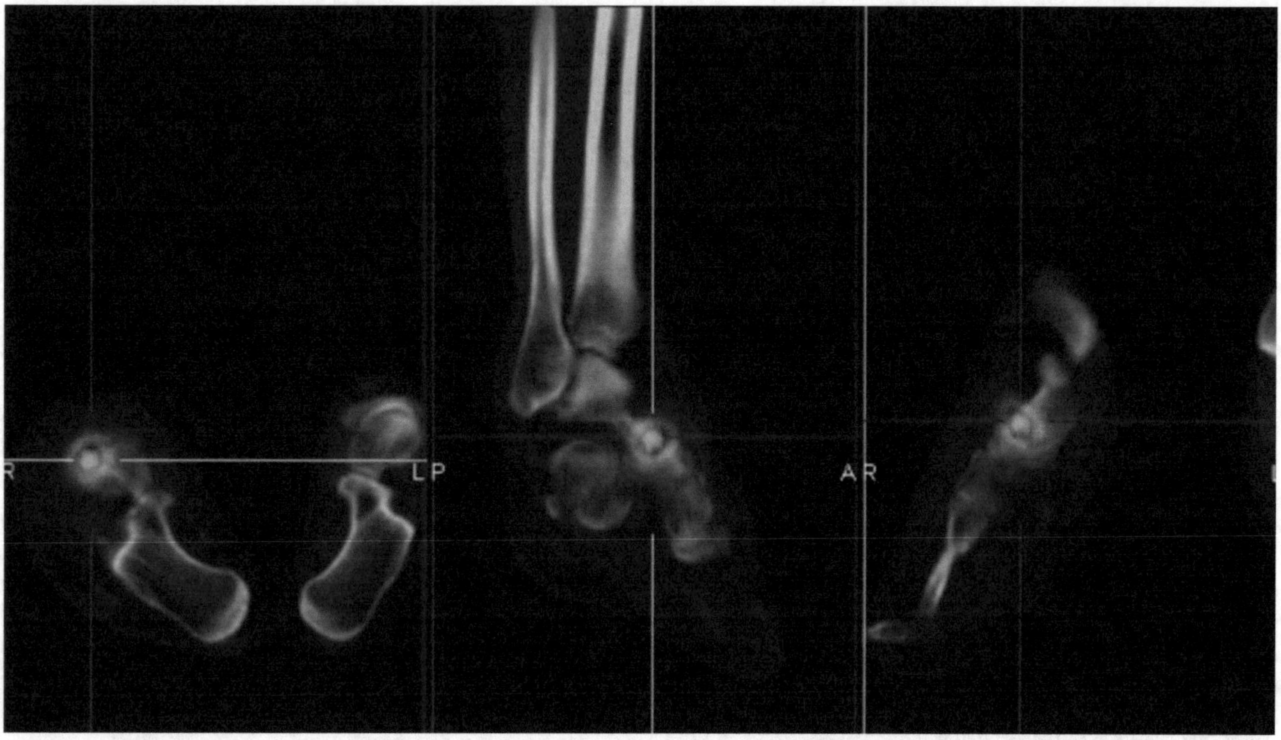

Fig. 3.34 ^{99m}Tc-HMPAO scintigraphy. Fused SPECT/CT images (transaxial, *left*; sagittal, *middle*; coronal, *right*) of feet 4 h p.i. of labeled leukocytes. The images show a focal uptake of labeled leukocytes in right talo-navicular joint consistent with septic arthritis

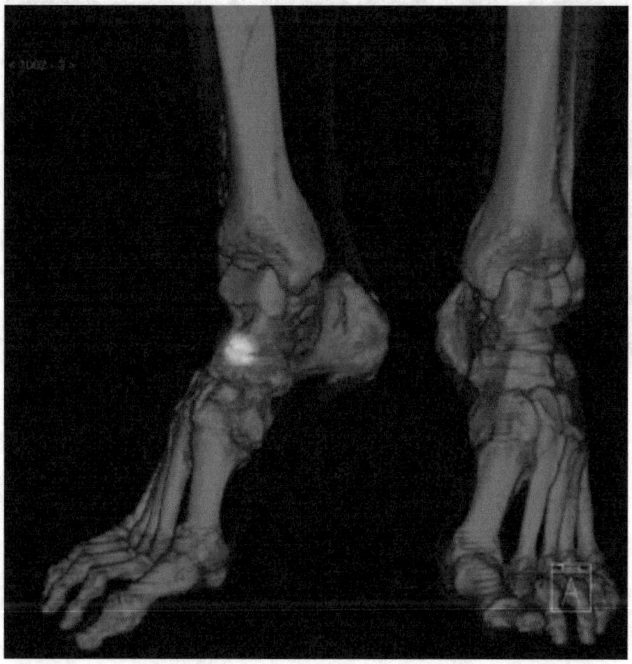

Fig. 3.35 ^{99m}Tc-HMPAO scintigraphy. 3D surface volume rendering of SPECT/CT imaging, showing focal accumulation of labeled leukocytes in the right talo-navicular joint without CT signs of bone structure changes

[^{18}F]FDG PET/CT was performed to confirm the presence of spondylodiscitis and also to evaluate with whole-body imaging potential septic embolism. Increased [^{18}F]FDG uptake was observed in the cervical spine, involving C5, C6, and C7; furthermore, unexpected bilateral pleural effusion was found, with mild tracer accumulation (Fig. 3.37).

The follow-up [^{18}F]FDG PET/CT scan performed after 2 months of antimicrobial therapy showed considerable reduction of [^{18}F]FDG uptake both at the cervical region and in the bilateral pleural effusion (Fig. 3.38), indicating partial response to therapy.

Suspected Site of Infection

Cervical spine.

Radiopharmaceutical Activity

[^{18}F]FDG, 276 MBq.

Imaging

[^{18}F]FDG PET/CT acquired 60 min post-injection, including CT scout view (120 kV, 10 mA), whole-body CT scan (140 kV, 80 mA), and PET (3 min/FOV). Images were reconstructed with and without attenuation correction using the low-dose transmission CT scan.

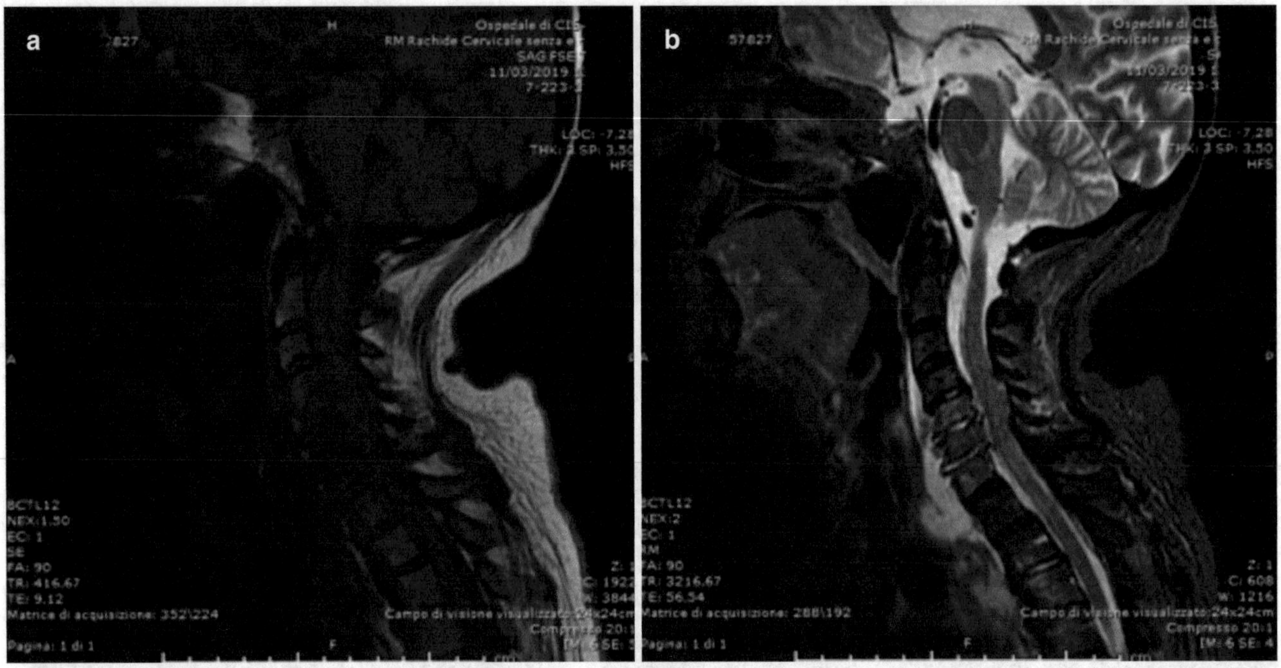

Fig. 3.36 MRI: Sagittal T1 image (**a**) with low signal intensity, and sagittal STIR image (**b**) with high signal intensity in the C5–C7 spine region. These findings are consistent with infection

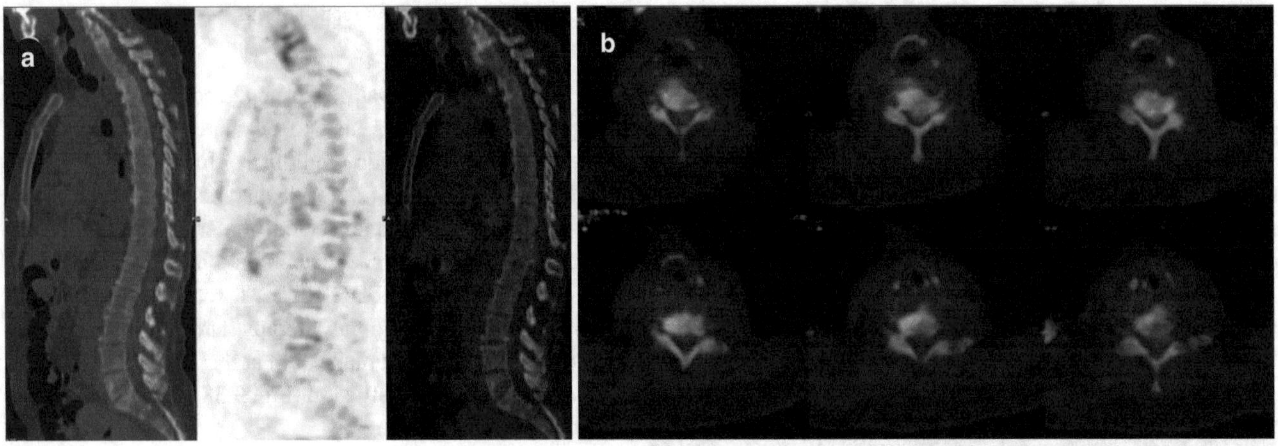

Fig. 3.37 [^{18}F]FDG PET/CT. The sagittal images (CT *left*; PET *middle*; fused *right*) of the skeleton (**a**) show increased [^{18}F]FDG uptake in the region C5–C7 and mild increase of uptake at the T3–T4 space. The transaxial fused images (**b**) show the extension of pathological uptake of [^{18}F]FDG at the cervical vertebral bodies. These findings confirm the presence of infection of the cervical spine and the suspicion of thoracic spine involvement

Conclusion/Teaching Point

[^{18}F]FDG PET/CT confirmed the clinical suspicion of cervical spine infection and ruled out septic embolism. The persistence of [^{18}F]FDG uptake in the cervical spine during the follow-up PET/CT scan (although reduced versus the baseline scan) does not permit to establish a sure differential diagnosis between persistence of infection and presence of inflammation only.

Case 3.4

Elena Lazzeri

Background

A 36-year-old man with fever, pain at the left gluteal region, and positive blood culture for *Staphylococcus aureus*. MRI of the lumbar spine showed the presence of a median hernia

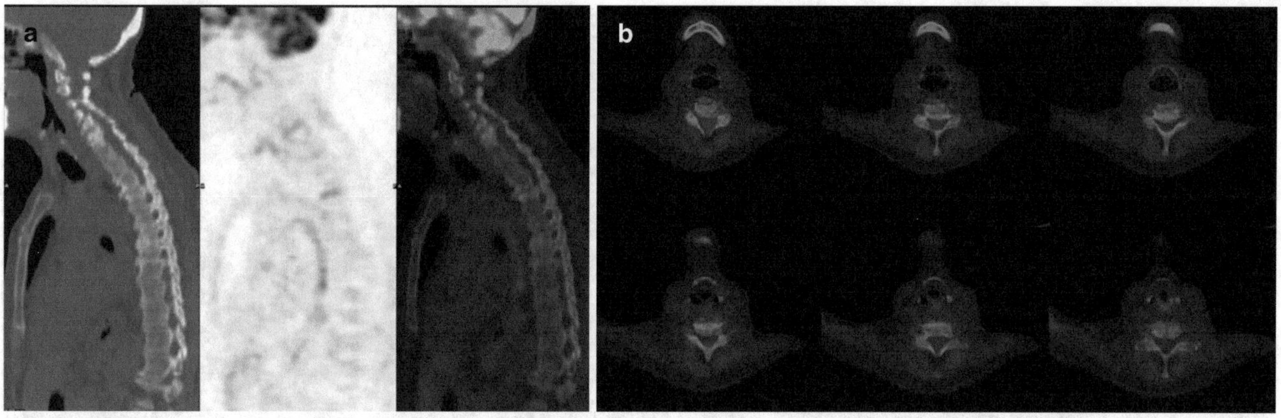

Fig. 3.38 [^{18}F]FDG PET/CT. The follow-up [^{18}F]FDG PET/CT sagittal images (CT *left*; PET *middle*; fused *right*) (**a**) performed 3 months later during antibiotic therapy, show a significant reduction of [^{18}F]FDG uptake in the C5–C7 region and the persistence of mild tracer uptake at the T3–T4 space. The transaxial fused images (**b**) confirm the marked decrease of pathological uptake of [^{18}F]FDG at the cervical vertebral bodies. These findings are consistent with a good response to therapy for the cervical spine infection and allow to diagnose the presence of inflammatory disease at the T3–T4 region

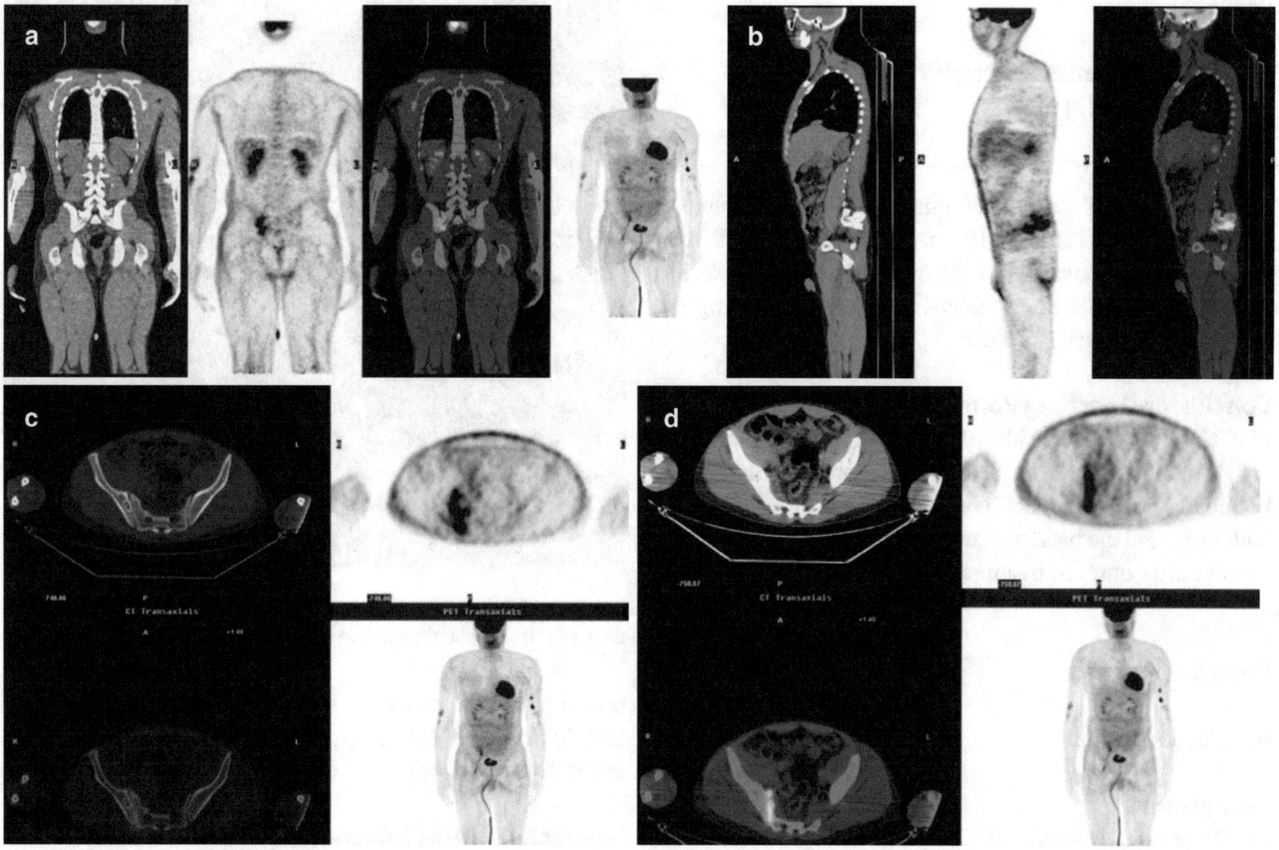

Fig. 3.39 [^{18}F]FDG PET/CT. The coronal (**a**), sagittal (**b**), and transaxial (**c, d**) images (CT, PET, and fused) show increased [^{18}F]FDG uptake at the right sacroiliac joint, with involvement of the anterior soft tissues of the pelvic plane

at L5–S1 with limited cord and spinal compression without evidence of infection and/or pathology of cauda.

PET/CT with [^{18}F]FDG was performed to definitely rule out the clinical suspicion of spondylodiscitis. The PET/CT scan was negative for infection of the lumbosacral spine, whereas markedly increased [^{18}F]FDG uptake was observed in the right sacroiliac joint and the adjacent soft tissues (Fig. 3.39). These findings suggest the presence of infection of the right sacroiliac joint with involvement of adjacent soft tissues. A repeat MRI scan performed 1 week later became positive for infection/inflammation (Fig. 3.40).

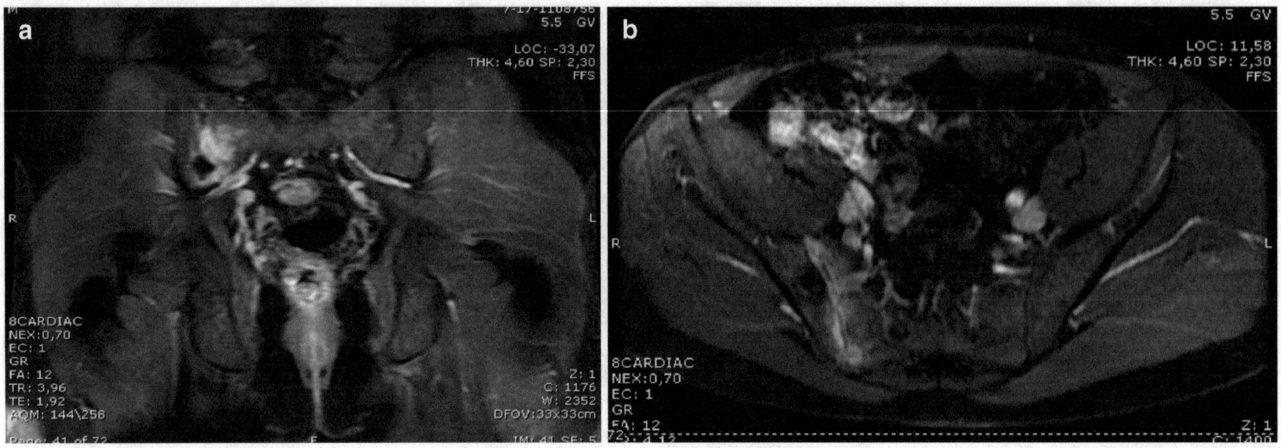

Fig. 3.40 MRI: Coronal (**a**) and transaxial (**b**) images show impaired signal and contrast enhancement of articular surfaces of the right sacroiliac joint, with edema of the soft tissues consistent with inflammatory reaction

Suspected Site of Infection

Lumbosacral spine.

Radiopharmaceutical Activity

[^{18}F]FDG, 260 MBq.

Imaging

[^{18}F]FDG PET/CT acquired 60 min post-injection, including CT scout view (120 kV, 10 mA), whole-body CT scan (140 kV, 80 mA), and PET (3 min/FOV). Images were reconstructed with and without attenuation correction using the low-dose transmission CT scan.

Conclusion/Teaching Point

PET/CT with [^{18}F]FDG identified the etiology of fever, leading to establish a final diagnosis of right infective sacroiliitis. Following high-dose antibiotic treatment (linezolid i.v.), both fever and the back pain markedly declined within about 15 days after onset of treatment.

Case 3.5

Napoleone Prandini

Background

A 77-year-old woman with polyarthritis and rheumatoid arthritis presenting with fever and pain at both shoulders and both knees. The patient was referred for PET/CT with [^{18}F] FDG, which demonstrated increased tracer uptake in both shoulders (but predominant in left shoulder) and in left wrist (Fig. 3.41), indicating the presence of infection and/or inflammation at these sites.

^{99m}Tc-HMPAO-WBC scintigraphy was then performed to better characterize the multiple sites of increased [^{18}F]FDG uptake. Abnormal accumulation of labeled leukocytes was observed in both shoulders (predominantly in left shoulder) and both knees (of mild degree), but not in left wrist (Figs. 3.42 and 3.43).

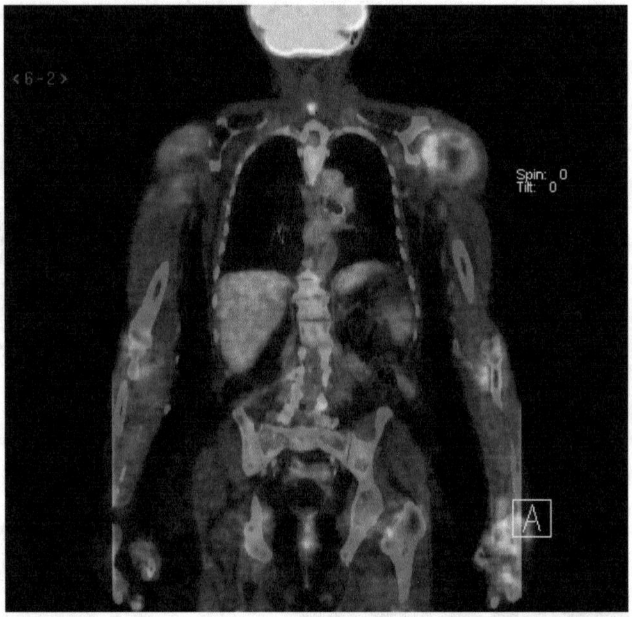

Fig. 3.41 [^{18}F]FDG PET/CT showed increased tracer uptake predominantly in the left shoulder and in left wrist

Suspected Site of Infection

Both shoulders and both knees.

Radiopharmaceutical Activities

[^{18}F]FDG, 270 MBq.

^{99m}Tc-HMPAO-WBC, 740 MBq.

Imaging

[^{18}F]FDG PET/CT acquired 60 min post-injection, including CT scout view (120 kV, 10 mA), whole-body CT scan

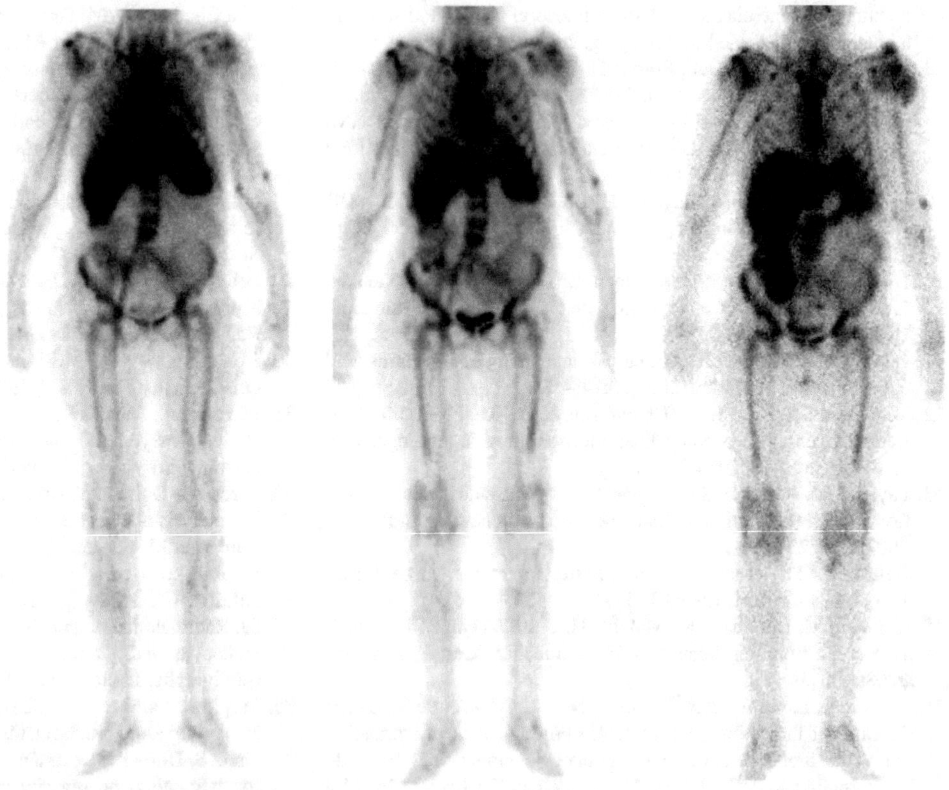

Fig. 3.42 ^{99m}Tc-HMPAO-WBC scintigraphy: total-body scan 1 h, 4 h, and 20 h p.i. The images show significantly increased accumulation of labeled leukocytes in the articular cavity of both shoulders and knees

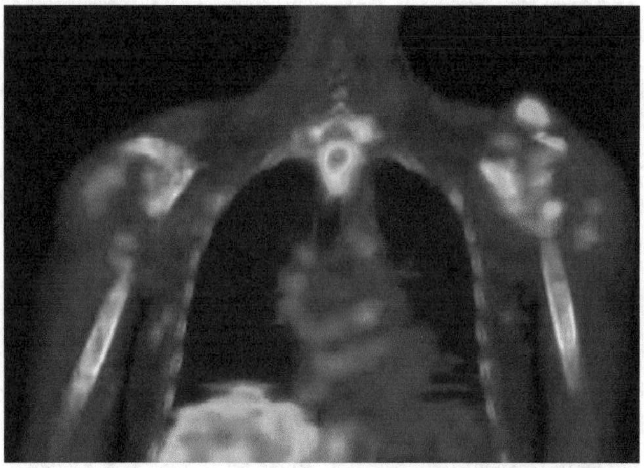

Fig. 3.43 ^{99m}Tc-HMPAO-WBC scintigraphy. SPECT/CT acquisition of the shoulders obtained at 4 h showed increased accumulation of labeled leukocytes in the left joint shoulder cavity, indicating septic arthritis

(140 kV, 80 mA), and PET (3 min/FOV). Images were reconstructed with and without attenuation correction using the low-dose transmission CT scan.

^{99m}Tc-HMPAO-WBC scintigraphy: acquisition of planar images at 1 h, 4 h, and 20 h; SPECT/CT acquisition at 4 h.

Conclusions/Teaching Point

PET/CT with [^{18}F]FDG showed high tracer uptake in both shoulders and left wrist (because of technical malfunction, the knees were not included in the scan). ^{99m}Tc-HMPAO-WBC scintigraphy showed increased leukocyte accumulation predominantly in left shoulder, with no accumulation at all in left wrist. The most likely diagnosis in this patient was infective arthritis of left shoulder, with concomitant inflammation of right shoulder, left wrist, and both knees.

References

1. Lew DP, Waldvogel FA. Osteomyelitis. Lancet. 2004;364:369–79.
2. Jutte P, Lazzeri E, Sconfienza LM, Cassar-Pullicino V, Trampuz A, Petrosillo N, et al. Diagnostic flowcharts in osteomyelitis, spondylodiscitis and prosthetic joint infection. Q J Nucl Med Mol Imaging. 2014;58:2–19.
3. Ochsner P, Bodler P-M, Eich G, Hefti F, Maurer T, Notzli H, et al. Infections of the musculoskeletal system. Grandvaux: Swiss Orthopaedics In-house Publisher; 2014.
4. Korim MT, Payne R, Bhatia M. A case-control study of surgical site infection following operative fixation of fractures of the ankle in a large U.K. trauma unit. Bone Joint J. 2014;96-B:636–40.
5. Malhotra AK, Goldberg S, Graham J, Malhotra NR, Willis MC, Mounasamy V, et al. Open extremity fractures: impact of delay in operative debridement and irrigation. J Trauma Acute Care Surg. 2014;76:1201–7.
6. Glaudemans AWJM, Jutte PC, Cataldo MA, Cassar-Pullicino V, Gheysens O, Borens O, et al. Consensus document for the diagnosis of peripheral bone infection in adults: a joint paper by the EANM, EBJIS, and ESR (with ESCMID endorsement). Eur J Nucl Med Mol Imaging. 2019;46:957–70.
7. Lazzeri E, Bozzao A, Cataldo MA, Petrosillo N, Manfrè L, Trampuz A, et al. Joint EANM/ESNR and ESCMID-endorsed consensus

document for the diagnosis of spine infection (spondylodiscitis) in adults. Eur J Nucl Med Mol Imaging. 2019;46:2464–87.
8. Signore A, Scofienza ML, Borens O, Glaudemans AWJM, Cassar-Pullicino V, Trampuz A, et al. Consensus document for the diagnosis of prosthetic joint infections: a joint paper by the EANM, EBJIS, and ESR (with ESCMID endorsement). Eur J Nucl Med Mol Imaging. 2019;46:971–88.
9. Elgazzar AH, Abdel-Dayem HM, Clark JD, Maxon HR III. Multimodality imaging of osteomyelitis. Eur J Nucl Med. 1995;22:1043–63.
10. Aliabadi P, Tumeh SS, Weissman BN, McNeil BJ. Cemented total hip prosthesis: radiographic and scintigraphic evaluation. Radiology. 1989;173:203–6.
11. Chau CL, Griffith JF. Musculoskeletal infections: ultrasound appearances. Clin Radiol. 2005;60:149–59.
12. Venkatesh SK, Riederer B, Chhem RK, et al. Reactivation in post-traumatic chronic osteomyelitis: ultrasonographic findings. Can Assoc Radiol J. 2003;54:163–8.
13. Fayad LM, Carrino JA, Fishman EK. Musculoskeletal infection: role of CT in the emergency department. Radiographics. 2007;27:1723–36.
14. Beltran J. MR imaging of soft-tissue infection. Magn Reson Imaging Clin N Am. 1995;3:743–51.
15. Chianelli M, Boerman OC, Malviya G, Galli F, Oyen WJ, Signore A. Receptor binding ligands to image infection. Curr Pharm Des. 2008;14:3316–25.
16. Signore A, Jamar F, Israel O, Buscombe J, Martin-Comin J, Lazzeri E. Clinical indications, image acquisition and data interpretation for white blood cells and anti-granulocyte monoclonal antibody scintigraphy: an EANM procedural guideline. Eur J Nucl Med Mol Imaging. 2018;45:1816–31.
17. Weon YC, Yang SO, Choi YY, Shin JW, Ryu JS, Shin MJ, et al. Use of Tc-99m HMPAO leukocyte scans to evaluate bone infection: incremental value of additional SPECT images. Clin Nucl Med. 2000;25:519–26.
18. Gemmel F, Van den Wyngaert H, Love C, Welling MM, Gemmel P, Palestro CJ. Prosthetic joint infections: radionuclide state-of-the-art imaging. Eur J Nucl Med Mol Imaging. 2012;39:892–909.
19. Palestro CJ, Love C, Tronco GG, Tomas MB, Rini JN. Combined labeled leukocyte and technetium 99m sulfur colloid bone marrow imaging for diagnosing musculoskeletal infection. Radiographics. 2006;26:859–70.
20. Pakos EE, Koumoulis HD, Fotopoulos AD, Ioannidis JP. Osteomyelitis: antigranulocyte scintigraphy with ^{99m}Tc radiolabeled monoclonal antibodies for diagnosis—meta-analysis. Radiology. 2007;245:732–41.
21. Dyke JP, Garfinkel JH, Volpert L, Sanders A, Newcomer M, Dutruel SP, et al. Imaging of bone perfusion and metabolism in subjects undergoing total ankle arthroplasty using ^{18}F-fluoride positron emission tomography. Foot Ankle Int. 2019;40:1351–7.
22. Rini JN, Palestro CJ. Imaging of infection and inflammation with ^{18}F-FDG-labeled leukocytes. Q J Nucl Med Mol Imaging. 2006;50:143–6.
23. Domínguez ML, Lorente R, Rayo JI, Serrano J, Sánchez R, Infante JR, et al. SPECT-CT with ^{67}Ga-citrate in the management of spondylodiscitis. Rev Esp Med Nucl Imagen Mol. 2012;31:34–9.
24. Sathekge M, Maes A, D'Asseler Y, Vorster M, Van de Wiele C. Nuclear medicine imaging in tuberculosis using commercially available radiopharmaceuticals. Nucl Med Commun. 2012;33:581–90.
25. Grane P, Josephsson A, Seferlis A, Tullberg T. Septic and aseptic postoperative discitis in the lumbar spine—evaluation by MR imaging. Acta Radiol. 1998;39:108–15.
26. Van Goethem JWM, Parizel PM, van den Hauwe L, Van de Kelft E, Verlooy J, De Schepper AM. The value of MRI in the diagnosis of postoperative spondylodiscitis. Neuroradiology. 2000;42:580–5.
27. Longo M, Granata F, Ricciardi K, Gaeta M, Blandino A. Contrast-enhanced MR imaging with fat suppression in adult-onset septic spondylodiscitis. Eur Radiol. 2003;13:626–37.
28. Carragee EJ. Single-level posterolateral arthrodesis, with or without posterior decompression, for the treatment of isthmic spondylolisthesis in adults. A prospective, randomized study. J Bone Joint Surg Am. 1997;79:1175–80.
29. Felix SC, Mitchell JK. Diagnostic yield of CT-guided percutaneous aspiration procedures in suspected spontaneous infectious diskitis. Radiology. 2001;218:211–4.
30. Honan M, White GW, Eisenberg GM. Spontaneous infectious discitis in adults. Am J Med. 1996;100:85–9.
31. Perronne C, Saba J, Behloul Z, Salmon-Céron D, Leport C, Vildé JL, et al. Pyogenic and tuberculous spondylodiskitis (vertebral osteomyelitis) in 80 adult patients. Clin Infect Dis. 1994;19:746–50.
32. Torda AJ, Gottlieb T, Bradbury R. Pyogenic vertebral osteomyelitis: analysis of 20 cases and review. Clin Infect Dis. 1995;20:320–8.
33. Raghavan M, Lazzeri E, Palestro CJ. Imaging of spondylodiscitis. Semin Nucl Med. 2018;48:131–47.
34. Palestro CJ, Kim CK, Swyer AJ, Vallabhajosula S, Goldsmith SJ. Radionuclide diagnosis of vertebral osteomyelitis: indium-111-leukocyte and technetium-99m-methylene diphosphonate bone scintigraphy. J Nucl Med. 1991;32:1861–5.
35. Turpin S, Lambert R. Role of scintigraphy in musculoskeletal and spinal infections. Radiol Clin N Am. 2001;39:169–89.
36. Gratz S, Dorner J, Oestmann JW, et al. ^{67}Ga citrate and ^{99}Tc^{m}-MDP for estimating the severity of vertebral osteomyelitis. Nucl Med Commun. 2000;21:111–20.
37. Modic MT, Feiglin DH, Piraino DW, Boumphrey F, Weinstein MA, Duchesneau PM, et al. Vertebral osteomyelitis: assessment using MR. Radiology. 1985;157:157–66.
38. Sonmezoglu K, Sonmezoglu M, Halac M, Akgün I, Türkmen C, Onsel C, et al. Usefulness of ^{99m}Tc-ciprofloxacin (infection) scan in diagnosis of chronic orthopedic infections: comparative study with ^{99m}Tc-HMPAO leukocyte scintigraphy. J Nucl Med. 2001;42:567–74.
39. Lazzeri E, Erba P, Perri M, Tascini C, Doria R, Giorgetti J, et al. Scintigraphic imaging of vertebral osteomyelitis with ^{111}in-biotin. Spine (Phila Pa 1976). 2008;33:198–204.
40. Lazzeri E, Erba P, Perri M, Doria R, Tascini C, Mariani G. Clinical impact of SPECT/CT with In-111 biotin on the management of patients with suspected spine infection. Clin Nucl Med. 2010;35:12–7.
41. Tigges S, Stiles RG, Roberson JR. Appearance of septic hip prostheses on plain radiographs. AJR Am J Roentgenol. 1994;163:377–80.
42. Perry D, Stewart N, Benton N, Robinson E, Yeoman S, Crabbe J, et al. Detection of erosions in the rheumatoid hand; a comparative study of multidetector computerized tomography versus magnetic resonance imaging. J Rheumatol. 2005;32:256–67.
43. Ostergaard M, Dohn UM, Ejbjerg BJ, McQueen FM. Ultrasonography and magnetic resonance imaging in early rheumatoid arthritis: recent advances. Curr Rheumatol Rep. 2006;8:378–85.
44. Demertzis JL, Rubin DA. MR imaging assessment of inflammatory, crystalline-induced, and infectious arthritis. Magn Reson Imaging Clin N Am. 2011;19(2):339–63.
45. Weber U, Østergaard M, Lambert RG, Maksymowych WP. The impact of MRI on the clinical management of inflammatory arthritis. Skelet Radiol. 2011;40:1153–73.
46. Craig JG, Amin MB, Wu K, Eyler WR, van Holsbeeck MT, Bouffard JA, et al. Osteomyelitis of the diabetic foot: MR imaging pathologic correlation. Radiology. 1997;203:849–55.

Radionuclide Imaging of Miscellaneous Bone and Joint Conditions

4

Giovanni D'Errico, Emanuele Casciani, and Saadi Sollaku

Contents

Learning Objectives

- To optimize and select the diagnostic imaging procedure (radionuclide imaging, CT, and MRI) as being the most appropriate and useful in a series of musculoskeletal conditions (inflammatory, traumatic, infectious, and neoplastic) which affect the bone and large or small joints and which, although very frequent, are sometimes considered not to be of "high priority"
- To help the reader to better define which nuclear medicine imaging method to use for faster and more accurate diagnosis in the musculoskeletal conditions indicated above
- To describe the radionuclide imaging methods to be employed in the different bone and joint conditions
- To provide indications for the use of the different radionuclide imaging methods according to the specific condition suspected on clinical ground or based on prior imaging with non-radionuclide modalities

4.1 Introduction

A number of the inflammatory, traumatic, infectious, or neoplastic musculoskeletal conditions that affect the bone and large or small joints often (but not always) arise with pain and may exhibit atypical clinical symptoms that make the diagnosis difficult, especially in the early stages of disease.

This chapter summarizes how musculoskeletal conditions (infectious, neoplastic, or traumatic) associated with increased blood perfusion and increased local bone remodeling can be assessed with nuclear medicine imaging [1–

G. D'Errico (✉) · E. Casciani · S. Sollaku
Department of Nuclear Medicine, Private Hospital "Pio XI", Rome, Italy

E. Lazzeri et al. (eds.), *Radionuclide Imaging of Infection and Inflammation*, https://doi.org/10.1007/978-3-030-62175-9_4

4]. In particular, we describe two cases with abnormalities of the dentomaxillofacial region [5–7], a case of uncertain diagnosis of patella stress fracture in a volley player (it was instead bipartite patella) [8, 9], stress micro-fracture of the fibula with bone marrow involvement [10–13], osteomyelitis due to surgical insertion of ischiocrural muscles in hamstring syndrome [14], a case of spondylosis with Modic changes [15–18], tennis player with os trigonum syndrome and exacerbated posterior ankle pain (as a result of an overuse injury of the posterior ankle caused by repetitive plantar flexion stress associated with his sport) [10, 19–23], pseudoarthrosis of the left tail and tendonosis of the left peroneal ligament [24–28], incidental radiological finding of space-occupying lesion, hypointense on MRI, and in the left femur during a CT performed for recent fracture of the ipsilateral tibial plateau (it was non-ossifying fibroma) [28, 29].

The aim of this chapter is to direct the reader to better define which nuclear medicine imaging procedure to use for a more prompt and accurate diagnosis in these musculoskeletal conditions. Thus, the reader will be able to better define which imaging procedure (more emphasis will be placed on nuclear medicine procedures) to use for a faster and more accurate diagnosis.

By providing a physiological assessment, nuclear medicine tests can be valuable and sometimes be the initial test of choice; in general, they are particularly useful for solving some diagnostic problems, particularly in patients with underlying medical conditions that may limit the use of other imaging modalities [30–32].

Key Learning Points

- Numerous inflammatory, traumatic, infectious, or neoplastic conditions can affect the bone and/or joints (large or small) and often arise with pain, with atypical clinical symptoms that make diagnosis difficult, especially in the early stages of disease.
- Nuclear medicine imaging tests may be able to evaluate these conditions if, as often happens, associated with increased vascularization and local bone remodeling.
- By providing a physiological assessment, nuclear medicine tests can be valuable and sometimes be the initial test of choice; they are particularly useful for solving certain diagnostic problems, especially in patients with underlying medical conditions that may limit the use of other imaging modalities.

4.2 General Background on Non-infection Imaging for Miscellaneous Bone/Joint Conditions

When pain and/or functional impairment are present in patients in whom conventional radiological imaging yields little or no diagnostic result, nuclear medicine imaging can be a valid support for an accurate diagnosis [1, 2, 5, 11, 30, 32–35].

In case of suspicion or clear indication of altered bone turnover, or if conventional radiology or MRI is impractical (due to the presence of contraindications), bone scintigraphy with hybrid SPECT/CT is very sensitive in the diagnostic pathway of many skeletal conditions. This method is based on the use of a radiotracer that evaluates the distribution of active bone formation; the most commonly used radiopharmaceuticals are ^{99m}Tc-labeled bisphosphonates that, injected intravenously, are absorbed on the hydroxyapatite crystals in amounts that are proportional to local blood perfusion and osteoblastic activity.

Approximately 50–60% of the injected radiotracer binds to the skeleton over the first 3 h, while most of the remaining fraction is excreted in the urine and a small percentage (about 5–6%) remains in circulating blood. Therefore, it is appropriate to perform bone scintigraphy at 2–3 h after tracer injection, when the maximum accumulation relative to soft tissues is reached within a logistically optimal time window for imaging.

Bone scintigraphy is performed with different sequential imaging modalities to evaluate in their entirety the pathological conditions of bone and joints: (1) three-phase bone scintigraphy; (2) spot planar images; (3) planar whole-body images; (4) SPECT/CT imaging; (5) post-acquisition processing as three-dimensional reconstruction and volume rendering [1].

Bone scintigraphy with ^{99m}Tc-methylene-diphosfonate (^{99m}Tc-MDP) is widely used for the diagnosis and management of various bone diseases due to its low cost and its simple use and because it provides crucial information on bone turnover. The main drawback of this imaging procedure is that its very high sensitivity is associated with a relatively low specificity.

Three-phase bone scintigraphy is a first-line test in the evaluation of many bone or joint disease, in particular in case of doubtful/suspected osteomyelitis and tendonosis.

The double-head gamma-camera is placed in such a way that the area to be evaluated is fully included in the field of view [11, 33–35], and the ^{99m}Tc-MDP bone scan is performed with the following steps: (a) intravenous injection, preferably in an antecubital vein, of 740 MBq of ^{99m}Tc-MDP with simultaneous dynamic acquisition for 2–3 min (120–180 frames of 1 s) on the region of interest; (b) planar acquisition at 3–5 min for 2 min to evaluate the blood pool phase; (c) new planar acquisition, with the same geometry, at the tenth min for 2 min for the focal study of radiopharmaceutical distribution, according to the EANM practice guidelines for bone scintigraphy [1]; (d) delayed whole-body scan and planar spot views at about 150 min; and finally (e) SPECT/CT imaging immediately following the 3-h planar acquisition.

As mentioned above, hybrid multimodality SPECT/CT imaging provides an exact anatomical correlation between pathological ^{99m}Tc-MDP (HDP) bone uptake and anatomical, structural bone changes [27, 28, 33]. Although CT imaging per se does not have 100% diagnostic accuracy in cases where bone turnover is predominant, its association with SPECT (that provides information on bone turnover and clearly demonstrates locally increased tracer absorption) provides morphological information and thus makes hybrid SPECT/CT imaging an increasingly used diagnostic procedure in patients with a variety of musculoskeletal conditions. For SPECT/CT imaging in patients with musculoskeletal conditions, the CT component must imply reconstruction of high-resolution images and an appropriate field of view.

As reported by different authors [35–37], sometimes skeletal lesions that had been classified as inflammatory or neoplastic changes on CT or MRI alone are reclassified as occult-fractures or micro-fractures on the basis of SPECT/CT imaging.

In some complex anatomical situations such as the ankle, foot, and knee or in the case of occult fractures or for the differential diagnosis between benign and malignant disease, SPECT/CT imaging allows accurate identification of the area of the skeleton responsible for pain.

Key Learning Points

- In case of suspicion or clear indication of alteration of bone turnover, or if conventional radiology or magnetic resonance imaging are impractical (due to the presence of contraindications), the SPECT/CT hybrid bone scan (with non-diagnostic low-dose multi-slice CT) constitutes a milestone for the diagnosis of many skeletal conditions, as a very sensitive method, also improving the lack of specificity of bone scan.
- Three-phase bone scintigraphy integrated with SPECT/CT hybrid imaging is a first-line test in the evaluation of many bone or joint disease, due its low cost, simple use, and because it provides information on bone turnover.
- Because of markedly improved specificity over planar imaging alone, hybrid SPECT/CT imaging is often crucial for the diagnosis of many skeletal conditions, changing classification of skeletal lesions assessed as inflammatory or neoplastic on CT or MRI into benign conditions such as occult fractures or micro-fractures.

4.3 General Background on Infection Imaging for Miscellaneous Bone/Joint Conditions

In case of infection (suspected or already established), nuclear medicine imaging continues to play a very important role in the diagnosis, localization and extent of infection, and evaluation of treatment response. It remains therefore the first-line test when other imaging procedures yield equivocal or inconclusive/non-diagnostic information.

Skeletal infection is a rather common clinical condition, and early and accurate diagnosis is vital to the most appropriate treatment strategy; therefore, clinical and laboratory tests (often nonspecific for bone infection) and a series of imaging methods are employed. Plain X-ray and CT have low sensitivity (50–75% and 43%, respectively) and relatively low specificity (75–83% and 75%, respectively) [27, 28] for the diagnosis of osteomyelitis.

Early assessment of functional impairment due to the infectious process is crucial for the most appropriate treatment strategy of skeletal infection. With regard to single-photon emission imaging, scintigraphy with radiolabeled autologous white blood cells (either ^{111}In-oxine-WBS or, more recently, ^{99m}Tc-HMPAO-WBC), including both planar and hybrid SPECT/CT imaging, is currently the preferred imaging procedure, representing the gold standard method to diagnose, localize, define the extent of infection, as well as to evaluate response to treatment.

One of the main features of an infectious process is increased vascular permeability (which leads to loss of fluid and small molecules at the affected site) associated with transudation or diapedesis of leukocytes with subsequent focal accumulation of these cells. The process of leukocyte migration to sites of infection must be considered the most important factor for targeting/imaging of infection foci. Autologous leukocytes, obtained by blood sampling and cell separation, are most frequently labeled with ^{99m}Tc-HMPAO using a ^{99m}Tc activity ranging between 740 and 1000 MBq [32, 37–40]. Such an in vitro procedure maintains most of the chemotactic properties of the activated leukocytes, thus constituting the basis of the most widely used method for investigating infections with radionuclide imaging.

The ^{99m}Tc-HMPAO-WBC images are acquired by using preferably a double-head gamma-camera equipped with high-resolution collimators, in the anterior and posterior (sometimes lateral or oblique) views of the area of investigation after ^{99m}Tc-HMPAO-WBC reinfusion at different time points: 2–5 min to evaluate in vivo biodistribution, 50–60 min for early images, 180–240 min for late images, and 22–24 h for the final, delayed images. Timing of acquisition will depend on the clinical requirements (to be evaluated in the individual patient), but will always be correct for radioactive decay. SPECT/CT imaging can be acquired between early and late imaging, and/or after planar imaging after the final 22–24 h imaging [41, 42].

While SPECT imaging provides functional information and localization of all the foci of leukocyte accumulation, CT images provide exact anatomical delineation of the infection sites visualized by SPECT imaging. Thus, multimodality imaging with SPECT/CT identifies the morphological abnormalities that correspond to the areas of increased activity on the radionuclide images [38].

The main indications for the imaging of infection with autologous radiolabeled leukocytes in patients with various bone joint conditions, as derived from the most recent procedural guidelines on the matter, can be summarized as follows: diagnosis, location, extent of infection, and evaluation of the response to treatment [42].

Key Learning Points

- Early assessment of functional impairment due to skeletal infection (a rather common clinical problem) is crucial for choosing the most appropriate treatment strategy.
- By identifying the morphological changes that correspond to the areas of greatest activity on the radionuclide images, hybrid SPECT/CT multimodality imaging with ^{99m}Tc-HMPAO-WBC (or less commonly ^{111}In-oxine-WBC) is the preferred imaging procedure based on single-photon emission, currently representing the gold standard method for diagnosing, locating, defining the extent of infection, and evaluating the response to treatment in case of suspected infection or in case of infection clearly established.

4.4 Conclusions

By combining anatomical and functional imaging, hybrid SPECT/CT imaging during ^{99m}Tc-MDP/HDP bone scintigraphy or during ^{99m}Tc-HMPAO-WBC/^{111}In-oxine-WBC scintigraphy improves anatomical localization and provides more accurate identification of bone abnormalities compared to the diagnostic yield of each imaging test considered separately.

Findings of the bone scan with hybrid SPECT/CT imaging with ^{99m}Tc-MDP/HDP imaging are very sensitive in identifying sport injuries or inflammatory conditions or benign/malignant tumors (dento-maxillofacial region, knees, feet, ankles, occult fractures, or microfractures).

Hybrid SPECT/CT imaging with radiolabeled autologous leukocytes enable to identify the morphological changes that correspond to the areas of greatest activity on the radionuclide images. It constitutes therefore for single-photon emission imaging, the preferred diagnostic procedure not only to establish the diagnosis of infection per se, but also to locate the infection site, define its extent, and evaluate the response to treatment in case of suspected infection or in case of infection clearly established.

Acknowledgments The authors express their gratitude to Drs. Alessandro Carbonara and Dario Di Luzio (Department of Radiology of the "Pio XI" Private Hospital, Rome, Italy) for their precious contribution.

Clinical Cases

Case 4.1

Background

A 42-year-old woman submitted to dental graft. The CT scan performed before the dental graft showed complete normalization of bone thickness on the mandibular bone (in the right hemimandible, edentula at site 45, or lower right second premolar). An osteolucency area is present in the lower portion of the root tip of 45, with extension of the tooth beyond the entrance of the mandibular canal.

A three-phase bone scan with ^{99m}Tc-MDP (integrated with SPECT/CT imaging) was performed to exclude the productive inflammatory nature of the aforementioned area, and it showed no asymmetry of vascularization and no abnormal tracer accumulation in the blood pool phase in area 45 (not shown in the figure); no significant tracer uptake was detected at 3 h in the planar view nor in the SPECT/CT images (coronal SPET, CT, and fused SPECT/CT sections in the upper panel and sagittal sections in the lower panel) (Fig. 4.1).

Conclusion/Teaching Point

The radionuclide imaging procedure has solved the diagnostic problem about the possible presence of a productive inflammatory process at the site of radiolucency.

Three-phase bone scintigraphy, integrated with SPECT/CT imaging, excluded the presence of a productive inflammatory disease (based on the absence of abnormalities in the blood pool image and in the osteoblastic phase).

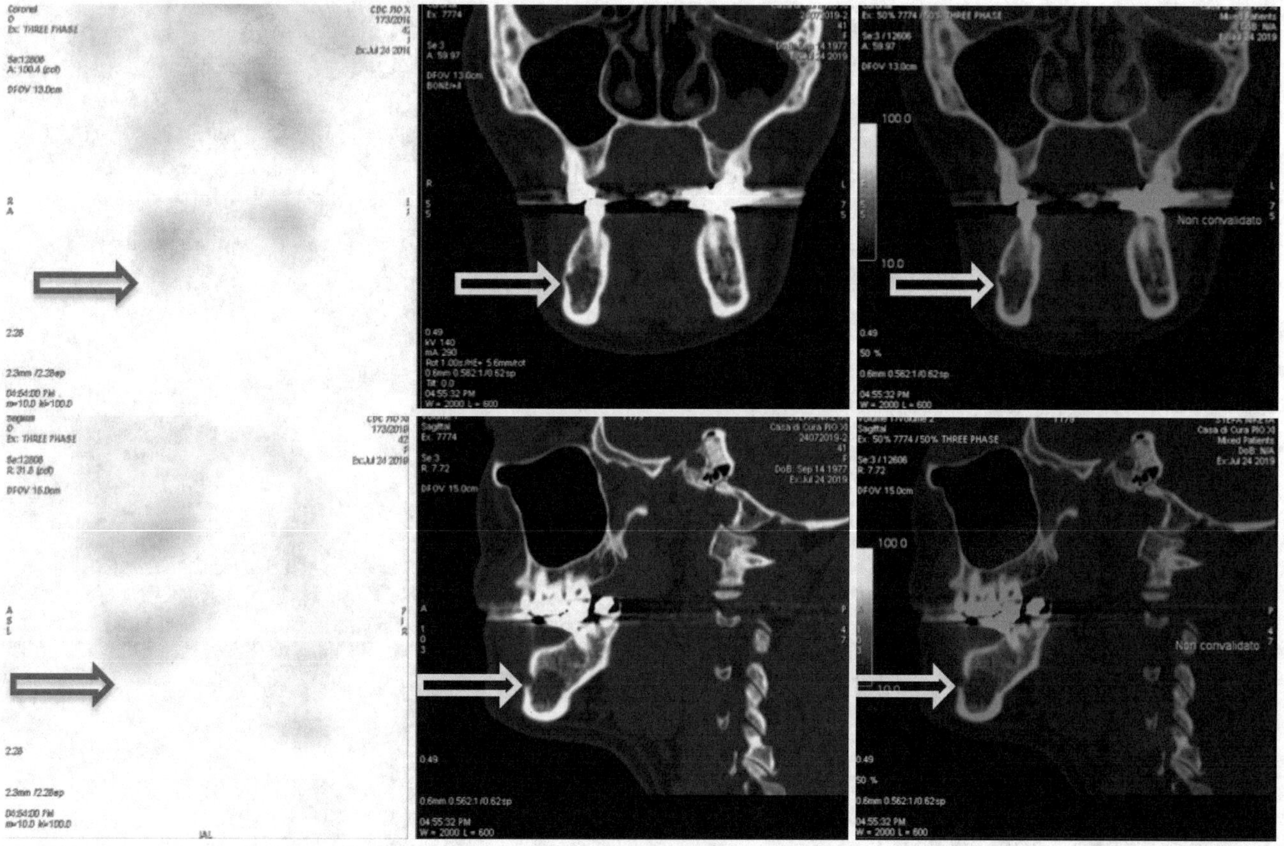

Fig. 4.1 See text

Case 4.2

Background

A 27-year-old woman who had suffered 2 years earlier of right subcondylar mandibular fracture treated with segment removal. Surgery was followed by fistulization. Microbiology of the fistula discharge grew antibiotic-resistant *Staphylococcus aureus*, and the patient received high-dose antibiotics for 7 months; the wisdom teeth were also removed. The antibiogram, performed in the fistula, showed staph resistant, and therefore, the patient has executed an antibiotic therapy for 7 months. The wisdom teeth have been removed.

The patient was referred for ^{99m}Tc-HMPAO-WBC scintigraphy (with SPECT/CT imaging) because of suspected osteomyelitis of the mandibular angle; planar spot images were recorded at 1 h, 3 h, and 22 h post-administration of the radiolabeled leukocytes, with additional SPECT/CT acquisition immediately after acquiring the delayed planar image.

The fused SPECT/CT images (two adjacent coronal section in the upper panel and two adjacent sagittal sections in the lower panel) demonstrate accumulation of the radiolabeled leukocytes in the right sub-condylar mandible, thus confirming osteomyelitis in this area (Fig. 4.2).

Conclusion/Teaching Point

The radionuclide imaging procedure solved the clinical problem about the presence or not of osteomyelitis and about its size/extent, confirming that there is indeed osteomyelitis localized in the right sub-condylar area, at the mandible angle.

Case 4.3

Background

A 30-year-old woman, a professional volleyball player, complained of left knee pain; clinical suspicion of sport-related stress fracture of the left knee patella was raised, and the patient was referred for three-phase bone scintigraphy with ^{99m}Tc-MDP, integrated with SPECT/CT imaging. After acquisition of the dynamic phase for 120 s, a static spot

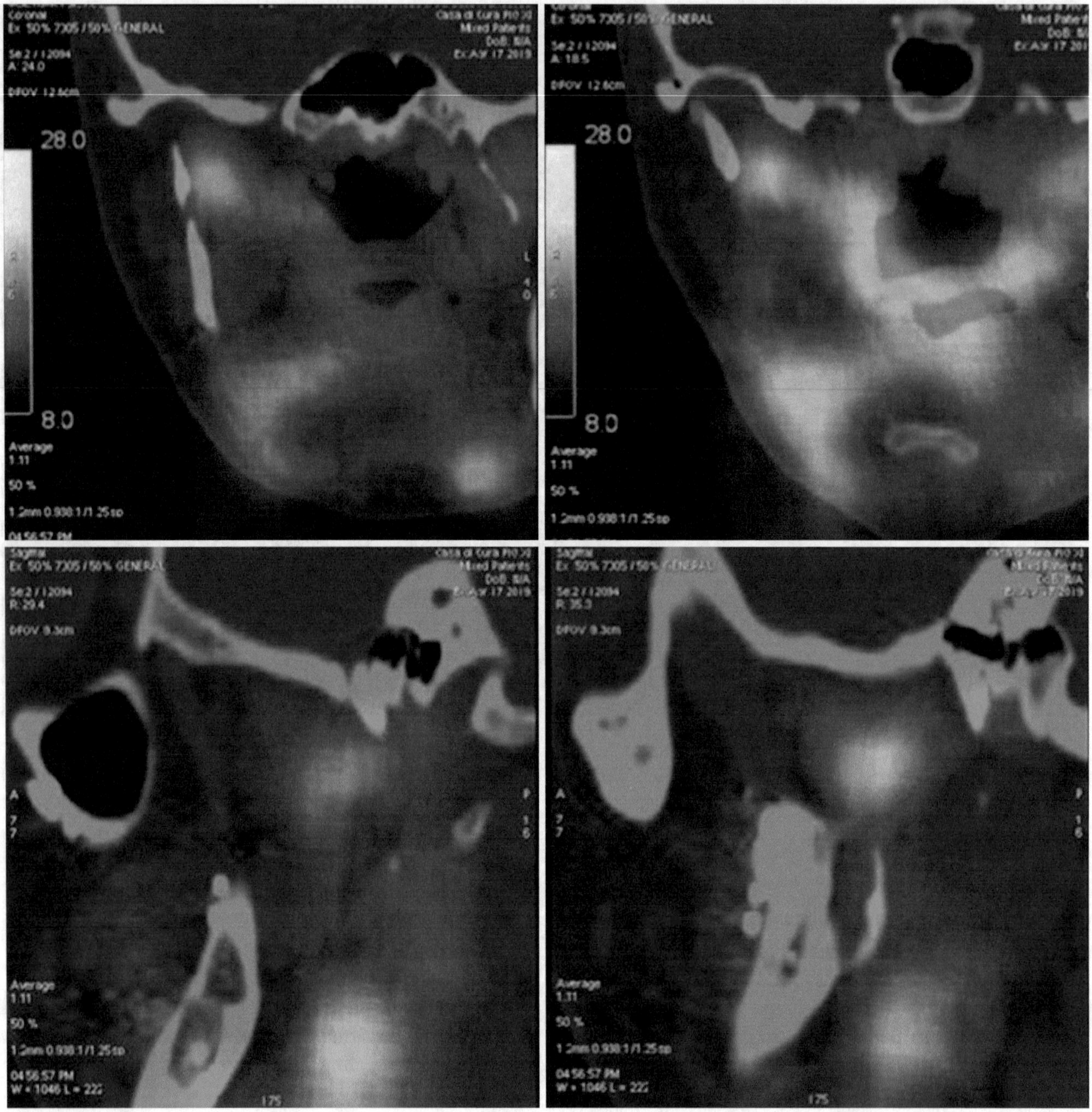

Fig. 4.2 See text

acquisition was recorded at 10 min, then again at 3 h after tracer injection (anterior views in the center panel). SPECT/CT imaging was acquired after recording the planar 3-h image.

The activity/time curve over the lower-medial portion of the left patella (red line in the upper panel) showed increased blood perfusion compared to the upper-external portion of the same patella (blue curve). Static imaging in the blood pool phase at 10 min showed increased radioactivity accumulation at the same site, which on delayed planar imaging (osteoblastic phase) exhibited frankly increased tracer uptake at the left knee patella (anterior views in center panel), without a clear dividing line between the upper portion and the lower portion of the patella and with distribution of the increased tracer uptake predominantly to the medial portion of the patella.

The fused volume rendering SPECT/CT images (lower panel, together with 3D volume rendering of the CT component) demonstrated that the focus of markedly increased ^{99m}Tc-MDP uptake was localized in the medial portion of the left patella; this finding, associated with the CT appearance of the patella, is consistent with chronic inflammation in a subject with "bipartite patella," a con-

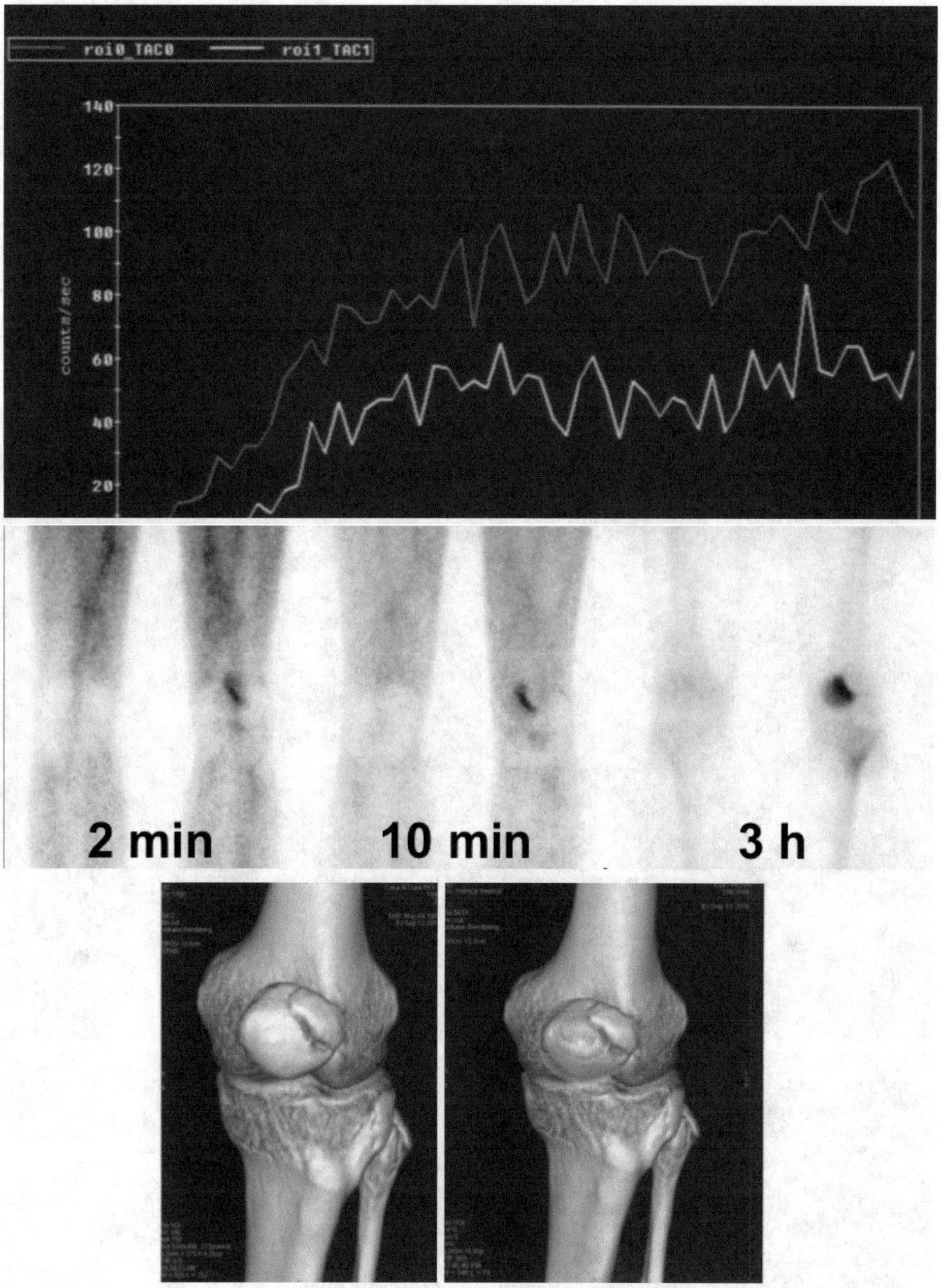

Fig. 4.3 See text

dition due to repeated trauma—as it typically occurs in sport-related bone injuries (Fig. 4.3).

Conclusion/Teaching Point

The radionuclide imaging procedure solved the clinical problem in this patient, by clearly defining within a small bone (the left knee patella) the sites of active bone remodeling associated with this sport-related bone injury. Post-acquisition processing with three-dimensional reconstruction and fused SPECT/CT volume rendering was especially useful in this case, by demonstrating the presence of "bipartite patella" rather than of a fracture stress.

Case 4.4

Background

A 27-year-old woman, a professional soccer player, complained since about 5 months of pain in the middle third of left fibula.

MR imaging (T1- and T2-weighted sequences with fat suppression) visualized focal hyperintense areas in the spongious bone at the middle third of left fibula, extending for about 7.5 cm; this finding is consistent with edema of the spongious bone. Homogeneous hyperintensity close to the bone marrow was also noted, possibly related to bone marrow involvement. Furthermore, persistent fluid level in the peroneal muscles was detected. The patient was referred for a three-phase bone scintigraphy with 99mTc-MDP (integrated with SPECT/CT imaging), in order to exclude the presence of bone marrow inflammation. After acquisition of the dynamic phase for 120 s, a static spot acquisition was recorded at 10 min, then again at 3 h after tracer injection (not shown). SPECT/CT imaging was acquired after recording the planar 3-h image.

No relevant abnormalities were detected in the early dynamic phase and in the blood-pool phase. The SPECT/CT images acquired about 3 h after injection of ^{99m}Tc-MDP focal revealed a restricted, focal area of increased ^{99m}Tc-MDP uptake involving the cortex of the middle-distal third of the left fibula (upper panel). Zooming of this area of interest (lower panel) helped to better identify a small fracture in the cortical bone, at the middle-distal third of the left fibula (Fig. 4.4).

Conclusion/Teaching Point

In this case, the added value of ^{99m}Tc-MDP three-phase bone scintigraphy integrated with SPECT/CT acquisition was the

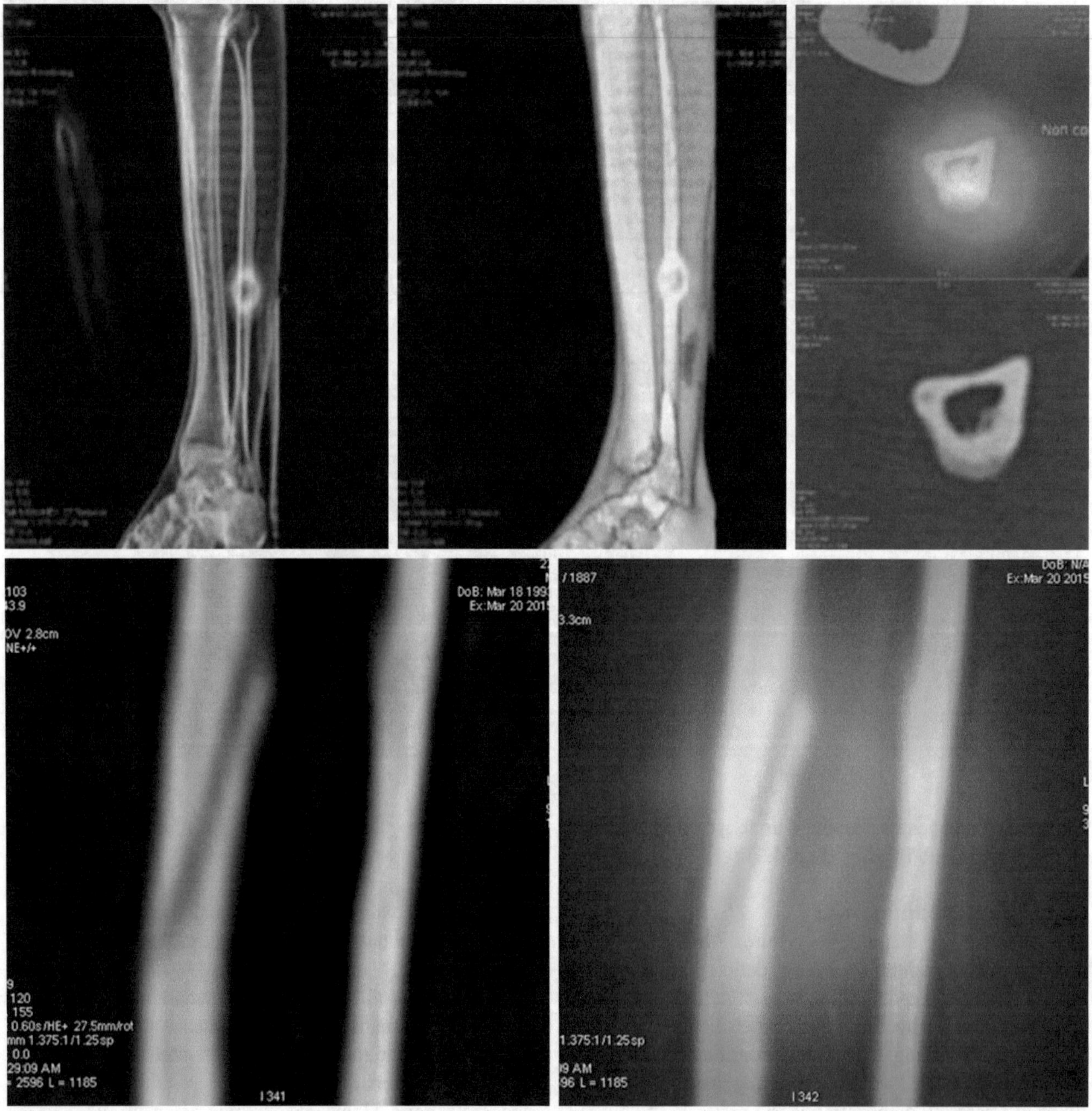

Fig. 4.4 See text

targeted use of CT data in the area characterized by increased tracer uptake. In particular, hybrid SPECT/CT imaging excluded the presence of bone marrow inflammation.

Case 4.5

Background

About 2 months before being referred for the radionuclide imaging procedure, this 27-year-old man, a professional athlete, had been submitted to surgery because of proximal "hamstring syndrome" (also known as the ischio-crural syndrome, a condition often occurring in high-level athletes). Surgery consisted of tendon release, that is, cutting the ischio-crural muscle and reinserting its tendon into the femoral bone. The patient was referred for a ^{99m}Tc-HMPAO-WBC scintigraphy because of infection with fluid collection near the left iliac bone; the serum markers of infection/inflammation were negative. Purpose of the scan was to ascertain the presence of osteomyelitis and, if present, its extension. Planar spot images were recorded at 1 h, 3 h, and 22 h after administration of the radiolabeled leukocytes (not shown), with additional SPECT/CT acquisition immediately after acquiring the delayed planar image.

The fused SPECT/CT images (sagittal sections in the upper panel and coronal sections in the lower panel) display abnormally increased accumulation of the radiolabeled leukocytes in the left femur, thus confirming the clinical suspicion of osteomyelitis due to surgical insertion of the ischio-crural muscle (Fig. 4.5).

Conclusion/Teaching Point

^{99m}Tc-HMPAO-WBC scintigraphy played a key role in this patient, by confirming the presence of infection due to surgical insertion of the ischio-crural muscle (even with normal values of the serum markers of infection/inflammation and in defining the exact extension of the infectious focus).

Case 4.6

Background

This 63-year-old woman complained of long-lasting back pain. MR imaging (T1- and T2-weighted sequences with fat suppression) visualized spondylosis in the mid-thoracic spine with Modic-1 changes affecting the anterior edges of T8–T9, consistent with reflex sympathetic dystrophy. Modic changes adjacent to a degenerated intervertebral disc have three generally interchangeable types, thus suggesting that

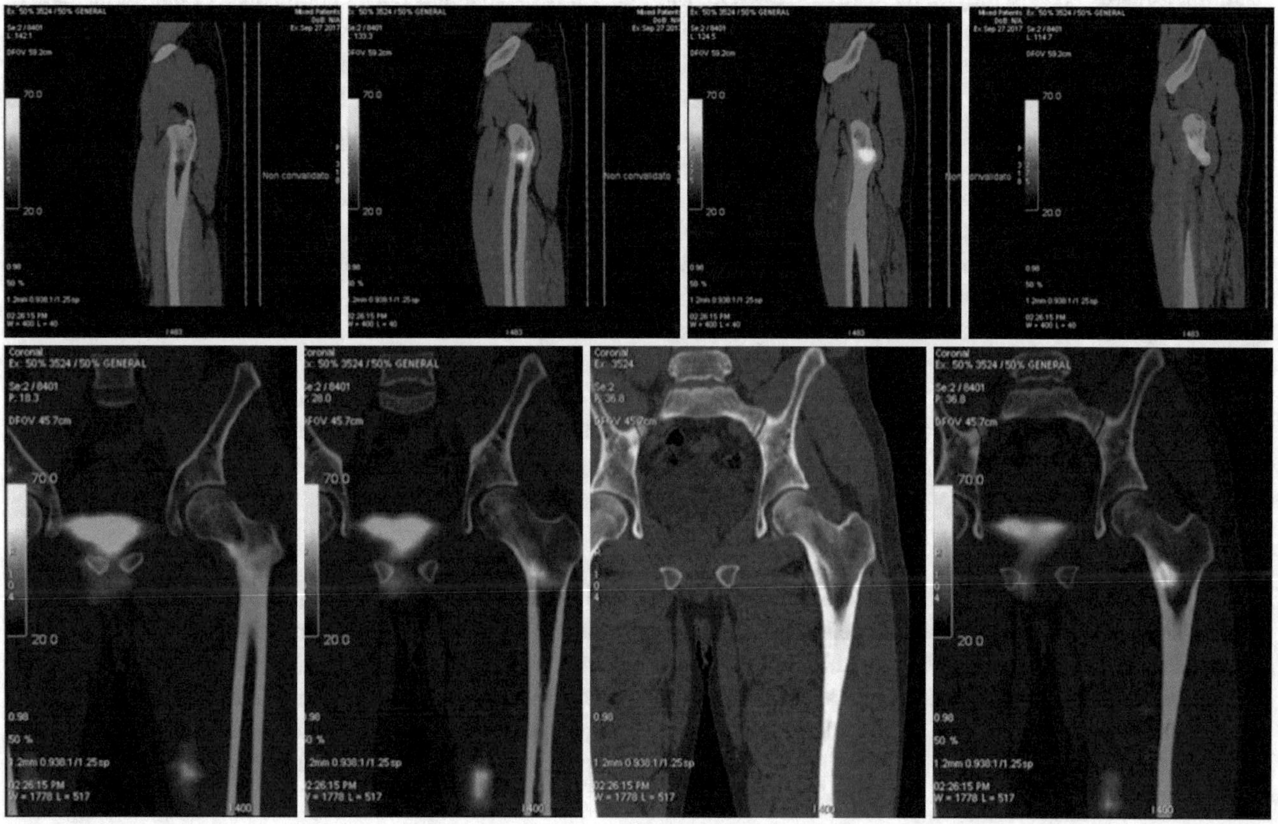

Fig. 4.5 See text

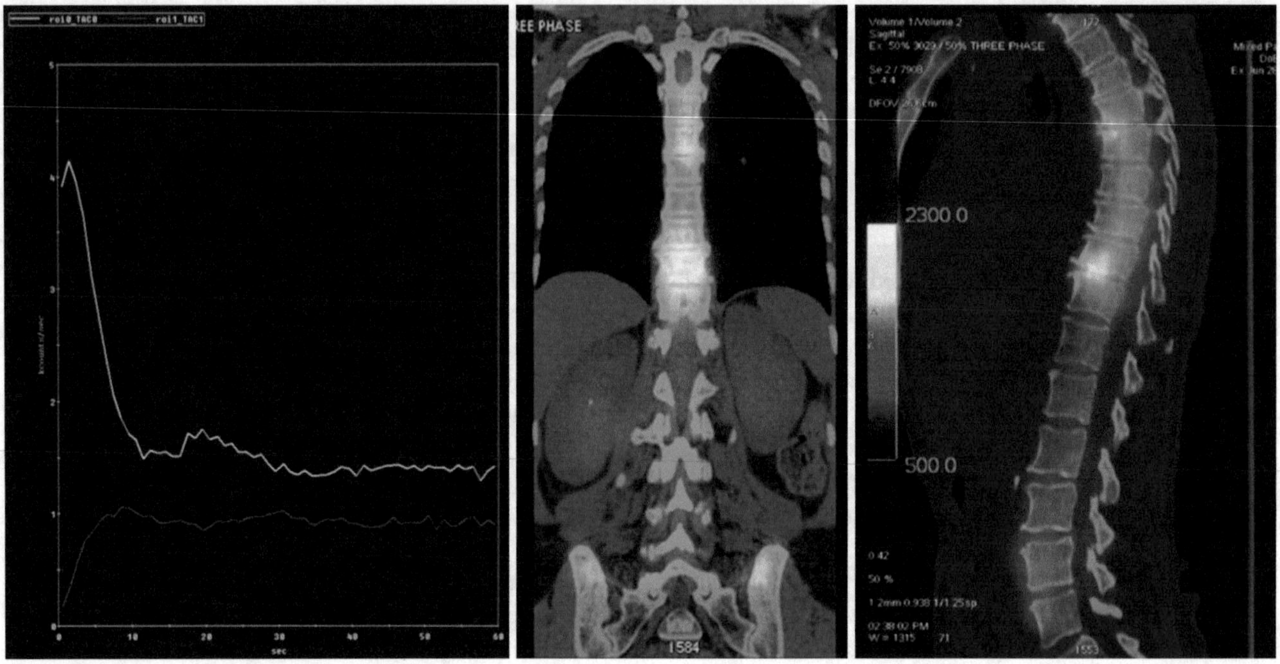

Fig. 4.6 See text

the different Modic change types actually represent different stages of the same pathological process, which is characterized by inflammation, increased bone turnover, and fibrosis.

A three-phase bone scintigraphy with ^{99m}Tc-MDP was performed to better characterize the patient, recording a dynamic phase for 120 s (upper panel), a static spot acquisition at 10 min, then again at 3 h after tracer injection (not shown). SPECT/CT imaging was acquired after recording the planar 3-h image.

The activity/time curve corresponding to the region of interest in the thoracic spine (red curve in upper left panel) showed frankly increased blood perfusion when compared to the lumbar spine (white curve). The planar 3-h spot image (not shown), and especially the SPECT/CT images (fused coronal section in the center panel and fused sagittal section in the right panel) demonstrated markedly increased tracer uptake in the thoracic spine, both above the T6–T7 region and below such level (T10–T11, with even greater ^{99m}Tc-MDP uptake) (Fig. 4.6).

Conclusion/Teaching Point

Hybrid SPECT/CT imaging during bone scintigraphy correctly assessed Modic changes and degenerative disc disease at T6–T7 and mostly at T10–T11 in this patient with back pain, thus allowing better characterization of the patient with reference to the clinical suspicion raised by the neurosurgeon.

Case 4.7

Background

A 19-year-old tennis player complained of pain at the base of the left foot for the past 4 months, following a sprained ankle on the same side. The patient was referred for a three-phase bone scintigraphy with ^{99m}Tc-MDP, integrated with SPECT/CT imaging, to ascertain the presence of pseudoarthrosis of the left talar bone with pain in the trigonum bone. After acquisition of the dynamic phase for 120 s, a static spot acquisition was recorded at 10 min, then again at 3 h after tracer injection (not shown). SPECT/CT imaging was acquired after recording the planar 3-h image.

The fused SPECT/CT images show markedly increased ^{99m}Tc-MDP uptake (indicating enhanced osteoblastic activity) in the left talus and in the ipsilateral ankle joint (left panel). Increased tracer uptake is also observed in the left talus-scaphoid-cuboid bones (center panel), as well as in the os trigonum (Fig. 4.7).

Conclusion/Teaching Point

In this patient, SPECT/CT imaging during bone scintigraphy with ^{99m}Tc-MDP enabled to correctly ascertain the origin of pain as the result of a sinus tarsi syndrome (pain in the lateral side of the hind foot) associated with os trigonum syndrome, pseudoarthrosis in the ankle joint, in the joint between talus, scaphoid and cuboid, and in the metatarsal joints.

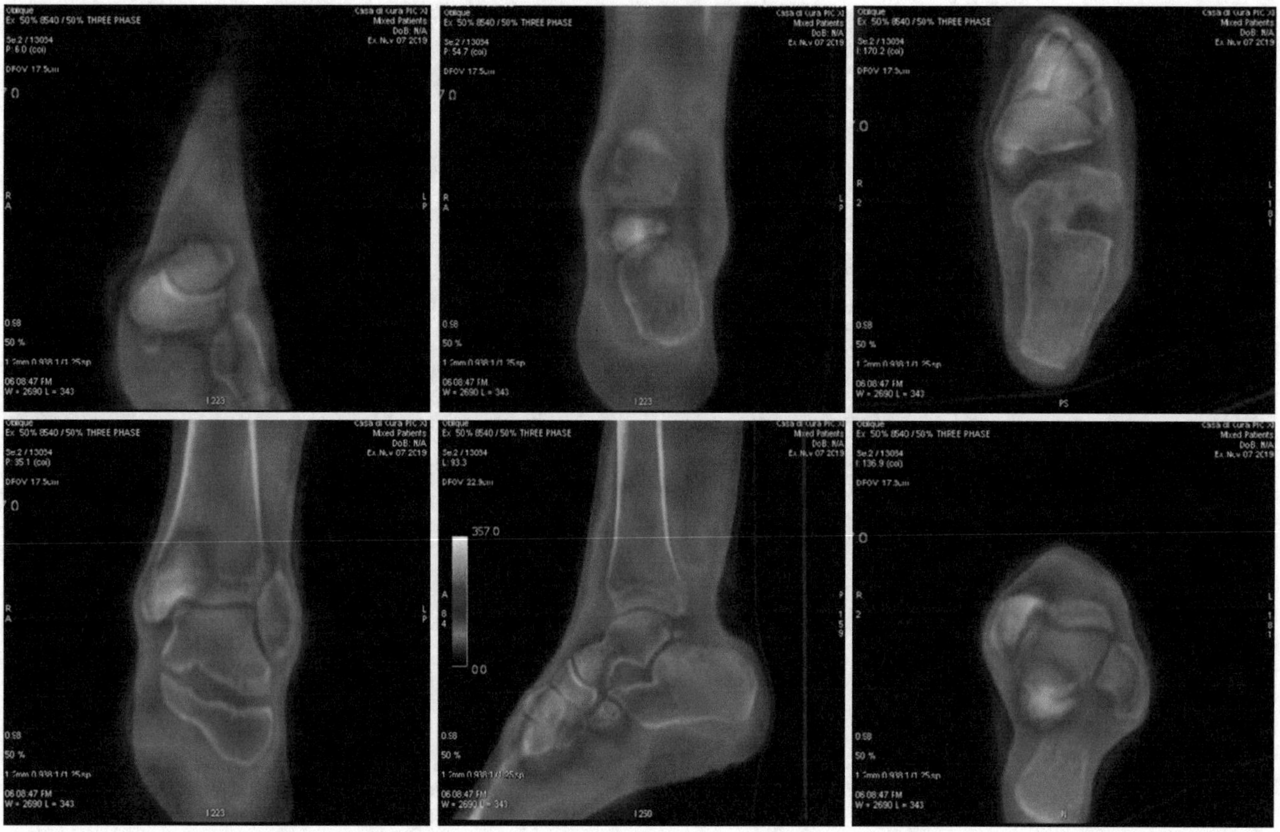

Fig. 4.7 See text

Case 4.8

Background

Because of a ski accident, a 40-year-old woman suffered a recent compound tibial fracture (external posterior plate of the left knee). The CT and MRI scans performed to assess healing of the tibial fracture visualized the incidental finding of a coarse, hypodense, oval-shaped mass located adjacent to the tibial head; the mass (12 mm in longitudinal diameter) had a hypodense edge on the medullary side, spiculated margins and discontinuity of the cortical bone. The patient was referred for three-phase bone scintigraphy with ^{99m}Tc-MDP, integrated with SPECT/CT imaging, in order to better characterize such incidentally detected lesion. After acquisition of the dynamic phase for 120 s, a static spot acquisition was recorded at 10 min, then again at 3 h after tracer injection (not shown). SPECT/CT imaging was acquired after recording the planar 3-h image.

The activity/time curves obtained over the knees from the dynamic acquisition did not detect significant differences between the two sides, and also the blood pool image acquired 10 min after injection of ^{99m}Tc-MDP was unremarkable (not shown). Markedly increased tracer uptake at the left knee was instead noted on the planar and SPECT/CT images acquired at 3 h post injection. In particular, the fused SPECT/CT images demonstrated that the focus of increased tracer uptake (reflecting increased osteoblastic activity) was localized at the site of the recent tibial fracture, whereas there was no ^{99m}Tc-MDP in the oval-shaped mass previously detected on CT and MRI, which was identified as a non-ossifying fibroma during subsequent surgery (CT components in upper row, corresponding fused SPEC/CT images in lower row) (Fig. 4.8).

Conclusion/Teaching Point

It was in particular hybrid SPECT/CT imaging acquired during bone scintigraphy that clarified the diagnostic doubt whether the mass incidentally found on radiologic imaging was a malignant tumor or a benign lesion. This diagnostic conclusion was consistent with the absence of abnormalities both in blood perfusion (dynamic phase of the scan) and in the blood pool phase of the scan, as well as with absent tracer uptake also in the late, osteoblastic phase of bone scintigraphy. Malignancy of the left tibial lesion was thus excluded.

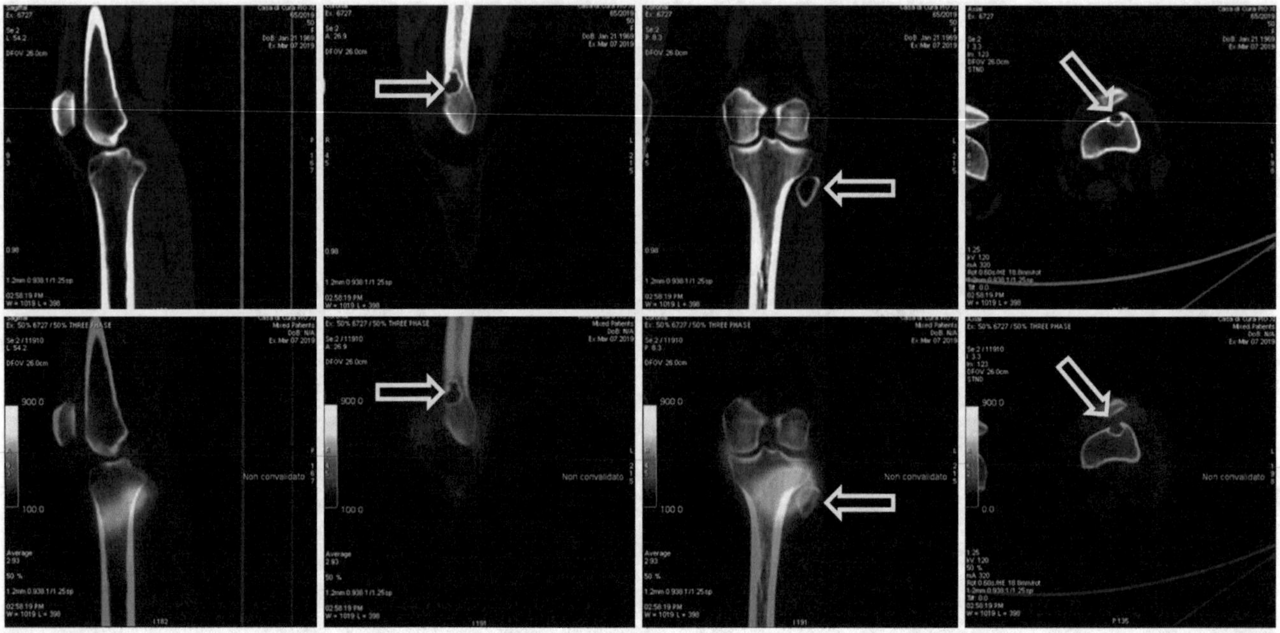

Fig. 4.8 See text

References

1. Van den Wyngaert T, Strobel K, Kampen WU, et al. EANM Bone & Joint Committee and the Oncology Committee. The EANM practice guidelines for bone scintigraphy. Eur J Nucl Med Mol Imaging. 2016;43:1723–38.
2. Glaudemans AWJM, Bosch P, Slart RHJA, et al. Diagnosing fracture-related infections: can we optimize our nuclear imaging techniques? Eur J Nucl Med Mol Imaging. 2019;46:1583–7.
3. Govaert GAM, Bosch P, IJpma FFA, et al. High diagnostic accuracy of white blood cell scintigraphy for fracture related infections: results of a large retrospective single-center study. Injury. 2018;49:1085–90.
4. Govaert G, Hobbelink M, Reininga Ihf, et al. The accuracy of diagnostic imaging techniques in patients with a suspected fracture-related infection (IFI) trial: study protocol for a prospective multicenter cohort study. BMJ Open. 2019;9(9):e027772.
5. Suh MS, Lee WW, Kim YK. Maximum standardized uptake value of ^{99m}Tc hydroxymethylene diphosphonate SPECT/CT for the evaluation of temporomandibular joint disorder. Radiology. 2016;280:890–6.
6. Wassef HR, Colletti PM. Nuclear medicine imaging in the dentomaxillofacial region. Dent Clin N Am. 2018;62:491–509.
7. Ferri J, Raoul G, Potier J, Nicot R. Temporomandibular joint (TMJ): condyle hyperplasia and condylectomy. Rev Stomatol Chir Maxillofac Chir Orale. 2016;117:259–65.
8. Oohashi Y, Koshino T. Bone scintigraphy in patients with bipartite patella. Knee Surg Sports Traumatol Arthrosc. 2007;15:1395–9.
9. Lu S-J, Ul Hassan F, Vijayanathan S, Gnanasegaran G. Radionuclide bone SPECT/CT in the evaluation of knee pain: comparing two-phase bone scintigraphy, SPECT and SPECT/CT. Br J Radiol. 2018;91(1090):20180168. https://doi.org/10.1259/bjr.20180168.
10. Mohan HK, Clarke SE, Centenara M, et al. Value of lateral blood pool imaging in patients with suspected stress fractures of the tibia. Clin Nucl Med. 2011;36:173–7.
11. Huellner MW, Strobel K. Clinical applications of SPECT/CT in imaging the extremities. Eur J Nucl Med Mol Imaging.2014; 41(Suppl 1):S50–8.
12. Pelletier-Galarneau M, Martineau P, Gaudreault M, Pham X. Review of running injuries of the foot and ankle: clinical presentation and SPECT-CT imaging patterns. Am J Nucl Med Mol Imaging. 2015;5:305–16.
13. Matcuk GR Jr, Mahanty SR, Skalski MR, et al. Stress fractures: pathophysiology, clinical presentation, imaging features, and treatment options. Emerg Radiol. 2016;23:365–75.
14. Martin HD, Khoury A, Schröder R, Palmer IJ. Ischiofemoral impingement and hamstring syndrome as causes of posterior hip pain: where do we go next? Clin Sports Med. 2016;35: 469–86.
15. Dudli S, Fields AJ, Samartzis D, et al. Pathobiology of Modic changes. Eur Spine J. 2016;25:3723–34.
16. Russo VM, Dhawan RT, Dharmarajah N, et al. Hybrid bone single photon emission computed tomography imaging in evaluation of chronic low back pain: correlation with Modic changes and degenerative disc disease. World Neurosurg. 2017;104:816–23.
17. Gardellin A, Cha J, Cho A, Mijin Y. Correlation of SPECT/CT findings and MRI Modic changes in endplate degenerative diseases. J Nucl Med. 2017;58(Suppl 1):1219.
18. Crockett MT, Kelly BS, van Baarsel S, Kavanagh EC. Modic type 1 vertebral endplate changes: injury, inflammation, or infection? AJR Am J Roentgenol. 2017;209:167–70.
19. Mandegaran R, Dhillon S, Jen H. Beyond the bone and joints: a review of ligamentous injuries of the foot and ankle on ^{99m}Tc-MDP-SPECT/CT. Br J Radiol. 2019;92(1104):20190506. https://doi.org/10.1259/bjr.20190506.
20. Huang J1, Servaes S, Zhuang H. Os trigonum syndrome on bone SPECT/CT. Clin Nucl Med. 2014;39:752–4.
21. Nault ML, Kocher MS, Micheli LJ. Os trigonum syndrome. J Am Acad Orthop Surg. 2014;22:545–53.
22. Usmani S, Abu Al Huda F, Al Kandari F. Three-phase ^{99m}Tc MDP bone scintigraphy and SPECT-CT in sinus tarsi syndrome. Clin Nucl Med. 2016;41:e208–10.

23. Biersack HJ, Wingenfeld C, Hinterthaner B, et al. SPECT-CT of the foot. Nuklearmedizin. 2012;51:26–31.
24. Roster B, Michelier P, Giza E. Peroneal tendon disorders. Clin Sports Med. 2015;34:625–41.
25. Sinha P, Kim A, Umans H, Freeman LM. Scintigraphic findings in peroneal tendonitis: a case report. Clin Nucl Med. 2000;25:17–9.
26. Stockton KG, Brodsky JW. Peroneus longus tears associated with pathology of the os peroneum. Foot Ankle Int. 2014;35:346–52.
27. Davda K, Malhotra K, O'Donnell P, et al. Peroneal tendon disorders. EFORT Open Rev. 2017;2:281–92.
28. Choi E, Wert M, Guerrieri C, Tucci J. A pathologic fracture of an intracortical chondroma masking as an osteoid osteoma. Orthopedics. 2010;33:845.
29. Herget GW, Mauer D, Krauß T, et al. Non-ossifying fibroma: natural history with an emphasis on a stage-related growth, fracture risk and the need for follow-up. BMC Musculoskelet Disord. 2016;17:147.
30. Simpfendorfer CS. Radiologic approach to musculoskeletal infections. Infect Dis Clin N Am. 2017;31:299–324.
31. Filippi L, Schillaci O. Usefulness of hybrid SPECT/CT in ^{99m}Tc-HMPAO-labeled leukocyte scintigraphy for bone and joint infections. J Nucl Med. 2006;47:1908–13.
32. Termaat MF, Raijmakers PG, Scholten HJ, et al. The accuracy of diagnostic imaging for the assessment of chronic osteomyelitis: a systematic review and meta-analysis. J Bone Joint Surg Am. 2005;87:2464–71.
33. Thang SP, Tong AK, Lam WW, Ng DC. SPECT/CT in musculoskeletal infections. Semin Musculoskelet Radiol. 2014;18:194–202.
34. Linke R, Kuwert T, Uder M, et al. Skeletal SPECT/CT of the peripheral extremities. AJR Am J Roentgenol. 2010;19:W329–35.
35. Allainmat L, Aubault M, Noël V, et al. Use of hybrid SPECT/CT for diagnosis of radiographic occult fractures of the wrist. Clin Nucl Med. 2013;38:e246–51.
36. Saha S, Burke C, Desai A, et al. SPECT-CT: applications in musculoskeletal radiology. Br J Radiol. 2013;86(1031):20120519. https://doi.org/10.1259/bjr.20120519.
37. Palestro CJ. Radionuclide imaging of musculoskeletal infection: a review. J Nucl Med. 2016;57:1406–12.
38. Connolly CM, Donohoe KJ. Nuclear medicine imaging of infection. Semin Roentgenol. 2017;52:114–9.
39. Glaudemans AW, de Vries EF, Vermeulen LE, et al. A large retrospective single-centre study to define the best image acquisition protocols and interpretation criteria for white blood cell scintigraphy with ^{99m}Tc-HMPAO-labelled leucocytes in musculoskeletal infections. Eur J Nucl Med Mol Imaging. 2013;40:1760–9.
40. Love C, Palestro CJ. Nuclear medicine imaging of bone infections. Clin Radiol. 2016;71:632–46.
41. Erba PA, Glaudemans AW, Veltman NC, et al. Image acquisition and interpretation criteria for ^{99m}Tc-HMPAO-labelled white blood cell scintigraphy: results of a multicentre study. Eur J Nucl Med Mol Imaging. 2014;41:615–23.
42. Signore A, Jamar F, Israel O, et al. Clinical indications, image acquisition and data interpretation for white blood cells and anti-granulocyte monoclonal antibody scintigraphy: an EANM procedural guideline. Eur J Nucl Med Mol Imaging. 2018;45:1816–31.

Nuclear Medicine Imaging of Joint Prosthesis Infections and Peripheral Bone Infections

5

Napoleone Prandini and Andrea Bedini

Contents

Learning Objectives

- To acquire basic knowledge on the management of early and late complications after joint arthroplasty
- To understand the pathophysiologic bases of infection in joint prostheses
- To become familiar with the diagnosis of periprosthetic joint infection with the most frequently used radionuclide imaging techniques
- To become familiar with the signs and the interpretation criteria of bone scintigraphy in unstable or infected painful prosthesis
- To acquire basic knowledge of the interpretation criteria of multi-phase ^{99m}Tc-HMPAO-leukocyte scintigraphy
- To understand how to use the different imaging modalities in the management of prosthetic infections and of peripheral bone infections

Replacement of failing or injured joints with artificial prosthetic components is commonly employed to reduce the pain and disability associated with many orthopedic conditions including arthritis, congenital deformities, trauma, and other diseases of bone and joint tissues. The most successful type of joint replacement procedure is the replacement of both sides of a diseased joint (total joint arthroplasty, TJA). Other types of joint replacement include hemi-arthroplasty and surface arthroplasty, where the surface of the joint is covered with a foreign material that provides a smooth articulating surface.

The joints most commonly replaced are hips and knees: the results are now excellent, with 10-year survival rates of 91.5% for hips and 96.5% for knees [1]. Although the materials used in prosthetic implants (stainless steel, cobalt-chrome, molybdenum alloy, titanium-aluminum-vanadium alloy, and ceramics) are considered biocompatible, they still represent a foreign body. These components usually articulate with plastic components (often composed of ultra-high molecular polyethylene), which may have a metal backing.

Over the last few decades, the number of primary TJA procedures has increased considerably, and it is estimated that, by 2030, two million of total hip or total knee arthroplasties will be performed in the USA every year [2].

With the increment of joint prosthetic replacements, the number of postoperative complications has also increased. Joint replacement failure may be due to the failure of structural materials, such as fatigue fracture of a metal prosthetic

N. Prandini (✉)
Nuclear Medicine Department, Azienda Ospedaliero-Universitaria di Modena, Modena, Italy

A. Bedini
Infectious Diseases Unit, Department of Medical and Surgical Sciences for Children and Adults, University Hospital "Policlinico di Modena", Modena, Italy

E. Lazzeri et al. (eds.), *Radionuclide Imaging of Infection and Inflammation*, https://doi.org/10.1007/978-3-030-62175-9_5

stem, or the rapid destruction of a polyethylene cup. But a more common cause of arthroplasty failure is aseptic loosening of the implant. This complication is usually associated with late implant failure, occurring several years after the implant has been in situ and functioning reasonably. Both mechanical and biological factors contribute to the pathogenesis of aseptic loosening.

The incidence of periprosthetic joint infection (PJI) is lower than aseptic loosening, but it is more serious and complex complication following arthroplasty [3]. The diagnosis of PJI can be challenging because its definition is not standardized. In general, the diagnosis rests on a combination of factors including history and physical examination, synovial fluid analysis, serum inflammatory markers, culture data, and intraoperative findings.

5.1 Infection of Joint Prostheses

Periprosthetic joint infection (PJI) occurs in 1–2% of primary and in 4% of revision arthroplasties [4–7]. The infection can originate by three pathways: (1) during the perioperative period, most commonly through intraoperative inoculation; (2) by the hematogenous route (which can occur at any time after implantation) by a microorganism that comes from any infection site (e.g., pneumonia, urinary tract infection); and iii) by direct contact with a nearby infection (e.g., infected soft tissue) [8].

PJIs are often classified as early onset (<3 months after surgery), delayed onset (3–12 months after surgery), and late onset (>12 months after surgery); nevertheless, these definitions are controversial and not always clear-cut, particularly for patients in whom the diagnosis is delayed [9].

For optimal management of the patient with the infection, the most useful classification is based on time of appearance of the infection's symptoms. This information provides a direct correlation with the maturation stage of the biofilm and is crucial for choosing the optimal treatment. Biofilm is a complex community of microorganisms embedded in an extracellular matrix that forms on the surfaces of prosthesis and that can resist to antibiotic treatments when it is well structured.

When the biofilm is removed early, within 4 weeks from the implant or within 3 weeks from the appearance of signs of infection, the immature biofilm can be surgically eradicated without removing prosthesis (DAIR approach: Debridement, Antibiotics, Implant Retention). Otherwise, the mature biofilm adheres so firmly to the prosthesis that it is necessary to remove the implant in order to achieve eradication of the infection.

In conclusion, PJIs are classified as:

Acute PJI

- <4 weeks after the surgery (early, perioperative origin)
- <3 weeks of symptoms (hematogenous origin)
- Immature biofilm, high-virulence microorganisms (i.e., *Staphylococcus aureus*, *Enterobacteriaceae* species)
- Signs of an acute infection (pain, erythema, edema, wound effusion)
- Treatment: debridement, retention of implant, long course of antibiotics

Chronic PJI

- ≥4 weeks after surgery (delayed/low grade)
- ≥3 weeks of symptoms (hematogenous origin)
- Mature biofilm, low-virulence microorganisms (i.e., coagulase-negative staphylococci, *Cutibacterium* spp.)
- Signs: chronic pain, loosening of the prosthesis, sinus tract (fistula).
- Treatment: removal of prosthesis (1- or 2-stage approach), antibiotics.

Acute infections typically present with an acute onset of joint pain, effusion, erythema, and warmth at the implant site, and fever; they are most commonly caused by virulent microorganisms, such as *Staphylococcus aureus* and gram-negative bacilli (e.g., *Escherichia coli*, *Klebsiella* spp., *Pseudomonas aeruginosa*). Surgical treatment consists in debridement and retention of the prosthesis (replacement of mobile parts is recommended).

Patients with chronic (low-grade) infection usually present with subtle signs and symptoms, such as implant loosening, persistent joint pain, and sinus tract (fistula). The infections are usually caused by less virulent microorganisms, such as coagulase-negative staphylococci, *Cutibacterium* spp. [10, 11]. In chronic infection, complete removal of prosthesis (in 1 or 2 stages) is recommended.

Early diagnosis is a favorable factor to maintain the prosthesis in place, therefore also joint function. A number of radiological, nuclear medicine and laboratory investigations, such as erythrocyte sedimentation rate and C-reactive protein, provide a guide as to whether arthroplasty loosening may be due to sepsis; however, in general, there is no single laboratory test which has proved sensitive or specific enough to distinguish reliably between aseptic and septic loosening [12]. The criteria proposed by European Bone and Joint Infection Society (EBJIS) greatly increase sensitivity in the diagnosis of PJI.

Diagnosis of PJI must be considered if at least one of the following four criteria is fulfilled:

- Clinical features: sinus tract or visible purulence.
- Histology in periprosthetic tissue: acute inflammation (defined as ≥2 granulocytes per high-power field).
- Microbiology (culture): synovial fluid or tissue samples or sonication fluid (≥50 CFU/mL). For highly virulent microorganisms, already one positive sample confirms infection. Under antibiotics and for anaerobes, <50 colony-forming unit (CFU)/mL can be significant.

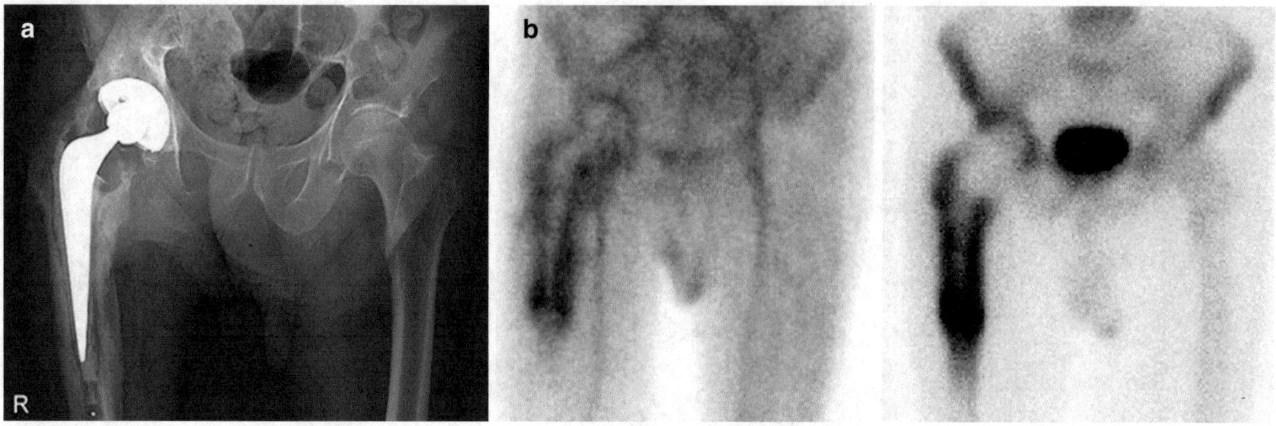

Fig. 5.1 X-ray and three-phase bone scintigraphy (vascular pool and late phase) in a patient with infection of the right hip prosthesis

- Leukocyte count in synovial fluid: >2000/μL leukocytes or >70% granulocytes (limitations: leukocyte cut-off levels can be equivocal within 6 weeks of surgery, in rheumatic joint disease, periprosthetic fracture or luxation. Leukocyte count should be determined within 24 h; clotted specimens are treated with 10 μL hyaluronidase).

The only clinical signs confirming infection are the presence of a sinus tract (fistula) or visible purulence around the prosthesis. Histological examination of biopsy aspirates and specimens of periprosthetic tissues can distinguish between septic and aseptic loosening; the histological findings are of value post-operatively when they can be used to confirm the preoperative diagnosis of septic or aseptic loosening. However, distinguishing between septic and aseptic loosening in a clinical context is crucial for the choice of treatment options.

Surgical treatment is the gold standard treatment for prosthetic joint infections [13]. Acute PJIs, in the setting of a well-fixed prosthesis, are routinely managed with debridement and prosthesis retention, as removal of the implant can result in bone loss, non-negligible blood loss, and increased pain. Otherwise, chronic PJIs (those presenting at >4 weeks following index surgery or an inciting hematogenous event) demand implant removal and replacement via a one- or two-stage approach [13, 14]. One-stage prosthetic replacement is offered to relatively healthy patients with adequate bone stock and soft tissues, and easily treatable infecting pathogens [15]. Two-stage prosthetic replacement involves removal of the prosthesis and all its components, debridement of devitalized soft tissue, and profuse irrigation, but provides for a "prosthesis holiday" with a temporary antibiotic delivery device inserted instead of another prosthesis. Reimplantation of the new prosthesis is performed when infection is supposed to have been eradicated based upon clinical judgment.

Radiographic imaging can be of value, but usually does not provide a definitive diagnosis of PJI. In general, plain radiographs should be performed in the setting of suspected PJI; these are useful to screen for prosthetic loosening and fracture, but lack sensitivity and specificity for the diagnosis of PJI [16] (Fig. 5.1a).

Key Learning Points

- The increase in early bone perfusion and late accumulation all around the acetabulum and the prosthetic stem is the most characteristic sign of PJI.
- This finding must be confirmed by the more specific leukocyte scintigraphy.

On the other hand, the interpretation of cross-sectional imaging modalities (CT and MRI) can be hampered by the artifacts due to the presence of prosthetic devices.

5.2 Nuclear Medicine Imaging for Periprosthetic Joint Infection

5.2.1 Three-Phase Bone Scintigraphy for Periprosthetic Joint Infection

Bone scintigraphy with ^{99m}Tc-labeled diphosphonates is highly sensitive for detecting bone remodeling around prosthetic joints. Increased periprosthetic activity on bone scintigraphy reflects increased bone mineral turnover, which can be caused by any number of conditions besides infection. In infection of hip prostheses, the bone scan shows an increase in early perfusion and a delayed metabolic tracer accumulation all around the prosthesis, marking out its contour (Fig. 5.1b). Three-phase bone scintigraphy has a sensitivity of about 80% in hip prosthesis infection [17]. In the case of simple instability (without infection), there is no

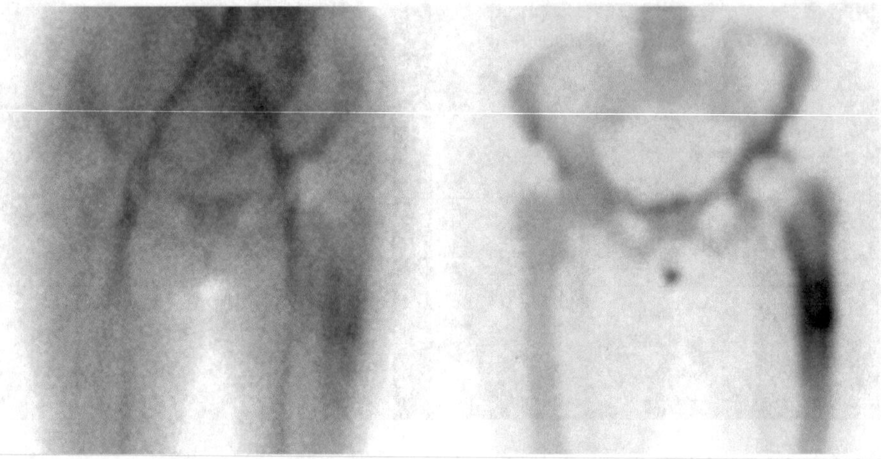

Fig. 5.2 Three-phase bone scintigraphy (vascular pool and late phase) in a patient with mobilized left hip prosthesis

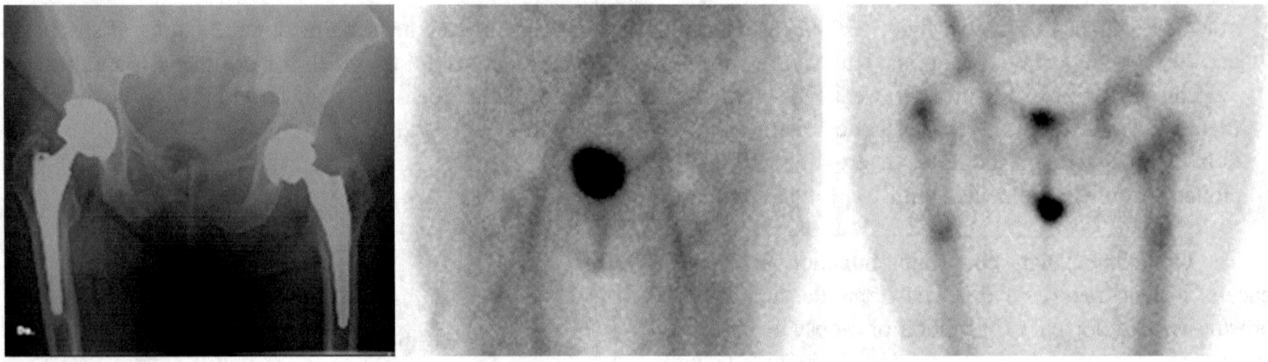

Fig. 5.3 X-ray and three-phase bone scintigraphy (vascular pool and late phase) in a patient with bilateral hip prostheses

early increase in perfusion, while the delayed tracer accumulation is typically concentrated in the load-bearing points at the top of the acetabulum, in the minor and major trochanter and at the top of the prosthesis stem (Fig. 5.2). Periarticular heterotopic calcifications limit mobility and cause joint pain: the bone scan evaluates the metabolic activity of calcifications and the possible need for their removal (Fig. 5.3).

Key Learning Points

- The most common cause of painful prosthesis is prosthetic mobilization.
- The increase in perfusion and bone uptake is less obvious and concentrated near the stem and the prosthetic apex.
- In cases like this, replacement of the mobilized prosthesis must be preceded by a leukocyte scintigraphy to exclude an infection.
- Only when the bone scan findings are completely normal, a PJI can be excluded.
- Periarticular calcifications that form as a deposit of calcium in the granulomas after the release of the wear material of the prosthesis, limit joint movement and cause pain.
- In this case, the vascular phase of the bone scan is perfectly normal, but there are signs of late phase mobilization in both prostheses in the large and the small trochanter, at the apex of the stem and at the acetabulum.
- There is focal accumulation in the right trochanter at the point where the calcifications almost form a bridge with the acetabulum.
- In this case, it is necessary to surgically remove the calcifications when they have a high metabolism, a sign of rapid growth and ongoing conflict.

In knee prosthesis, the periprosthetic uptake patterns are extremely variable, with asymptomatic patients often demonstrating persistent periprosthetic activity for several years after implantation (Fig. 5.4); the role of three-phase bone scintigra-

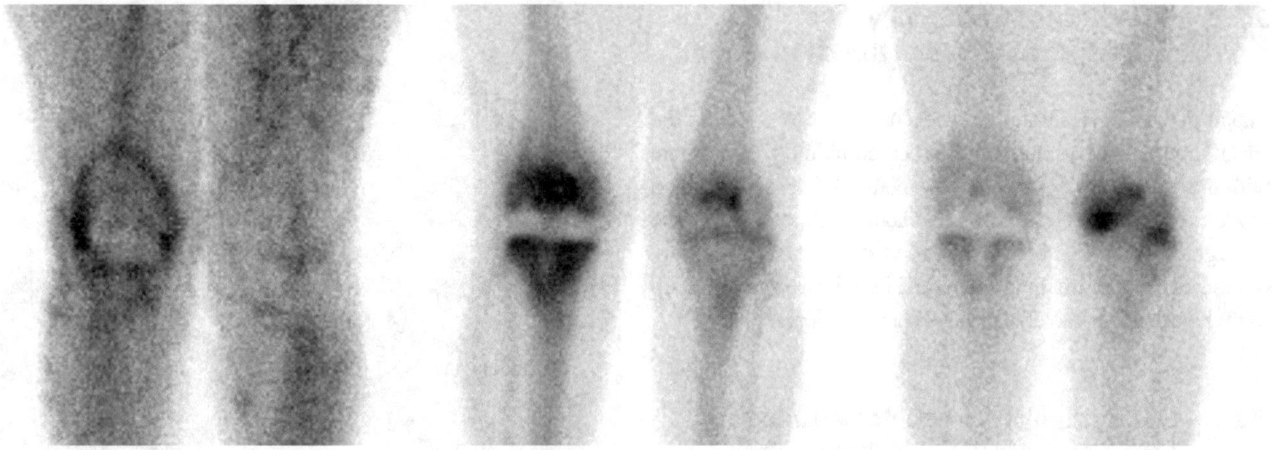

Fig. 5.4 Painful right knee prosthesis. Left and center panel: perfusion and late phase of a three-phase bone scintigraphy, respectively, acquired 9 months after implantation of the knee prosthesis. Right panel: late image of the same patient 2 years later. The first scan shows clearly increased perfusion and late periprosthetic uptake. In the second scan, the periprosthetic activity has normalized and signs of joint overload in the left knee have appeared

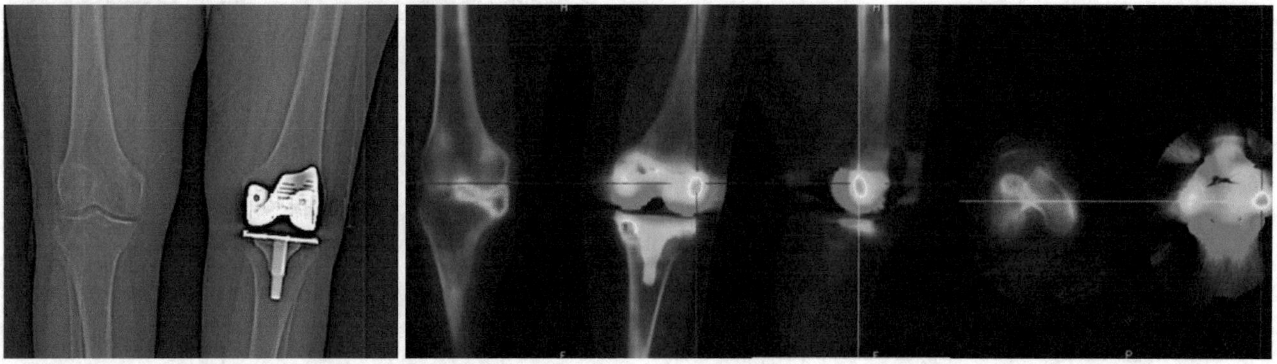

Fig. 5.5 X-ray and bone scan SPECT/CT of a painful left knee prosthesis. The greater intensity of uptake of the lateral femoral condyle compared to the medial tibial condyle, for example, is a sign of prosthetic mobilization [20]

phy is less definite, and it is more difficult to distinguish instability from infection [18]. Adding to the difficulty is the fact that about two thirds of all joint replacement infections occur during the first year after implantation, when, regardless of the type or location of the prosthesis, periprosthetic uptake is so variable that only a bone scan with normal findings provides useful information. SPECT/CT imaging during bone scintigraphy provides exact anatomical correlation of pathological tracer uptake. In many cases, SPECT increases the sensitivity and CT the specificity of the bone scan study, thus increasing confidence in the final diagnosis over planar imaging alone [19]. Hirschmann et al. highlighted the clinical value of a standardized diagnostic algorithm including SPECT/CT in patients with problems after total knee arthroplasty. With this specific algorithm, the authors aim to identify typical distribution patterns and intensity thresholds of bone tracer uptake, which reflect conditions such as mechanical loosening, instability, component malposition, or patella femoral problems [20] (Fig. 5.5).

Key Learning Points

- In the first 2 years after implantation of a joint prosthesis (especially knee prosthesis), bone scintigraphy is useless because it is positive even in the absence of a prosthetic infection.
- In these cases, infection can only be ruled out with leukocyte scintigraphy.
- SPET/CT improves the accuracy of planar bone scan, especially in knee prostheses, because it allows evaluation of correct positioning of the prosthesis and of metabolic activity of the different joint compartments and of the patella.

5.2.2 ^{67}Ga-Citrate Scintigraphy for Periprosthetic Joint Infection

Imaging with ^{67}Ga-citrate has been proposed to enhance the specificity of bone scintigraphy. When combining ^{67}Ga-citrate with the bone scan, the accuracy is about 70–80%, with only a modest improvement over bone imaging alone. ^{67}Ga-citrate scintigraphy is now less frequently used, because of these drawbacks and because imaging agents and imaging techniques with more favorable characteristics have been developed [18, 21].

5.2.3 Scintigraphy with Labeled Autologous Leukocytes for Periprosthetic Joint Infection

Autologous leukocyte scintigraphy is obtained by labeling in vitro the autologous leukocytes with either ^{111}In-oxyquinoline or ^{99m}Tc-HMPAO. After the development of successful labeling of leukocytes with ^{99m}Tc-HMPAO, the use of ^{99m}Tc-labeled white blood cells (^{99m}Tc-HMPAO-WBC) has virtually replaced ^{111}In-oxine-WBC for most indications, because of more favorable imaging characteristics and lower radiation burden to patients [22]. The normal biodistribution of labeled leukocytes includes the reticuloendothelial system and blood pool for both types of labeled leukocytes (Fig. 5.6). Moreover, the distribution of hematopoietically active marrow is extremely variable, due to blood overflow and reparative processes after prosthetic implant surgery. In adults with prosthetic infections, surgery may induce a peripheral displacement of the bone marrow toward surrounding spaces, which may then be mistakenly interpreted as septic (Fig. 5.7).

Key Learning Points

- The normal distribution of labeled leukocytes includes the red marrow, liver, and spleen.
- Metabolites of ^{99m}Tc-HMPAO are excreted in part via the urinary tract (bladder), with a small extent being excreted via the intestinal route.
- Displacement of the bone marrow is one of the most frequent causes of false positivity of leukocyte scintigraphy.
- It can be seen that the image of the right knee does not increase in intensity with respect to the activity of the iliac crest and does not change shape in the three acquisitions.
- The presence of activity in the ascending colon and in the cecum is very frequent in the late image at 20–24 h.
- In equivocal cases, SPECT/CT imaging is useful to study the pelvis.

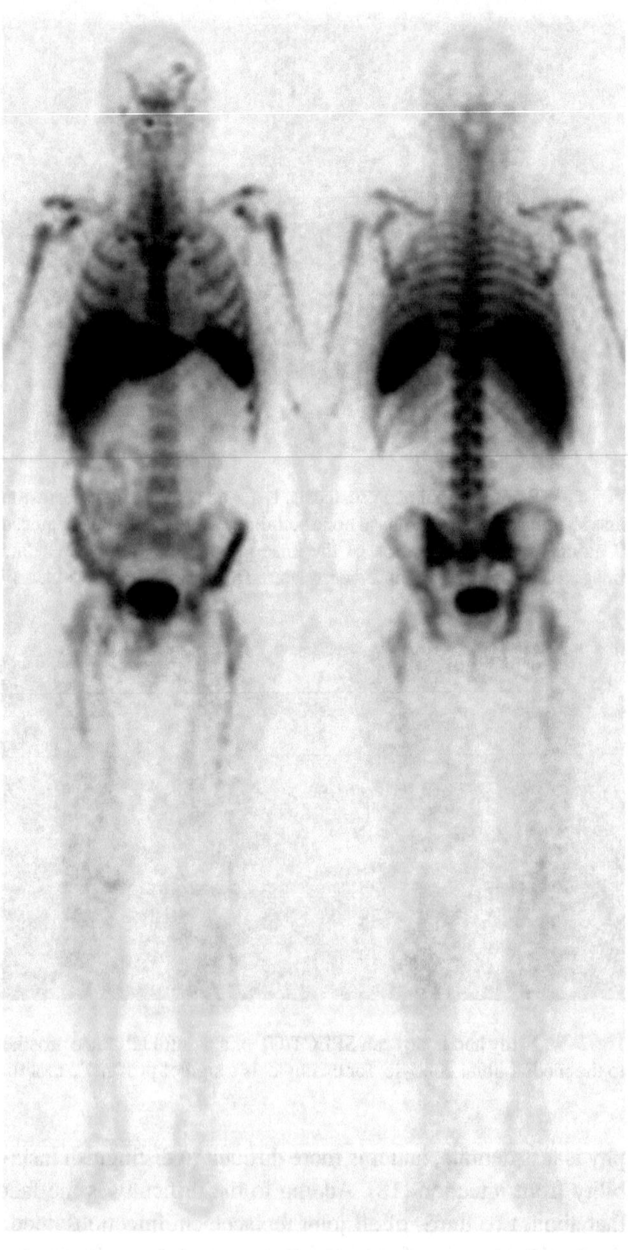

Fig. 5.6 Normal biodistribution of leukocyte scintigraphy 4 h post administration of ^{99m}Tc-HMPAO-WBC

In cases with equivocal/inconclusive leukocyte scintigraphy, Palestro et al. [23] suggested to correlate the findings of ^{111}In-oxine-WBC scintigraphy with a bone marrow scan with ^{99m}Tc-sulfur colloid. A discrepancy between the two scintigraphic images (leukocyte accumulation greater than radiocolloid uptake) more accurately identifies the presence of infection. When leukocyte scintigraphy is combined with bone marrow scintigraphy, no significantly increased specificity was found, but sensitivity decreases compared to leukocyte scintigraphy alone.

The optimal acquisition protocol requires a comparison of multiple sequential acquisitions, at 1–4 h and 20–24 h, respectively. When using this acquisition protocol, visual qualitative

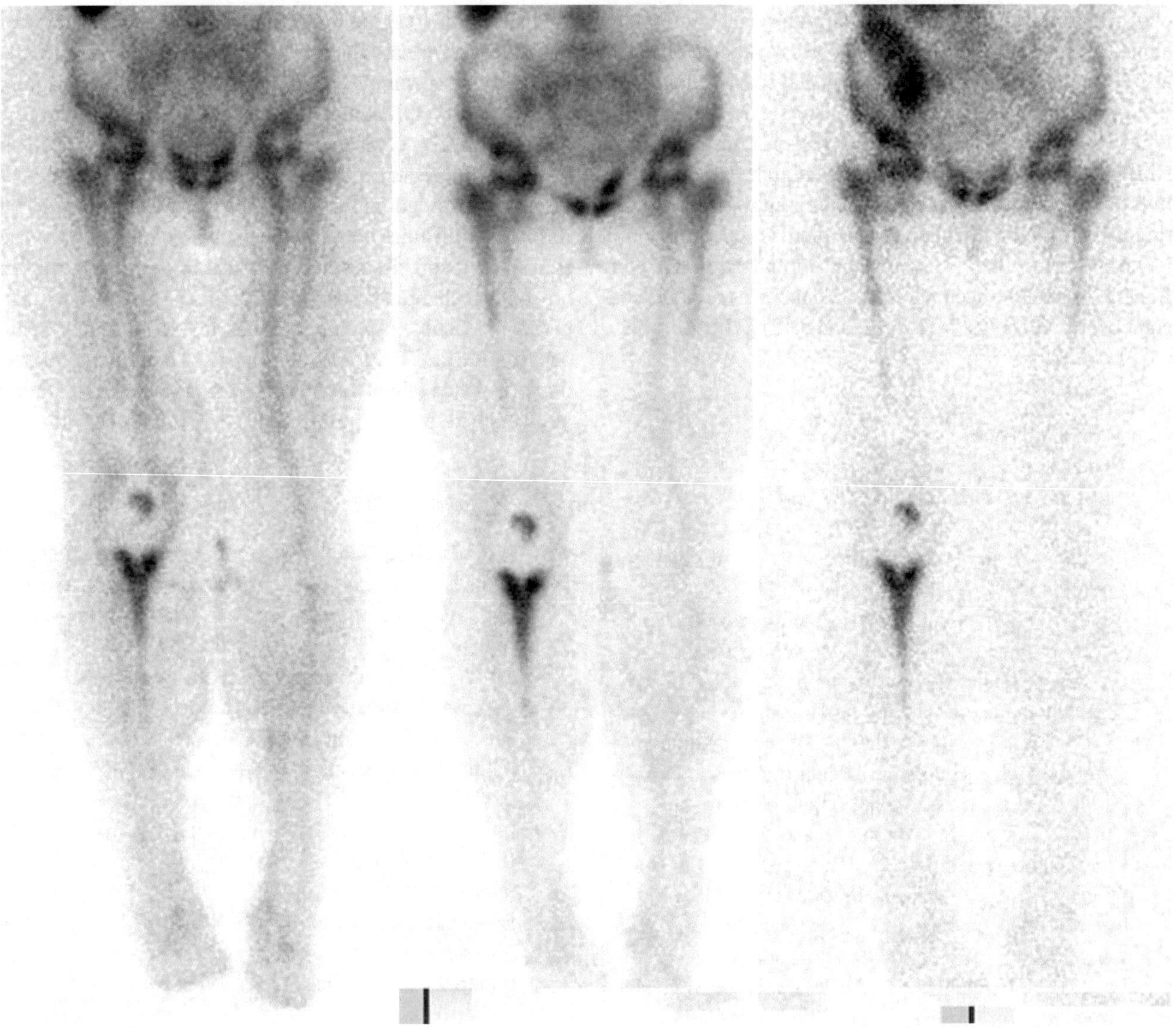

Fig. 5.7 ^{99m}Tc-HMPAO-WBC scintigraphy of the lower limbs 1 h, 4 h, and 20 h after administration in a patient with a right knee prosthesis. Activity in the patella and in the tibia is due to the surgical trauma associated with implant the prosthesis, causing expansion of the red marrow in the same limb. The bone marrow activity remains constant over time, while the vascular activity gradually declines

interpretation yields a sensitivity of 85.1%, specificity of 97.1%, and overall diagnostic accuracy of 94.5% [24–26] (Fig. 5.8a). In patients with chronic infection or undergoing long-term antibiotic treatment, scintigraphy should be postponed until at least 2 weeks after the end of therapy (Fig. 5.8b).

Key Learning Points

- Comparison of the images reveals a significant difference between the image at 1 h (only bone marrow activity) and the 20-h image, where there is an additional accumulation due to PJI.

- Leukocyte scintigraphy can be used to assess response to antibiotic therapy.
- In these patients, the scan must be acquired at least 2–3 weeks after the end of therapy, in order to avoid interference of circulating antibiotics with diapedesis of the granulocytes (risk of false-negative findings).

In patients with suspected PJI, leukocyte scintigraphy should include a whole-body scan, which may reveal infections in unexpected locations (Fig. 5.9). Whether combined with bone marrow scintigraphy or not, leukocyte scintigraphy improves specificity compared with bone scintigraphy alone (Figs. 5.4 and 5.10). Radiolabeled leukocytes localize at infected sites via chemotaxis and diapedesis: their accumulation depends on maintained chemotaxis, number and types of cells labeled, and cellular response to a particular stimulus. Since labeled neutrophils migrate by diapedesis into the infection site, leukocyte scintigraphy is able to distinguish prosthetic infection (where there is accumulation of leukocytes over time) from prosthetic mobilization or a bone fracture (where the accumulation of leukocytes remains constant over time) (Figs. 5.11, 5.12, and 5.13) [27].

Key Learning Points

- The total body scan should always be acquired to search for metastatic infectious foci.
- They must also be reported, because otherwise the infection can recur after the prosthesis is reimplanted.
- SPECT/CT imaging increases the diagnostic accuracy of planar scintigraphy by demonstrating the close correlation between the accumulation of labeled leukocytes and the prosthesis.
- Correct localization of the site of leukocyte accumulation allows guidance for bone biopsy, and possible for drainage of the collection.
- In full-blown cases, simple visual comparison of the leukocyte scintigraphy images obtained in different phases that can be defined as medullary (1 h), late (4 h), and delayed (20 h) is sufficient to diagnose infection.
- A 20–24 h imaging is mandatory to distinguish infection from simple sterile inflammation.
- Leukocytes tend to form collections in soft tissues along the muscle bands and in the joint cavities, usually along a gravity gradient.
- The same three-stage acquisition protocol is also used for peripheral fractures with delayed consolidation, clearly visualizing progressive accumulation of leukocytes at the site of infection and also in ipsilateral inguinal lymph nodes.
- Bone marrow activity of the iliac crest serves as a reference to distinguish peripheral accumulation from bone marrow displacement.

SPECT/CT imaging increases the diagnostic accuracy of planar leukocyte scintigraphy and is currently considered the best imaging technique for the diagnosis of bone and joint infections [28, 29]. Adding a SPECT/CT acquisition to planar scintigraphy considerably improves anatomic localization of the infected site(s) and definition of the extent of disease. A pathognomonic sign of prosthetic infections is the formation of fistulas between the prosthetic infection and the surrounding soft tissues, but also within the joint cavity in hip and knee prostheses (Figs. 5.14, 5.15, and 5.16). In peripheral bones, osteomyelitis has the same scintigraphic pattern on SPECT/CT imaging; in these conditions, formation of a fistula (sinus tract) is possible, as also the formation of ulcers with bone exposure (Figs. 5.17, and 5.18) [30].

Key Learning Point

- Bone fractures typically exhibit a certain degree of leukocyte accumulation, without however increase over time as typically observed in case of infection.
- SPECT/CT imaging during leukocyte scintigraphy in hip replacement infections helps to distinguish a superficial infection from a PJI.
- A superficial infection can be treated with simple debridement, whereas in PJI replacement of the prosthesis takes place in two stages with a prolonged loss of patient mobility and two surgical interventions.
- Leukocyte scintigraphy with SPECT/CT imaging also serves to exclude or demonstrate a pelvic infection that can complicate a PJI.

5.2.4 Antigranulocyte Scintigraphy for Periprosthetic Joint Infection

^{99m}Tc-labeled antigranulocyte antibodies (anti-G mAb) allow in vivo labeling of WBCs. The biodistribution is similar to that of ^{99m}Tc-HMPAO-WBCs, but with a higher intensity of bone marrow uptake. Thus, antigranulocyte scintigraphy is less specific than scintigraphy with in-vitro labeled leukocytes [31].

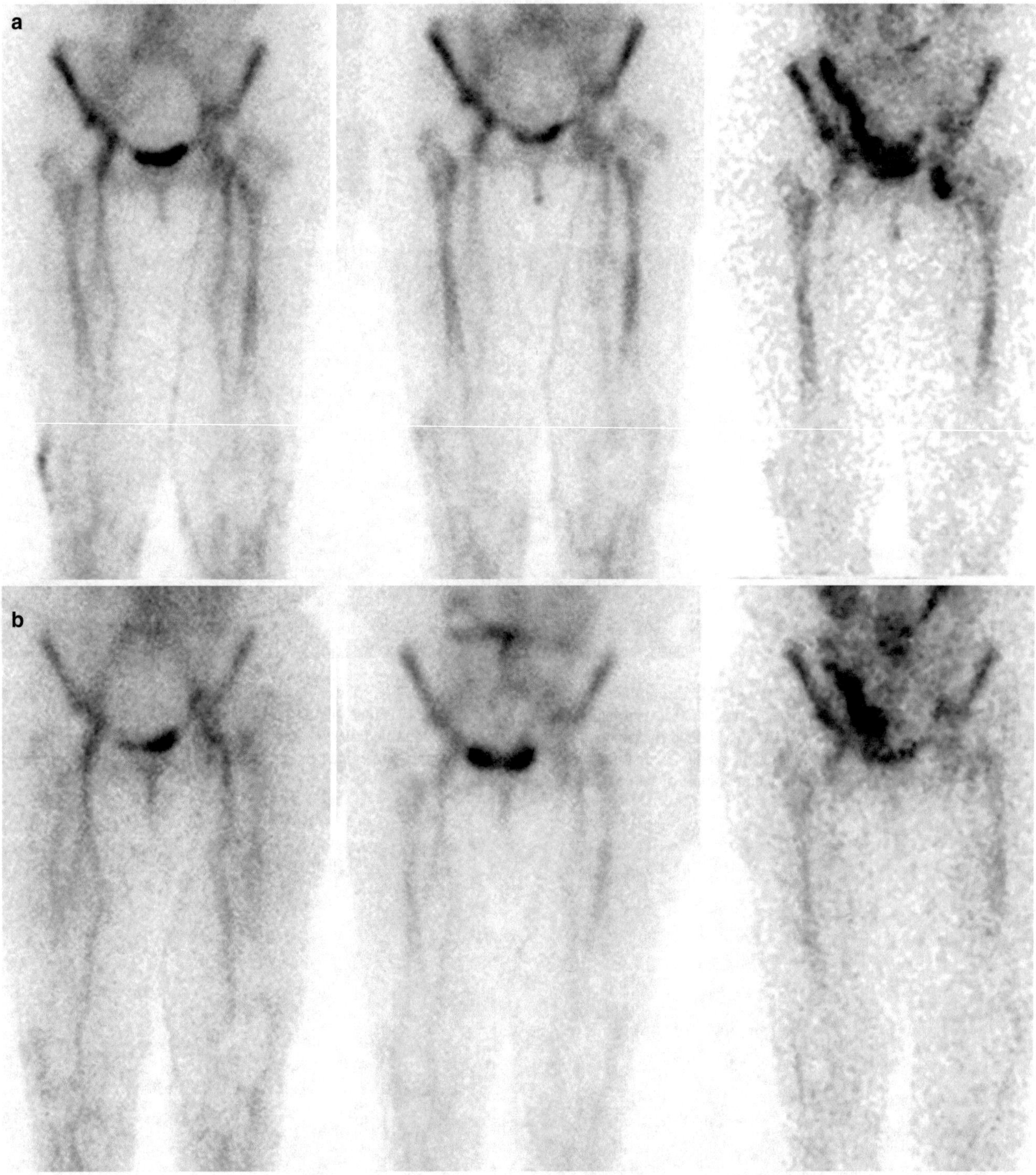

Fig. 5.8 (**a**) (upper row) ^{99m}Tc-HMPAO-WBC scintigraphy of the lower limbs 1 h, 4 h, and 20 h after administration in a patient with left hip prosthesis. A focal accumulation of leukocytes is clearly seen in the inferior-internal portion of the acetabulum in the 20-h images. (**b**) (lower row) the same patient 2 months later after 6-week course of antibiotic treatment: there are no more signs of periprosthetic infection

Key Learning Point

- In obviously positive cases as in this case, the late 20-h acquisition can safely be omitted, because it does not add useful information.
- SPECT/CT imaging after planar leukocyte scintigraphy is often crucial in equivocal cases.
- Leukocyte accumulation in the soft tissues outside and in connection with the medullary cavity is a certain sign of persistent infection.

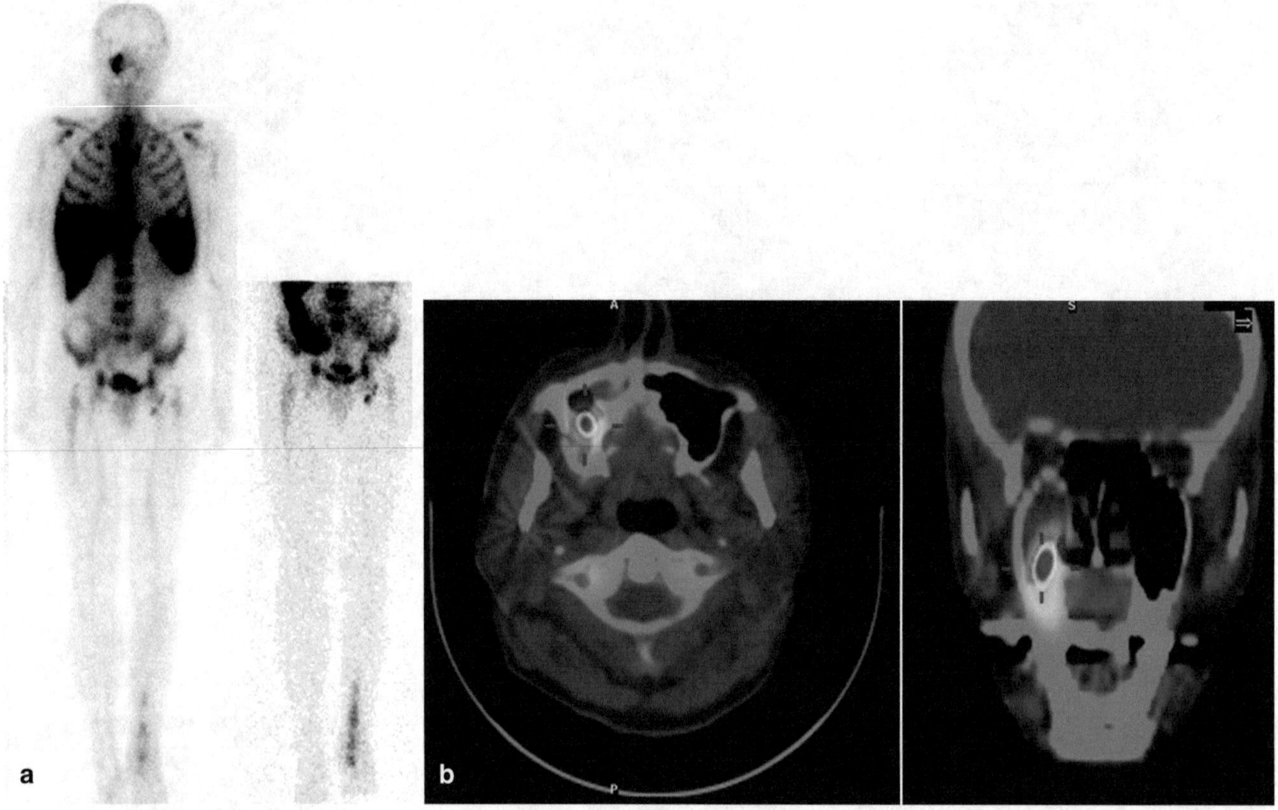

Fig. 5.9 (**a**) Whole-body ^{99m}Tc-HMPAO-WBC scintigraphy 4 h after administration and scan of the lower limbs at 20 h in a patient with exposed fracture of left tibia. (**b**) SPECT/CT images of the head, transverse and coronal views, obtained after the planar acquisition at 4 h. In the whole-body image, there is an accumulation of leukocytes in the head, that SPECT/CT imaging proves to be due to an infection of the right maxillary sinus. In the late image, accumulation of leukocytes around the intramedullary nail of the left tibia and in the inguinal lymph nodes of the same side is enhanced because of peripheral bone infection

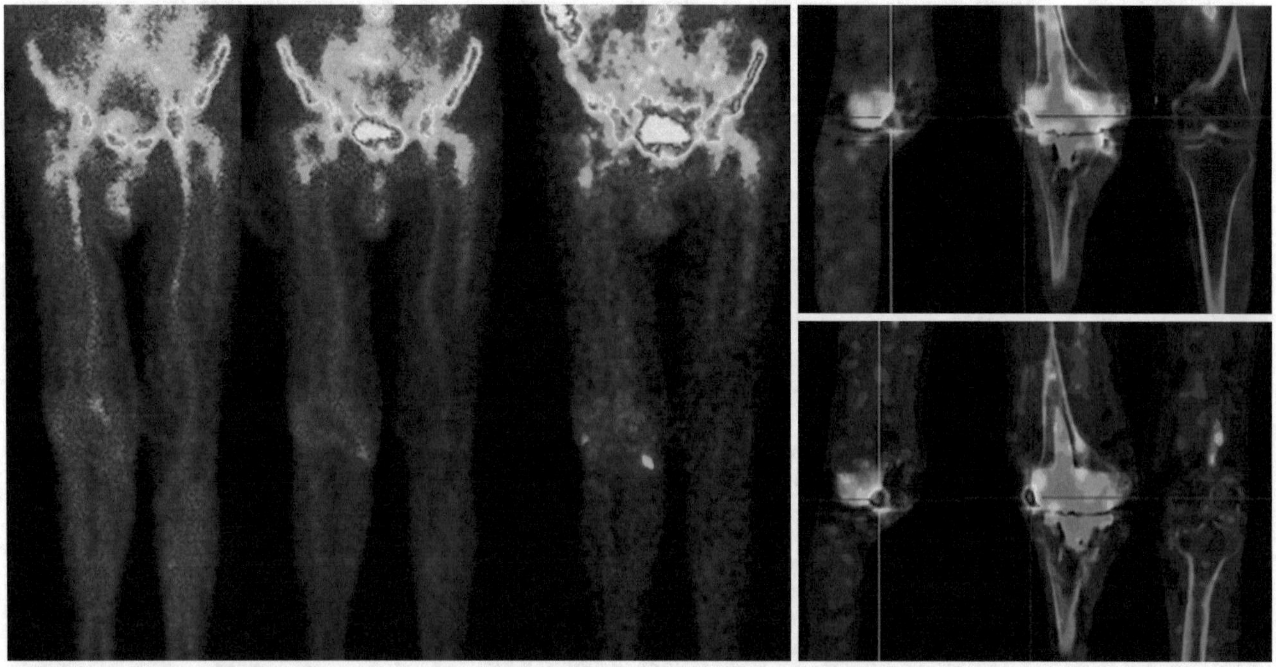

Fig. 5.10 Whole-body ^{99m}Tc-HMPAO-WBC scintigraphy 1 h, 4 h, and 20 h after administration, and SPECT/CT imaging of the lower limbs (at 20 h) in a patient with infection of the right knee prosthesis. In the whole-body image, there is a progressive faint accumulation of leukocytes in the internal compartment of the articular space, which is well localized in the SPECT/CT images

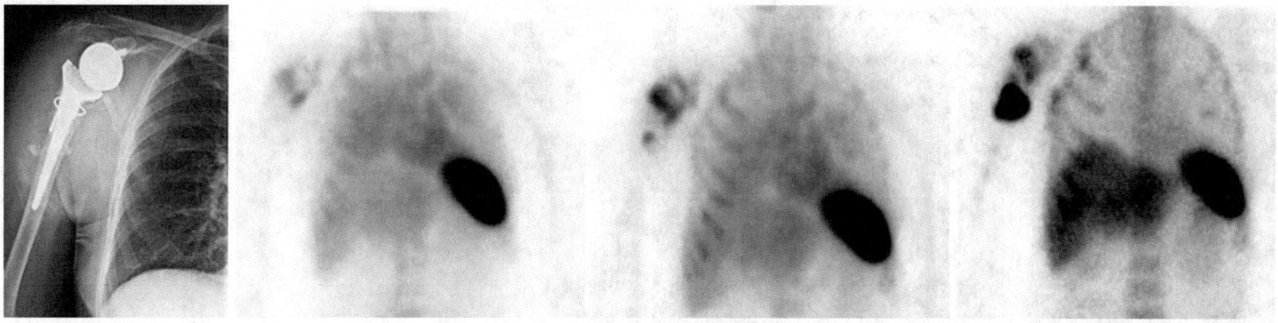

Fig. 5.11 X-ray and ^{99m}Tc-HMPAO-WBC scintigraphy 1 h, 4 h, and 20 h after administration in a patient with infection of the right shoulder inverted prosthesis. There is progressive intense accumulation of leukocytes in the right arm both at the 4-h and at the 20-h images. Faint uptake in axillary ipsilateral lymph nodes is well detectable in the 20-h acquisition

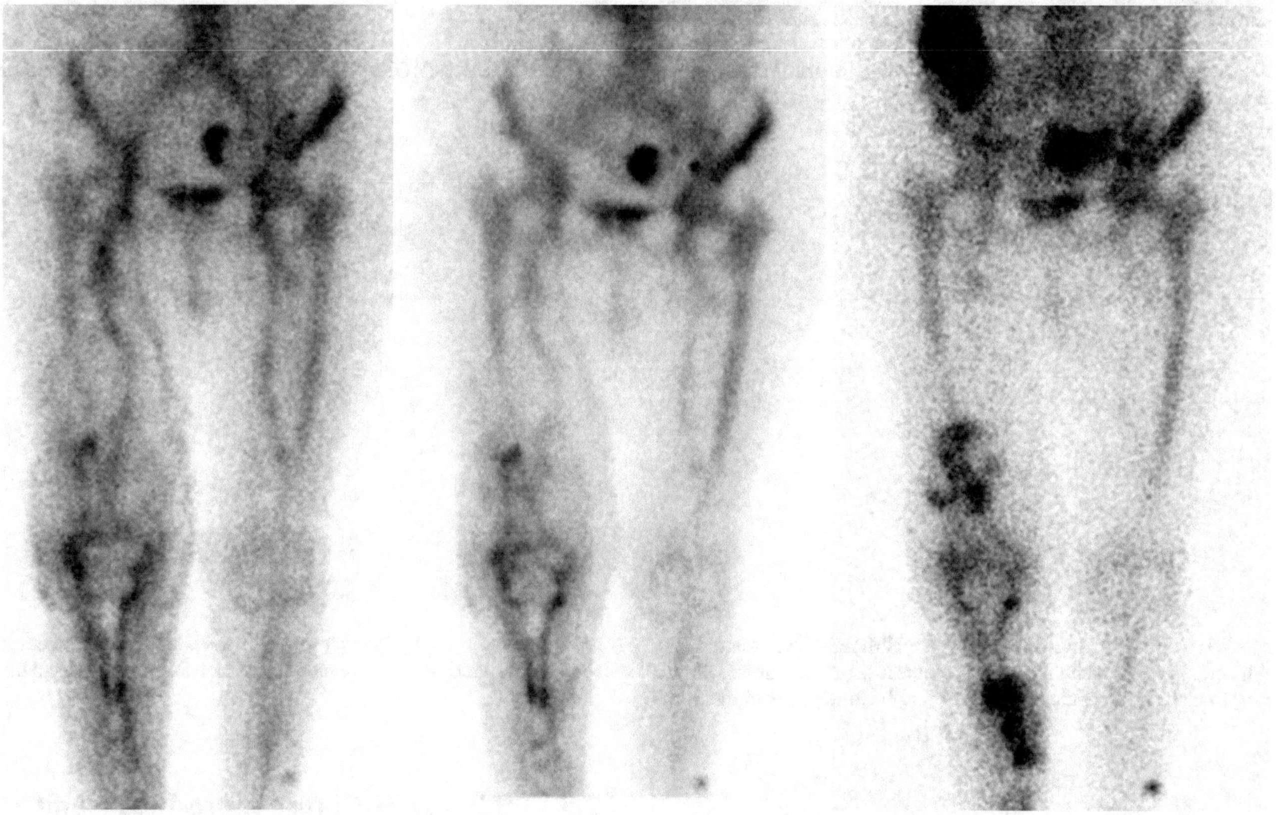

Fig. 5.12 ^{99m}Tc-HMPAO-WBC scintigraphy 1 h, 4 h, and 20 h after administration in a patient with an infection of the right replaced knee prosthesis. There is a progressive intense accumulation of leukocytes in the right thigh and right leg, around both the femoral and the tibial components of the prosthesis. In the late image, the accumulation of leukocytes is massive and distal to the site of the prosthesis. A small metastatic focus of leukocyte accumulation is also shown in the distal portion of left leg

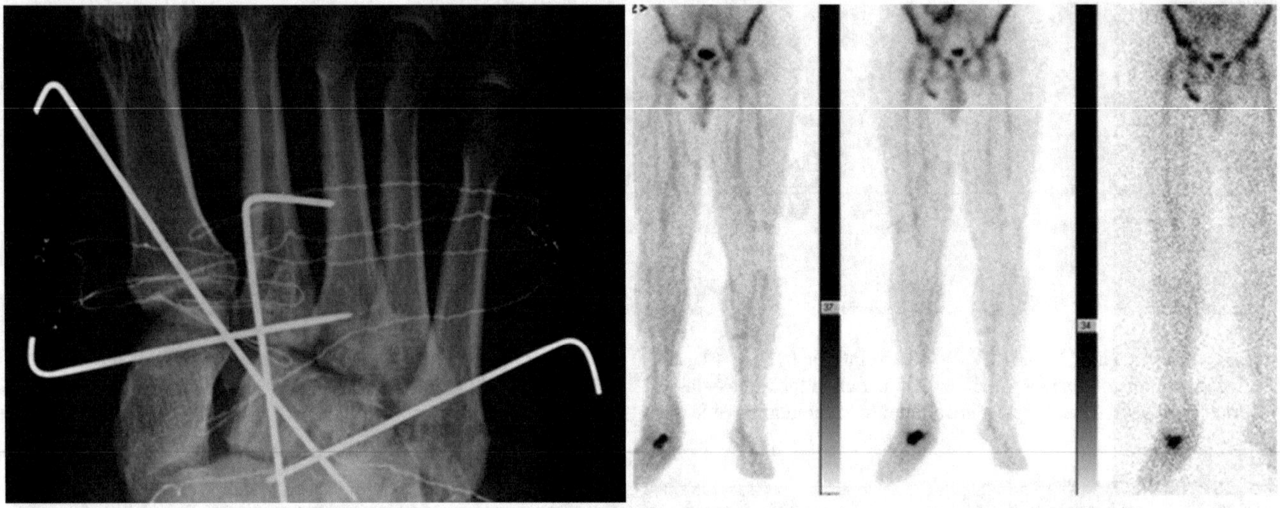

Fig. 5.13 X-ray of an unconsolidated fracture of the first and second metatarsals. ^{99m}Tc-HMPAO-WBC scintigraphy 1 h, 4 h, and 20 h after administration in a patient with infection of the right foot

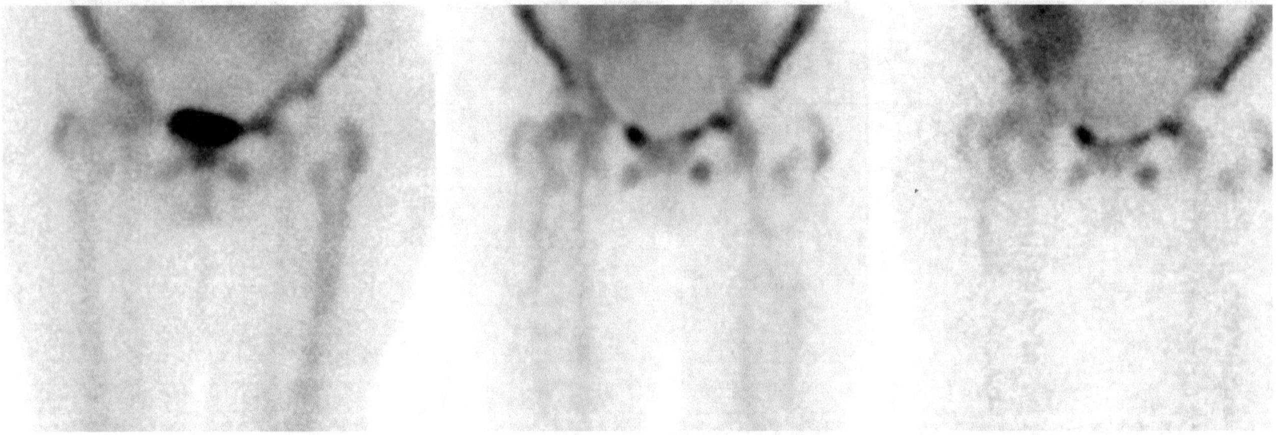

Fig. 5.14 Bone scintigraphy and ^{99m}Tc-HMPAO-WBC scintigraphy 4 h and 20 h after administration in a patient with bilateral fractures of iliac branch and ischiatic branch. The four fracture points of the pelvis (masked on the right by bladder activity) show increased leukocyte accumulation, which however remains constant between the 4-h and the 20-h images

Key Learning Points

- The most suitable imaging modality for the differential diagnosis between infection and pseudoarthrosis is leukocyte scintigraphy, because of its high specificity.
- In fractures with bone exposure, infection is a constant and almost invariably occurring complication.

5.2.5 [^{18}F]FDG PET/CT for Periprosthetic Joint Infection

PET/CT with [^{18}F]FDG is being increasingly used for the diagnosis of prosthesis joint infections, especially regarding hip arthroplasty. At variance with leukocyte scintigraphy, [^{18}F]FDG accumulation in infections does not depend on leukocyte migration, but it is mainly related to the gly-

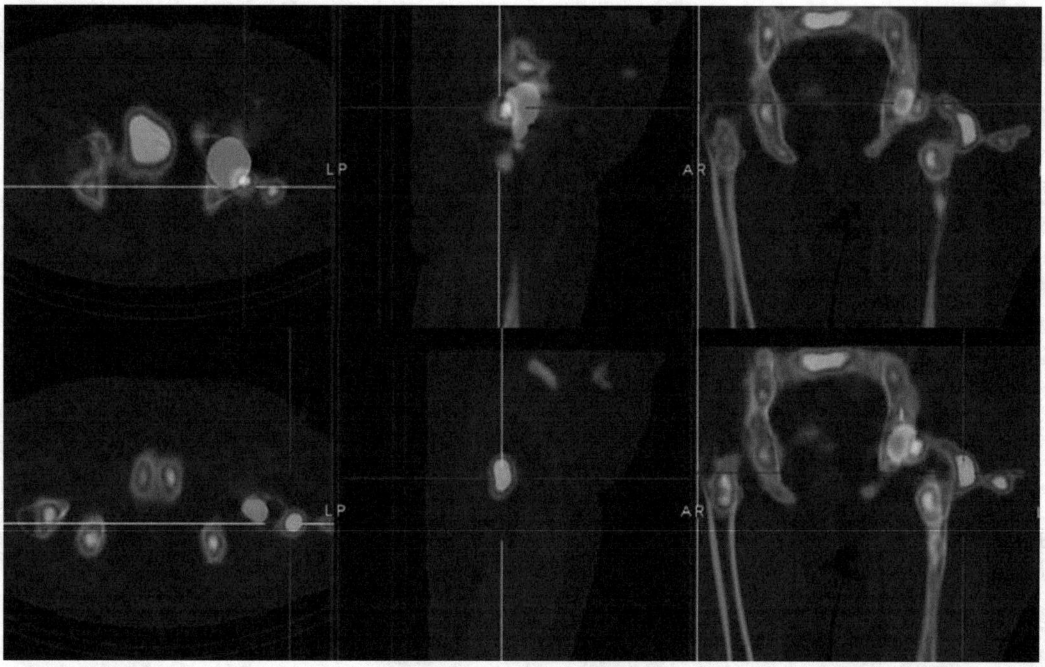

Fig. 5.15 ^{99m}Tc-HMPAO-WBC scintigraphy 4 h after administration in a patient with infected left hip prosthesis: transaxial, sagittal, and coronal reconstructions (two rows). The sites of leukocyte accumulation are in contact and behind the prosthesis and expand into the soft tissues to form a cutaneous fistula

colytic activity of the cells involved in the inflammatory response [32]. Compared with leukocyte scintigraphy, [^{18}F]FDG PET/CT offers advantages such as time efficiency, increased resolution, and the use of low-dose CT [33, 34]. Tracer uptake along the bone–prosthesis interface of the femoral component is considered the most reliable indicator for periprosthetic hip infection; it should be noted, however, that tracer uptake around the head, neck, and distal tip of the prosthesis can remain for up to 2 years after implantation [35].

Nonetheless, in most cases, a repeat PET scan after antibiotic treatment can be useful to confirm the diagnosis of the PJI and to assess response to the antibiotic treatment or to surgical removal of the joint prosthesis (Figs. 5.19 and 5.20). [^{18}F]FDG PET has good sensitivity (91–100%) for diagnosing infection of joint hip arthroplasty, although it is less specific for diagnosing periprosthetic knee infection. Specificity of [^{18}F]FDG PET in patients with metallic implants, however, is based on both localization and intensity of [^{18}F]FDG uptake, and it depends on the positivity criteria used [28]. The accumulation of [^{18}F]FDG in the soft tissues adjacent to a joint prosthesis or a fracture of the peripheral bone constitutes one of the most certain signs of infection diagnosed with PET (Fig. 5.21). When both leukocyte scintigraphy and [^{18}F]FDG PET/CT are available, it can be useful to reserve the PET scan for the most serious and acute cases, such as the elderly's fever.

Key Learning Points

- [^{18}F]FDG PET/CT is the gold standard in patients with fever of unknown origin, because of its high sensitivity and overall diagnostic accuracy.
- PET is quick to perform and better tolerated, making it the first choice test in elderly and seriously ill patients with suspected infection.
- [^{18}F]FDG PET is less specific than leukocyte scintigraphy for identifying infection, but it can direct biopsy to confirm the diagnosis.
- Alternatively, by repeating the PET scan after antibiotic therapy, infection can be confirmed in most cases.
- Detection of periprosthetic [^{18}F]FDG uptake is one of the most certain signs of infection.
- [^{18}F]FDG PET/CT is also useful to assess response to antibiotic therapy.
- A completely negative PET rules out an infection and can be used as an alternative to leukocyte scintigraphy before implanting the new prosthesis.
- Focal [^{18}F]FDG uptake near the synthesis hardware is a sign of probable infection.
- A rim-shaped [^{18}F]FDG uptake surrounding a central cold area is typical of an abscess, where the peripheral part is rich in viable cells while the central liquid collection is less metabolically active.

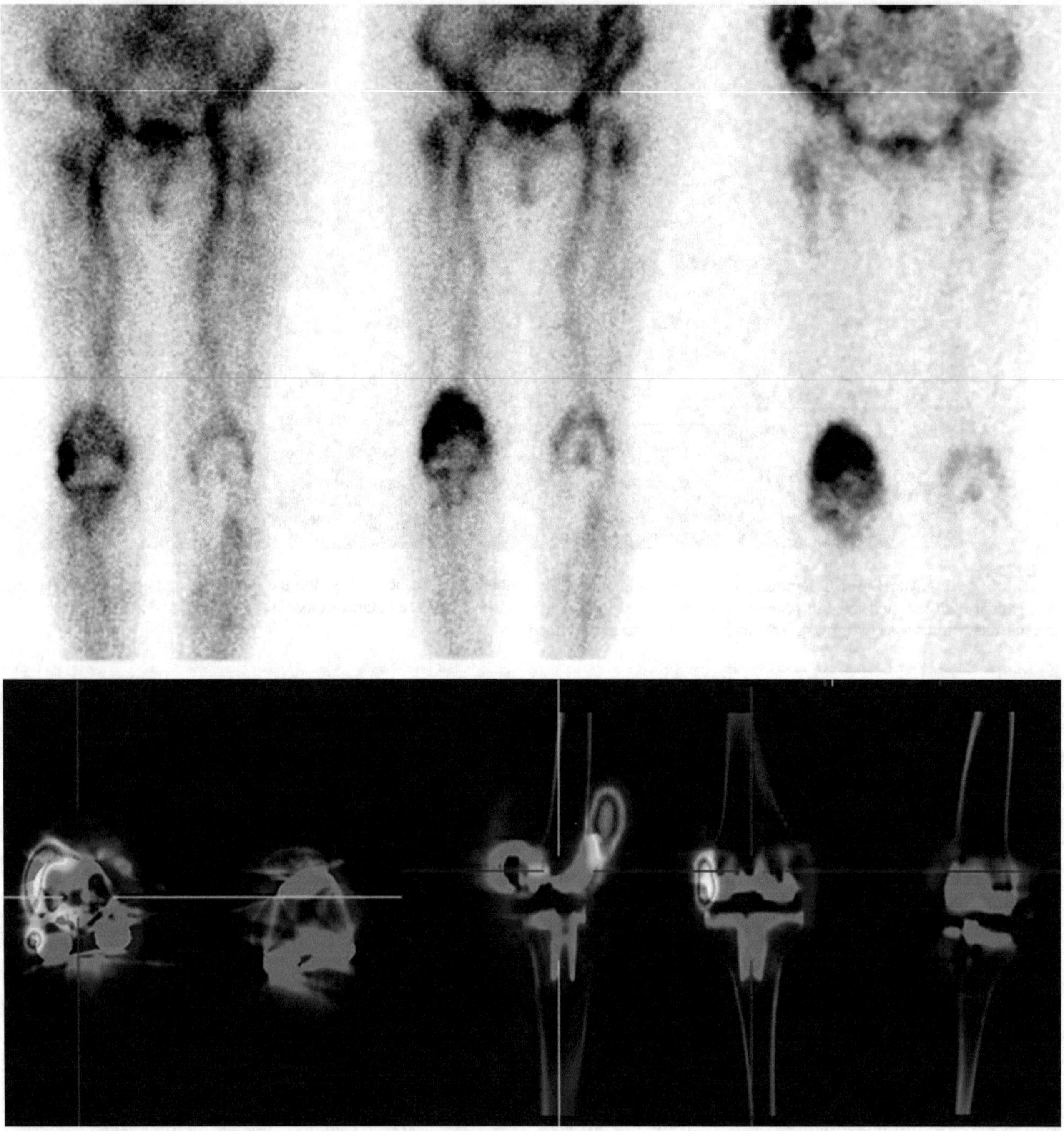

Fig. 5.16 ^{99m}Tc-HMPAO-WBC scintigraphy 1 h, 4 h, and 20 h after administration in a patient with bilateral knee prostheses and infection in the right prosthesis (upper row). SPET/CT of the same patient at the 4-h acquisition: transaxial, sagittal, and coronal sections of the right knee. Clear and progressive accumulation of labeled leukocytes in the joint capsule and articular space (retropatellar and lateral spaces) is correctly demonstrated already at the 4-h time point

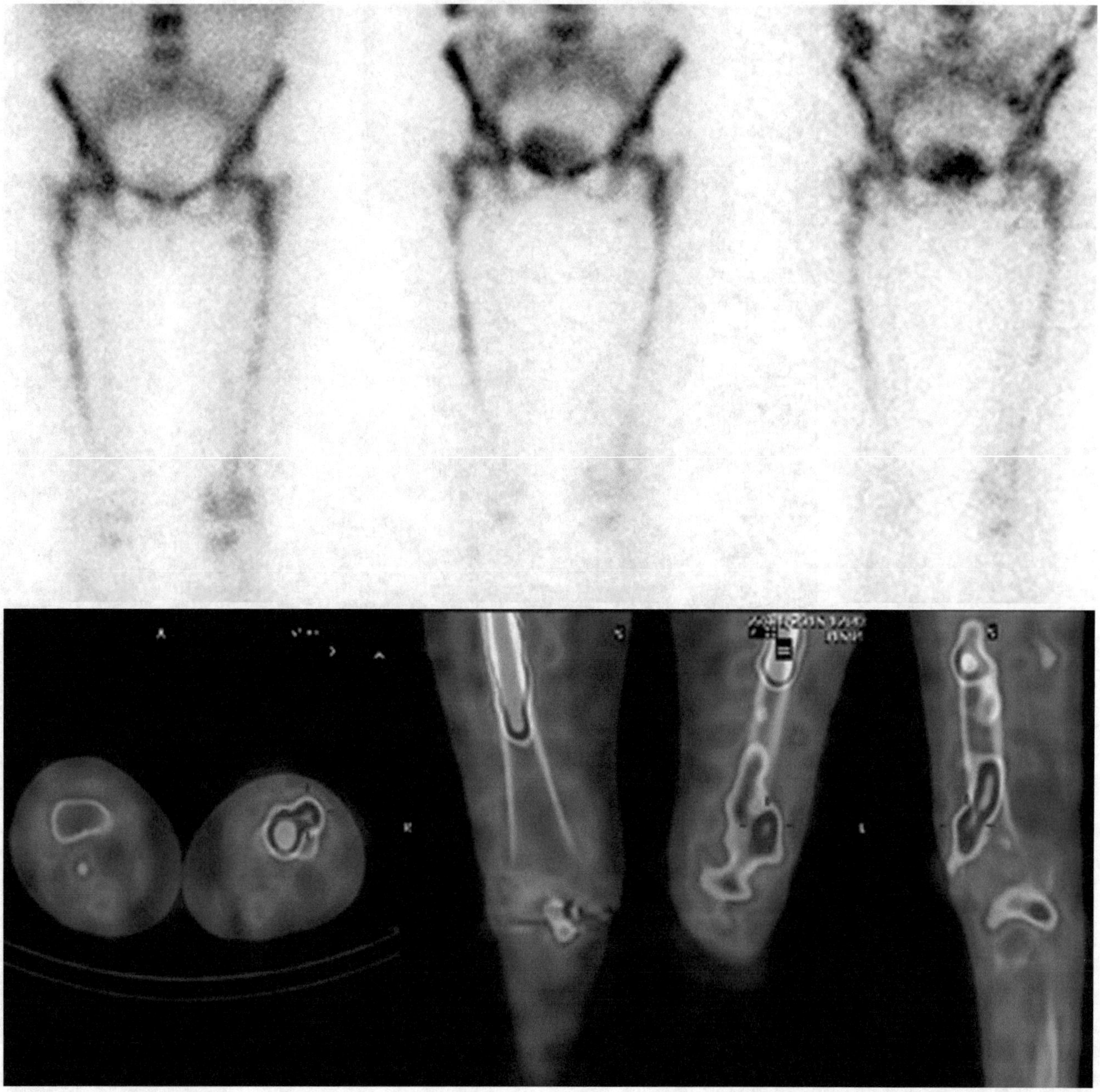

Fig. 5.17 ^{99m}Tc-HMPAO-WBC scintigraphy 1 h, 4 h, and 20 h after administration in a patient with infection of the left knee joint prosthesis infection during two-stage replacement (before reimplantation in the upper row). Mild leukocyte accumulation is detectable in the soft tissues of the left knee. SPECT/CT imaging (transaxial, coronal, and sagittal sections) of the left knee acquired at 4 h better demonstrates leukocyte accumulation in the antero-lateral soft tissues of the thigh and in the knee joint cavity

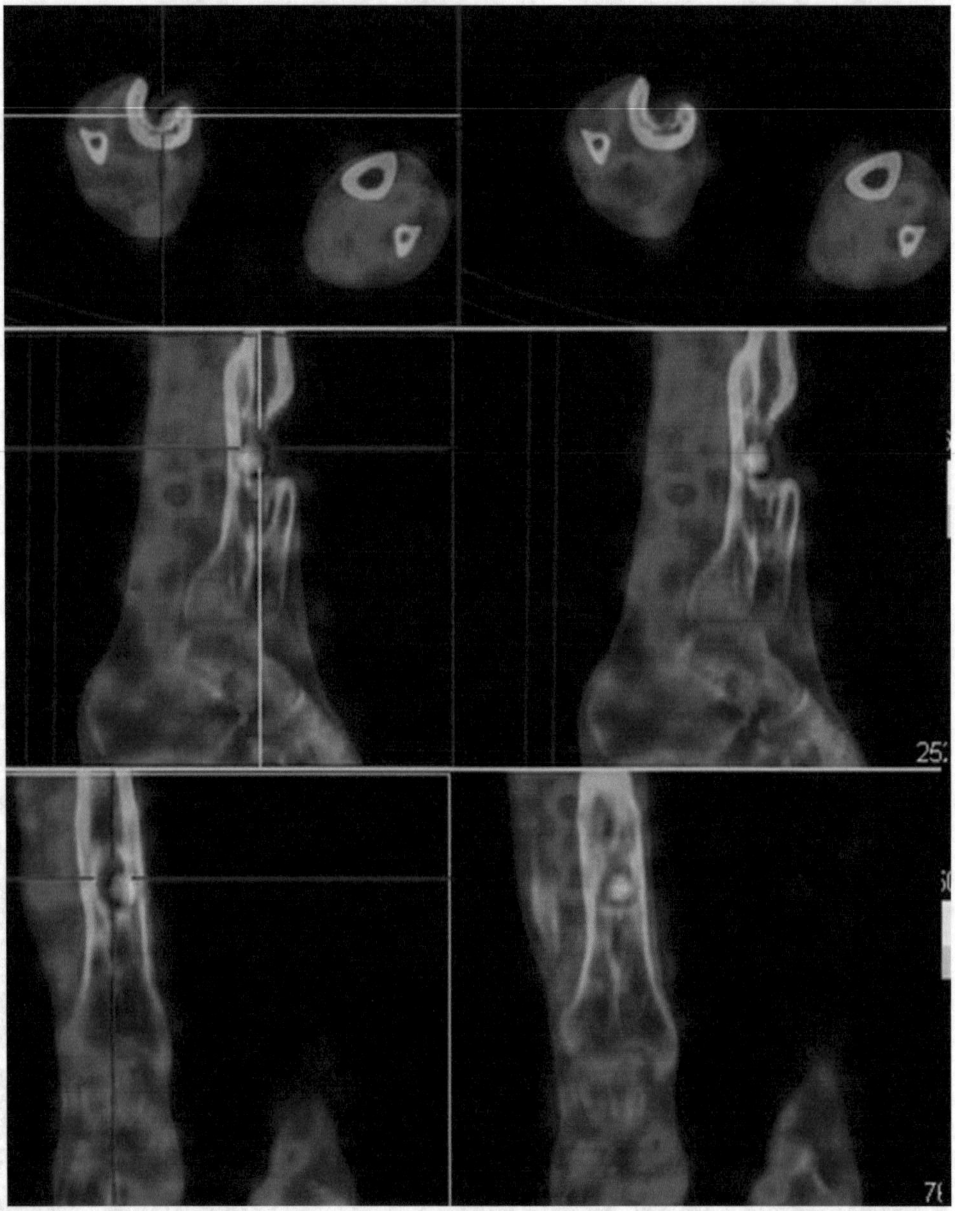

Fig. 5.18 SPECT/CT of the right leg acquired during ^{99m}Tc-HMPAO-WBC scintigraphy: transaxial (upper row), sagittal (middle row), and coronal sections (lower row). Infection of an exposed fracture resulted in ulcer and loss of substance and persistence of bone infection

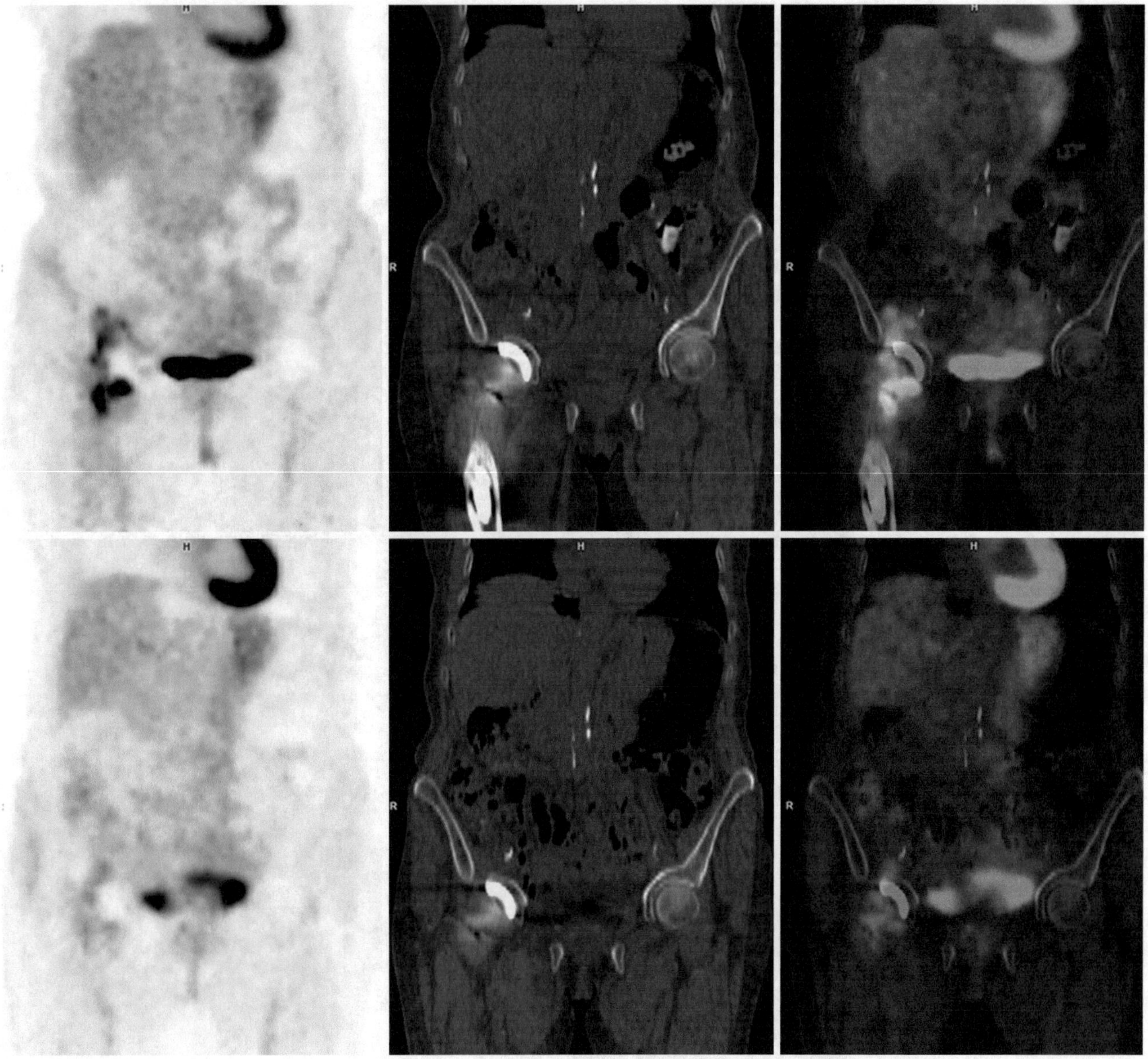

Fig. 5.19 [^{18}F]FDG PET/CT: coronal reconstruction of PET, CT, and fused images in a patient with fever of unknown origin (upper row), and the same patient after 4 weeks of antibiotic therapy (lower row). The high [^{18}F]FDG uptake around the right hip prosthesis observed in the baseline scan (upper row) disappears after antibiotic treatment

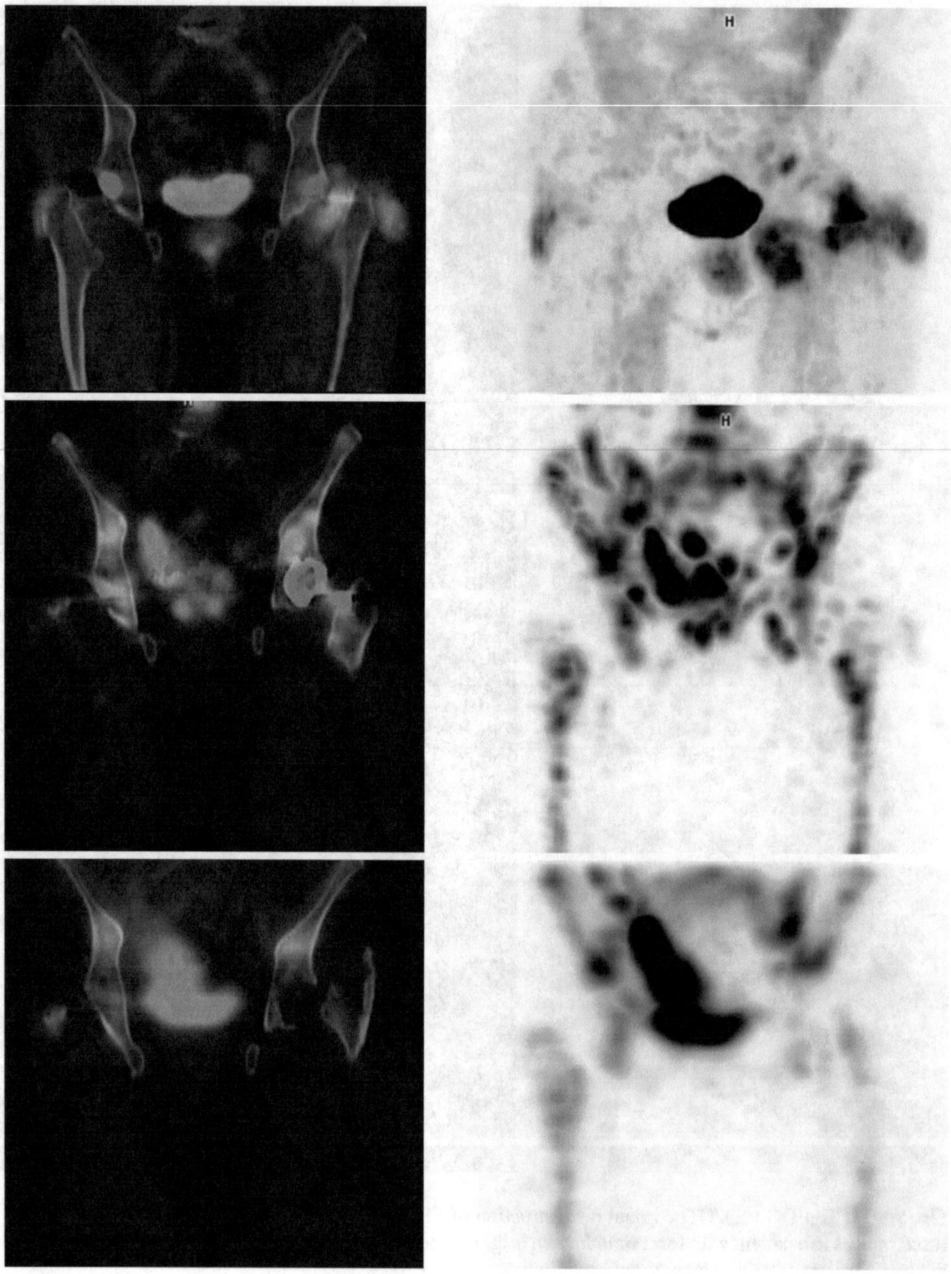

Fig. 5.20 [^{18}F]FDG PET/CT: coronal section of the fused images and MIP in a patient with fever of unknown origin (upper row), and the same patient after 4 weeks of antibiotic therapy (center row). Lower row: fused coronal SPECT/CT sections of ^{99m}Tc-HMPAO-leukocyte scintigraphy of the same patient 2 months after the removal of the PJI of the left hip and prior to the implantation of the new prosthesis. The high [^{18}F]FDG uptake in a collection at the inner root of the thigh and in the soft tissues surrounding the greater trochanter shown in the upper row disappears after antibiotic treatment (center row). Negative leukocyte scintigraphy confirms the success of antibiotic therapy after removing the infected prosthesis

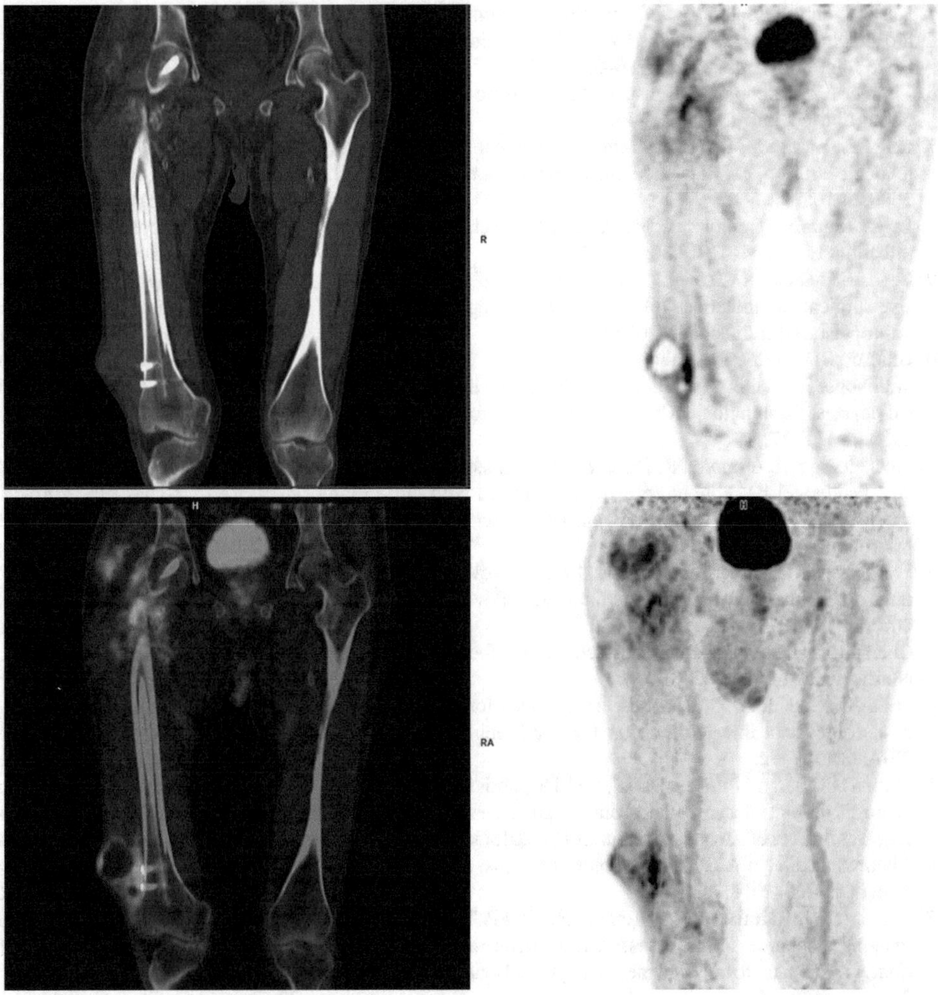

Fig. 5.21 [^{18}F]FDG PET/CT: coronal CT and PET sections (upper row), fused PET/CT image, and MIP (lower row) in a patient with a right femur infection following osteosynthesis because of fracture. Typical [^{18}F]FDG uptake in soft tissues both at the root of the thigh near the metallic plate and at the distal lateral surface adjacent to the screws that fix the intramedullary nail

5.3 Conclusions

In patients with a painful joint prosthesis and normal laboratory tests, a negative three-phase bone scan excludes infection. In the case of positive bone scintigraphy, however, it is necessary to perform a more specific scintigraphy with labeled leukocytes, completed by SPECT/CT imaging in the hip prostheses. This procedure visualizes the spread of the infection in periprosthetic soft tissues and avoids false-positive uptake of labeled leukocytes in bone marrow or in the periarticular calcifications.

In the case of painful prostheses with positive or suspected laboratory parameters for infection or in prostheses implanted since less than 2 years, the search for prosthetic infections must be based on leukocyte scintigraphy or on [^{18}F]FDG PET/CT.

PET/CT is quick to perform and allows exploration of the whole body in search for any foci of infection but also enables to exclude other causes of fever such as tumors. In these cases, the probability of infection is high, and it is important to start the appropriate treatment quickly. Leukocyte scintigraphy, on the other hand, is employed to confirm or exclude a chronic prosthetic infection, as well as in case of a doubtful or non-conclusive PET scan, or in excluding an infection by replanting a prosthesis joint explanted by PJI or mobilization [36].

References

1. Report of R.I.P.O. Regional register of orthopaedic prosthetic implantology in Emilia Romagna. https://ripo.cineca.it/authzssl/pdf/report_eng_2017.pdf.
2. Sloan M, Premkumar A, Sheth NP. Projected volume of primary total joint arthroplasty in the U.S., 2014 to 2030. J Bone Joint Surg Am. 2018;100:1455–60.
3. Ulrich SD, Seyler TM, Bennett D, et al. Total hip arthroplasties: what are the reasons for revision? Int Orthop. 2008;32:597–604.
4. Corvec S, Portillo ME, Pasticci BM, et al. Epidemiology and new developments in the diagnosis of prosthetic joint infection. Int J Artif Organs. 2012;35:923–34.

5. Kurtz S, Ong K, Lau E, et al. Projections of primary and revision hip and knee arthroplasty in the United States from 2005 to 2030. J Bone Joint Surg Am. 2007;89:780–5.
6. Zimmerli W, Trampuz A, Ochsner PE. Prosthetic-joint infections. N Engl J Med. 2004;351:1645–54.
7. Ong KL, Kurtz SM, Lau E, et al. Prosthetic joint infection risk after total hip arthroplasty in the Medicare population. J Arthroplast. 2009;24:105–9.
8. Li C, Renz N, Trampuz A. Management of periprosthetic joint infection. Hip Pelvis. 2018;30:138–46.
9. Lewis SS, Dicks KV, Chen LF, et al. Delay in diagnosis of invasive surgical site infections following knee arthroplasty versus hip arthroplasty. Clin Infect Dis. 2015;60:990–6.
10. Brause BD. Infected orthopedic prostheses. In: Bisno AL, Waldvogel FA, editors. Infections associated with indwelling medical devices. Washington, DC: American Society for Microbiology; 1989. p. 111–27.
11. Steckelberg JM, Osmon DR. Prosthetic joint infections. In: Bisno AL, Waldvogel FA, editors. Infections associated with indwelling medical devices. 3rd ed. Washington, DC: American Society for Microbiology; 2000. p. 173–209.
12. Trampuz A, Steckelberg JM, Osmon DR, et al. Advances in the laboratory diagnosis of prosthetic joint infection. Rev Med Microbiol. 2003;14:1–14.
13. Chen AF, Heller S, Parvizi J. Prosthetic joint infections. Surg Clin North Am. 2014;94:1265–81.
14. Suda AJ, Cieslik A, Grützner PA, et al. Flaps for closure of soft tissue defects in infected revision knee arthroplasty. Int Orthop. 2014;38:1387–92.
15. Osmon DR, Berbari EF, Berendt AR, et al. Diagnosis and management of prosthetic joint infection: clinical practice guidelines by the Infectious Diseases Society of America. Clin Infect Dis. 2013;56:e1–e25.
16. Abad CL, Haleem A. Prosthetic joint infections: an update. Curr Infect Dis Rep. 2018;20:15.
17. Verberne SJ, Raijmakers PG, Temmerman OPP. The accuracy of imaging techniques in the assessment of periprosthetic hip infection. A systematic review and meta-analysis. J Bone Joint Surg Am. 2016;98:1638–45.
18. Duus BR, Boeckstyns M, Kjaer L, Stadeager C. Radionuclide scanning after total knee replacement: correlation with pain and radiolucent lines. A prospective study. Investig Radiol. 1987;22:891–4.
19. Huellner MW, Strobel M. Clinical applications of SPECT/CT in imaging the extremities. Eur J Nucl Med Mol Imaging. 2014;41(Suppl 1):S50–8.
20. Hirschmann MT, Konala P, Iranpour F, et al. Clinical value of SPECT/CT for evaluation of patients with painful knees after total knee arthroplasty—a new dimension of diagnostics? BMC Musculoskelet Disord. 2011;4:12–36.
21. Verlooy H, Victor J, Renson L, et al. Limitations of quantitative radionuclide bone scanning in the evaluation of total knee replacement. Clin Nucl Med. 1993;18:671–4.
22. Elgazzar AH, Abdel-Dayem HM, Clark JD, et al. Multimodality imaging of osteomyelitis. Eur J Nucl Med. 1985;22:1043–63.
23. Palestro CJ, Kim CK, Swyer AJ, et al. Total-hip arthroplasty: periprosthetic indium-111-labeled leukocyte activity and complementary technetium-99m-sulfur colloid imaging in suspected infection. J Nucl Med. 1990;31:1950–5.
24. Prandini N, Feggi LM, Massari L. ^{99m}Tc-HMPAO-WBC three phases scintigraphy in secondary osteomyelitis. Q J Nucl Med. 1996;40(Suppl 1):55.
25. Glaudemans AW, de Vries EF, Vermeulen LE, et al. A large retrospective single-Centre study to define the best image acquisition protocols and interpretation criteria for white blood cell scintigraphy with ^{99m}Tc-HMPAO-labelled leucocytes in musculoskeletal infections. Eur J Nucl Med Mol Imaging. 2013;40:1760–9.
26. Signore A, Sconfienza LM, Borens O, et al. Consensus document for the diagnosis of prosthetic joint infections: a joint paper by the EANM, EBJIS, and ESR (with ESCMID endorsement). Eur J Nucl Med Mol Imaging. 2019;46:971–88.
27. Love C, Tomas MB, Marwin SE, et al. Role of nuclear medicine in diagnosis of the infected joint replacement. Radiographics. 2001;21:1229–38.
28. Van der Bruggen W, Bleeker-Rovers CP, Boerman OC, et al. PET and SPECT in osteomyelitis and prosthetic bone and joint infections: a systematic review. Semin Nucl Med. 2010;40:3–15.
29. Kim HO, Na SJ, Oh SJ, et al. Usefulness of adding SPECT/CT to ^{99m}Tc-hexamethyl-propylene amine oxime (HMPAO)-labeled leukocyte imaging for diagnosing prosthetic joint infections. Comput Assist Tomogr. 2014;38:313–9.
30. Filippi L, Schillaci O. Usefulness of hybrid SPECT/CT in ^{99m}Tc-HMPAO-labeled leukocyte scintigraphy for bone and joint infections. J Nucl Med. 2006;47:1908–13.
31. Gemmel F, Van den Wyngaert H, Love C, et al. Prosthetic joint infections: radionuclide state-of the-art imaging. Eur J Nucl Med Mol Imaging. 2012;39:892–909.
32. Jamar F, Buscombe J, Chiti A, et al. EANM/SNMMI guideline for ^{18}F-FDG use in inflammation and infection. J Nucl Med. 2013;54:647–58.
33. Zoccali C, Teori G, Salducca N. The role of FDG-PET in distinguishing between septic and aseptic loosening in hip prosthesis: a review of literature. Int Orthop. 2009;33:1–5.
34. Manthey N, Reinhard P, Moog F, et al. The use of [^{18}F]fluorodeoxyglucose positron emission tomography to differentiate between synovitis, loosening and infection of hip and knee prostheses. Nucl Med Commun. 2002;23:645–53.
35. Zhuang H, Chacko TK, Hickeson M, et al. Persistent non-specific FDG uptake on PET imaging following hip arthroplasty. Eur J Nucl Med Mol Imaging. 2002;29:1328–33.
36. Prandini N, Lazzeri E, Rossi B, et al. Nuclear medicine imaging of bone infections. Nucl Med Commun. 2006;27:633–44.

Nuclear Medicine Imaging of Vascular Prosthesis Infections

6

Giovanni D'Errico, Emanuele Casciani, and Saadi Sollaku

Contents

Learning Objectives

- To understand the different indications for imaging of vascular infection
- To evaluate the different pros and cons of each nuclear medicine imaging technique
- To acquire basic knowledge of nuclear medicine imaging of vascular prosthesis infection
- To become familiar with the most frequent imaging findings in vascular infection

6.1 Introduction

Vascular graft infection (VGI) is a severe complication that can occur after vascular surgery. It is characterized by high morbidity and mortality rates (around 50% and 25–75%, respectively) and represents one of the most challenging issues for both diagnosis and treatment. Its incidence depends on several risk factors, with reported rates ranging from 1.5% up to 2% for extracavitary grafts and from 1% up to 5% for intracavitary grafts. Moreover, aortic graft erosion or fistulous communication into the duodenum (or generally in the bowel) occurs in 1–2% of patients after aortic reconstruction. The risk of infection is also linked to the fact that more and more patients with comorbidities, such as diabetes mellitus, undergo vascular surgery [1].

G. D'Errico (✉) · E. Casciani · S. Sollaku
Department of Nuclear Medicine, Private Hospital "Pio XI", Rome, Italy

E. Lazzeri et al. (eds.), *Radionuclide Imaging of Infection and Inflammation*, https://doi.org/10.1007/978-3-030-62175-9_6

6.2 Clinical Presentations of Vascular Graft Infections

The clinical presentation depends on the intracavitary or extracavitary localization of infection [2, 3]. Extracavitary VGIs occur in the groin or less frequently in the popliteal fossa or more distantly in the leg. Early onset VGIs (<2 months after surgery) are characterized by fever, leukocytosis, and other signs of sepsis such as erythema, abscess, anastomotic rupture with hemorrhage. Late-onset VGIs (>2 months after surgery) show less typical signs of systemic sepsis and often have a more indolent course.

The intracavitary localization of graft infection represents the most insidious complication, due to lack of physical manifestation and the possibility of clinical onset several months or years after surgery. Intra-abdominal VGIs may present with pain, fever, leukocytosis, failure to thrive, and sepsis. Moreover, the aortic graft can erode into the duodenum with the possibility of important gastrointestinal bleeding and intermittent polymicrobial bacteremia [4].

For the intra-thoracic localization of VGIs, signs and symptoms can mimic infective endocarditis with fever, chills, heart failure, and disruption of anastomotic suture line. Moreover, septic emboli can reach the central nervous system (CNS) or distant peripheral vessels [5].

6.3 Microbiology of Vascular Graft Infections

The use of prophylaxis with antibiotics before vascular surgery has lowered the incidence of VGI. On the other hand, the microorganisms involved in VGI have changed over the years, and it is not rare to find multidrug resistant microorganisms in the site of infection, such as methicillin-resistant *Staphylococcus aureus* (MRSA). The most represented flora consists of Gram-positive cocci (up to 75%) and Gram-negative cocci, *Pseudomonas aeruginosa* being the most frequent (up to 10%) [6].

6.4 Diagnosis of Vascular Graft Infections

Management of infected vascular graft depends on several factors including the position of the infected prosthesis, the extent of infection, and underlying microorganism. The diagnosis is difficult as there is no single diagnostic procedure that has 100% accuracy. The most appropriate diagnostic path should include a physical examination, laboratory tests, and different imaging techniques. Patients with suspected graft infection usually present with local pain, redness, a palpable lump, and/or secretion in the area of the surgical wound, associated with abnormal blood chemistry values. Microbiological cultures (obtained by CT-guided needle aspiration, when technically feasible) may confirm the diagnosis.

Diagnosis is generally difficult on clinical ground alone. In fact, patients may show nonspecific symptoms and signs, and the assessment of the extent of the infection is often the most difficult challenge. Furthermore, blood chemistry parameters can only show moderately elevated white blood cell (WBC) counts, erythrocyte sedimentation rate (ESR), and/or C-reactive protein (CRP) values, which constitute a common and nonspecific finding. When clinical signs are minimal or absent because of low-grade infection, the diagnosis of VGI is uncertain. Nevertheless, it is critically important to avoid complications such as sepsis, aneurysmatic ruptures, gastrointestinal bleeding and suture line disruption. Early and accurate diagnosis is required for the correct choice of treatment, which may include an aggressive surgical procedure with dissection and graft revision in order to remove the infected material. Delay in treatment can lead to sepsis and/or bleeding, with a mortality rate of virtually 100% for gastrointestinal hemorrhage.

Imaging studies are routinely required to confirm or exclude the diagnosis of VGI. Early diagnosis requires highly sensitive and specific imaging modalities, since the consequences of a false-positive result may lead to unnecessary surgery. On the contrary, a false-negative result may be associated with high-risk morbidity and even mortality.

In the case of a potentially infected vascular graft based on clinical features and/or inflammatory markers, the diagnostic approach should begin with imaging technique that are readily available in all healthcare institution (mainly angio-CT and Ultrasounds (US)). Radionuclide imaging studies are usually complementary to radiologic imaging and are reserved to those cases with equivocal conventional imaging or to those where cooperation between vascular surgeon and nuclear medicine physicians allows accurate assessment of the vascular prosthesis status [7].

6.5 Ultrasonography for Detecting Vascular Graft Infections

Ultrasonography with color flow Doppler is the first-line imaging procedure to identify an infected prosthetic vascular graft. This noninvasive, highly cost-effective technique does not involve any risk of contrast allergy and nephrotoxicity and does not expose the patient to ionizing radiation. Unfortunately, in case of an aortic graft, its predictive value is limited by air content in the intestinal lumen and sometimes by abundant subcutaneous fat [8].

6.6 Computed Tomography (CT) for Detecting Vascular Graft Infections

CT is widely available and not only provides diagnostic information but also is useful for surgical planning and guidance for aspiration biopsy. It has 94% sensitivity and 85% specificity. Unfortunately, detection of gas bubbles around the graft, a diagnostic sign of infection, has good specificity but rather low sensitivity (about 50%). Despite several advantages (high specificity, guidance for needle aspiration and microbiological analyses, speed of execution), CT imaging suffers from some limitations such as low sensitivity in detecting low-grade and early post-surgical infections—along with a non-negligible radiation burden to patients [8].

6.7 Magnetic Resonance Imaging for Detecting Vascular Graft Infections

The diagnostic role of magnetic resonance imaging (MRI) in patients with suspected VGI is still unclear. In particular, its sensitivity in detecting peri-graft infection has not been thoroughly investigated and is probably similar to that of CT. Furthermore, MRI suffers from the same limitations as CT imaging for the differential diagnosis of peri-prosthetic fluid accumulation in the first weeks after surgery. Nevertheless, this noninvasive imaging modality provides multiparametric information, which is particularly useful for tissue characterization [8].

6.8 Nuclear Medicine Imaging for Detecting Vascular Graft Infections

Nuclear medicine techniques are characterized by high accuracy in detecting VGI in patients with aortic graft and without specific signs of infection (low-grade stages), even though the possibility of false-positive results must be kept in mind when the infection is localized in the proximity of the prosthesis.

Scintigraphy with ^{99m}Tc-HMPAO-WBC should be performed when morphological imaging (CT and/or MRI) provides equivocal or inconclusive results for the evaluation of VGI, especially in immune-competent patients. Scintigraphy with ^{99m}Tc-antigranulocyte antibodies also has high diagnostic accuracy (95%) when images are acquired both early and late post-injection, although it carries the generic risk of inducing production of human anti-mouse antibodies (HAMA).

The sensitivity of ^{99m}Tc-HMPAO-WBC scintigraphy is very high (reportedly close to 100%), while variable specificity has been reported in different studies (ranging between 62 and 100%). The increasing use of hybrid SPECT/CT scanners enables exact anatomical localization of the focus of infection and thus improves both sensitivity and specificity. ^{99m}Tc-HMPAO-WBC scintigraphy is the nuclear medicine imaging modality of choice for VGI and should be performed (if available) regardless of the results of conventional radiologic imaging. It is important to mention the utility of acquiring a short dynamic sequence of images immediately after injection in order to visualize the vascular blood flow. Subsequently, if SPECT/CT is not available, several projections are required to avoid the background activity of the spine and gut [8, 9].

Limitations of ^{99m}Tc-HMPAO-WBC scintigraphy are its long examination time, which requires the patient's collaboration and a certain time delay before achieving a definite diagnostic information. Moreover, concomitant therapy with antibiotics could lower the diagnostic performance of ^{99m}Tc-HMPAO-WBC scintigraphy [8].

PET/CT with the metabolic tracer [^{18}F]FDG is a well-established nuclear medicine imaging modality, mostly used in the clinical practice to characterize oncologic patients [10]. More recently, the role of [^{18}F]FDG PET/CT has expanded, and this imaging modality is now routinely used for the diagnosis of inflammatory and infectious processes. This hybrid technique provides not only morphological information as that obtained with CT or ultrasonography but can also distinguish active infection from reparative tissue reaction [11].

Recent studies report values of sensitivity and specificity for [^{18}F]FDG PET/CT of 92% and 63%, respectively [12]. A limitation of [^{18}F]FDG are false-positive results from aseptic inflammatory processes in the proximity of vascular prosthesis that lead to the rather low value of specificity [13]. The reason behind these false-positive results is the [^{18}F]FDG uptake in neutrophils and macrophages located in a sterile inflammation site. In fact, synthetic grafts, implanted devices, or surgical bio-glue can trigger a foreign-body reaction resulting in sterile inflammation [14, 15]. The standardized uptake value (SUV) has not been validated in inflammation and infection. There are no general criteria published for inflammatory and infectious disorders. Some authors have reported 6.3 SUV as a good cut-off value for differential diagnosis of these two processes [12].

The main characteristics of ^{99m}Tc-HMPAO-WBC scintigraphy and [^{18}F]FDG PET/CT are illustrated in Table 6.1.

Key Learning Points

- The first-line approach in VGI includes ultrasonography and CT for acute infection.
- Labeled-leukocyte scintigraphy (generally ^{99m}Tc-HMPAO-WBC) is the modality of choice for VGI and should be performed regardless of the results of radiologic imaging.
- Late onset complication should be assessed with [^{18}F]FDG PET/CT.
- Pitfalls of [^{18}F]FDG PET/CT imaging include false-positive associated with sterile inflammatory processes.

Table 6.1 Main characteristics of ^{99m}Tc-HMPAO-WBC scintigraphy and [^{18}F]FDG PET/CT for infection imaging

	^{99m}Tc-HMPAO-WBC scintigraphy	[^{18}F]FDG PET/CT
Sensitivity	Moderate	High
Specificity	High	Moderate
Effective radiation dose[a]	11.0 μSv/MBq (185–370 MBq per exam)	19.0 μSv/MBq (175–350 MBq per exam)
Required imaging time	2–24 h	1–2 h
Image quality	Low, moderate with hybrid imaging	High
Main limitations	Need for trained operator for in vitro labeling Long acquisition and labeling time	Possible false positives in case of sterile inflammation

[a]Source: EANM "Guidelines for the labeling of leukocytes with ^{99m}Tc-HMPAO" and "EANM/SNMMI Guideline for [^{18}F]FDG use in inflammation and infection"

Acknowledgments The authors express their gratitude to Cristina De Angelis, MD (Department of Radiological Sciences, Oncology and Anatomo-Pathology, "Sapienza" University of Rome, Italy) and Giacomo Gambaretto (Department of Radiology of the Private Hospital "Pio XI", Rome, Italy) for their precious contribution.

Clinical Cases

Case 6.1

Background

A 61-year-old patient with aorto-bisiliac prosthesis implanted 6 years before and recent development of fever. CT angiography performed 2 months previously revealed only a slight iodinated contrast endoleak without sign of infection in the prosthesis. In the same period, a blood test showed high level of ESR, C-reactive protein, and leukocytes count.

Scintigraphy with ^{99m}Tc-HMPAO-WBC was performed 5 min (early acquisition, Fig. 6.1a) and 1 h (late acquisition, Fig. 6.1b) post-injection. The late acquisition showed abnormal WBC accumulation in the common right iliac artery (arrow). CT angiography (Fig. 6.1c) did not reveal any morphologic abnormality, while the fused SPECT/CT image (Fig. 6.1d) confirmed the localization of WBC hyperaccumulation in the distal portion of the right iliac component of the vascular prosthesis (arrow).

Suspected Site of Disease

Aorto-bisiliac vascular prosthesis.

Radiopharmaceutical Activity

^{99m}Tc-HMPAO-WBC, 540 MBq.

Imaging

Planar acquisitions at 5 min and 1 h after administration of the radiolabeled leukocytes. SPECT/CT imaging acquired immediately after acquisition of the 1-h planar image.

Conclusion/Teaching Points

A patient with strong clinical suspicion of infection but negative CT angiography should undergo a ^{99m}Tc-HMPAO-WBC scintigraphy to exclude or confirm with certainty infection of the vascular prosthesis.

Case 6.2

Background

A 69-year-old patient with endovascular aorto-bisiliac prosthesis, recent onset of fever, and increased serum levels of ESR, C-reactive protein, and leukocytes count.

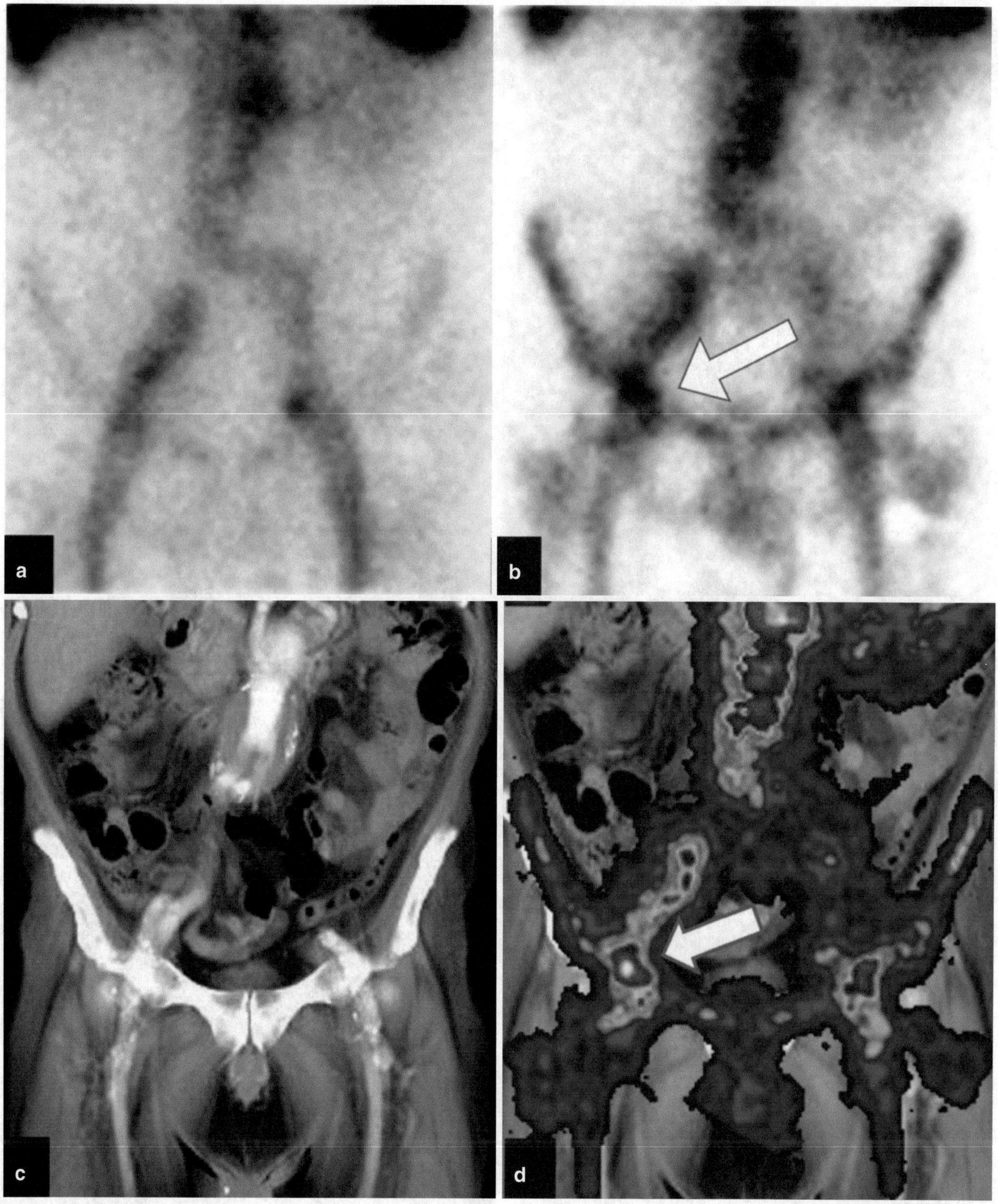

Fig. 6.1 See text

Scintigraphy with ^{99m}Tc-HMPAO-WBC was acquired 5-min (early acquisition, Fig. 6.2a) and 1 h (late acquisition, Fig. 6.2b, c). Anterior and right anterior oblique views of late acquisition (Fig. 6.2b, c) showed a focus of pathologic accumulation of WBC in the median abdominal region (arrow). CT angiography (Fig. 6.2d) revealed a peri-aortic abscess collection medially to the psoas muscle (arrowhead). The fused SPECT/CT fused image (Fig. 6.2e) localized the focus

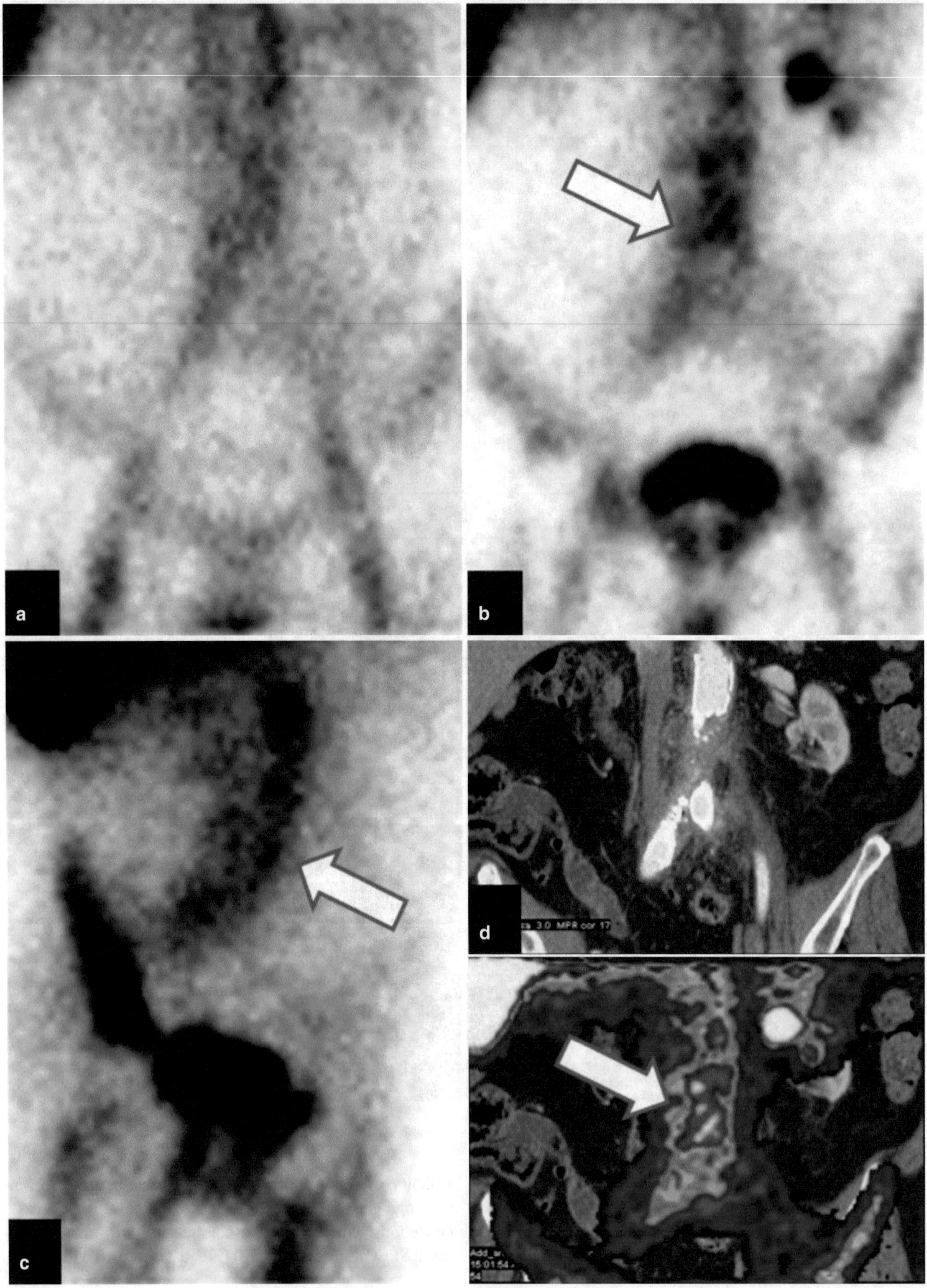

Fig. 6.2 See text

of WBC hyperaccumulation in the aortic component of the vascular prosthesis (arrow).

Suspected Site of Disease

Endovascular aorto-bisiliac prosthesis.

Radiopharmaceutical Activity

^{99m}Tc-HMPAO-WBC, 540 MBq.

Imaging

Planar acquisitions at 5 min and 1 h after administration of the radiolabeled leukocytes. SPECT/CT imaging acquired immediately after acquisition of the 1-h planar image.

Conclusion/Teaching Points

The use of hybrid imaging SPECT/CT offers great help not only in detecting the presence of infectious foci but also in localizing precisely the anatomical site of infection.

Case 6.3

Background

A 59-year-old patient with endovascular aorto-bisiliac prosthesis implanted 1 year earlier. CT angiography performed 1 month previously showed confluent corpuscular fluid collections with air bubbles adjacent to the endoprosthesis throughout its entire course. The most bulky collection was located on the left side expanding in part in the psoas muscle and adjacent to L4.

Scintigraphy with ^{99m}Tc-HMPAO-WBC was performed 5 min (early acquisition, Fig. 6.3a) and 1 h post-injection (late acquisition, Fig. 6.3b, c). The planar anterior and right anterior-oblique late views showed a focal accumulation of labeled leukocytes (arrow) in the vascular prosthesis (dashed red line) adjacent to the left edge of the lumbar column. The fused SPECT/CT image (Fig. 6.3d) localized WBC hyperaccumulation in the aortic component of the vascular prosthesis (arrow).

Suspected Site of Disease

Aorto-bisiliac vascular prosthesis.

Radiopharmaceutical Activity

^{99m}Tc-HMPAO-WBC, 550 MBq.

Imaging

Planar acquisitions at 5 min and 1 h after administration of the radiolabeled leukocytes. SPECT/CT imaging acquired immediately after acquisition of the 1-h planar image.

Conclusion/Teaching Points

The use of hybrid SPECT/CT imaging is crucial for identifying exact anatomical location of the infection.

Case 6.4

Background

A 71-year-old patient with aorto-bifemoral by-pass implanted 4 years earlier. The patient was admitted to the hospital after the recent onset of fever and appearance of a lump located in the left groin. A CT angiography scan revealed a corpuscular fluid collection adjacent to the left distal vascular prosthesis. This collection reached the left iliac fossa and superficially the left groin.

Scintigraphy with ^{99m}Tc-HMPAO-WBC was performed 5 min (early acquisition, Fig. 6.4a) and 1 h (late acquisition, Fig. 6.4b, c) post-injection. The planar anterior early acquisition showed faint accumulation of labeled leukocytes (arrowhead). The anterior and left anterior oblique late views (Fig. 6.4b, c) showed a more definite focus of abnormally increased accumulation of labeled WBC in the left iliac fossa and in the ipsilateral groin region (arrows). The fused SPECT/CT image (Fig. 6.4d) localized WBC hyperaccumulation along the left branch and the distal anastomosis of the aorto-bifemoral bypass previously implanted (arrows).

Suspected Site of Disease

Aorto-bifemoral bypass.

Radiopharmaceutical Activity

^{99m}Tc-HMPAO-WBC, 535 MBq.

Imaging

Planar acquisitions at 5 min and 1 h after administration of the radiolabeled leukocytes. SPECT/CT imaging acquired immediately after acquisition of the 1-h planar image.

Conclusion/Teaching Points

The use of hybrid imaging CT/SPECT is crucial for identifying exact anatomical location of the infection.

Case 6.5

Background

A 51-year-old patient with rheumatic fever and secondary annulo-aortic ectasia treated with aortic composite valve graft about 18 months earlier. Approximately 1 year later, the patient was treated for an episode of endocarditis caused by *Enterococcus faecalis*, complicated with inferior limb ischemia. A few months later, the patient was admitted to the hospital after the onset of fever preceded by chills, peaks of 38 °C, dysuria, myalgia, and increased inflammation indexes. A relapsed endocarditis was suspected; this clinical suspicion was then confirmed with blood cultures and transesophageal echocardiography, which showed an iso-echogenic mass adherent to the aortic prosthetic valve.

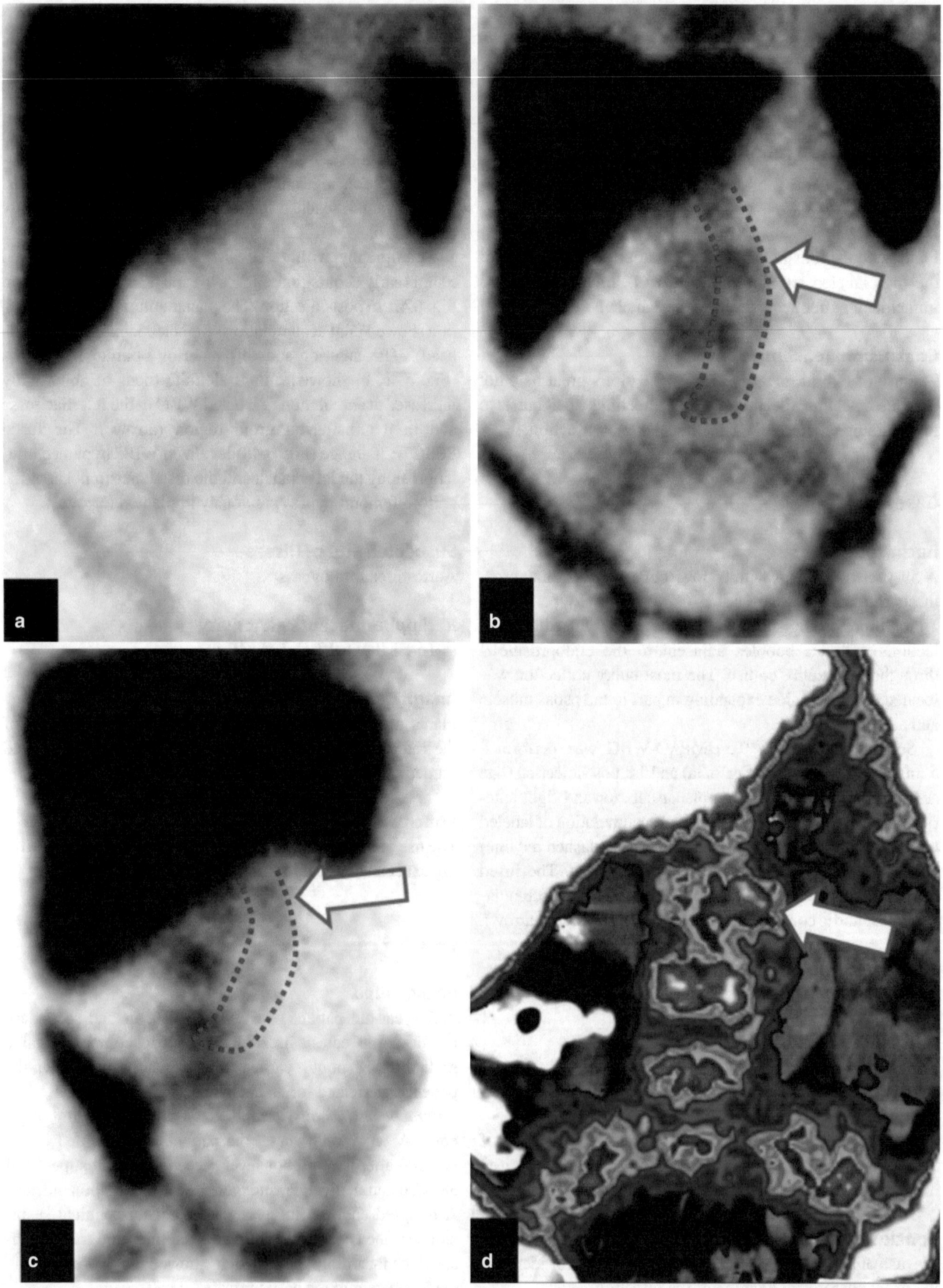

Fig. 6.3 See text

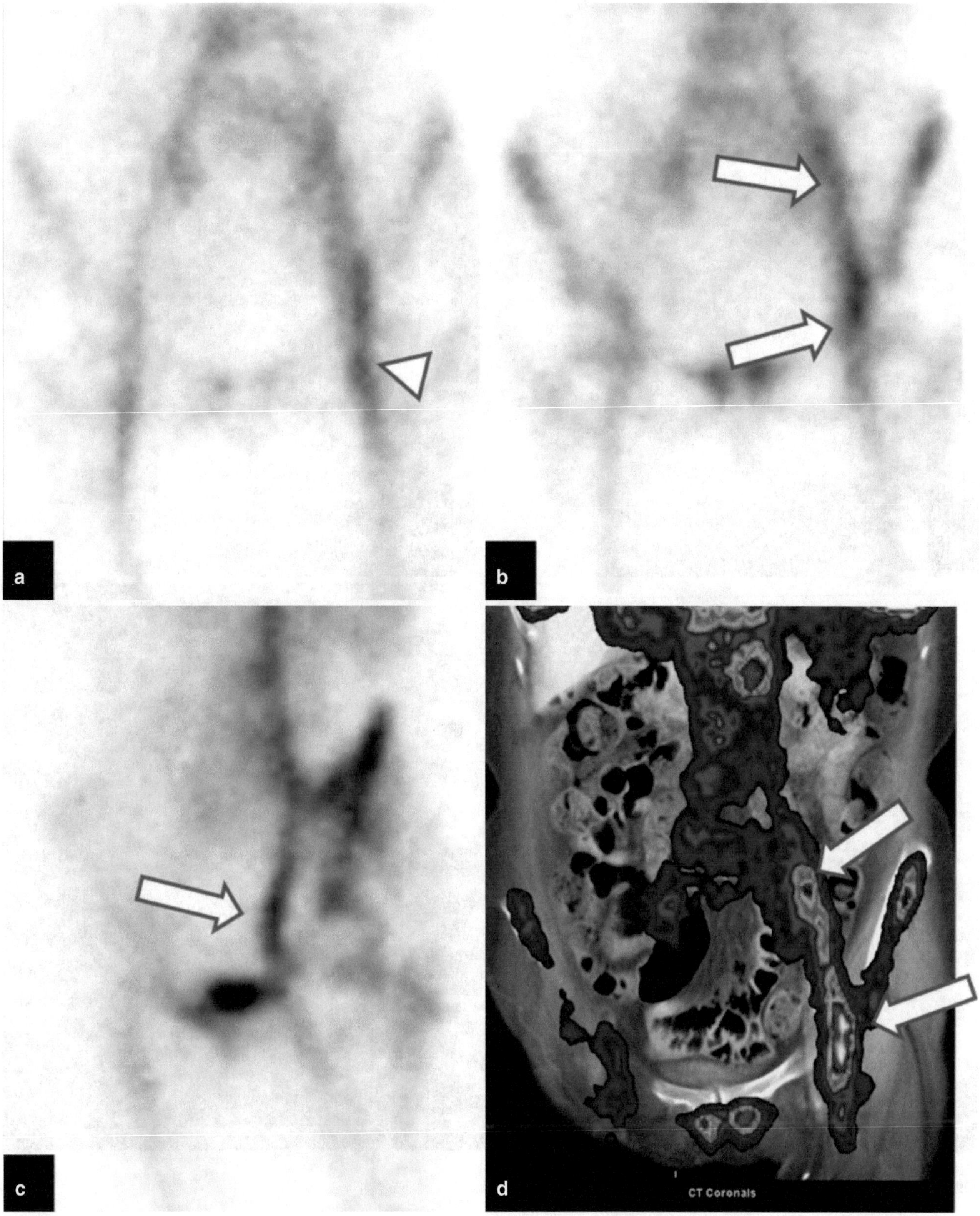

Fig. 6.4 See text

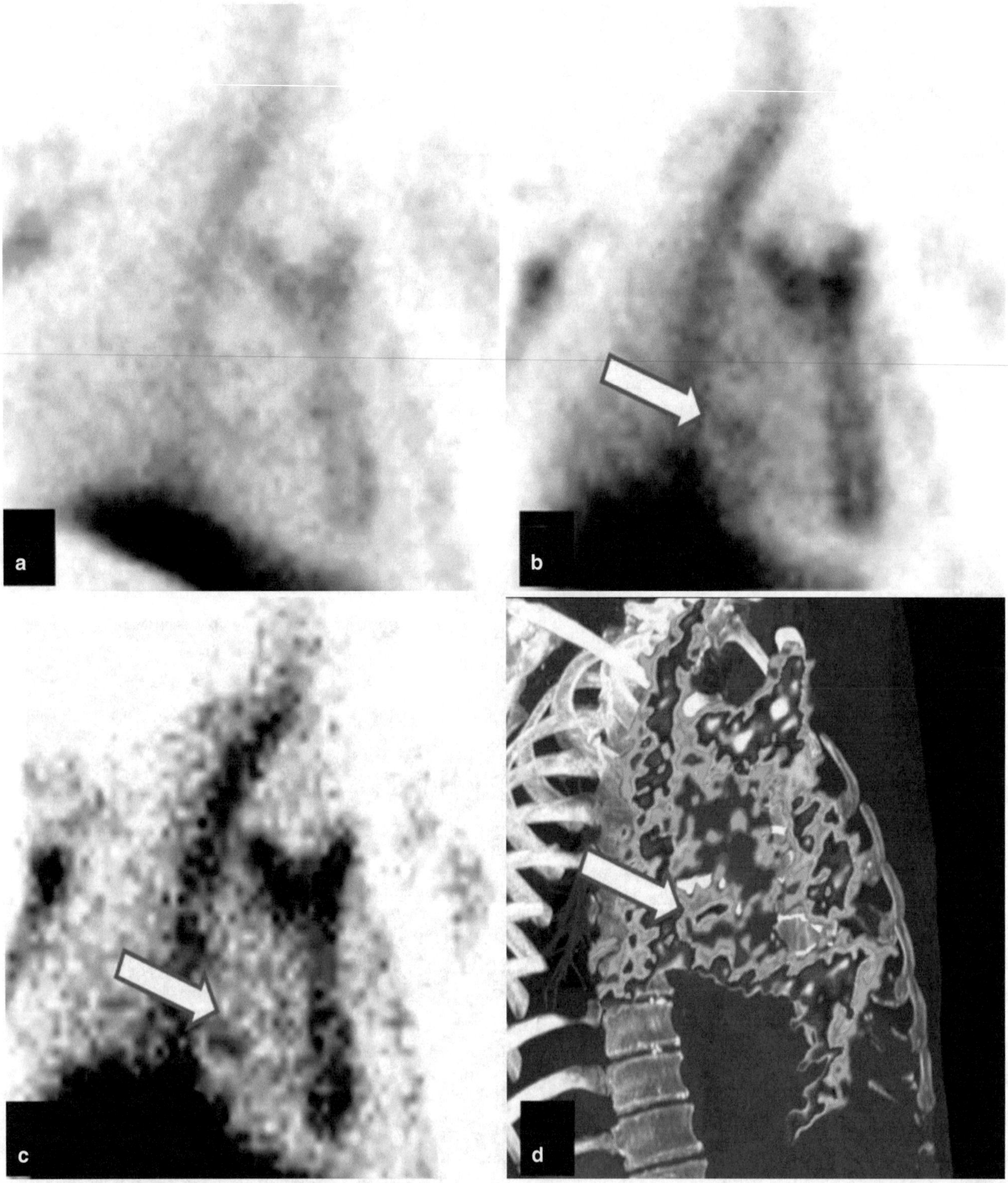

Fig. 6.5 See text

^{99m}Tc-HMPAO-WBC whole-body scintigraphy was performed without discontinuing high-dose antibiotic therapy and resulted in a negative scan (Fig. 6.5a). Two months later, the scintigraphy was repeated without the interference of antibiotics, with acquisitions at 3 h (Fig. 6.5b) and at 24 h (Fig. 6.5c). The scan revealed a focal area of increased accumulation of labeled leukocytes in the mediastinum (arrow). The fused SPECT/CT image confirmed localization of the focus of infection in the aortic graft (arrow).

Suspected Site of Disease
Infection of the aortic composite valve graft.

Radiopharmaceutical Activity
^{99m}Tc-HMPAO-WBC, 530 MBq.

Imaging
Planar acquisitions at 3 and 24 h after administration of the radiolabeled leukocytes. SPECT/CT imaging acquired after acquisition of planar images.

Conclusion/Teaching Points
When planning scintigraphy with labeled autologous leukocytes, attention must be paid to the current therapy administered to the patient. Several antibiotics can alter leukocytes motility, thus increasing the risk of a false-negative result. When clinical signs strongly suggest the presence of an infectious focus, a negative ^{99m}Tc-HMPAO-WBC scintigraphy should be repeated after withholding antibiotic therapy for an adequate period.

Case 6.6

Background
An 84-year-old man with aortic graft implanted 6 months earlier and recent development of fever, pre-sternal fluid collection, and high level of ESR, C-reactive protein, and leukocyte count.

[^{18}F]FDG PET/CT was performed because of clinical suspicion of infection of the aortic graft. Tomographic sections of the chest at different levels in the transaxial (Fig. 6.6a–c), coronal (Fig. 6.6d), and sagittal (Fig. 6.6e) planes, and 3D surface volume rendering of PET/CT fused with angiography (Fig. 6.6f) show aortic valve and distal graft (white arrow in Fig. 6.6a, d, f) focal uptakes (SUV_{max} 5.5) associated with sternum and soft tissues fluid collection (black arrow in Fig. 6.6c–e) and mediastinum fistula (arrowhead in Fig. 6.6b, c, e) uptakes (SUV_{max} 4.8).

Suspected Site of Disease
Aortic graft, sternum.

Radiopharmaceutical Activity
[^{18}F]FDG, 330 MBq.

Imaging
Unenhanced CT and PET images were acquired consecutively 60 min after injection of 330 MBq of [^{18}F]FDG using a PET/CT system combining a multislice spiral CT scanner with a full-ring PET scanner. Arterial contrast-enhanced CT was obtained after the injection of 135 mL iodinated contrast media.

Conclusion/Teaching Points
The use of [^{18}F]FDG PET/CT and CT angiography with fusion imaging offers great help not only for detecting the presence of infectious foci but also for localizing precisely the site(s) of infection.

Case 6.7

Background
A 2-year-old child affected by immune deficiency because of chromosome 22q11.2 deletion (DiGeorge syndrome) with conotruncal heart defects was treated with implantation of a BioPulmonic® valve in the right ventricular outflow tract. Fever and increased serum levels of the inflammation indexes suggested to perform [^{18}F]FDG PET/CT, after a CT angiography yielded inconclusive findings.

Tomographic sections in the transaxial (Fig. 6.7a, b) and coronal (Fig. 6.7c) planes, and 3D surface volume rendering of PET/CT fused with angiography (Fig. 6.7d, e) show focally increased [^{18}F]FDG uptake in the bioconduit valve (dashed red line in **a** and **c**) (SUV_{max} 4, arrow), thus confirming the clinical suspicion of infection.

The BioPulmonic® valve was replaced, and microbiology of the explanted valve confirmed infection due to *Staphylococcus aureus*, *Staphylococcus epidermidis*, and saccharomyces.

Suspected Site of Disease
BioPulmonic® valve.

Radiopharmaceutical Activity
[^{18}F]FDG, 55 MBq.

Imaging
After sedation, unenhanced CT and PET images were acquired consecutively 60 min after injection of [^{18}F]FDG using a PET/CT system combining a multislice spiral CT scanner with a full-ring PET scanner. For post-acquisition processing, the [^{18}F]FDG PET/CT and arterial-phase contrast-enhanced CT images were fused using a dedicated workstation, in order to define the precise anatomical position of the site(s) of focally increased [^{18}F]FDG uptake.

Conclusion/Teaching Points
A patient with prior cardiovascular prosthesis and clinical suspicion of infection should undergo [^{18}F]FDG PET/CT to look for infection of vascular prosthesis after an inconclusive CT angiography. Post-acquisition processing for fusion imaging can help to localize more precisely the site of infection in particular settings such as a child with biologic prosthesis.

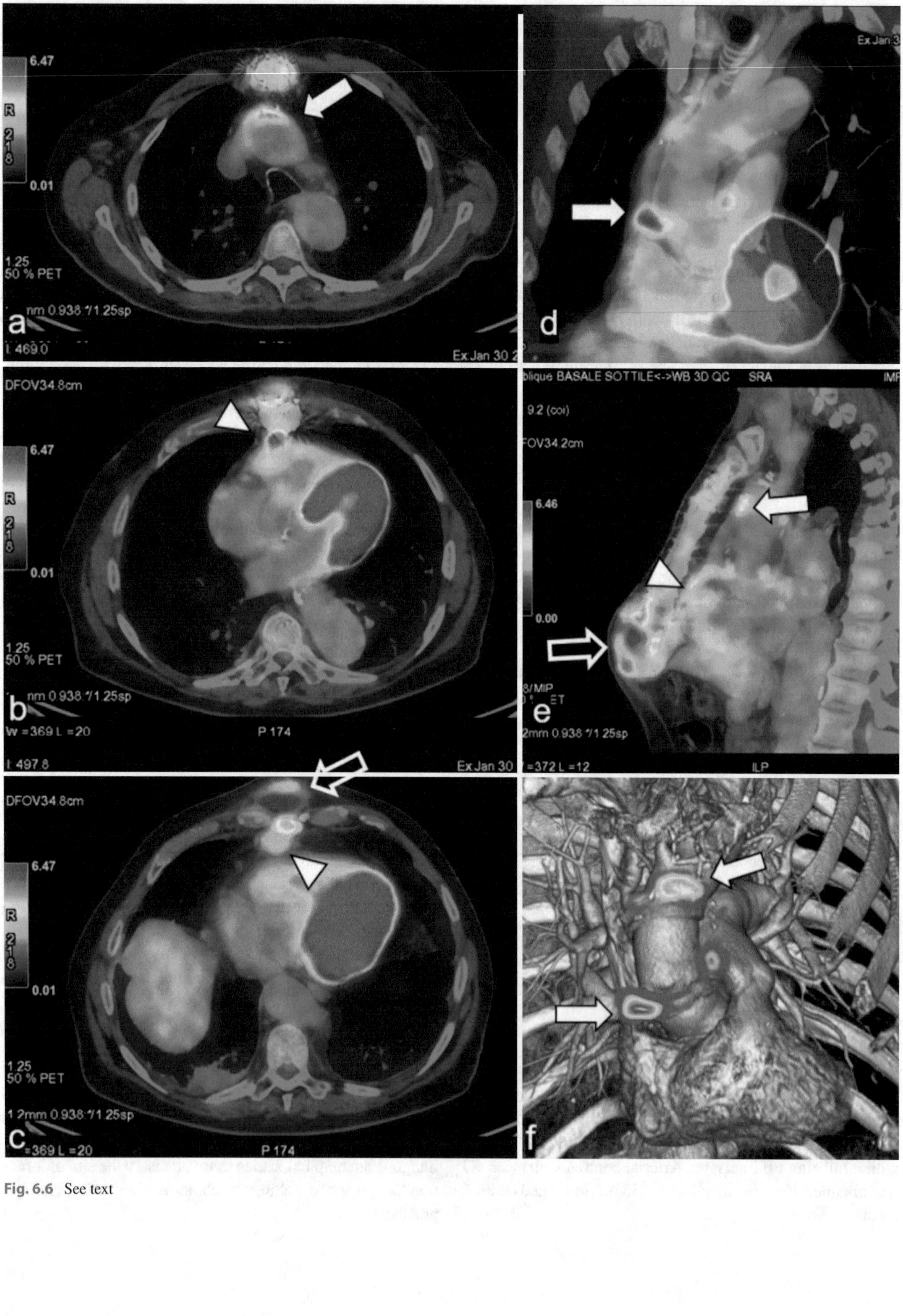

Fig. 6.6 See text

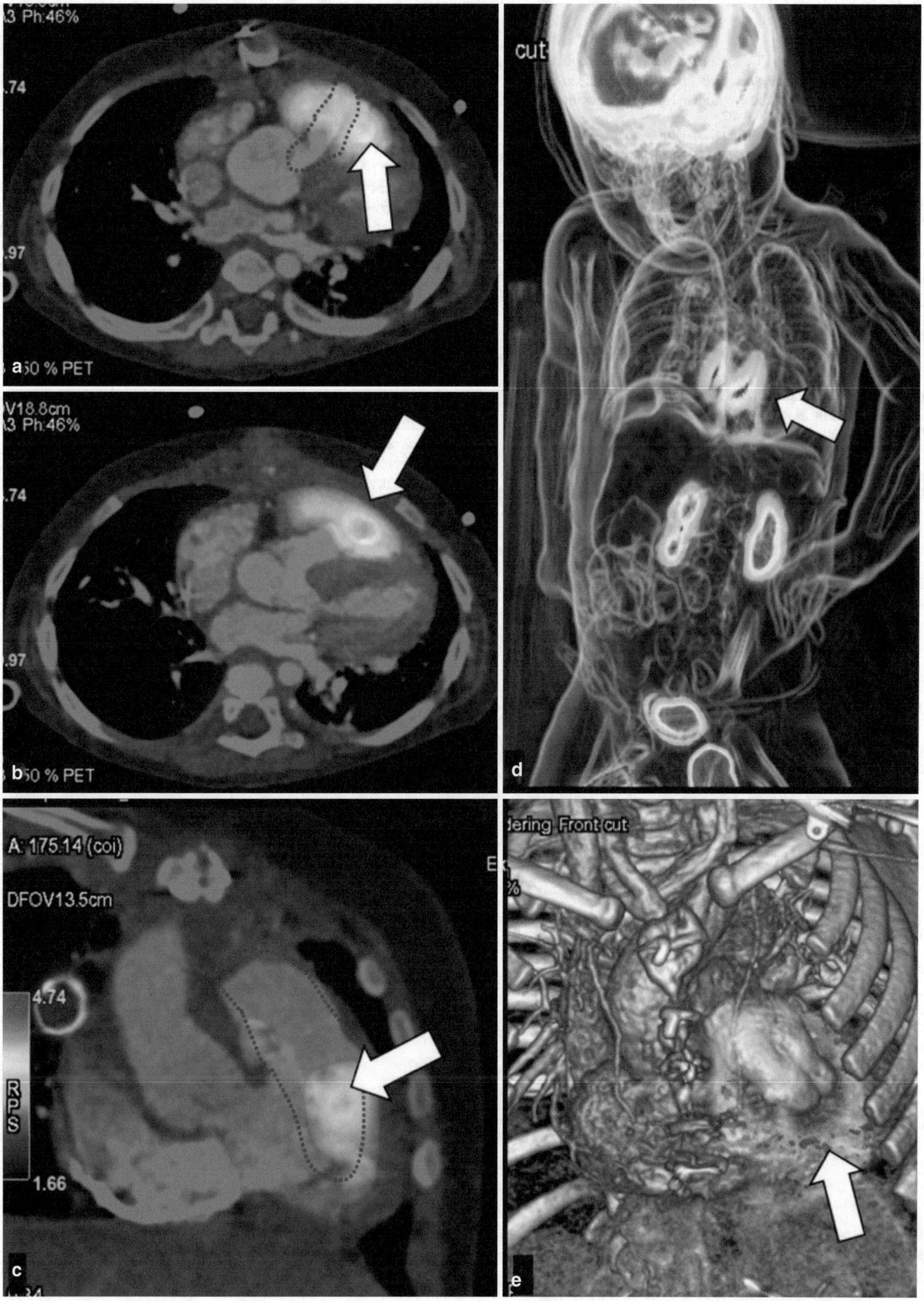

Fig. 6.7 See text

References

1. Wilson WR, Bower TC, Creager MA, et al. Vascular graft infections, mycotic aneurysms, and endovascular infections: a scientific statement from the American Heart Association. Circulation. 2016;134:e412–60.
2. Lyons OT, Baguneid M, Barwick TD, et al. Diagnosis of aortic graft infection: a case definition by the management of aortic graft infection collaboration (MAGIC). Eur J Vasc Endovasc Surg. 2016;52:758–63.
3. Zetrenne E, Wirth GA, McIntosh BC, Evans GR, Narayan D. Managing extracavitary prosthetic vascular graft infections: a pathway to success. Ann Plast Surg. 2006;57:677–82.
4. Swain TW 3rd, Calligaro KD, Dougherty MD. Management of infected aortic prosthetic grafts. Vasc Endovasc Surg. 2004;38:75–82.
5. Bianco V, Kilic A, Gleason TG, Arnaoutakis GJ, Sultan I. Management of thoracic aortic graft infections. J Card Surg. 2018;33:658–65.
6. Gharamti A, Kanafani ZA. Vascular graft infections: an update. Infect Dis Clin N Am. 2018;32:789–809.
7. Li HL, Chan YC, Cheng SW. Current evidence on management of aortic stent-graft infection: a systematic review and meta-analysis. Ann Vasc Surg. 2018;51:306–13.
8. Spacek M, Jindrak V, Spunda R, et al. Current trends in the diagnosis of vascular prosthesis infection. Acta Chir Belg. 2012;112:405–13.
9. Medricka M, Janeckova J, Koranda P, Buriankova E, Bachleda P. ^{18}F-FDG PET/CT and ^{99m}Tc-HMPAO-WBC SPECT/CT effectively contribute to early diagnosis of infection of arteriovenous graft for hemodialysis. Biomed Pap Med Fac Univ Palacky Olomouc Czech Repub. 2019;163:341–8.
10. Rojoa D, Kontopodis N, Antoniou SA, Ioannou CV, Antoniou GA. ^{18}F-FDG PET in the diagnosis of vascular prosthetic graft infection: a diagnostic test accuracy meta-analysis. Eur J Vasc Endovasc Surg. 2019;57:292–301.
11. Fukuchi K, Ishida Y, Higashi M, et al. Detection of aortic graft infection by fluorodeoxyglucose positron emission tomography: comparison with computed tomographic findings. J Vasc Surg. 2005;42:919–25.
12. Mitra A, Pencharz D, Davis M, Wagner T. Determining the diagnostic value of ^{18}F-fluorodeoxyglucose positron emission/computed tomography in detecting prosthetic aortic graft infection. Ann Vasc Surg. 2018;53:78–85.
13. Youngstein T, Tombetti E, Mukherjee J, et al. FDG uptake by prosthetic arterial grafts in large vessel vasculitis is not specific for active disease. JACC Cardiovasc Imaging. 2017;10:1042–52.
14. Dilsizian V, Chandrashekhar Y. Distinguishing active vasculitis from sterile inflammation and graft infection: a call for a more specific imaging target. JACC Cardiovasc Imaging. 2017;10:1085–7.
15. Schouten LR, Verberne HJ, Bouma BJ, van Eck-Smit BL, Mulder BJ. Surgical glue for repair of the aortic root as a possible explanation for increased F-18 FDG uptake. J Nucl Cardiol. 2008;15:146–7.

Nuclear Medicine Imaging of Non-orthopedic or Cardiovascular Implantable Device Infection

7

Paola Anna Erba, Francesco Bartoli, Roberta Zanca, and Martina Sollini

Contents

P. A. Erba (✉) · F. Bartoli · R. Zanca
Department of Translational Research and Advanced Technologies in Medicine and Surgery, Regional Center of Nuclear Medicine, University of Pisa, Pisa, Italy
e-mail: paola.erba@unipi.it

M. Sollini
Department of Biomedical Sciences, Humanitas University, Pieve Emanuele, Italy

Humanitas Clinical and Research Center - IRCCS, Rozzano, Italy

Learning Objectives

- To become familiar with the most relevant devices currently used in clinical practice
- To understand the clinical problem of device-related infections

E. Lazzeri et al. (eds.), *Radionuclide Imaging of Infection and Inflammation*, https://doi.org/10.1007/978-3-030-62175-9_7

- To learn the process of biofilm formation on devices and its implication in the treatment of device-related infections
- To understand the requirements of an imaging procedure to be used in the diagnostic algorithm of device-related infections
- To learn the clinical features of the most relevant implantable device-related infections of interest to nuclear medicine
- To understand the most adequate diagnostic strategy for each implantable device-related infection, with particular regard to the role of nuclear medicine imaging in the diagnostic algorithm

7.1 Introductory Background

The use of implantable medical devices (IMDs) has increased in "modern" medical and surgical practice [1]. Such devices may be utilized only over a short time, or intermittently (months/years), or permanently. These devices are associated with a small but clinically important risk of foreign body infections [2–4], as the presence of any foreign body significantly increases the risk of infection [5].

The total number of medical devices implanted each year in the United States, the risk of infection associated with first-time insertion of medical devices, and ascribed mortality are reported in Table 7.1 [6]. These data illustrate that there are major differences in the impact of infections associated with various medical devices. For instance, the number of indwelling bladder catheters inserted each year in the United States exceeds that of central venous catheters (CVCs) by at least sixfold, and the overall rate of catheter-related urinary tract infection is higher than that of bloodstream infection associated with CVCs [7]. However, the vast majority of cases of catheter-related urinary tract infection involve only the lower urinary tract and have a low expected mortality rate (<5%), whereas 5–25% of patients, particularly those critically ill [8], may not survive an episode of vascular catheter-related bloodstream infection (moderate mortality). Infections of all intravascular medical devices, including vascular grafts, cardiac pacemakers, mechanical heart valves, and left-ventricular assist devices are considered life-threatening, prosthetic valve endocarditis being associated with the highest risk of mortality (>25%) [9]. However, also when mortality of infections associated with certain devices is low, such infections can result in major morbidity. For instance, infections of medical devices implanted in sexual organs, including mammary [10] and penile [11] implants, can cause major disfigurement and serious psychological trauma although they rarely result in death. Moreover, the true rates of device-associated infection may be higher than those reported because (1) the rate of infection associated with reimplanted devices exceeds that of first-time implants by several-fold [12], (2) the rates of device-associated infection are also usually higher in patients in whom the infected implants have been only partially explanted [13], and (3) microbiology results might have relatively low yield because of inadequate culture sampling [14], failure to culture organisms located in the biofilm, and use of antibiotics before the appropriate diagnostic cultures are obtained, thereby possibly yielding false-negative results [15].

Over the next decades, exacerbation of this problem can be expected as vulnerability to microbial pathogens increases in elderly, immuno-compromised, and hospitalized populations. In fact, the risk for device-related infections is not uniformly distributed. The overall risk of device-related infection (DRI) across a population is around 1%. However, the risk of infection is not uniformly spread with this average value uniformly across all individuals (i.e., everyone would have the same 1% chance of developing an infection). Rather, and more realistically, there is a highly nonuniform model of risk distribution according to which 90% of the population is at very low risk (approximately zero) while 10% of the population is vulnerable. Individuals in this susceptible decile of the population each have a 10% risk of developing infection. Therefore, in this simplified and hypothetical scenario, individuals in the risk-free group would be those without any risk factors, whereas individuals in the high-risk group would be those with one or more risk factors. While reality is certainly more complex, it seems likely that the distribution of risk for DRI is highly skewed. Some estimate for the size of the vulnerable subpopulation

Table 7.1 Total number of medical devices inserted each year in the United States, risk of infection associated with first-time insertion of medical devices, and attributable mortality (modified from [6])

Device	Estimates number insert in US/year	Rate of infections (%)	Mortality
Bladder catheters	>3,000,000	10–30	Low
Central venous catheters	5,000,000	3–8	Moderate
Fracture fixation devices	2,000,000	5–10	Low
Dental implants	1,000,000	5–10	Low
Joint prosthesis	600,000	1–3	Low
Vascular graft	450,000	1–5	Moderate
Cardiac PM	300,000	1–7	Moderate
Mammary implants (pairs)	130,000	1–2	Low
Mechanical heart valves	85,000	1–3	High
Penile implants	15,000	1–3	Low
Heart assist devices	700	25–50	High

Table 7.2 Summary of statistically significant risk factors for biofilm infections for all devices

	N	$P < 0.1$	%	OR
Immunomodulation/steroid	11	10	91	4–98
Renal disease	9	8	89	2–24
Diabetes	21	15	71	3–31
Smoking	11	6	55	3–64
BMI	12	6	50	3–16
Age	15	7	47	–

N = number of studies in which a particular risk factor was examined; $P < 0.1$ = number of these studies in which the p-value for significance of the risk factor was less than 0.1; % = percentage of studies with significance for the risk factor; OR = odds ratio

Table 7.3 Frequencies of comorbidities in total patient populations receiving an implanted device

	N	Mean ± SD
Smoking	11	21.2 ± 13.6
High BMI	8	17.7 ± 8.0
Diabetes	13	12.7 ± 8.4
Immunomodulation/steroid	3	6.7 ± 4.8
Alcohol abuse/cirrhosis	1	2.5
Renal disease/hemodialysis	6	2.3 ± 1.4

The uncertainty indicated for the mean is the standard deviation. N = number of the studies reporting a frequency value

has been recently provided by an analysis of the frequency of co-morbidities [16]. This size ranged from as low as 2% for renal disease to 21% for smoking. Across all risk factors included in Table 7.2, the mean at-risk population size was 11%. This analysis oversimplifies the real world, which includes individuals receiving the same device who have different risk factors and individuals with multiple risk factors (see Table 7.3).

Device-related infection results from the multifaceted interaction of bacterial, device, and host factor. Loss of integrity of the body surface as a consequence of implantable medical device implants constitutes the direct/indirect route of access of microorganisms [17]. The plastic materials, which devices are made of, are easily colonized by either bacteria and/or fungi [18]. Multiresistant nosocomial pathogens are the most common organisms colonizing the surface of catheters where they can proliferate with high speed (with rates up to 0.5 cm/h) [1, 19].

Thorough understanding of how a biofilm forms on the surface of medical devices is crucial to understand the pathogenesis of their infection. A biofilm is not a static, film-like slime layer, but rather is a living organism composed of multiple species of bacteria and their secreted polysaccharide matrix, as well as components deposited from body fluids [20–22]. Biofilm formation is a multi-step process, in which bacteria first adhere to the surface (initial attachment phase) and subsequently form cell–cell aggregates (microcolonies), developing a young biofilm followed by differentiation of structured mature biofilm and dispersal (accumulative phase) [23, 24]. The first step in the formation of a device-associated biofilm is the deposition of a conditioning film on the surface. The nature of this conditioning film depends on the type of fluid present around the device. For example, vascular catheters rapidly acquire a sleeve of fibrin and fibronectin, while urinary catheters become encrusted with proteins, electrolytes, and other organic molecules from the host's urine [21, 22, 25]. Once the catheter has acquired a conditioning film, the features of the underlying catheter surface may be partially or completely altered. Therefore, the conditioning film favors microbial attachment [20]. Other factors that influence attachment include hydrophobic and electrostatic forces, cell-surface structures such as pili or flagella, and shear stress from the fluid environment [20, 25–27]. Under unfavorable environmental conditions, microorganisms can detach from the biofilm and become free-floating, or "planktonic" [22]. The presence of planktonic organisms in the bloodstream or urine can lead in turn to symptomatic host infection.

Biofilms have major medical significance because (1) they reduce susceptibility to antimicrobial agents, and (2) microbiology laboratory results based on planktonic organisms may not apply to sessile organisms embedded within a biofilm. The reduced susceptibility to antimicrobial agents within a biofilm arises from multiple factors including physical barrier to diffusion of antimicrobial agents, reduced bacterial growth rates, and local alterations of the microenvironment that may impair activity of the antimicrobial agent [28, 29]. Bacteria in biofilms are 100–1000 times more resistant to antibiotics than "planktonic" cells [30, 31].

As mentioned above, the incidence of infection varies according to the medical device involved, the clinical setting (i.e., nosocomial setting), and the patient population [32]. The most relevant among all the IMDs available are listed here below, and in this chapter we describe those of interest to nuclear medicine.

Intravascular devices:

- Peripheral catheters (venous, arterial).
- Midline catheters.
- Central venous catheters (CVCs).
  - Non-tunneled catheters (Cook, Arrow).
  - Tunneled catheters (Hickman, Broviac, Groshong).
- Pulmonary artery catheters.
- Totally implanted ports (Port-a-Cath, MediPort, Infuse-port).

Neurosurgical devices:

- Ventricular shunts.
- Ommaya reservoirs.
- Intracranial pressure devices.
- Implantable neurological stimulators.

Respiratory devices:

- Endotracheal tubes.
- Tracheotomy.
- Nasal masks.

Abdominal devices:

- Mesh used for hernioplasty.
- Peritoneal dialysis catheters.

Urological devices:

- Urinary catheters.
- Inflatable penile implants.

Gynecological devices:

- Breast implants.

Otolaryngological devices:

- Cochlear implants.
- Middle-ear implants.

Opthalmological devices:

- Intraocular lenses.
- Glaucoma tubes.

Dental devices:

- Dental implants.

Key Learning Points

- The use of IMDs has increased in "modern" medical and surgical practice.
- There are major differences in the impact of infections associated with different medical devices.
- Implantable device-related infections are associated with high mortality; despite low mortality in the case of certain devices, such infections can result in major morbidity.
- Exacerbation of DRI can be expected as vulnerability to microbial pathogen increases in elderly, immunocompromised, and hospitalized populations.
- Infection rates vary among device type, with an overall across population around 1%; however, the risk of infection is not uniformly spread with this average value uniformly across all individuals.
- Device-related infection results from the multifaceted interaction of bacterial, device, and host factor.
- Multiresistant nosocomial pathogens are the most common organisms colonizing the surface of devices, where they can proliferate.
- Biofilm formed on the surface of medical devices is a crucial factor in the pathogenesis of the infection.
- Biofilms reduce susceptibility to antimicrobial agents, as well as the sensitivity of microbiological testing.

7.2 Infections of Central Venous Catheters

Central venous catheters (CVCs) are used for various indications in patients with cancer, such as the administration of chemotherapeutics and other medications, the substitution of blood components, parenteral nutrition, and blood withdrawal. CVCs can remain in place for either short term or long term. Different types of long-term CVCs are currently used: peripherally inserted CVCs (PICCs), tunneled catheters, and implanted port catheter systems. Single-lumen, double-lumen, or triple-lumen catheters are available. Several catheters have special characteristics, such as the presence of a cuff or the impregnation with heparin, antibiotics, or antiseptics. Although the use of CVCs provides important benefits, their use is sometimes counterbalanced by a certain potential for inducing local and systemic complications. Early complications are usually related to the catheter insertion and include hematoma, arterial puncture, misplacement of the catheter tip, air embolism, and pneumothorax. In contrast, catheter dysfunction, CVC-related thrombosis, and CVC-related infection are the most common complications over the long term [33]. The incidence of CVC-related infections has been estimated to be as high as 2.7 per 1000 catheter-days using classical non-cuffed CVCs. The risk of infections can be substantially lowered to 1.6 per 1000 catheter-days with the use of cuffed and tunneled CVCs and to 0.2 per 1000 catheter-days with the use of implantable port systems [33]. Use of PICCs is also associated with a low incidence of infectious complications (1.1 per 1000 catheter days), which is however counterbalanced by an increased risk of thrombotic complications [34]. Infections can be restricted to the insertion site; however, colonization of the catheter may also result in systemic bloodstream infection. Cancer patients who receive intensive chemotherapy and those who undergo bone marrow transplantation are at high risk for developing life-threatening infectious complications.

Different strategies have been implemented to prevent CVC-related infections, including an aseptic insertion technique, education of patients and healthcare providers on how to handle CVCs, early removal of catheters no longer required, and technological approaches (e.g., antimicrobial coating and lock solutions) [35]. The routine use of antibiotics given intravenously before catheter insertion did not reduce the incidence of tunnel or pocket infections and is therefore not recommended [36]. In contrast, recent studies have demonstrated that CVCs impregnated with antimicrobials reduce CVC colonization and lower the risk of infection [37]. On the basis of the current evidence, the ASCO guidelines recommend the use of these catheters especially in high-risk patients, such as patients with recurrent infections, bone marrow transplant recipients, or leukemia patients [33].

CVC-related infections are most frequently caused by coagulase-negative Staphylococcus species. However, other microorganisms can also cause CVC-related infections, including *Staphylococcus aureus*, gram-negative Enterobacteriaceae, *Escherichia coli*, *Pseudomonas aeruginosa*, and Candida species [38]. Most CVC-related infections are caused by colonization of the skin flora at the catheter's external surface. Localized infections at the catheter insertion site, tunnel, and pocket infections are usually caused by pyogenic bacteria, such as *Staphylococcus aureus* [39]. Alternatively, microorganisms can be transferred from the patient's skin or the hand of a health professional to the catheter hubs, resulting in intraluminal colonization, which is a mechanism more common to long-term catheter use. Other rare causes of colonization include contaminated infusions or hematogenous seeding from another infection site or from the gut [39].

Infection of an insertion site can be diagnosed on the basis of local erythema, pain, swelling, increased warmth, tenderness, a palpable cord indicating phlebitis, or the discharge of pus around the CVC insertion site. Sensitivity of clinical symptoms in predicting infection is low [39]. The diagnosis must be confirmed by blood cultures and subsequent microbiological analysis before initiating antibiotic therapy. In a recent study on patients with *Staphylococcus aureus* (BSI) infection among patients with CVC-related *Staphylococcus aureus* bacteremia (SAB), the time the first positive blood culture was drawn, onset of clinical symptoms, and microbiological confirmation (cultures of catheter tips positive for *Staphylococcus aureus*) were close as compared to patients with infective endocarditis or vertebral osteomyelitis, in whom the onset of clinical symptoms most often preceded the time the first positive blood culture was drawn (median time = −1.5 days, interquartile range (IQR) −4; 0 and 4 days, IQR −11; −1, respectively), and imaging confirmation was most frequently obtained subsequent to the SAB diagnosis [40]. Patients with CVC-related infection rarely developed further infective foci, whereas this was observed in more than half the patients with infective endocarditis and ventricular overload, respectively [40].

Imaging modalities are usually not necessary, or irrelevant in this condition [31], as the CT findings in patients with catheter and/or pocket infections are frequently normal [31]. Nevertheless, in selected cases, radiological examinations may be useful to detect thrombosis [38, 41, 42] or foci of septic embolism [43], particularly in patient with CVC or arterial catheter-related bloodstream infections. This is important for subsequent patient management since the presence of septic complications or metastatic infection (e.g., endocarditis) requires immediate removal of the catheter. In addition, infections with virulent microorganisms, such as methicillin-resistant *Staphylococcus aureus* (MRSA), *Pseudomonas aeruginosa*, or Candida species require removal of the catheter because of their potential to cause recurrent infection and fatal complications. Data from a recent prospective interventional trial in neutropenic patients with a long-term CVC in situ and BSI showed that an ultrasonography-driven strategy seems to offer advantages over a clinically driven strategy, enabling effective control of BSI and demonstrating overall survival rate at 30 days significantly higher (95%) as compared to the historical cohort (80%). Patients not protected by ultrasonographic surveillance had a 17% risk of infection-related mortality, with the majority of events occurring relatively early [44].

Limited experience has been reported with nuclear medicine imaging for the diagnosis of intravascular catheter-related infection. Only a few reports suggested the possible use of either ^{67}Ga-citrate or radiolabeled leukocytes to identify such infection [45–49]. On the other hand, more recent reports emphasize the role of [^{18}F]FDG PET for identifying intravascular catheter-related infection [50, 51], especially CVC infections [50, 52]. In particular, during severe neutropenia, there was a clear correlation between [^{18}F]FDG uptake in the CVC tract and septic thrombophlebitis of the subclavian vein. The presence of [^{18}F]FDG uptake in the CVC tract was not related to clinical signs of exit site or tunnel infection, preceding ultrasound findings which become positive at later time-point. Therefore, increased [^{18}F]FDG uptake in the CVC tract in patients with febrile neutropenia should not be ignored as it might have important consequences in CVC management, e.g., line removal, particularly when persistent bacteremia is diagnosed [53]. Therefore, [^{18}F]FDG PET/CT represents a rapid and reliable test that helps diagnose and manage intravascular catheter-related infections. Besides the potential role of [^{18}F]FDG PET/CT in early detection and managing of specific infectious complications during febrile neutropenia, its high negative predictive value may help in avoiding unnecessary diagnostic investigations and therapy.

Key Learning Points

- CVCs are used for various indications in patients with cancer, and their use is sometimes counterbalanced by a certain potential for inducing local and systemic complications.
- Early complications are usually related to the catheter insertion.
- Catheter dysfunction, CVC-related thrombosis, and CVC-related infection are the most common long-term complications.
- The incidence of CVC-related infections is as high as 2.7 per 1000 catheter-days using non-cuffed CVCs and might be lowered to 1.6 per 1000 catheter-days for cuffed and tunneled CVCs and to 0.2 per 1000 catheter-days for implantable port systems.
- Cancer patients who receive intensive chemotherapy and those who undergo bone marrow transplantation are at high risk for developing life-threatening infectious complications.
- CVC-related infections are most frequently caused by coagulase-negative Staphylococcus species, although other microorganisms can also cause CVC-related infections such as *Staphylococcus aureus*, gram-negative Enterobacteriaceae, *Escherichia coli*, *Pseudomonas aeruginosa*, and Candida species.
- Most CVC-related infections are mainly caused by colonization of the skin flora at the catheter's external surface or transferred from the patient's skin or the hand of a health professional to the catheter hubs, resulting in intraluminal colonization.
- Infection of an insertion site can be diagnosed on the basis of local erythema, pain, swelling, increased warmth, tenderness, a palpable cord indicating phlebitis or the discharge of pus around the CVC insertion site.
- Blood cultures and subsequent microbiological analysis before initiating antibiotic therapy are used to confirm the clinical suspicion.
- Imaging modalities are usually not necessary or irrelevant as the CT findings in patients with catheter and/or pocket infections are frequently normal.
- Radiological examinations may be useful in selected cases to detect thrombosis or foci of septic embolism, particularly in case of bloodstream infections.
- Limited experience has been reported with nuclear medicine imaging for the diagnosis of intravascular catheter-related infection, [^{18}F]FDG PET/CT being a rapid and reliable test that helps to diagnose and manage intravascular catheter-related infections.
- [^{18}F]FDG PET/CT has a role in early detection and managing of specific infectious complications during febrile neutropenia and its high negative predictive value may help in avoiding unnecessary diagnostic investigations and therapy.

7.3 Neurosurgical Infections

The incidence of neurosurgical infections is estimated between 1% and 7%, and the most common causative organisms are *Staphylococcus aureus*, *Staphylococcus epidermidis*, and *Propionibacterium acnes* [54]. Other pathogens may be involved in special situations, such as Candida in immunocompromised patients [55], *Streptococcus pneumoniae* and *Haemophilus influenzae* in patients with a cerebrospinal fluid (CSF) leak secondary to skull base fractures and the associated communication between nasal/oral cavities and the CNS [56].

Early diagnosis of postoperative CNS infections may be challenging. Often the symptoms are vague and nonspecific; headache, nausea, vomiting, photophobia, or neck stiffness may have existed prior to the operation or could be due directly to the underlying primary neurologic condition. Similarly, patients may have a depressed level of consciousness, preventing elucidation of symptoms and a detailed neurologic examination. The value of nonspecific laboratory markers such as C-reactive protein and procalcitonin is debated, some studies suggesting a benefit in diagnosing bacterial ventriculitis [57] and others finding it of limited value due to the proinflammatory state of critically ill neurologic patients and the high rate of concurrent systemic infections [58]. The CSF profile that we normally rely on to detect infection (such as CSF pleocytosis) may not be applicable to iatrogenic CNS infections [59]. Therefore, other methods have been proposed, such as trending the CSF white count [60] or measuring CSF lactate levels [61] mainly as a consequence that frequent CSF sampling per se increases the risk of secondarily introducing infection [62].

In certain instances, neuroimaging may support the diagnosis; however, it is often not definitive for confirming the diagnosis [63]. For example, magnetic resonance imaging (MRI) with gadolinium contrast may show meningeal/ventricular enhancement in patients with ventriculitis, while computed tomography (CT) imaging may show hydrocephalus in the setting of shunt malfunction. However, it may be difficult to ascertain whether the imaging findings are due to a postoperative infection, as they may be related to the original insult or to the procedure itself [64] (see also Table 7.4).

7.3.1 Craniotomy Infections

Infection after craniotomy, craniectomy, and cranioplasty can affect any layer between the skin and the ventricles. Bone flaps are separated from their blood supply and are therefore at a high risk for infection. Between 5% and 8% of craniotomies are complicated by infection, and the most commonly involved pathogens include *Staphylococcus aureus*, *Staphylococcus epidermidis*, and *Propionibacterium acnes* [66]. Prior radiotherapy, repeat surgery, CSF leak, and operation lasting >4 h are important risk factors for infection. Treatment involves flap removal, debridement, and anti-

Table 7.4 Summary of neurosurgical infections, adapted from [65]

Infection	Incidence	Specific risk factors	Pathogen	Treatment
Shunts (VP, VA, VPL)	4–17%	• Shunt revision procedure • Duration of operation • Use of neuroendoscope • Certain etiologies of hydrocephalus	• *S. aureus* • Coagulase-negative Staph • *P. acnes* • Gram negatives and anaerobes (for VPS)	• Vancomycin + cefepime/ceftazidime/meropenem for 10–14 days • Shunt removal
EVD	2–22%	• Frequency of manipulation/sampling • Duration of catheterization • Indication of placement • Multiple insertions • CSF leak	• *S. aureus* • Coagulase-negative Staph • Gram negatives are on the rise	• Vancomycin + cefepime/ceftazidime/meropenem for 10–14 days • EVD removal only when CSF is purulent or inadequate response to ABX
Craniotomy	5–8%	• Prior radiotherapy • Repeat surgery • CSF leak • Duration of operation >4 h	• *S. aureus* • *S. epidermidis* • *P. acnes*	• Flap removal, debridement • Antibiotics for 6 week to 12 month
Spinal	6%	• Duration of operation • Posterior surgical approach • Invasiveness of the procedure	• *S. aureus* • Coagulase-negative Staph	• Antibiotics • Bracing • Surgery if there is new neurologic deficit, spine instability, progressive deformity, or failed nonoperative treatment
DBS	0.6–14%	• Newer indications for DBS (Tourette's cluster headache, refractory partial epilepsy) pose higher risk than established indications such as PD	• *S. aureus* • *S. epidermidis* • *P. acnes*	• Generator removal if intracranial lead is not infected • Whole device removal if intracranial lead is infected • ABX for 2–6 week
Spinal cord stimulator	3.4–10%	• Decubitus ulcers • Poor hygiene • Urinary/fecal incontinence	• *S. aureus*	• Generator removal if spinal cord lead is not infected • Whole device removal if spinal cord lead is infected • ABX

biotics for an extended period of time, ranging from 6 weeks to 12 months [54]. For craniectomies, the risk of infection at cranioplasty increases when the bone flap is stored for a long period before replacement [67]. Cranioplasty in the presence of a ventriculo-peritoneal shunt (VPS) is associated with a higher rate of infection [68]. In a recent prospective study of 101 cranioplasty cases, there was no difference in the incidence of post cranioplasty surgical site infection using bone flaps stored either by cryopreservation or in subcutaneous pockets [69]. Several reports suggest that topical vancomycin, applied as a liquid solution intra-wound following open craniotomy, can reduce infection rates in both pediatric [70] and adult patients [71]. Imaging is essential in defining the extension of infection, in particular distinguishing between superficial and deep infection.

7.3.2 Infection of Ventricular Shunts

Primary cerebrospinal fluid (CSF) shunts (those implanted in patients with no prior neurosurgery) are most frequently placed in adults to treat idiopathic normal pressure hydrocephalus. Tumor, subarachnoid hemorrhage, head injury, and intraventricular hemorrhage are, instead, the most common causes of secondary shunt surgery. The estimated rate of shunt infection is 4–17% in adults [56]. Shunt infection can occur by iatrogenic introduction at the time of surgery (most commonly due to the skin flora *Staphylococcus aureus* and *Propionibacterium acnes*), by hematogenous spread (*Streptococcus pneumoniae* and *Hemophilus influenzae* for ventriculo-atrial shunts), or by contiguous spread (Gram negatives and anaerobes from peritonitis or bowel perforation for VPSs) [72]. Infection can develop at any time after shunt placement, either via hematogenous or contiguous dissemination, and the pathogen depends on etiology of the primary infection (Gram negatives, *Streptococcus pneumoniae*) [73]. Risk factors for developing shunt infections include a recent shunt revision procedure, duration of the operation, use of a neuroendoscope, and certain etiologies of hydrocephalus (purulent meningitis, hemorrhage, myelomeningocele) [56].

Shunt infection can present with nonspecific signs and symptoms such as headache, nausea/vomiting, neck stiffness, and mental status changes, which poses a diagnostic challenge as they have poor sensitivity and reliability [74]. The higher predictive value of fever versus other clinical symptoms and signs has been reported, and additional diagnostic clues include erythema close to the proximal end of the shunt, and peritonitis for VPSs [75]. The diagnosis of shunt-related infections is based on parameters similar to those of ventriculo-meningitis: CSF culture, Gram stain, chemistries, and cell count; blood cultures should always be performed [76]. In the case of shunt-related infection localized in the CNS (i.e., abscess), CT and MRI may be helpful to identify abnormal findings suggesting infection [77].

Scintigraphy with ^{111}In-oxine-leukocytes is highly accurate for the diagnosis of primary, post-traumatic and post-surgical infections (including patients with suspected VPS infections) [78]. Similar results have been reported for ^{99m}Tc-HMPAO-leukocyte scintigraphy to diagnose and manage skull neurosurgical infections including patients with intracerebral lesions, suspected postsurgical infections, suspected deep infection of the surgical wound, and suspected VPS infections [79]. In particular, ^{99m}Tc-HMPAO-leukocyte imaging correctly diagnosed VPS infections without any false-positive findings [79]. This procedure has therefore been suggested to optimize patient management, possibly impacting on the infection-related mortality and morbidity and reducing length of hospitalization and related costs. ^{67}Ga-citrate scintigraphy [80] and [^{18}F]FDG PET/CT [80, 81] have also been used in selected cases to detect VPS infection, with a high potential diagnostic role in patients with high clinical suspicion but equivocal/inconclusive standard diagnostic modalities.

7.3.3 Infections of Lumbar Drains

Lumbar drains (LDs), similar to external ventricular drains (EVDs), are connected to the subarachnoid space; however, they have a lower risk of infection, which may be related to the less infectious patient population they are used in (such as normal pressure hydrocephalus patients). The infection rate ranges from 4% to 7% [56]. For comparison, CNS infection after a lumbar puncture is estimated at 1 in 50,000 procedures according to one study [56], an observation that emphasizes that leaving an indwelling catheter in the subarachnoid space dramatically increases the infection rate.

7.3.4 Infections of Deep Brain Stimulators

Deep brain stimulators (DBS) are an effective option in the management of chronic pain and movement disorders, such as Parkinson's disease, dystonia, and essential tremor. Since the 1980s, it is estimates that >100,000 DBSs have been implanted worldwide [82, 83], and this number continues to grow since this technique is now approved by the US Food and Drug Administration for epilepsy, and there are many reports of its efficacy in psychiatric disorders and pain syndromes [82]. Infection rates vary widely in the literature, with rates from 0.62% to 25% [84, 85], reflecting differences in patient populations, surgical techniques adopted for DBS implant, and antimicrobial prophylaxis treatment; a certain variability exists also concerning the criteria to define infection (involvement of the hardware and/or superficial skin infections at the incision sites) [76, 86]. The most common pathogens isolated were microorganisms routinely found in the skin flora, *Staphylococcus aureus* being most common followed by *Staphylococcus epidermidis* [87]. Clinically, the infection may present with local signs like erythema and edema; however, focal neurological signs, including seizures, may be seen if an intracranial abscess develops [76]. Diagnosis of DBS infection is essentially based on clinical manifestations, but the identification of the microorganism responsible for infection is crucial to guide patient management [76]. Brain MRI and cultures may help in the diagnosis. Traditional management of DBS infections is systemic antibiotic therapy with wound incision and debridement (I&D) and removal of implanted DBS hardware [2, 4, 5]. If the intracranial lead is infected, the whole device should be removed and 6 weeks of antibiotics should follow [88]. Generator infections that do not involve the intracranial leads can be managed by 2 weeks of antibiotics in addition to removing the generator and the connecting wires (but keeping the intracranial leads in place for potential reimplantation of the generator after 3–6 months). Removal of a DBS can be very devastating for patients and sometimes infections can be managed without removal of hardware [4, 5]. Presurgical preparation with ethyl alcohol or use of intraoperative vancomycin showed to be effective in reducing infection rates in some studies; however, the results have been inconsistent [2, 17, 18]. There are conflicting studies as to whether infection rates are higher after de novo implantation surgery or battery replacement [19, 20]. Scintigraphy with ^{99m}Tc-labeled anti-granulocyte antibody fragments (^{99m}Tc-sulesomab) has been tested in patients with DBS implant for Parkinson's disease and persistent device-related skin erosion and/or infection [86]. Scintigraphy revealed infection also in areas that were clinically intact (i.e., without skin erythema and swelling, erosion, or purulent discharge) as a consequence of subcutaneous dissemination from the primary site of infection. ^{99m}Tc-sulesomab scintigraphy (with appropriate SPECT/CT acquisitions) proved therefore to impact on the treatment strategy of DBS-related infection because of its ability to accurately define the extent of infection and to identify the portion of DBS involved with the infectious process. Favorable results were also obtained in the evaluation of DBS-related infections during follow-up, since ^{99m}Tc-sulesomab scintigraphy facilitated the decision as to whether and when a reimplantation procedure would be appropriate [86].

7.3.5 Infection of Spinal Cord Stimulators and Medication Pumps

The incidence of spinal cord stimulator infections ranges from 3.4% to 10% [89]. Most cases are due to *Staphylococcus aureus* and affect the generator pocket [90]. For spinal cord medication pumps, the catheter tip is located in the intrathecal space; the incidence of infection is approximately 6% [91].

Risk factors for spinal cord stimulator infection include decubitus ulcers, diabetes, malnutrition, obesity, steroid use, preexisting infection, poor hygiene, and urinary/fecal incontinence. Similar to DBS stimulators, if the infection is confined to the generator, treatment entails antibiotics and taking out the generator while keeping the lead in place [90].

Key Learning Points

- The incidence of neurosurgical infections is between 1% and 7%.
- The most common causative microorganisms are *Staphylococcus aureus*, *Staphylococcus epidermidis*, and *Propionibacterium acnes*; other pathogens may be involved in special situations.
- Early diagnosis of postoperative CNS infections may be challenging since symptoms are vague and nonspecific.
- The value of nonspecific laboratory markers of infection/inflammation, such as C-reactive protein and procalcitonin is debated.
- The CSF profile may not be applicable to iatrogenic CNS infections.
- Neuroimaging may support the diagnosis; however, it is often inconclusive, and interpretation can be difficult because of confounding post-surgical changes.
- Infection after craniotomy, craniectomy and cranioplasty can affect any layer between the skin and the ventricles in about 5–8% of the procedures.
- The most commonly involved pathogens include *Staphylococcus aureus*, *Staphylococcus epidermidis*, and *Propionibacterium acnes*.
- Prior radiotherapy, repeat surgery, CSF leak, and operation lasting >4 h are important risk factors for infection.
- Treatment involves flap removal, debridement, and antibiotics for an extended period.
- Imaging is essential for defining the extension of infection, in particular for distinguishing between superficial and deep infection.
- Primary CSF shunts have an estimated infection rate of 4–17% in adults.
- Shunt infection can occur by iatrogenic introduction at the time of surgery (*Staphylococcus aureus* and *Propionibacterium acnes*), by hematogenous spread (*Streptococcus pneumoniae* and *Hemophilus influenzae* for ventriculo-atrial shunts) or by contiguous spread (Gram negatives and anaerobes from peritonitis or bowel perforation for VPSs).
- Risk factors for shunt infections include a recent shunt revision procedure, duration of the operation, use of a neuroendoscope, and certain etiologies of hydrocephalus (purulent meningitis, hemorrhage, myelomeningocele).
- The diagnosis of shunt-related infections is based on CSF culture, Gram stain, chemistries, and cell count; blood cultures should always be performed.
- In the case of shunt-related infection localized in the CNS, CT and MRI may be helpful to identify abnormal findings suggesting infection.
- Scintigraphy with ^{111}In-oxine-leukocytes or ^{99m}Tc-HMPAO-leukocytes is highly accurate for the diagnosis of primary, posttraumatic, and post-surgical infections.
- ^{67}Ga-citrate scintigraphy and [^{18}F]FDG PET/CT have also been used in selected cases with high clinical suspicion associated with equivocal/inconclusive results of other diagnostic modalities.
- LD infection rate ranges from 4% to 7%.
- DBS infection rates vary from 0.62% to 25%.
- The most common pathogens isolated are microorganisms routinely found in the skin flora, *Staphylococcus aureus* being most common followed by *Staphylococcus epidermidis*.
- Clinically, the infection may present with local signs such as erythema and edema; however, focal neurological signs, including seizures, may be seen if an intracranial abscess develops.
- Diagnosis of DBS infection is essentially based on clinical manifestations, but the identification of the microorganism responsible for infection is crucial to guide patient management; brain MRI and cultures may help for correct diagnosis.
- Management of DBS infections is systemic antibiotic therapy with wound incision, debridement, and removal of the implanted DBS hardware.
- Scintigraphy with ^{99m}Tc-sulesomab accurately defines the extent of infection and identifies the portion of DBS involved with the infectious process.
- The incidence of spinal cord stimulator infections is 3.4–10%.
- Most cases are due to *Staphylococcus aureus* and affect the generator pocket.
- Risk factors for spinal cord stimulator infection include decubitus ulcers, diabetes, malnutrition, obesity, steroid use, preexisting infection, poor hygiene, and urinary/fecal incontinence.

7.4 Infection of Respiratory Assistance Devices

Nosocomial pneumonia is often associated with the use of respiratory assistance devices, including endotracheal tubes, tracheotomy, nasal masks, and nebulization treatment with ventilator-associated pneumonia (VAP), the most common nosocomial infection in the intensive care unit for patients receiving prolonged (>48 h) mechanical ventilation. Also, tracheotomy is associated with VAP. Nasotracheal intubation is associated with sinusitis and otitis.

Key Learning Points

- VAP is the most common nosocomial infection in the intensive care unit for patients receiving prolonged (>48 h) mechanical ventilation.
- Tracheotomy is associated with VAP.
- Nasotracheal intubation is associated with sinusitis and otitis.

7.5 Infection of Peritoneal Dialysis Catheters

Infection of the peritoneal dialysis (PD) catheter may result in exit-site infections, tunnel infections, and peritonitis. Each technique of PD catheter insertion is related to a different incidence rate of infectious complication with higher rate 3 years after initiating PD. Bacterial peritonitis is the most frequent complication, but patients undergoing PD are more susceptible also to tuberculous peritonitis.

Key Learning Point

- PD catheter infections may result in exit-site infections, tunnel infections, and peritonitis.

7.6 Infection of Penile Devices

Since the 1960s, penile prosthesis implantation has played an important role in the treatment of end-stage erectile dysfunction [40], and inflatable penile prosthesis (IPP) has now become the gold standard treatment of choice for restoration of functional erections. Over the years, the IPP has undergone many improvements, making it a popular choice among urologists, with over 22,000 implants performed annually in the United States [92]. While mechanical malfunction is the most frequent complication of penile implants, infection continues to be the most dreaded complication [93, 94]. Prosthesis-associated infections often result in removal of the device, severe disability, loss of function, loss of tissue, and difficulty with subsequent implantation. Genital gangrene with extensive tissue loss is the most severe and dreaded manifestation of this difficult complication [95]. While the exact time of bacterial exposure to implanted prostheses remains controversial, most often these bacteria colonize prostheses at the time of implantation [96]. Bacteria may also come in contact with prosthetic materials through hematogenous or lymphatic spread [93]. Fishman et al. demonstrated that 56% of prosthesis infections occurred within 7 months of implantation, 36% between 7 and 12 months, and only 2.6% after 5 years [97]. Staphylococcus species, especially *Staphylococcus epidermidis*, are the most common microorganisms identified in penile prosthesis infection and have been isolated from 35% to 56% of infected penile prosthesis patients [95]. Gram-negative enteric bacteria may also be responsible for prosthetic infections more likely to occur at an earlier time, with an average time to infection of less than 1 month after implantation compared with 5.75 months in those patients infected with staphylococcal organisms [98]. Fungal infections represent 12% of all penile prosthesis infections and were seen mostly in diabetic or overweight patients [99]. Patients who have immune deficiency, severe/poorly controlled diabetes, or spinal cord injury or have had multiple surgical procedures increase their risk of post-prosthesis implantation infection and require increased attention to the principles of infection prevention [100]. Clinically apparent penile prostheses can be diagnosed from symptoms such as new onset of penile pain, erythema, and induration overlying a prosthesis part, fever, drainage, and ultimately device extrusion. While most of these infections occur in the early perioperative period, late device infections have been documented. Most infections within the first 24 months follow-up, however, are probably infections caused by bacterial colonization at the time of surgery with symptoms and signs beginning later. These infections are most often associated with *Staphylococcus epidermidis* infections on culture.

Subclinical prosthetic infections occur more frequently [93], most often present with chronic prosthesis-associated pain, and are difficult to diagnose and even more challenging to treat. Management of IPP infection usually includes antibiotic treatment, removal of all prosthetic components, and a thorough wash out of the retropubic space (or other ectopic reservoir location), scrotum, and corpora cavernosa. Attempted reimplantation may then be considered several months later, when the patient is rendered infection-free. Unfortunately, removal of the device will lead to fibrosis and scarring of the corporal bodies secondary to the inflammatory process involved. This fibrotic reaction results in penile shortening and makes subsequent insertion of a second IPP more challenging and prone to future infections and/or other complications [101, 102]. It is of utmost importance to recognize the earliest signs of IPP. Recognizing the different infection entity and picking up on early local and systemic signs that may indicate that severity could save the patient extensive morbidity. Imaging could be necessary to diagnose or plan surgery, while it should be noted that literature consistently reports that microbial cultures may not always be positive, despite clinical evidence of the presence of IPP [103]. Therefore, tissue swab and fluid (when present) should be obtained for microbiological culture. MRI may be helpful to detect signs of penile implant infection, representing the imaging modality of choice for the diagnosis of IPP due to a superior soft tissue contrast resolution and direct multiplanar capability. In the presence of an IPP, the soft tissue infection and inflammation appear as soft tissue thickening with T2 hyperintensity and hyper-enhancement in the vicinity of the device components. Abscess and infected fluid collections are suspected when a loculated fluid collection is present with a surrounding rim of soft tissue thickening and hyper-enhancement [104]. The clinical value of ultrasonography and CT in this setting is limited [105]. ^{67}Ga-citrate and ^{111}In-oxine-leukocyte scintigraphy has been successfully reported in the detection of penile implant infections—although in small series of patients [106, 107].

Key Learning Points

- Infection of penile prosthesis continues to constitute a serious complication.
- The majority of the infections occur within 7–12 months of implantation.
- Staphylococcus species, especially *Staphylococcus epidermidis* are isolated from 35% to 56% of patients with infected penile prosthesis.
- Gram-negative enteric bacteria may also be responsible for prosthetic infections more likely to occur at an earlier time.
- Fungal infections represent 12% of all penile prosthesis infections and occur mostly in diabetic or overweight patients.
- Immune deficiency, severe/poorly controlled diabetes, spinal cord injury, or prior multiple surgical procedures increase their risk of post-prosthesis implantation infection.
- Clinically apparent penile prosthesis infections can be diagnosed from symptoms.
- Subclinical prosthetic infections occur more frequently, presenting with chronic prosthesis-associated pain, and are challenging to diagnose.
- Management of IPP infection usually includes antibiotic treatment, removal of all prosthetic components, and a thorough wash out of the retropubic space (or other ectopic reservoir location), scrotum, and corpora cavernosa.
- Recognizing the different infection entity could save the patient extensive morbidity.
- Imaging could be necessary to diagnose the infection or to plan surgery.
- Tissue swab and fluid (when present) should be obtained for microbiological culture.
- MRI is the imaging modality of choice for the diagnosis of IPP, due to its superior soft tissue contrast resolution and direct multiplanar capability.
- The clinical value of ultrasonography, CT, and nuclear medicine procedures in this setting is limited.

7.7 Infection of Breast Implants

Augmentation mammoplasty with prosthetic breast implants is commonly performed for breast enlargement, for correction of asymmetries, or for reconstruction after mastectomy. Infection is the leading complication that occurs after breast implantation surgery, with variable incidence rates: 0.4–2.5% for augmentation mammoplasty, 1–35% for prosthetic breast reconstruction [108]. Besides prosthetic implant infections, additional surgery or removal of implant is often required for complications, such as capsular contractures (10-year incidence: 9.2% for augmentation, 14.5% for reconstruction), implant rupture (10-year incidence: 9%), implant malposition, asymmetry, wrinkling, or seromas (<5%). Periodic MRIs of breast implants are recommended to determine if implant rupture has occurred. Although risk factors for infection associated with breast implantation have not yet been carefully assessed, surgical technique and patient's clinical condition seem to be the most important factors [109]. Overall, neither the type of implant nor the surgical procedure seems to have a significant influence on the timing of infection onset. Potential sources of infection are a contaminated implant or saline, surgery or surgical environment, patient's skin or mammary ducts, or seeding of the implant from remote infection.

Acute infections occur between 6 days and 6 weeks after surgery [110]. Late infection usually results from secondary bacteremia or an invasive procedure at a site other than the breasts [109]. Management of breast implant infection usually entails prompt initiation of wide-spectrum antibiotic therapy, followed by a period of a few days of close observation to determine if implant removal or salvage is appropriate. Implant removal is often necessary to achieve cure especially in infections due to virulent pathogens, such as *Staphylococcus aureus* or fungi, or if rapid improvement of infection does not occur following antibiotic therapy.

Diagnosis of breast implant infection is largely clinical, based on local and systemic signs and symptoms, such as fever, spontaneous discharge from the incision, breast swelling, rapidly evolving breast pain, and erythema [111, 112]. Severe sepsis can also develop, but in the majority of cases, signs and symptoms remain non-specific [109]. Distinguishing breast implant infection from the red breast syndrome, cellulitis, and superficial surgical site infection is also important for clinical management. Superficial swabbing of draining fluid at the surgical site is not useful, due to contamination with skin flora. Ultrasound imaging and ultrasound-guided aspiration are recommended in cases with a suspected periprosthetic fluid collection; any aspirated fluid should be sent for standard aerobic and anaerobic bacteria, fungal, and mycobacterial cultures. Any debrided tissue and removed implants should be examined histologically and sent for culture [109]. Culture of internal content of the breast implant should be performed in case of surgical capsulotomy [113]. However, ultrasonography may be of limited value when examining the posterior side of the prosthesis and subjacent chest wall [109, 114]. MRI and contrast-enhanced CT scan are helpful to evaluate complications following breast implant, including fluid collections and abscesses, while infected fluid collections can be missed by mammography [114–118].

Nuclear medicine techniques can in principle be used to diagnose breast implant infection. However, a few data are currently available about their clinical application. ^{67}Ga-citrate and ^{111}In-oxine-leukocytes scans have been successfully used to confirm a breast peri-implant infection, as described in occasional case reports [119, 120]. Although [^{18}F]FDG PET has been shown to be useful to distinguish benign lesions from malignant lesions in patients with augmentation mammoplasty, it seems to be an unreliable method to accurately detect breast implant infection; this is because [^{18}F]FDG uptake can be observed in a variety of conditions other than infection (i.e., silicone granuloma, breast cancer) [121, 122] and the relative low specificity of the technique makes the differential diagnosis between sterile and infective process difficult [123, 124].

Key Learning Points

- Infection leads to complication of breast implantation surgery, with variable incidence rates: 0.4–2.5% for augmentation mammoplasty, 1–35% for prosthetic breast reconstruction.
- Surgical technique and patient's clinical condition seem to be the most important risk factors.
- Potential sources of infection are a contaminated implant or saline, surgery, or surgical environment, patient's skin or mammary ducts, or seeding of the implant from remote infection.
- Acute infections occur between 6 days and 6 weeks after surgery, whereas late infection usually results from secondary bacteremia or an invasive procedure at a site other than the breasts.
- Management of breast implant infection usually entails prompt initiation of wide-spectrum antibiotic therapy, followed by close observation to determine if implant removal or salvage is needed.
- Diagnosis of breast implant infection is largely clinical, based on local and systemic signs and symptoms.
- Distinguishing breast implant infection from superficial surgical site infection is important for clinical management.
- Ultrasound imaging and ultrasound-guided aspiration are recommended in cases with a suspected periprosthetic fluid collection.
- MRI and contrast-enhanced CT scan are helpful to evaluate complications following breast implant.
- Nuclear medicine imaging can in principle be used to diagnose breast implant infection, but few data are currently available.

7.8 Infection of Cochlear Implants

Cochlear implantation (CI) is currently a feasible treatment option in several conditions, including not only deafness but also patients with hearing still functioning in the low frequencies. Due to the benefits of binaural hearing, bilateral CI has become the standard treatment over the last decade, and recently, it also demonstrated benefits in case of unilateral deafness and severe tinnitus [125]. The most frequent CI complications are infections (1.7–16.6%) [126, 127] related to the biofilm covering the devices (even though they are made from well-tolerated materials) [128], to the spread of microorganism into the inner ear during surgery, or to bacteremia [129]. CI infections include cutaneous necrosis and surgical wound dehiscence (immediately after surgery or later), otitis, cerebritis, and meningitis [126, 127]. Even it has been demonstrated that abnormal cochlear or auditory canal anatomy is a risk factor for meningitis in CI, the increased incidence of CI-related meningitis entails the drafting of some recommendations, thereby prophylactic vaccination against *Streptococcus pneumoniae* has been scheduled before the implant [130].

The diagnosis of CI-related infection is essentially clinical [129]. When an acute otitis media is suspected, the middle-ear fluid should be obtained for culture, and, in case of clinical suspicion of meningitis, both middle-ear fluid and CFS cultures should be obtained [131].

Middle-ear mucosa biopsy specimens may also be obtained to diagnose biofilm-related otitis media [132]. Temporal bone radiographs are unsatisfactory in the detection of CI-related infection. In fact, although separation of the receiver/stimulator from the calvarium, a sign of the presence of underlying fluid, may be demonstrated on plain X-rays, this requires a tangential view necessitating careful patient positioning. In patients with suspected CI postoperative infection, CT is the technique of choice for detecting collections beneath the receiver/stimulator even though the images are masked by metallic artifacts [133].

Nuclear medicine imaging has a limited role for diagnosing CI infection, especially in the acute forms. However, ^{99m}Tc-diphosphonate scintigraphy and [^{18}F]FDG PET can be valuable tools in case of a late low-grade CI-related infection. In fact, in case of chronic osteomyelitis of the petrosal bone, since the presence of minimal signs of infection is undetectable by radiology, bone scintigraphy may reveal increased tracer uptake [134].

Key Learning Points

- The most frequent CI complications are infections, which can affect 1.7–16.6% of the devices.
- CI infections include cutaneous necrosis and surgical wound dehiscence, otitis, cerebritis, and meningitis.
- The diagnosis of CI-related infection is essentially clinical.
- In patients with suspected CI postoperative infection, CT is the imaging technique of choice.
- Nuclear medicine imaging has a limited role for diagnosing CI infection, especially in the acute forms.
- ^{99m}Tc-diphosphonate scintigraphy and [^{18}F]FDG PET can be used in case of a late, low-grade CI-related infection.

Clinical Cases

Case 7.1

Paola A. Erba

A 23-year-old women with LLC. Fever unresponsive to antipolymicrobial therapy. Negative blood culture, negative whole body US and CT.

Suspected Site of Infection

Unknown.

Radiopharmaceutical Activity

740 MBq of ^{99m}Tc-HMPAO-leukocytes.

Imaging

Whole-body, spot, and SPECT/CT images of the chest (Figs. 7.1, 7.2 and 7.3).

Conclusion/Teaching Point

This case identified the presence of port-a-chat infection. However, to obtain a diagnosis, SPECT/CT images were required since from the planar ones, it was impossible to detect any site of radiopharmaceutical uptake. This is a typical example of improved diagnostic accuracy using SPECT/CT.

Case 7.2

Martina Sollini

Man, 76 years. April 2005: significant stenosis (about 80%) of the right carotid artery treated with patch. February 2010: fever with increased CRP and ESR.

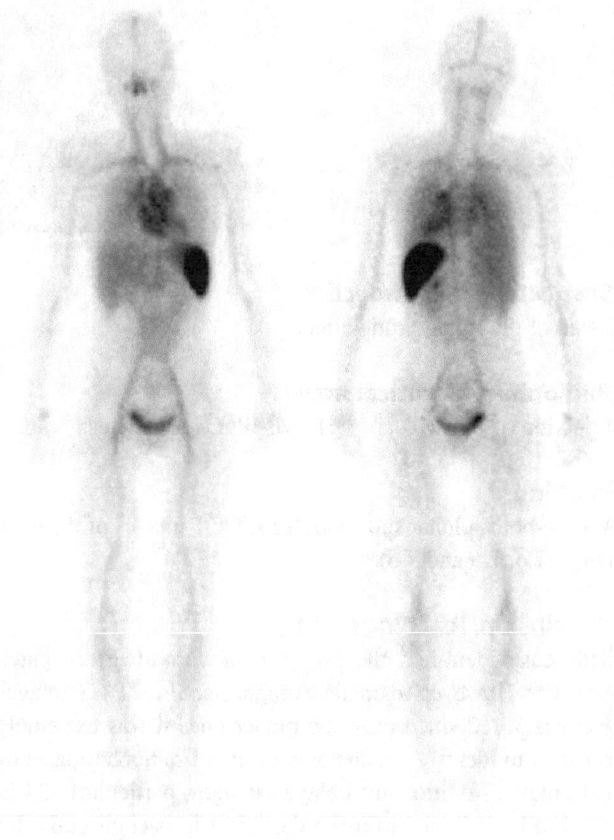

Fig. 7.1 Whole body radiolabeled leukocyte scan, 30 min after the ^{99m}Tc-HMPAO-leukocyte administration; anterior projection (left) and posterior projection (right). Normal distribution within the whole body

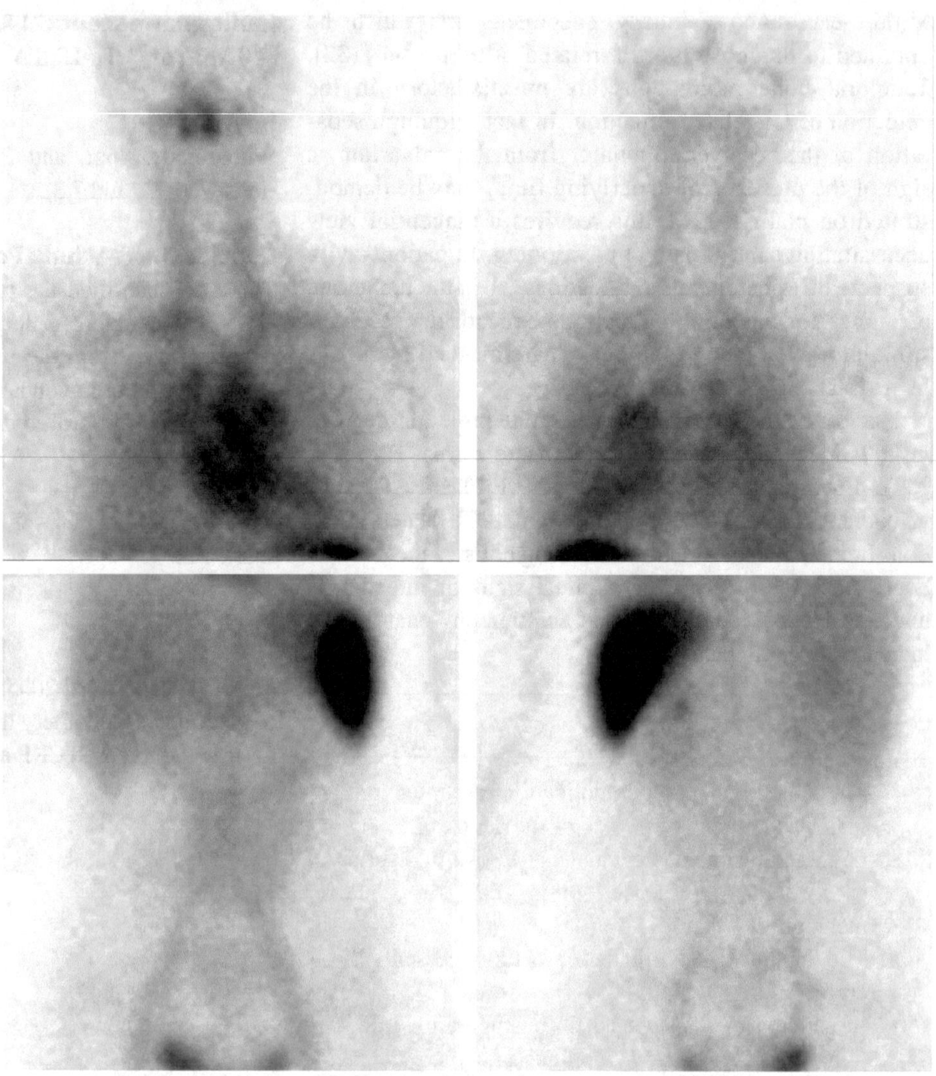

Fig. 7.2 Spot images of the thorax (upper) and abdominal (lower) regions obtained 6 h after labeled leukocyte administration, in the anterior (left) and posterior (right) positions. Images do not show significant sites of radioactivity accumulation. Based on this finding subsequent SPECT/CT images were acquired

Suspected Site of Infection
Patch of the right carotid artery.

Radiopharmaceutical Activity
Injection of 740 MBq of ^{99m}Tc-HMPAO-leukocytes.

Imaging
Whole-body, planar spot, and SPECT/CT images of the neck (Figs. 7.4, 7.5 and 7.6).

Conclusion/Teaching Point
This case identified the presence of carotid artery patch infection However, to obtain a diagnosis, SPECT/CT images were required since from the planar ones it was extremely difficult to identify the anatomical site of radiopharmaceutical uptake. Additionally, delayed images, particularly 24 h, need to be obtained to make the target to background ratio optimal for small vascular structure. After the examination, the patch was removed, infection was confirmed, and the patient was treated with common carotid-internal carotid bypass to minimize the risk of subsequent infections.

Case 7.3

Paola A. Erba

Woman, 62 years old. Allergy to iodinate contrast medium agents.

2009: Multiple right parietal meningiomas associated with left meningioma causing compression of the cerebral structures treated with craniotomy and patch.

Suspected Site of Infection
Frontal right osteomyelitis.

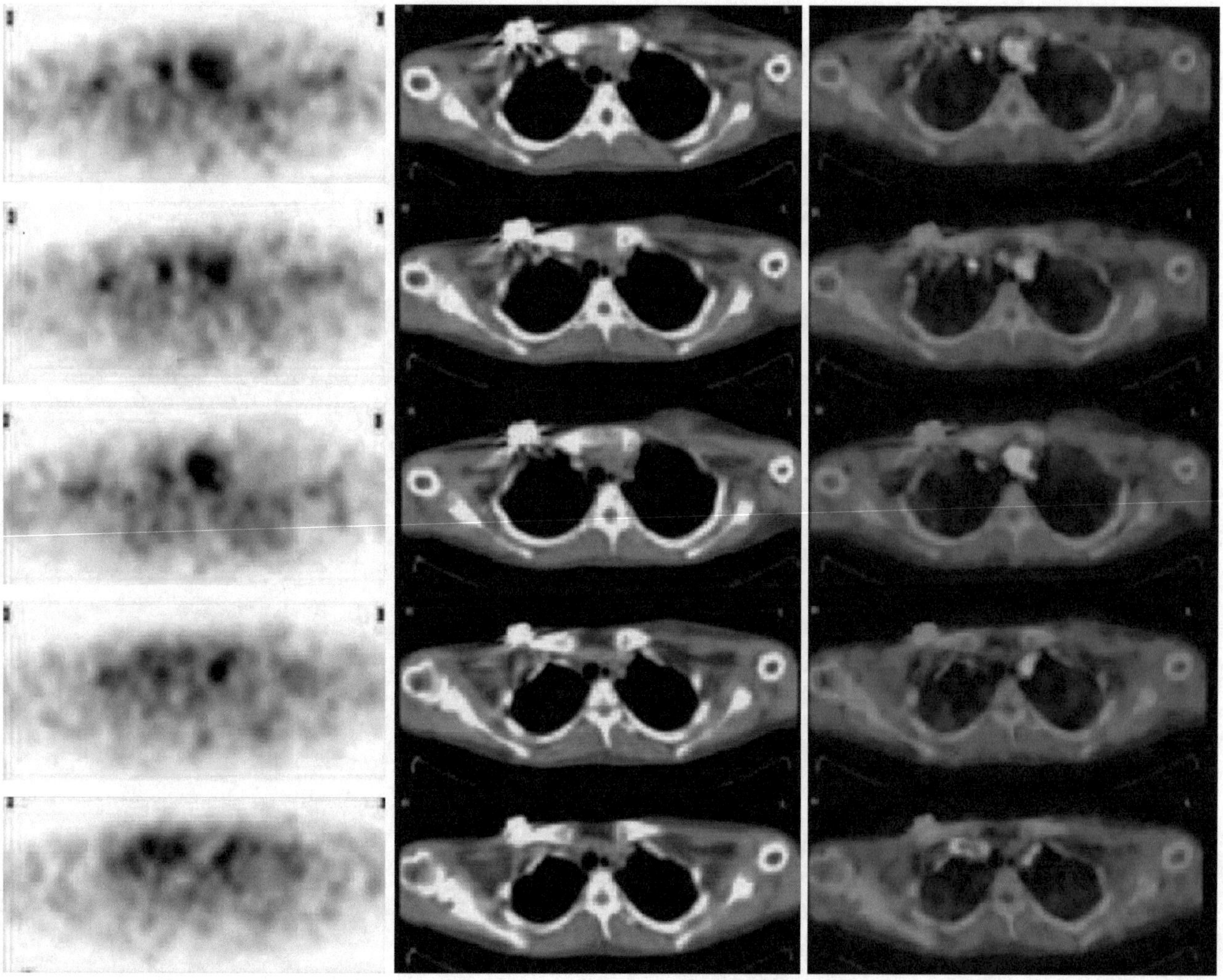

Fig. 7.3 SPECT/CT images SPECT (left), CT (middle) and fused SPECT/CT (right) of the thoracic regions, obtained 6 h after the radiolabeled leukocyte injection showed that the area of increased accumulation localized at the posterior region of the port-a-chat, continuing along the intravascular portion. Diagnosis of port-a-chat infection was formulated and confirmed after its removal

Radiopharmaceutical Activity

740 MBq of ^{99m}Tc-HMPAO-leukocytes.

Imaging

Whole-body, spot, and SPECT/CT images of the brain (Figs. 7.7, 7.8, 7.9, 7.10 and 7.11).

Conclusion/Teaching Point

Comparative evaluation between early and delayed images is necessary to define the presence of infection since the area of early uptake may be due only to inflammatory changes. SPECT/CT is mandatory to localize the site of infection and to exclude, in this case, involvement of CNS, soft tissue or native bone. Therefore, substitution of the patch may be planned.

Case 7.4

Roberto Boni

Man, 71 years old. February 2007: esophageal cancer treated with esophageal prosthesis, chemotherapy, and radiotherapy. Mediastinitis occurred after surgery, treated with antimicrobial treatment. September 2007: septic fever with increased CRP, ERS and pro-calcitonin values, and positive blood culture for MRSA that required intensive care assistance. However, CT scan excluded the presence of active mediastinitis at CT. Despite polyantimicrobial therapy, fever persisted.

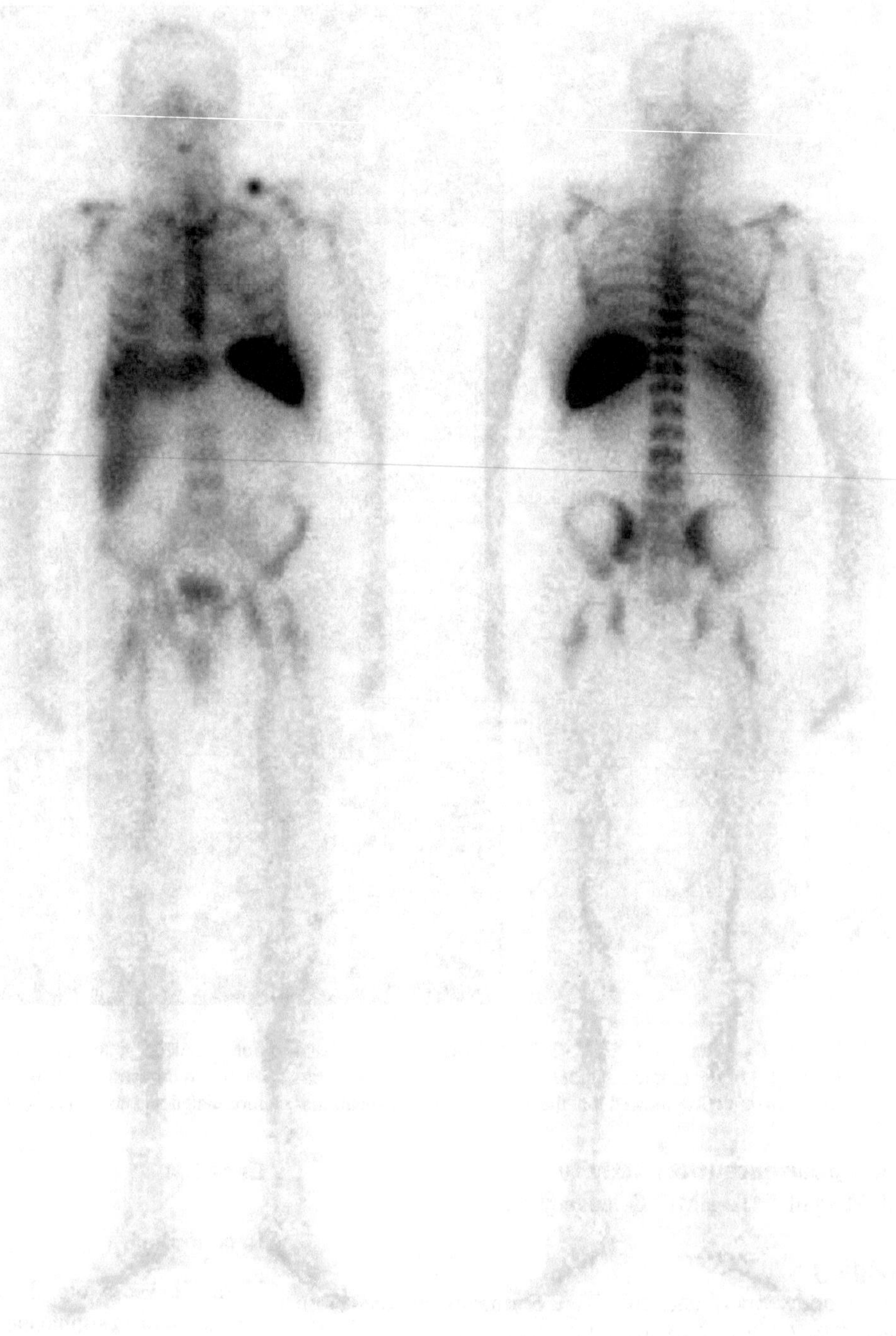

Fig. 7.4 Whole body radiolabeled leukocyte scan 30 min after the ^{99m}Tc-HMPAO-leukocyte administration showing the anterior projection (left) and the posterior projection (right). A normal radioactivity distribution within the whole body is seen. Note the site of injection at the base of the neck at the left, at site of CVC

Suspected Site of Infection

Unknown.

Radiopharmaceutical Activity

740 MBq of ^{99m}Tc-HMPAO-leukocytes.

Imaging

Whole-body, spot, and SPECT/CT images of the chest (Figs. 7.12, 7.13, and 7.14).

Conclusion/Teaching Point

This case identified, in a patient with septic fever of unknown origin, a site of infection in the initial part of prosthesis, excluding the presence of a recurrent mediastinitis. We were able to perform the examination despite the critical condition of the patient, who was admitted in intensive care unit. Interestingly, the scan showed a positive result despite the use of multi-antimicrobial treatment. Images show also a bilateral increased uptake of the radiolabeled leukocyte at

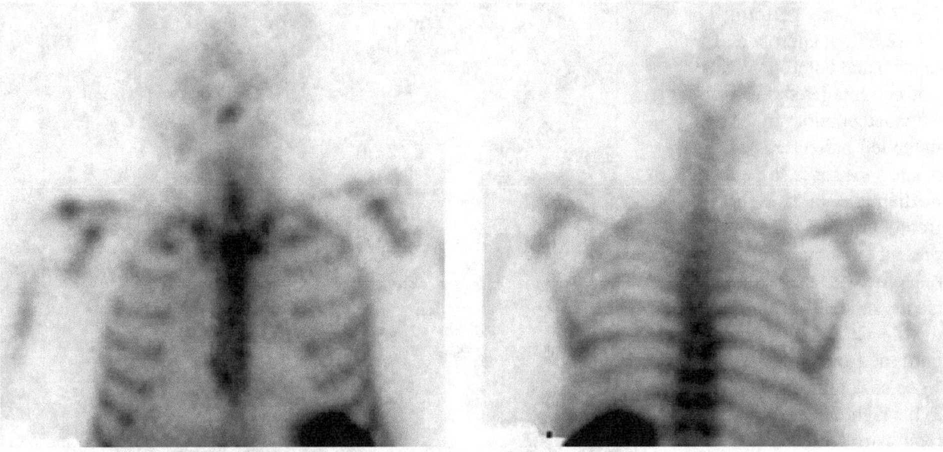

Fig. 7.5 Spot images of the head, neck and thorax obtained 6 h after ^{99m}Tc-HMPAO-leukocyte administration, in the anterior (left) and posterior (right). Images show a mild radioactivity accumulation in the right laterocervical region. Based on this finding subsequent SPECT/CT images were acquired, but due to the low uptake at this image we decided to acquire tomography at 24 h

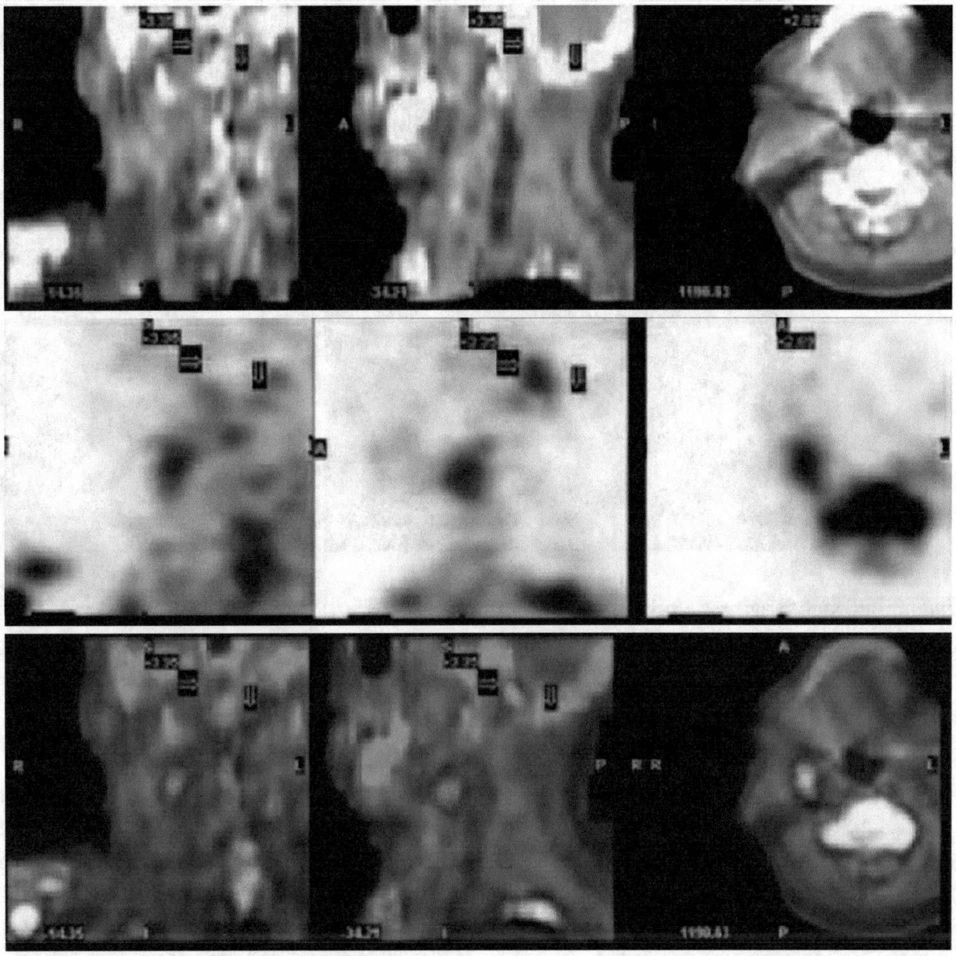

Fig. 7.6 SPECT/CT images CT (upper), SPECT (middle) and fused SPECT/CT images (lower) of the head and neck region, obtained 24 h after the radiolabeled leukocyte injection showed that the area of increased accumulation of labeled cells localized at right laterocervical region corresponds to anatomical site of vascular structures and is most likely consistent with an infection of the vascular patch

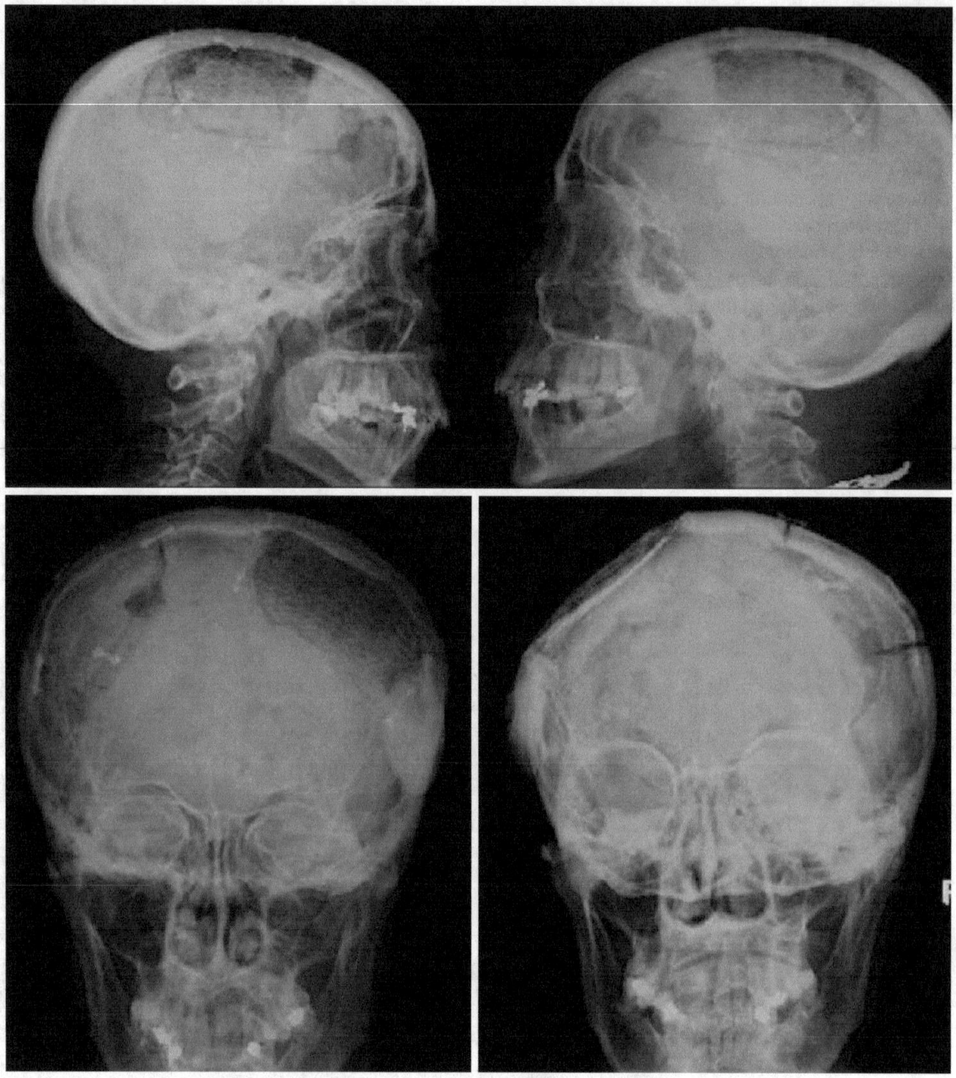

Fig. 7.7 X-ray performed on Jan 22, 2010; laterolateral (upper) and anteroposterior (lower). Images showed an extended craniotomy breach in the left parietal region that reaches the inner slope on the median line. In the right frontoparietal region the presence of craniotomy outcome with metal sutures is clearly evident (lower), so is the breach that is extending until the frontal region. No signs of definite osteomyelitis in the right lower frontal region are present

the lungs, persistent but stable as generally observed in presence of phlogistic reaction in ventilated assisted patients.

Case 7.5

Elena Lazzeri

Man, 51 years old. Pancreatectomy-splenectomy. Postsurgical fever.

Suspected Site of Infection

Unknown.

Radiopharmaceutical Activity

740 MBq of ^{99m}Tc-HMPAO-leukocytes.

Imaging

Whole-body, spot, and SPECT/CT images of the chest (Fig. 7.15).

Conclusion/Teaching Point

This case identified the presence of infection of a drainage catheter in the retropancreatic region in a patient with postsurgical fever. In this clinical, excluding the device infection is extremely important. In this clinical case, for the diagnosis, SPECT/CT images were required to localize the site of radioactivity accumulation at the tip of the drainage catheter. In fact, normal bone marrow activity at the ribs and the physiological uptake at the spleen required SPECT acquisition to differentiate the site of disease, whereas the CT component was necessary for the anatomical localization of the radiolabeled leukocyte at the tip of the drainage catheter.

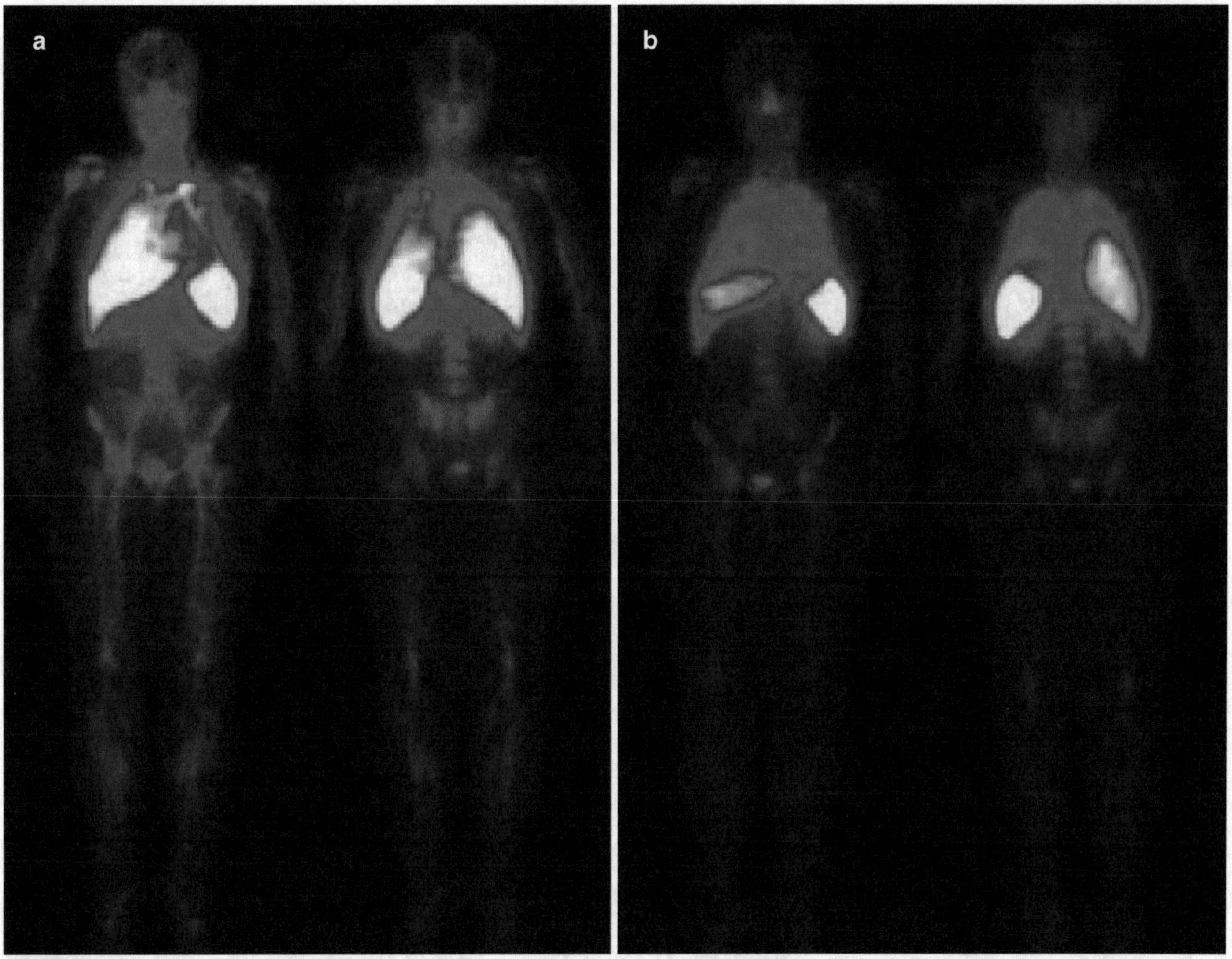

Fig. 7.8 Whole body radiolabeled leukocyte scan 30 min after administration in two different window levels (**a**, more contrasted; **b**, less contrasted) showing the anterior projection (left) and the posterior projection (right). A normal radioactivity within the whole body in present with slightly increased accumulation at the frontal region as is better depicted with the corresponding spot images (see Fig. 7.9)

Case 7.6

Paola A. Erba

Man, 69 years old. May 2008: prostatectomy and bilateral inguinal hernioplasty plus ileal resection; postsurgical fever.

Suspected Site of Infection

Unknown.

Radiopharmaceutical Activity

740 MBq of ^{99m}Tc-HMPAO-leukocytes.

Imaging

Whole-body, spot, and SPECT/CT images of the abdomen (Figs. 7.16, 7.17, 7.18 and 7.19).

Conclusion/Teaching Point

This case identified the presence of postsurgical infection localized at both the tip of the peritoneal drainage and the abdominal wall, at the site of the surgical wound. However, to obtain a correct diagnosis, SPECT/CT images were required. In fact, while for the abdominal wall infection, a lateral view as well as the standalone SPECT was sufficient to define the location of the infection, from the planar images it was extremely difficult to identify the infection at the tip of the drainage catheter as it is hampered by the normal bone marrow activity at the pelvic bones.

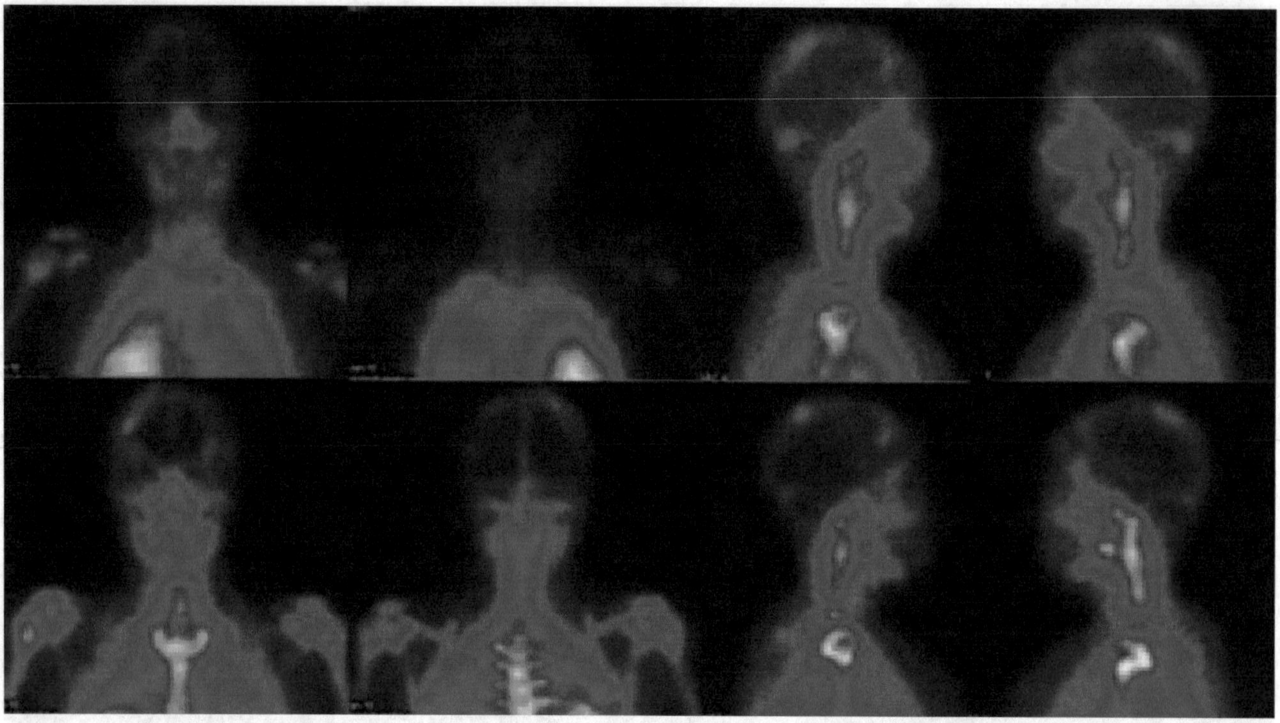

Fig. 7.9 Spot images of the brain obtained 30 min (upper panels) and 6 h (lower panels) after ^{99m}Tc-HMPAO-leukocyte administration, in the anterior, posterior and lateral views (from left to right, respectively). Images showed in the right frontal region that is present at early time point; however, over time accumulation of the radiolabeled leukocytes results in an intense area of activity clearly evident at 6 h. Based on this finding subsequent SPECT/CT images were acquired

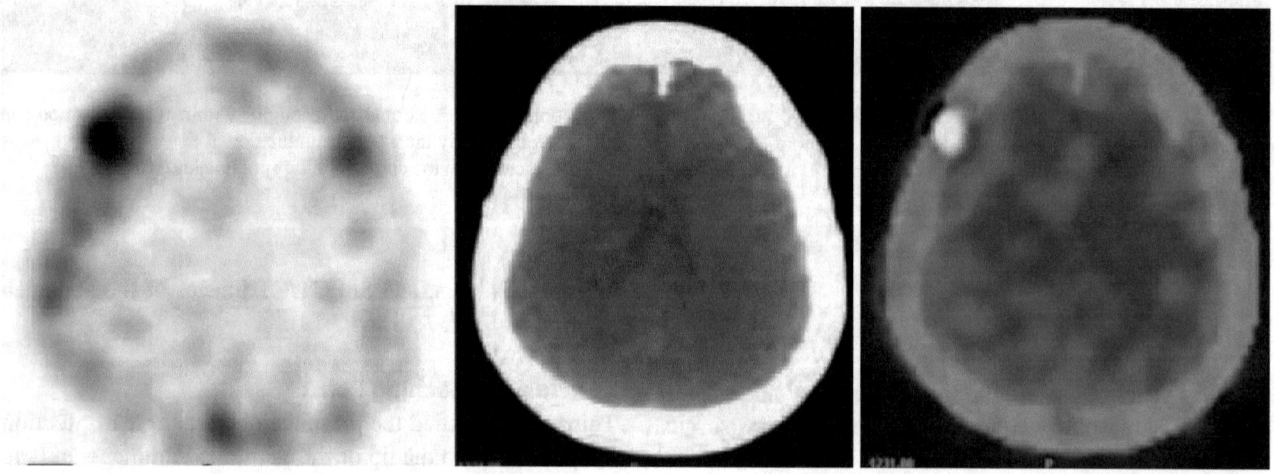

Fig. 7.10 Transaxial SPECT/CT images of the head SPECT image (left), CT image (middle), and fused SPECT/CT image (right) showed increased ^{99m}Tc-HMPAO-leukocyte accumulation in the right frontal region, corresponding to the anterior margin of the craniotomy patch at the bone level. No significant activity is evident around the patch either at the subcutaneous level or at the cerebral parenchyma

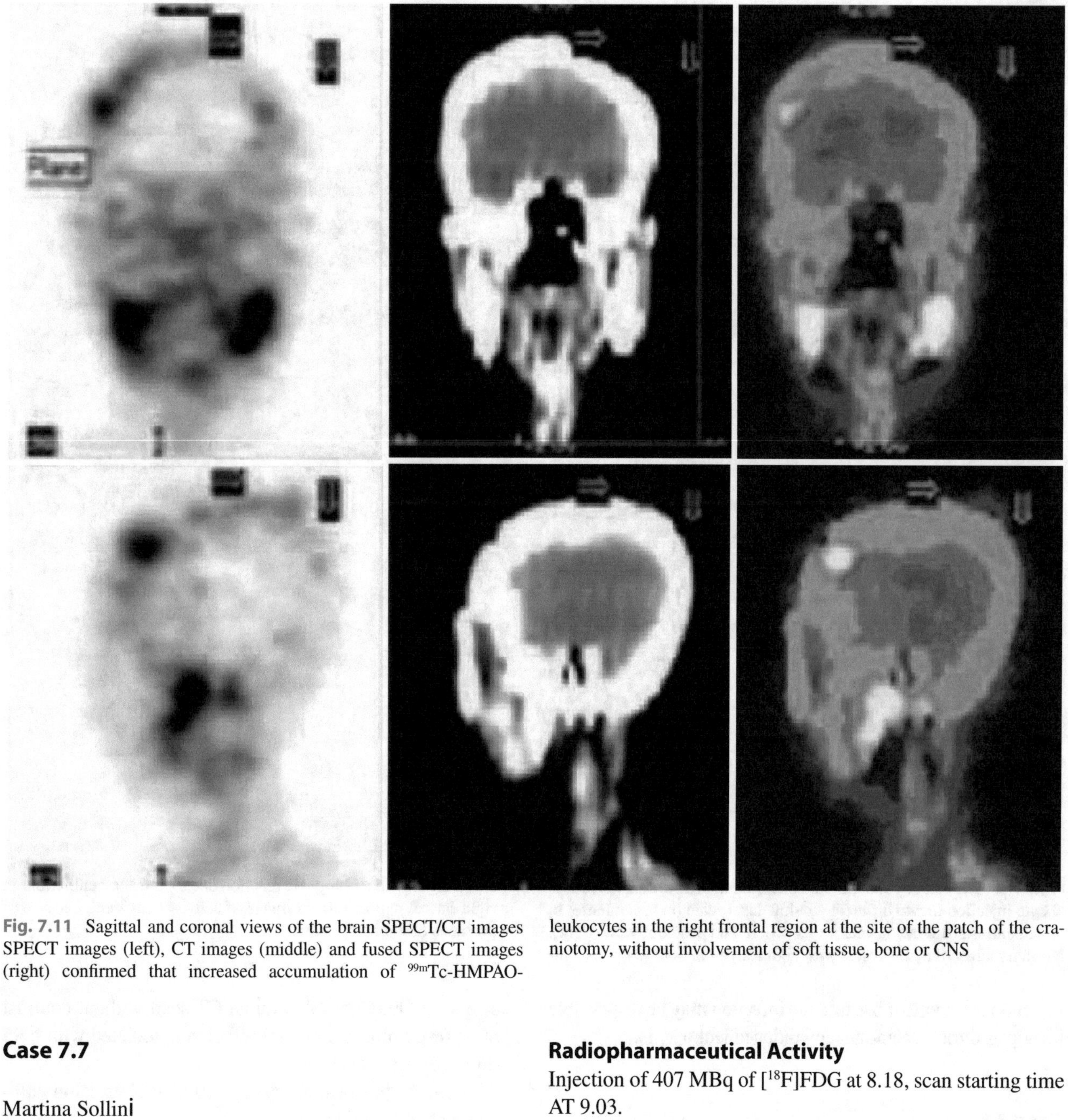

Fig. 7.11 Sagittal and coronal views of the brain SPECT/CT images SPECT images (left), CT images (middle) and fused SPECT images (right) confirmed that increased accumulation of ^{99m}Tc-HMPAO-leukocytes in the right frontal region at the site of the patch of the craniotomy, without involvement of soft tissue, bone or CNS

Case 7.7

Martina Sollini

Woman, 63 years (107 kg, 160 cm). Suspected neoplasm in patient with left leg deep venous thrombosis and implantation of a neurological stimulator fever and increased ESR. Suspected paraneoplastic syndrome that required PET/CT.

Suspected Site of Infection
Unknown.

Radiopharmaceutical Activity
Injection of 407 MBq of [^{18}F]FDG at 8.18, scan starting time AT 9.03.

Imaging
[^{18}F]FDG PET/CT 2D-mode (Figs. 7.20, 7.21, and 7.22).

Conclusion/Teaching Point
[^{18}F]FDG PET in this patient with fever, but low probability of infection, was able to depict both the primary tumor (a sarcoma) and an infection of the catheter of the neurological stimulator. In this specific patient, the discovery of a concomitant

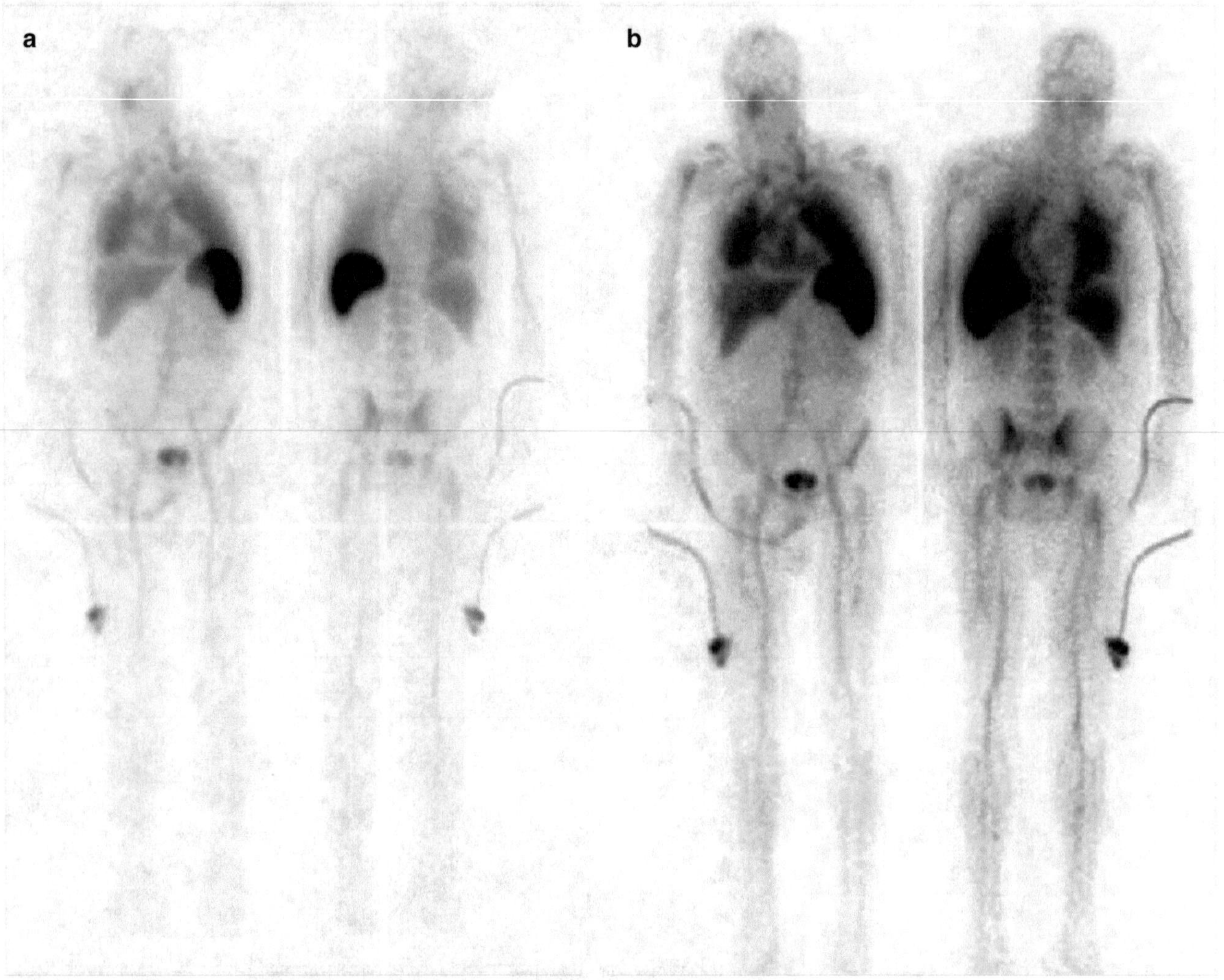

Fig. 7.12 Whole body Images obtained 30 min after radiolabeled leukocyte injection in two different window level scale (**a**, less intense; **b**, more contrasted) showing anterior view (left) and posterior view (right). Normal radioactivity is present with high activity in both lungs, as typical for patients with a phlogistic reaction due to assisted ventilation. In the right-lateral region a linear image of activity is evident, because of the presence of a urinary catheter

infection is important because the infection may be responsible for sepsis during chemotherapy induced leukopenia.

Case 7.8

Paola A. Erba

Man, 73 years old. Cardiac implantable electronic device (CIED); tracheotomy; cholecystectomy; CVC (January); acute pancreatitis (February 2009); and colitis due to *C. difficile* (March 2009); fever.

July 6, 2009: Chest/abdominal CT scan without contrast agent showed bilateral pleural effusion associated with both lower lobes subatelectasis.

July 13, 2009: Chest X-ray showed pleural effusion without lung abnormalities.

Suspected Site of Infection

Unknown.

Radiopharmaceutical Activity

Injection of 740 MBq of ^{99m}Tc-HMPAO-leukocytes.

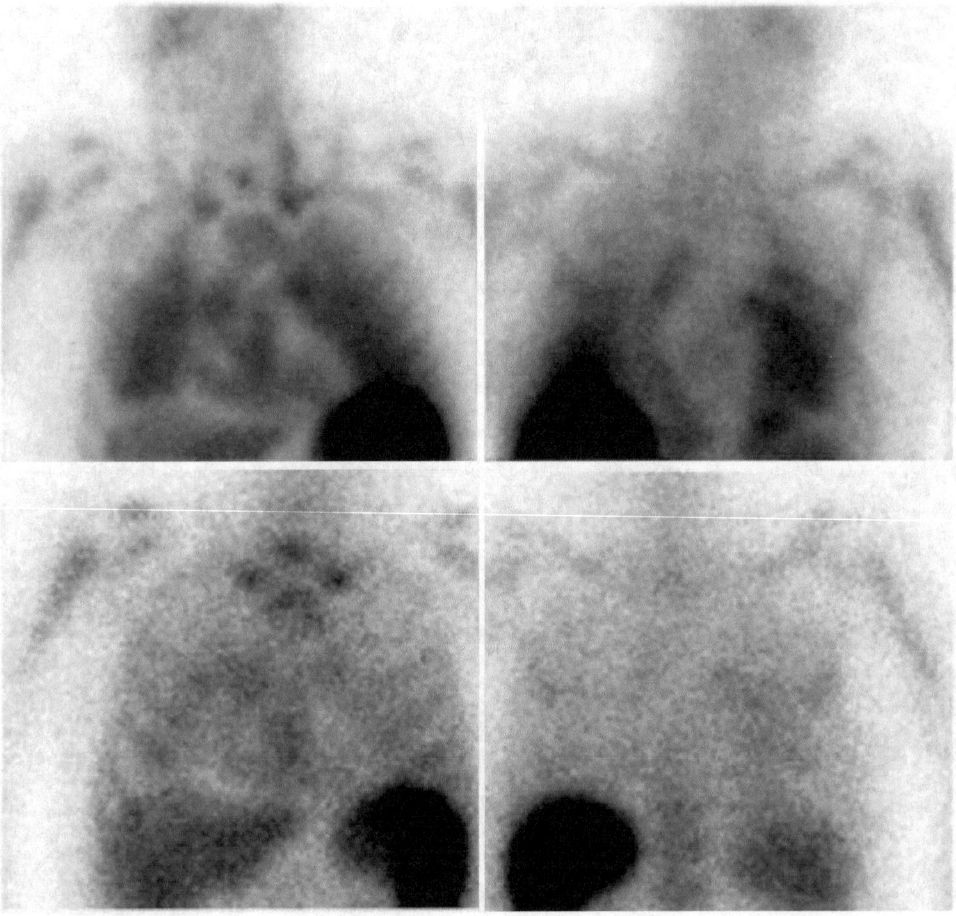

Fig. 7.13 Spot images of the chest at early time (30 min, upper) and delayed time (6 h) points (lower). Anterior view, left; posterior view, right Persistent, but stable in intensity accumulation of radiolabeled leukocyte at both lungs confirming the phlogistic origin. In the delayed anterior view an area of focal uptake localized at the lower cervical region becomes more intense as compared to early images, therefore suggesting infection. Indeed, based on this finding the region was evaluated with SPECT/CT

Imaging

Whole-body and spot images of the chest, 30 min after radiopharmaceutical administration, and spot images of chest and abdomen, 6 h after injection (Figs. 7.23, 7.24, 7.25, 7.26 and 7.27).

Conclusion/Teaching Point

Planar images were sufficient in a critical patient with fever, unresponsive to antipolymicrobial therapy to demonstrate the sites of radiolabeled leukocyte uptake and to diagnose lung infection. However, the image quality was suboptimal since the critical clinical condition of the patient prevented SPECT/CT acquisition. This may be considered to be one of the limitations of ^{99m}Tc-HMPAO-leukocyte scintigraphy in this specific clinical setting and thus suggests PET/CT as a possible candidate for both the shorter acquisition time and better spatial resolution of the images, as demonstrated in the next case.

Case 7.9

Elena Lazzeri

Man, 63 years old. Tracheotomy due to polytrauma. Septic fever and critical clinical condition, not responding to antipolymicrobial treatment.

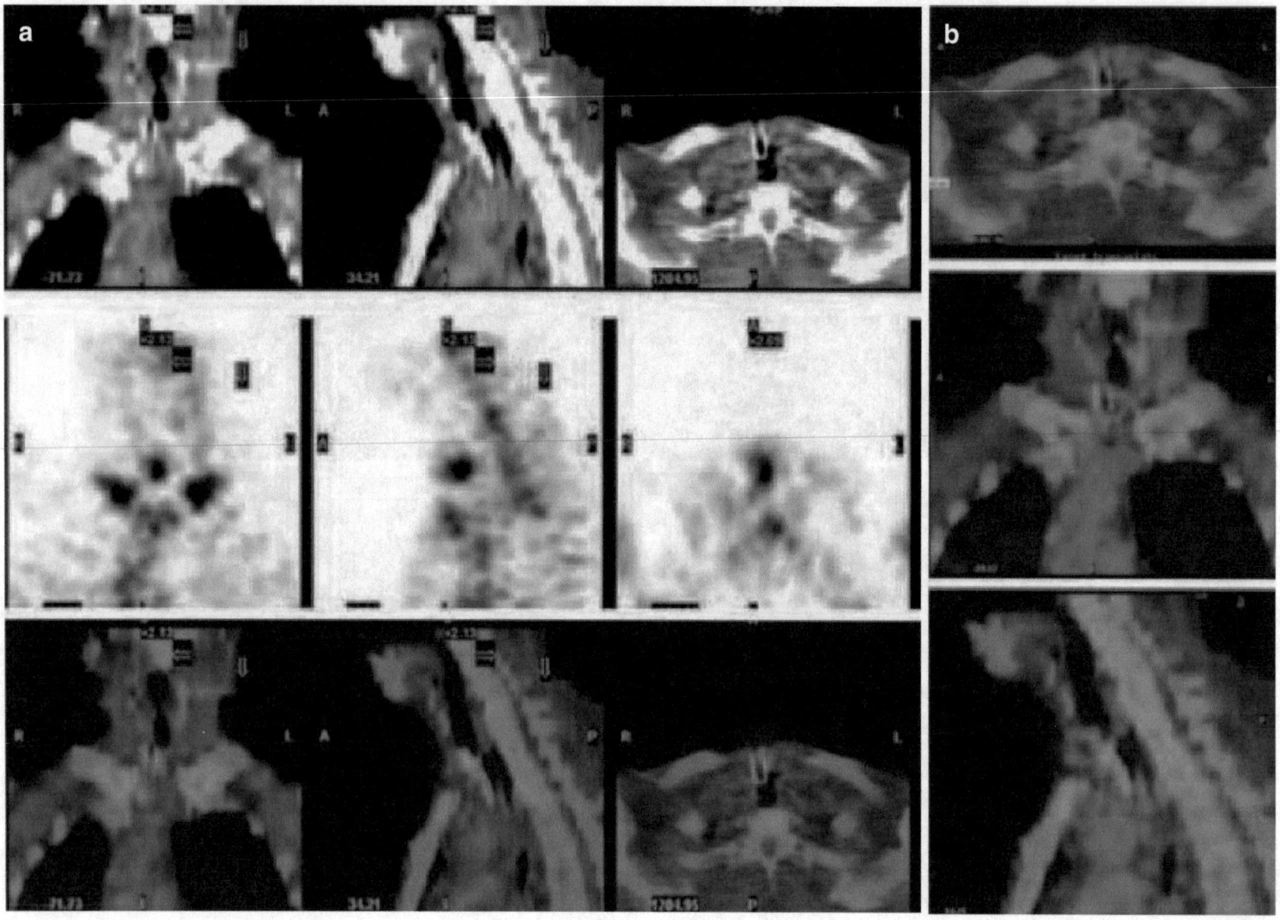

Fig. 7.14 (**a**) SPECT/CT images (CT slides upper panels, SPECT images middle panels and fused SPECT/CT images lower panels) showed that the site of increased labeled leukocyte accumulation corresponds to the initial portion of the esophageal prosthesis. (**b**) Fused SPECT/CT images (transaxial view, upper; coronal view, middle; sagittal view, lower) with a more clear definition of the site of infection

Suspected Site of Infection

Unknown.

Radiopharmaceutical Activity

Injection of 262 MBq of [^{18}F]FDG at 10.15, scan starting time at 11.09.

Imaging

[^{18}F]FDG PET/CT 3D mode (Figs. 7.28, 7.29 and 7.30).

Conclusion/Teaching Point

In this specific patient, [^{18}F]FDG PET/CT was preferred to other imaging modalities for the rapidity of the test, making it more appropriate in a very critical patient. The scan detected the lung as the site of infection.

Case 7.10

Roberta Zanca

Background

A 68-year-old man with acute renal failure treated with hemodialysis. The acute phase inflammatory serum markers were increased, and blood culture was positive for *Klebsiella pneumoniae*.

The patient was referred for [^{18}F]FDG PET/CT imaging, aimed at searching for and localizing infectious foci. The scan showed increased [^{18}F]FDG uptake in soft tissue of the right forearm, suggesting infection of the arterovenous fistula; a chronic expanding hematoma of the right thoracic wall (caused by prior trauma) was also observed, externally

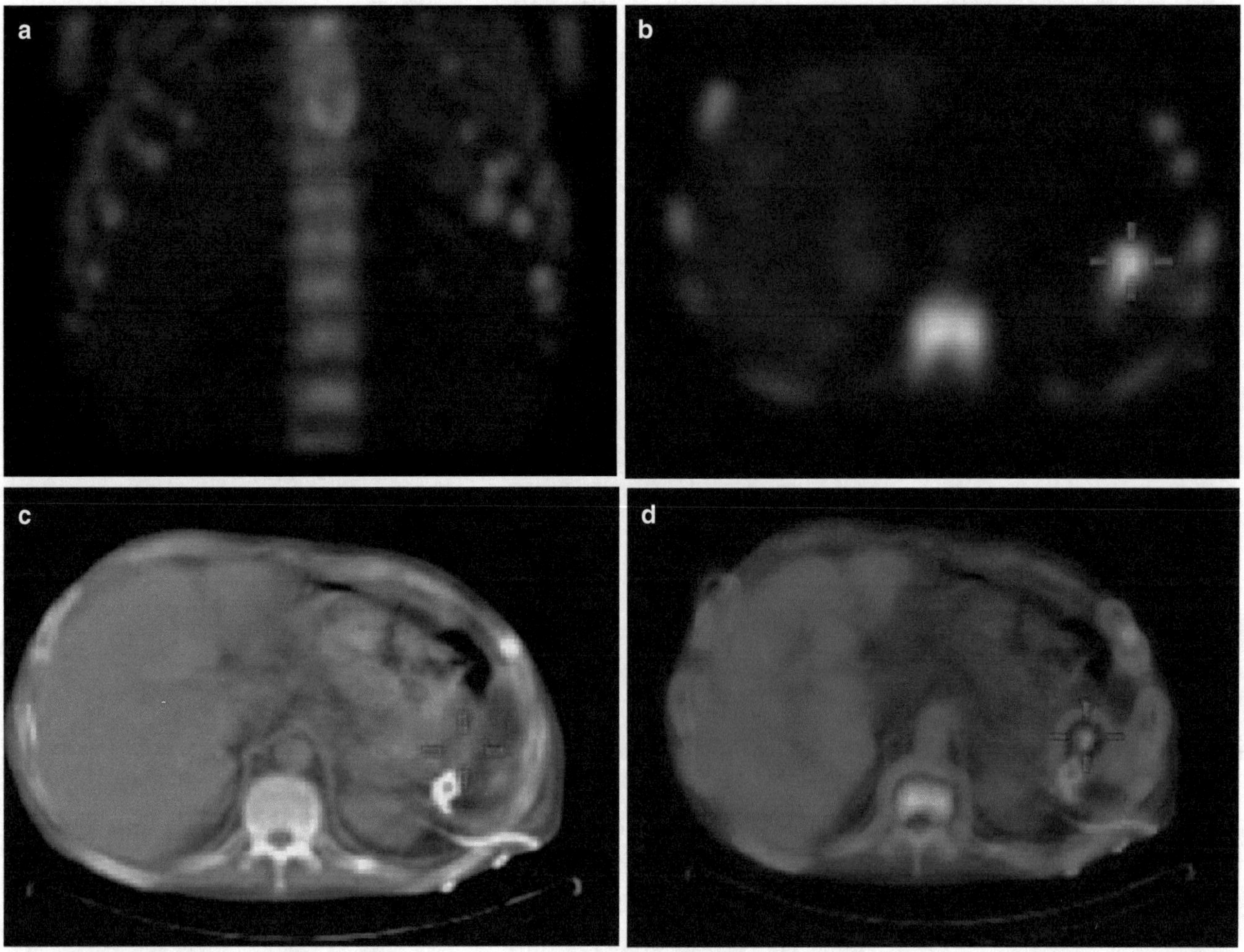

Fig. 7.15 SPECT/CT images of radiolabeled leukocyte scintigraphy obtained 6 h after admibistration. MIP image (**a**), transaxial SPECT (**b**), CT (**c**) and fused SPECT/CT image (**d**). Images showed labeled cell accumulation at the left hypochondrium, just below the lateral portion of the ribs (MIP image). Transaxial SPECT localized the site of accumulation to the posterolateral hypochondrium, which results in the fused SPECT/CT images localized near the drainage catheter in the retropancreatic region

of the ribcage, with mildly increased tracer uptake in the peripheral rim of the mass (Fig. 7.31).

Suspected Site of Infection

Arterovenous fistula and thoracic hematoma.

Radiopharmaceutical Activity

[^{18}F]FDG, 282 MBq.

Imaging

The PET/CT acquisition included scout CT view (120 kV, 10 mA), whole-body CT scan (140 kV, 80 mA), and PET (3D mode, 3 min/FOV). Images were reconstructed with and without attenuation correction using the low-dose transmission CT scan.

Conclusion/Teaching Point

[^{18}F]FDG PET/CT identified infection at the right forearm, corresponding to the arterovenous fistula.

Case 7.11

Roberta Zanca

Background

A 47-year-old woman submitted to surgery for right breast cancer about 18 months earlier (mastectomy and implant-based breast reconstruction), followed by adjuvant chemotherapy. A Port-a-Cath system was implanted for chemotherapy, which was still ongoing. The patient was

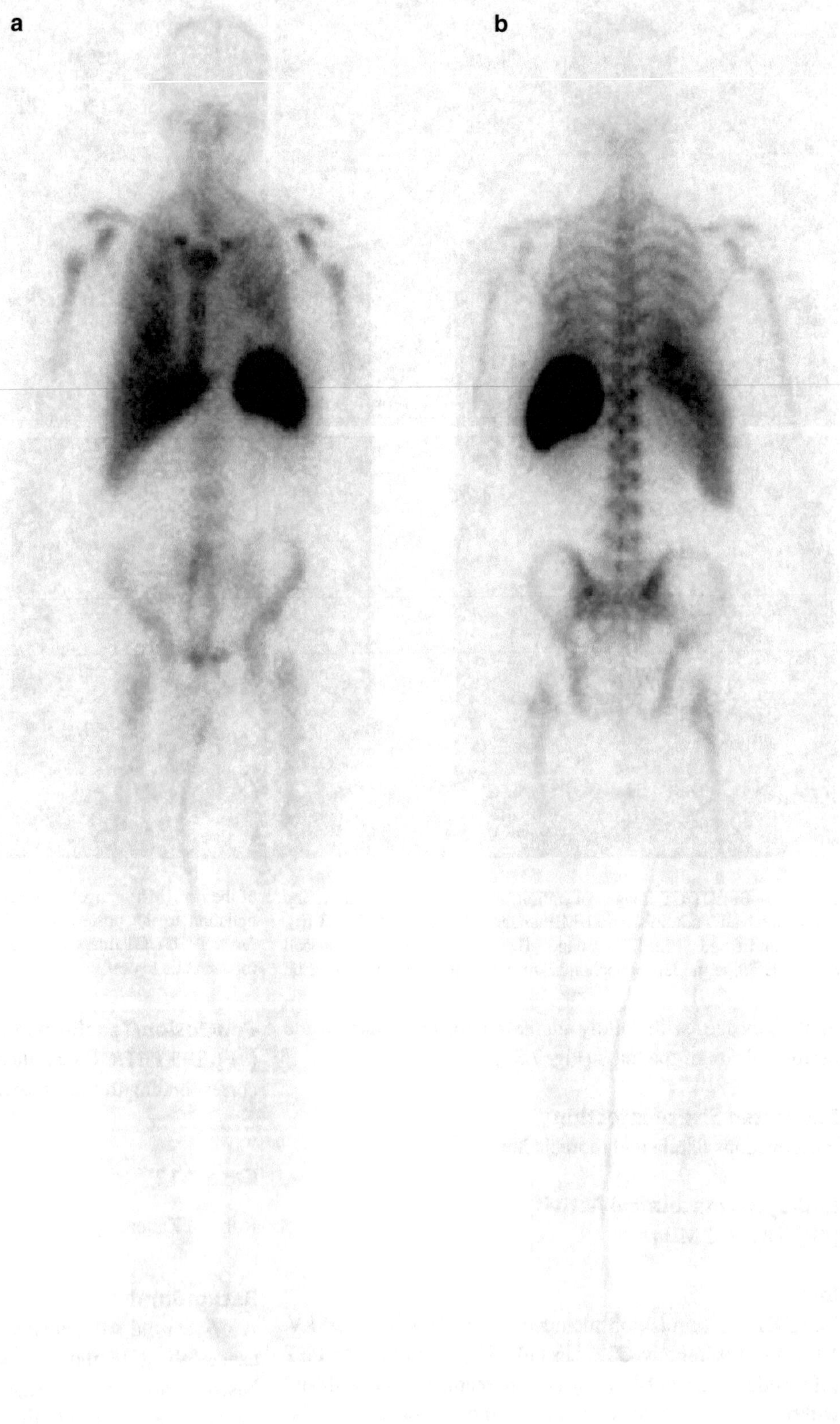

Fig. 7.16 Whole body radiolabeled leukocyte scan, 30 min after administration, showing the anterior projection (**a**) and the posterior projection (**b**). A normal labeled cell distribution within the whole body is present, with increased accumulation in the abdominal area, better depicted with the corresponding spot images (see Fig. 7.17)

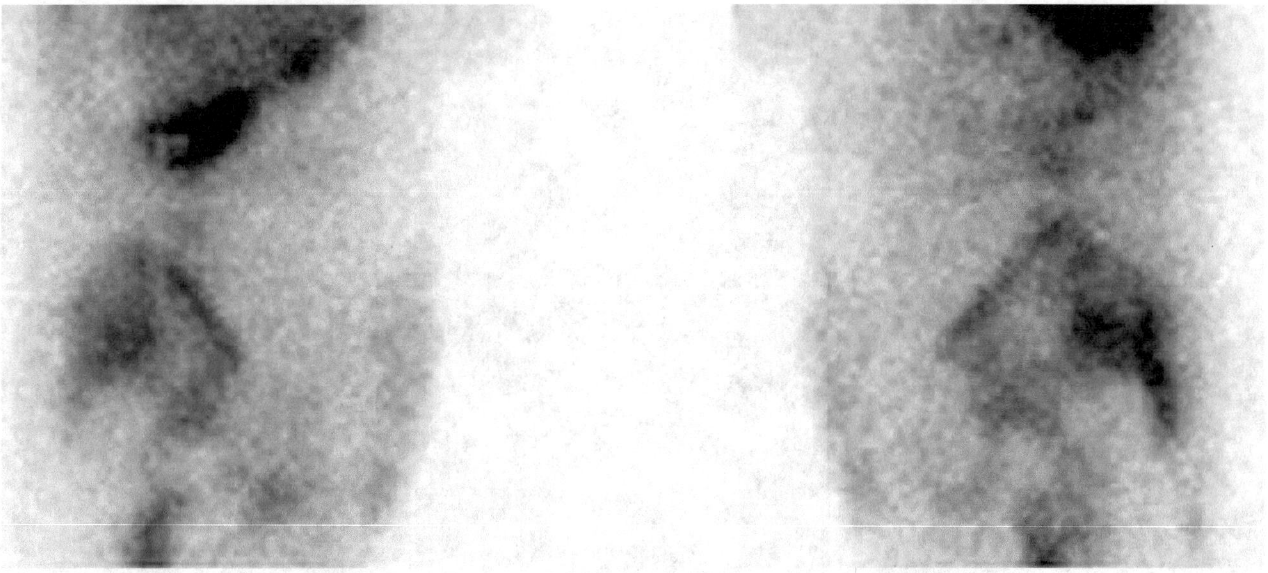

Fig. 7.17 Spot images of the abdomen obtained 30 min after ^{99m}TC-HMPAO-leukocyte administration, in the lateral view. Images showed labeled leukocyte accumulation in the abdominal region is anterior, involving the abdominal wall

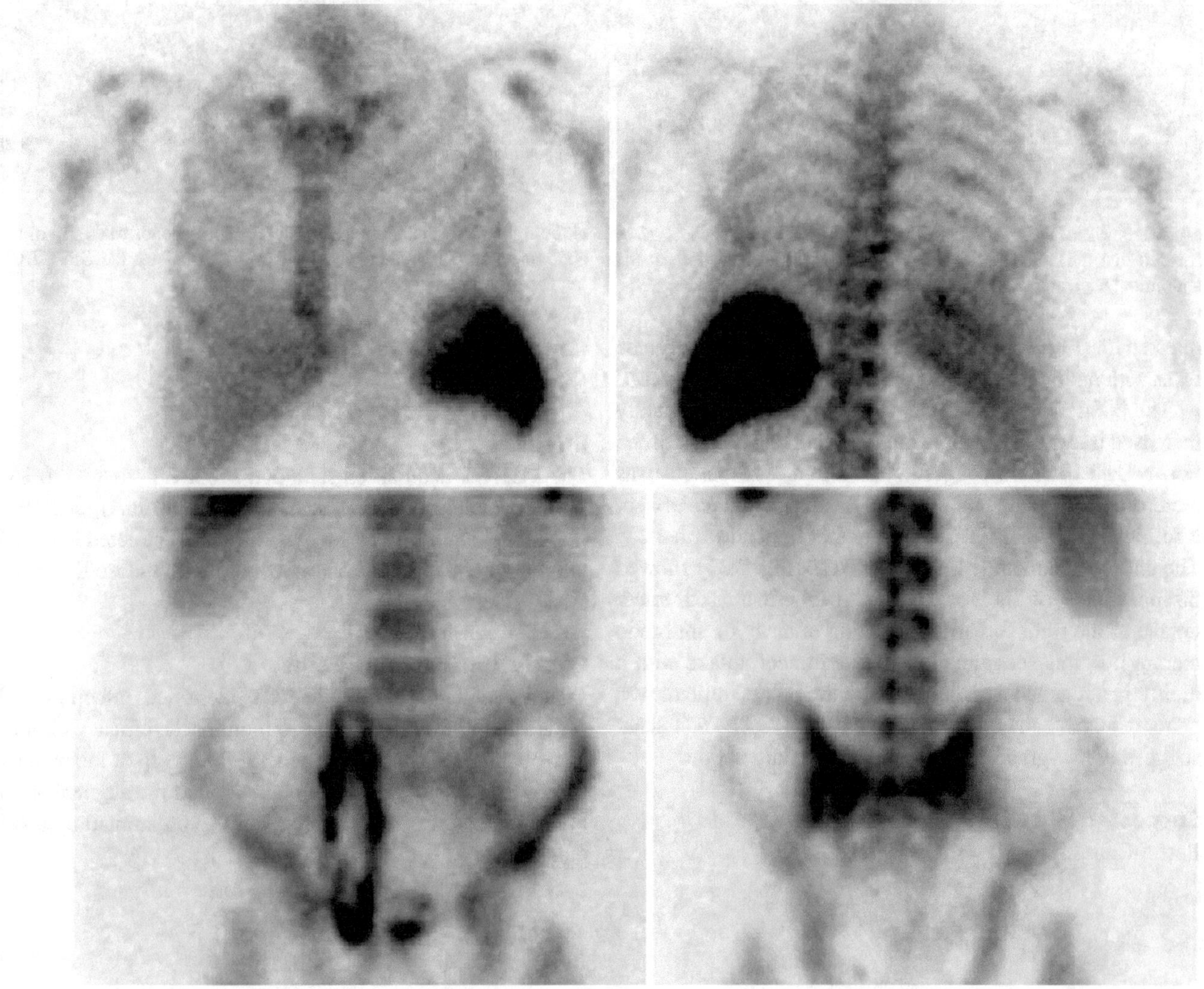

Fig. 7.18 Spot images of the thorax (upper) and abdomen (lower) obtained 6 h after labeled cell administration, in the anterior (left) and posterior views (right). Images confirm increased accumulation in the abdominal region, increased in intensity. Based on this finding, subsequent SPECT/CT images were acquired

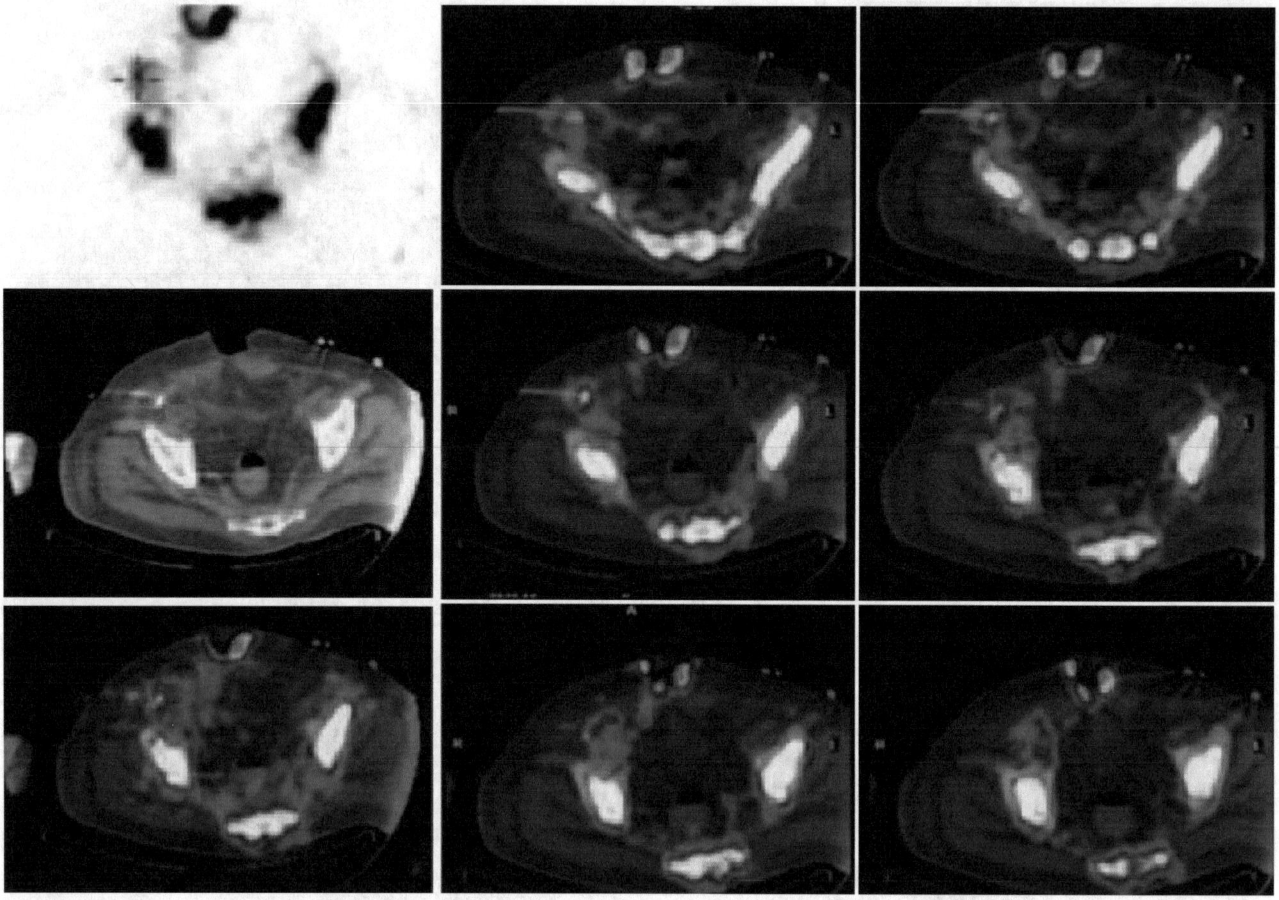

Fig. 7.19 SPECT/CT image (**a**, SPECT; **b**, CT and **c**, SPECT/CT) showed that the radioactivity accumulation was localized both at the abdominal wall, at the site of the surgical wound as well as in the pelvis, at the right site. This latter area of uptake corresponds to the tip of the abdominal drainage catheter, as clearly detected by the SPECT/CT images (**d**, transaxial SPECT/CT images)

referred for [^{18}F]FDG PET/CT because of persisting low-grade fever with mildly increased serum markers of inflammation.

The [^{18}F]FDG PET/CT scan (Fig. 7.32) showed markedly increased tracer uptake along the intra-thoracic portion of the Port-a-Cath catheter, suggesting infection. The patient was therefore treated with antimicrobial treatment, and underwent a further [^{18}F]FDG PET/CT scan and at the end of therapy. The end-of-treatment [^{18}F]FDG PET/CT (Fig. 7.33) showed disappearance of the focus of markedly increased tracer uptake at the right forearm (indicating efficacy of antibiotic therapy); in this scan, mildly increased tracer uptake with a highly heterogeneous pattern around the breast implant was better detectable than in the baseline [^{18}F]FDG PET/CT scan, suggesting low-grade ongoing infection/inflammation.

Suspected Site of Infection

Port-a-Cath.

Radiopharmaceutical Activity

[^{18}F]FDG, 264 MBq.

Imaging

The PET/CT acquisition included scout CT view (120 kV, 10 mA), whole-body CT scan (140 kV, 80 mA), and PET (3D mode, 3 min/FOV). Images were reconstructed with and without attenuation correction using the low-dose transmission CT scan.

Conclusion/Teaching Point

Imaging with [^{18}F]FDG PET/CT identified infection and provided helpful information to monitor the efficacy of antimicrobial treatment and for general follow-up of the patient. Mildly increased [^{18}F]FDG uptake around the augmentation breast implant was most likely related to inflammation rather than infection.

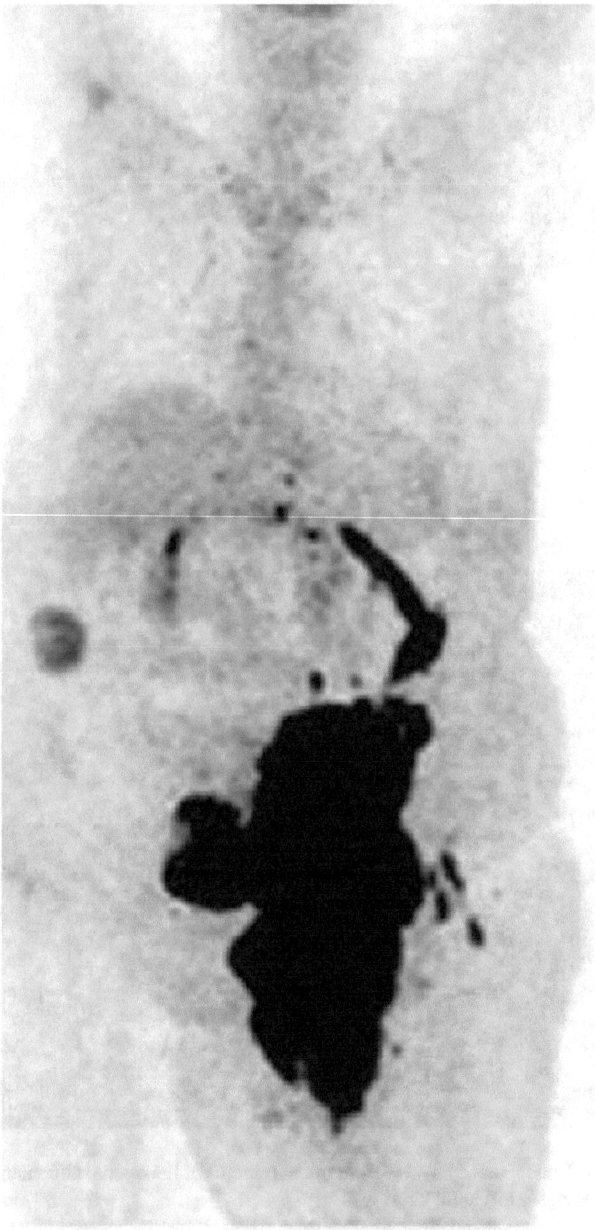

Fig. 7.20 [^{18}FDG PET/CT MIP images showing an intense and large area of radiopharmaceutical uptake extending from the pelvic region to the left thigh, which represents the primary tumor of the patient. Additional sites of [^{18}F]FDG uptake are also present. Particularly at the right abdominal flank where a round area of uptake is evident

Case 7.12

Martina Sollini

Background

A 45-year-old woman with recent diagnosis of tachy-brady syndrome (or "sick sinus" syndrome). Past medical history included prior treatment of urge incontinence with implantation (in the right gluteal region) of a sacral neurostimulation device, after failure of conservative treatments. Twenty days after removal of the sacral nerve neurostimulator and implant of an intracardiac electronic stimulation device, the patient presented with low-grade fever and increased serum markers of inflammation. She was therefore referred for [^{18}F]FDG PET/CT imaging with the clinical suspicion of possible infection related to recent implant of the intracardiac electronic stimulation device.

The [^{18}F]FDG PET/CT scan (Fig. 7.34) did not show any abnormal focus of increased tracer uptake related to the intracardiac electronic stimulation device. Instead, increased [^{18}F]FDG uptake was noted in the soft tissues of the right gluteal region, former site of the neurostimulator generator pocket.

Suspected Site of Infection

Related to intracardiac electronic stimulation device.

Radiopharmaceutical Activity

[^{18}F]FDG, 301 MBq.

Imaging

The PET/CT acquisition included scout CT view (120 kV, 10 mA), whole-body CT scan (140 kV, 80 mA), and PET (3D mode, 3 min/FOV). Images were reconstructed with and without attenuation correction using the low-dose transmission CT scan.

Conclusion/Teaching Point

[^{18}F]FDG PET/CT imaging ruled out the recent implantation of an intracardiac electronic stimulation device as the cause/site of infection, localizing instead the infectious focus at the former site of the sacral neurostimulation device (subcutaneous pocket).

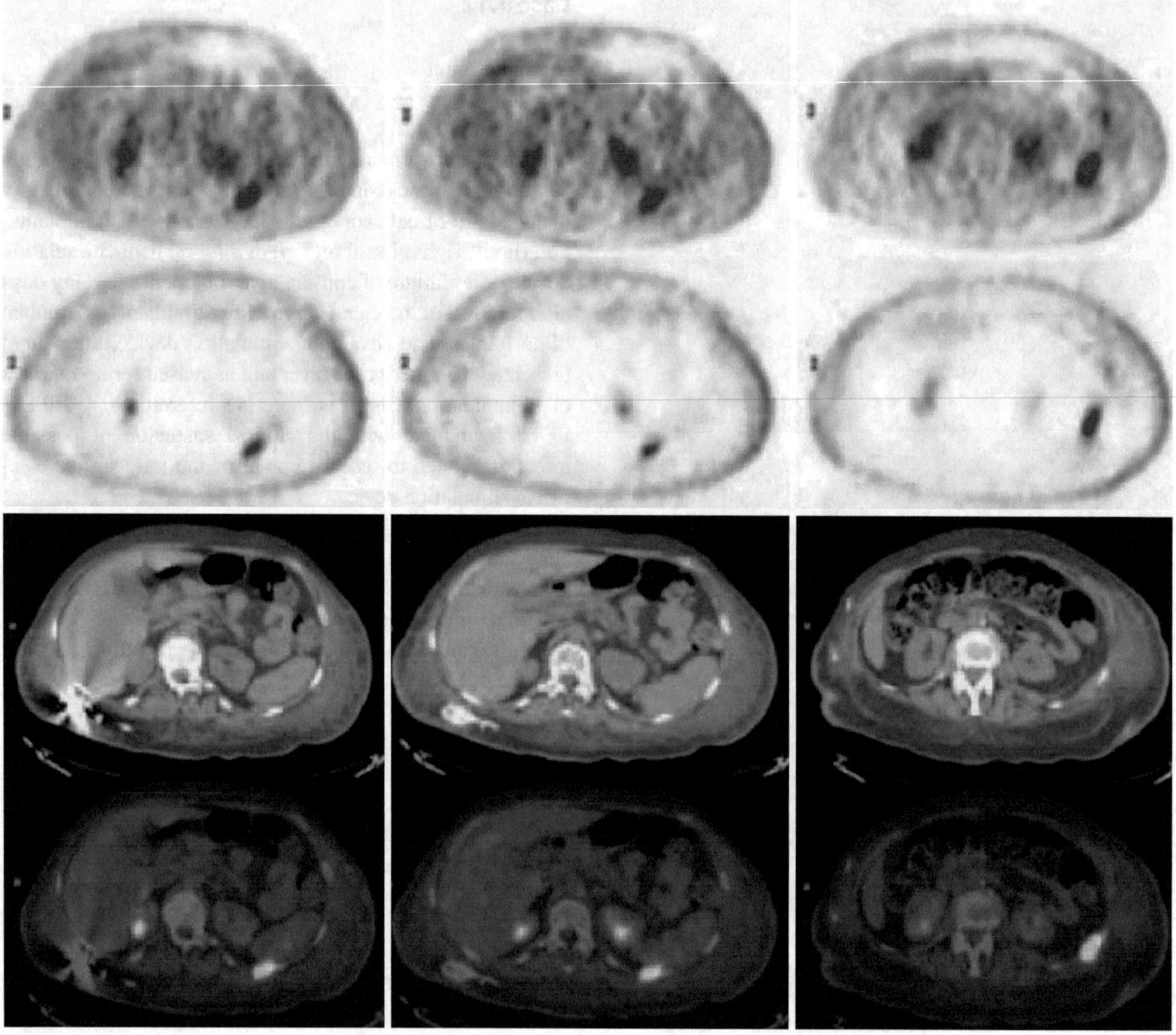

Fig. 7.21 [^{18}F]FDG PET attenuated corrected, PET nonattenuated corrected, CT and fused PET/CT (from top to bottom) of the middle abdomen showed no significant uptake at the site of the neurological device located at the posteriorlateral chest wall

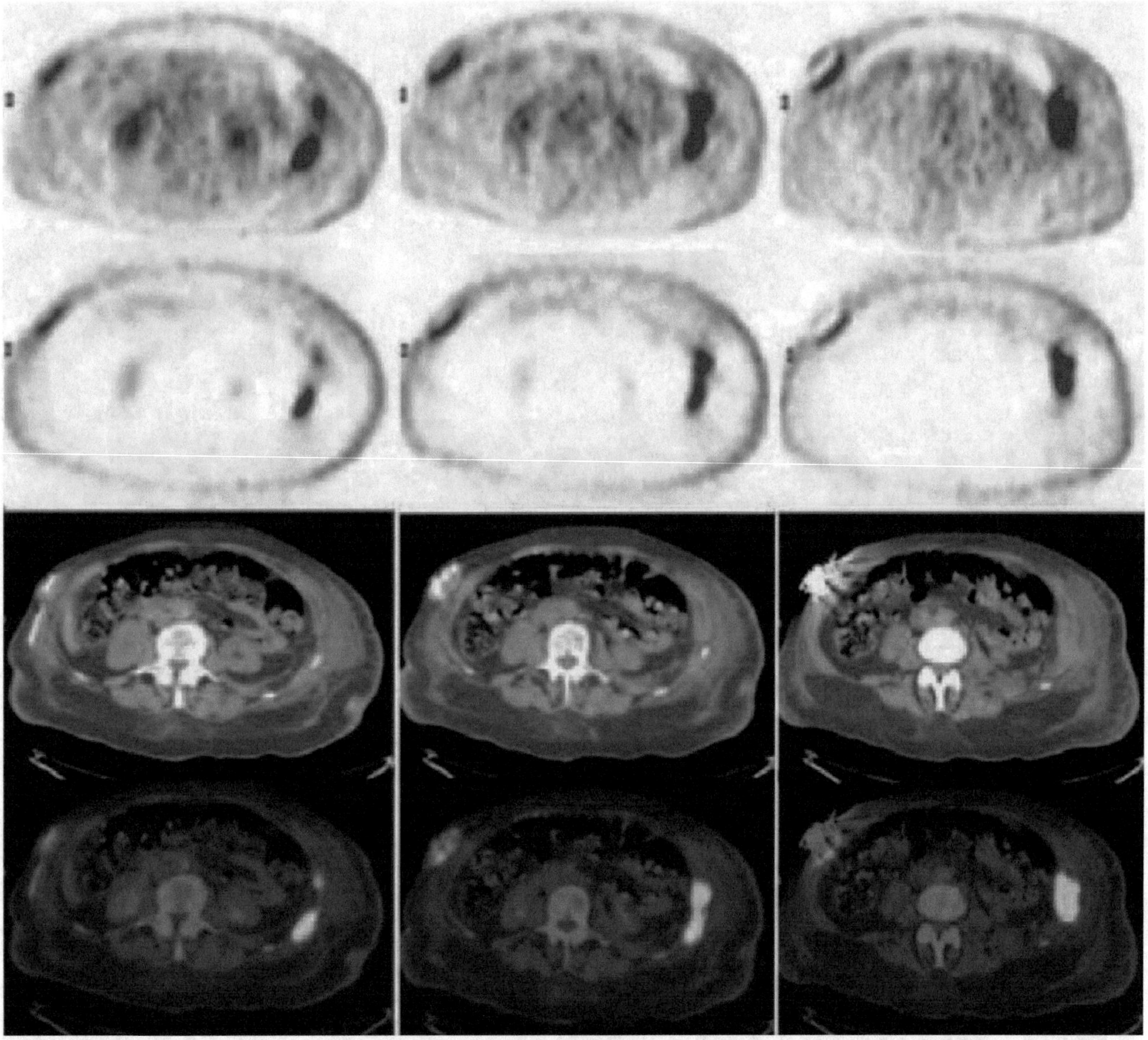

Fig. 7.22 [^{18}F] FDG PET attenuated corrected, PET nonattenuated corrected, CT and fused PET/CT (from top to bottom) of the middle abdomen showed an area of radiopharmaceutical uptake located at the right lateral abdominal wall, which is the site of the catheter of the neurological stimulator. Both the attenuated corrected and the nonattenuated corrected PET images presented the uptake

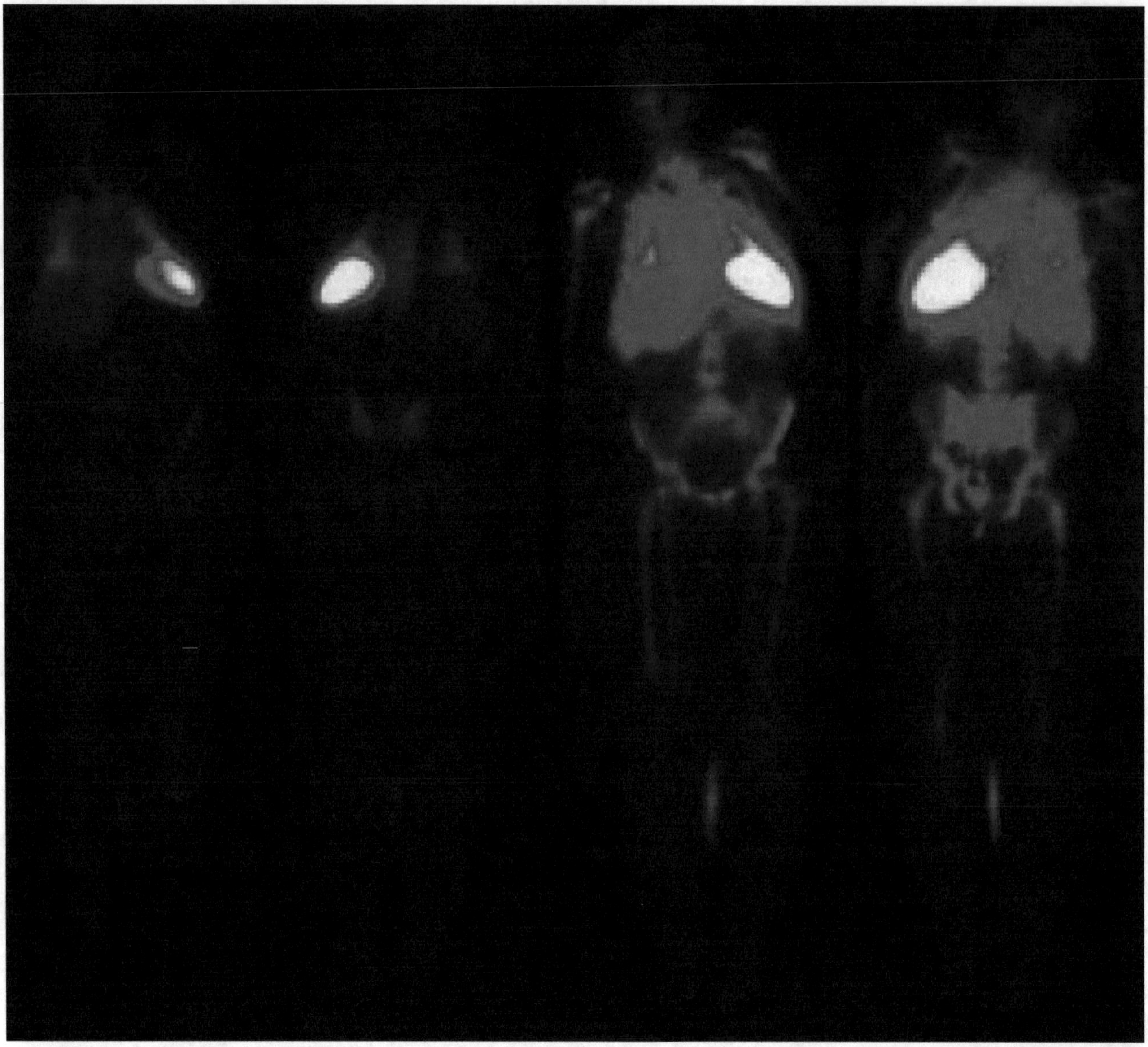

Fig. 7.23 Whole body images (anterior view, left; posterior view, right) showed increased accumulation of ^{99m}Tc-HMPAO-leukocytes in lower fields of both lungs

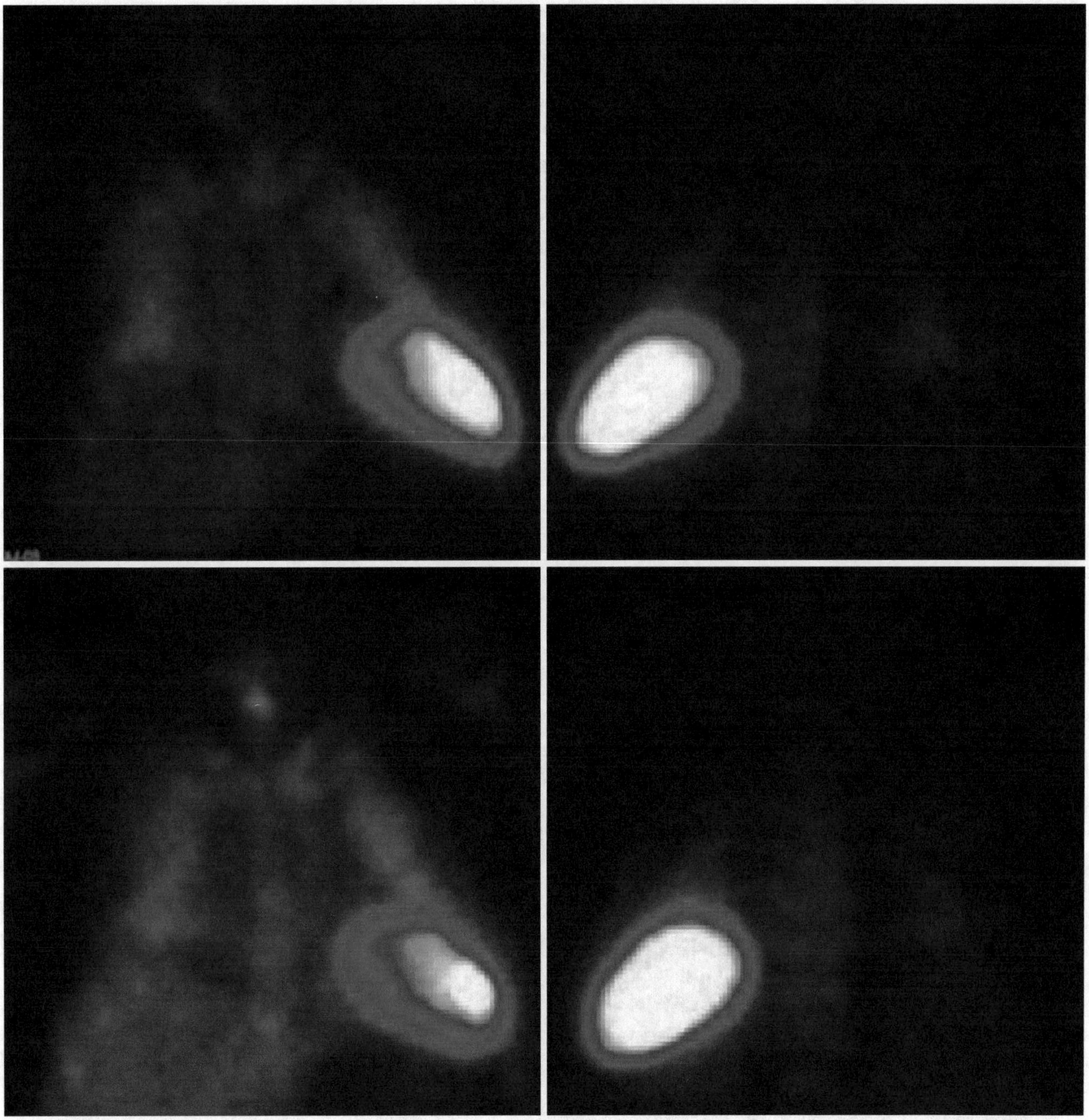

Fig. 7.24 Planar spots of the chest in anterior (right) and posterior (left) views obtained 30 min (upper) and 6 h (lower) after injection confirmed the presence of the increased radioactivity localization at the tracheotomy and in the basal posterior fields of the lungs

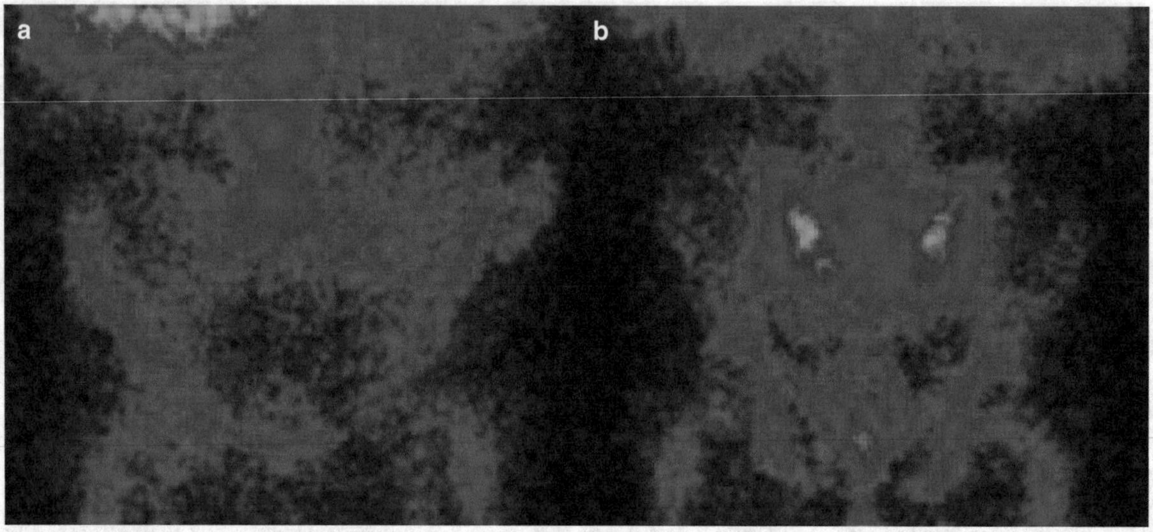

Fig. 7.25 Planar spots of the abdomen in anterior (**b**) and posterior (**a**) views obtained 6 h after injection demonstrated an additional site of increased accumulation at the posterior pelvis, most likely to be related to bedsores. In this patient we were not able to perform additional SPECT/CT images because of his critical condition

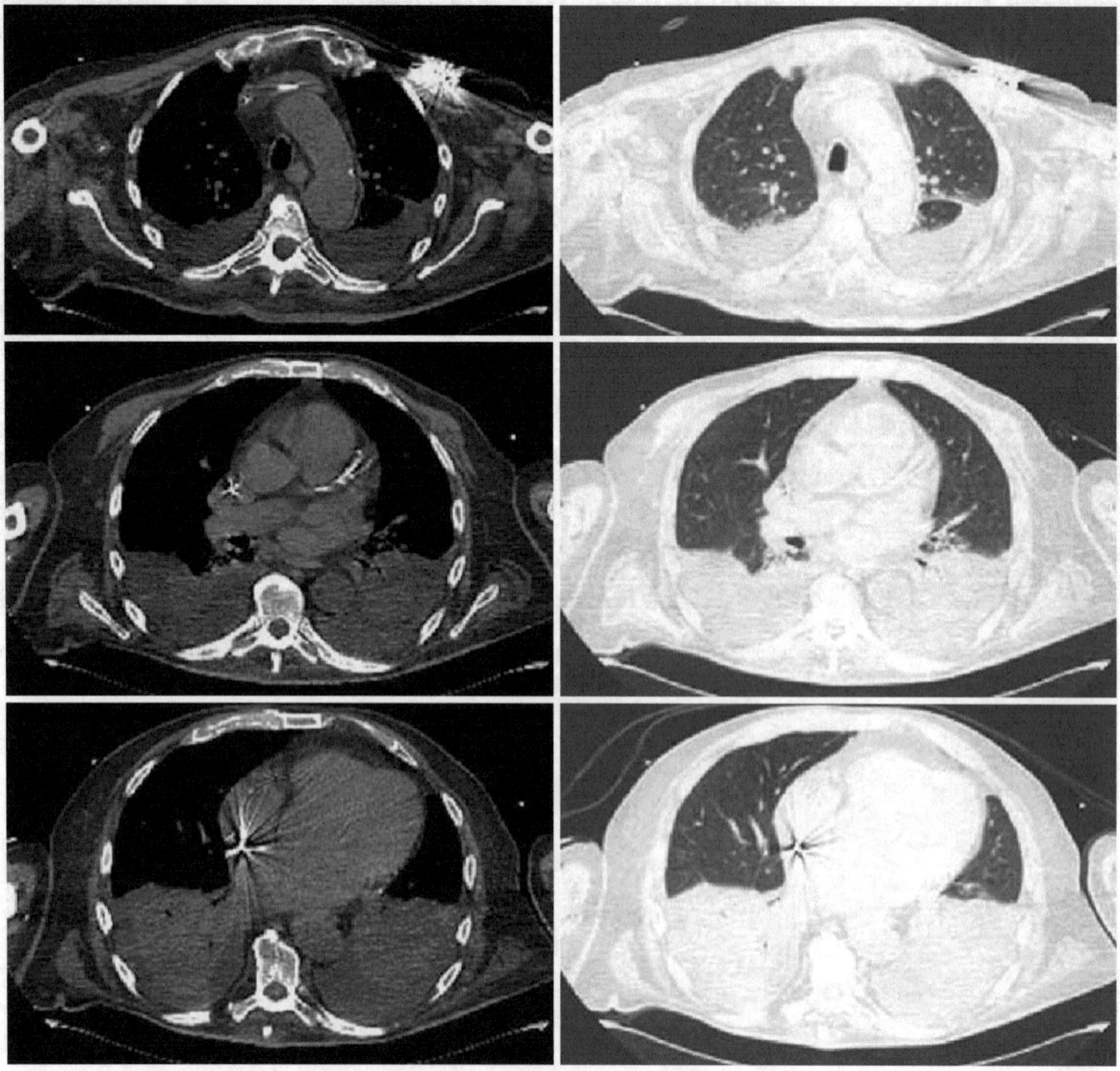

Fig. 7.26 Chest CT sections showed the presence of bilateral pleural effusion associated with atelectasis

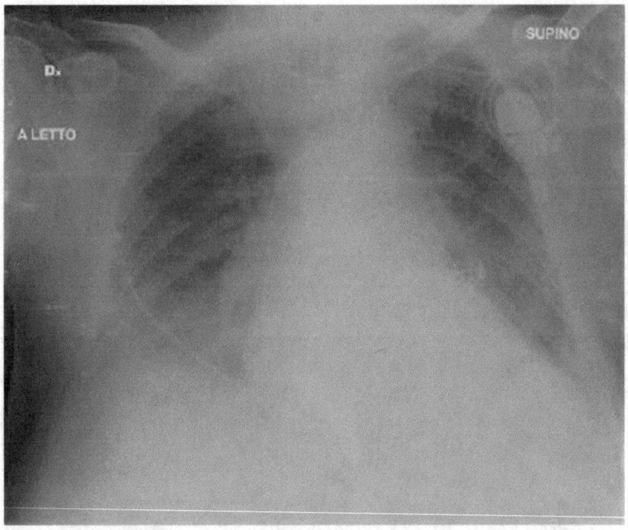

Fig. 7.27 Chest X-ray showed bilateral pleural effusion (right to left) associated with congestive aspect of both lung hilum and enlargement of mediastinum CVC in superior vena cava and endotracheal tube at D4 level. CIED in left upper chest

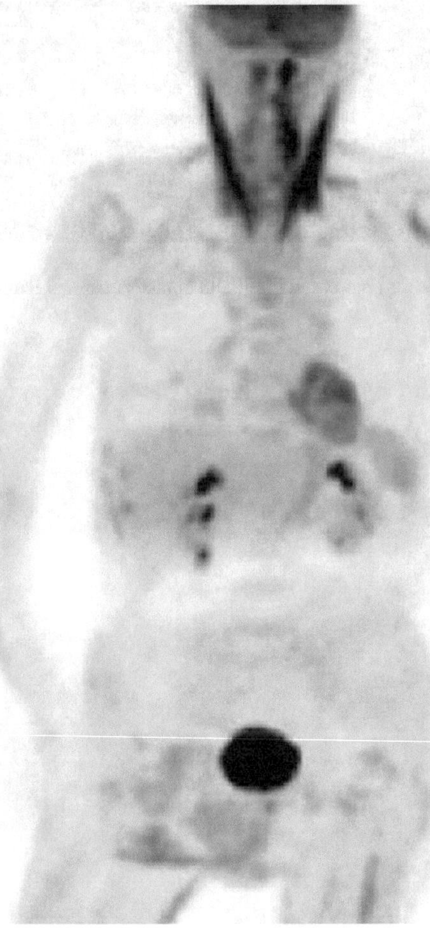

Fig. 7.28 MIP image showed intense [^{18}F]FDG uptake at neck muscle

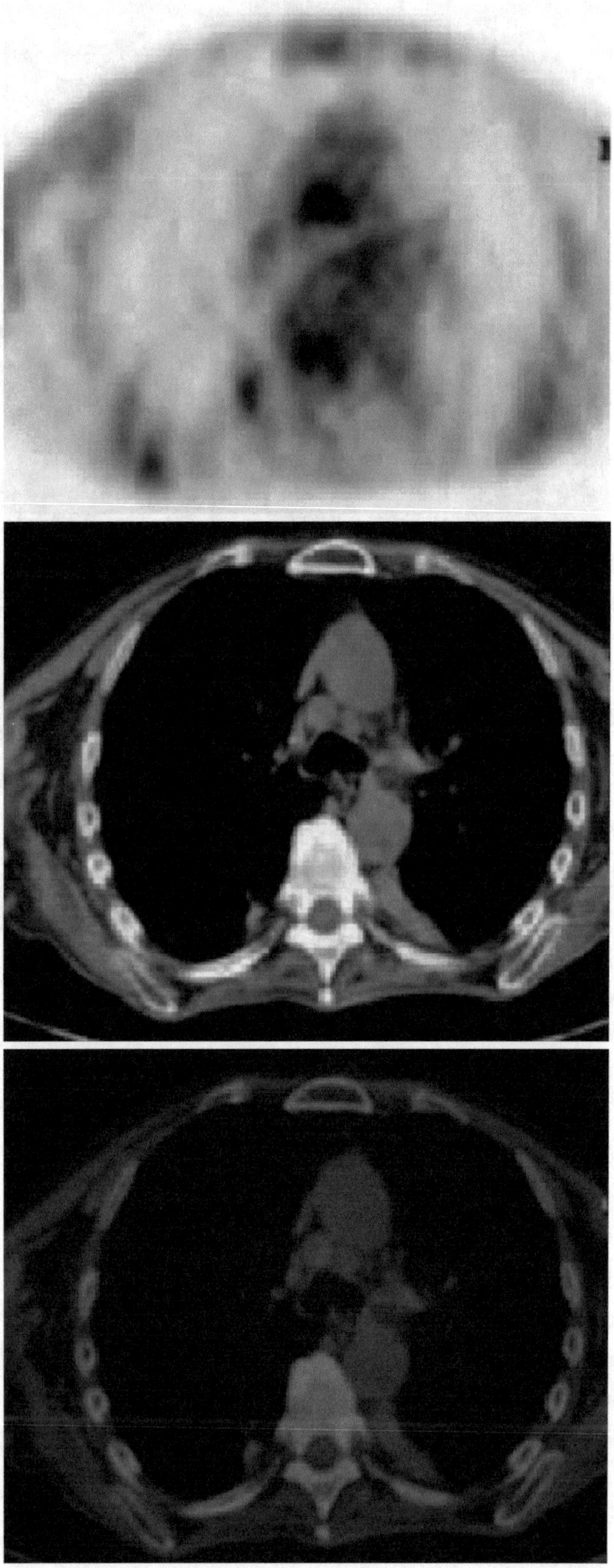

Fig. 7.29 Images (PET image, upper; CT slide, middle; fused PET/CT image, lower) showed increased [^{18}F]FDG uptake at carenal lymph nodes and right lung at mantle paravertebral region associated with CT lesion

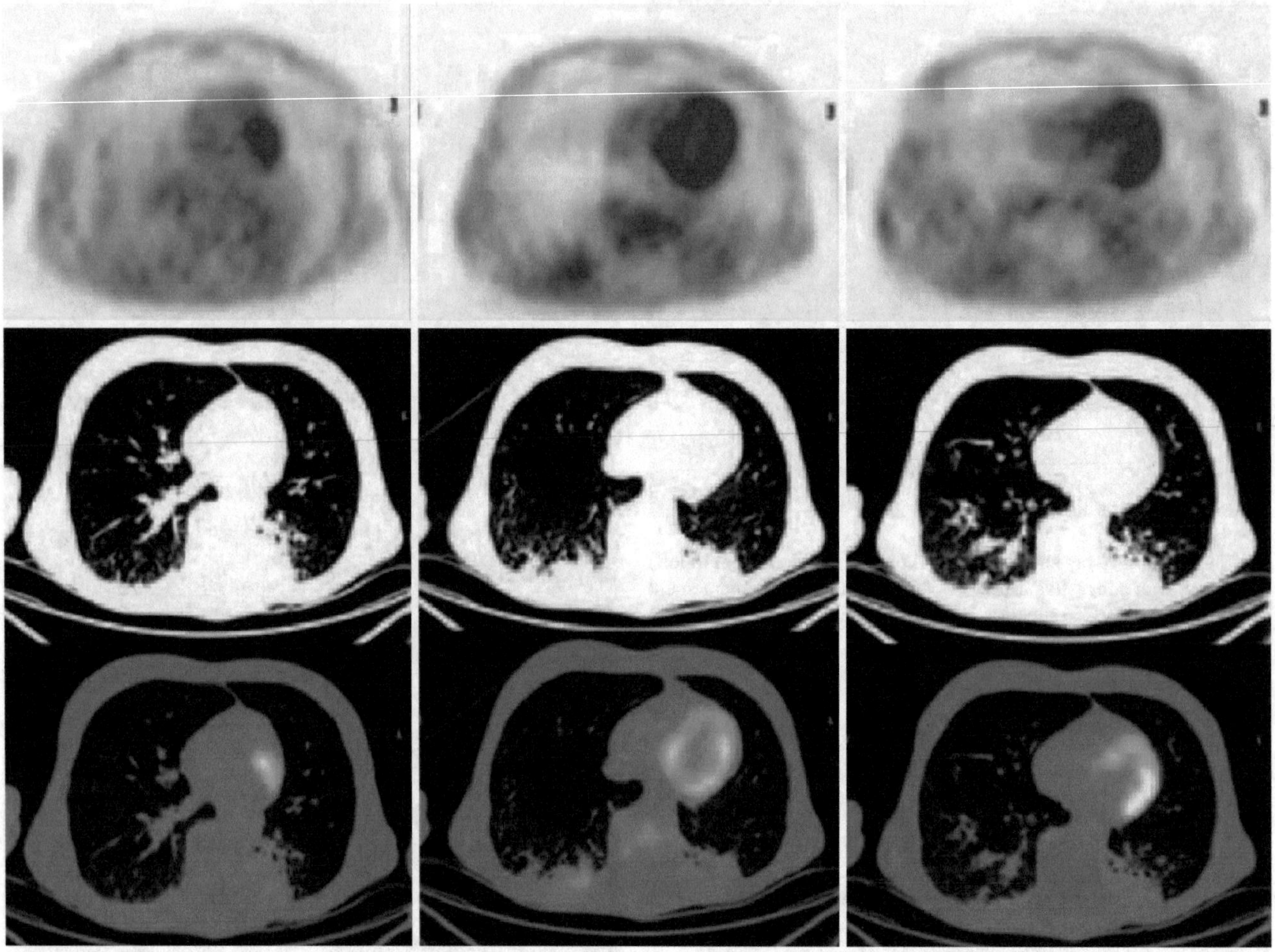

Fig. 7.30 Images (PET image, upper; CT slide, middle; fused PET/CT image, lower) showed increased [^{18}F]FDG uptake at carenal lymph nodes and right lung at mantle paravertebral region associated with CT lesion

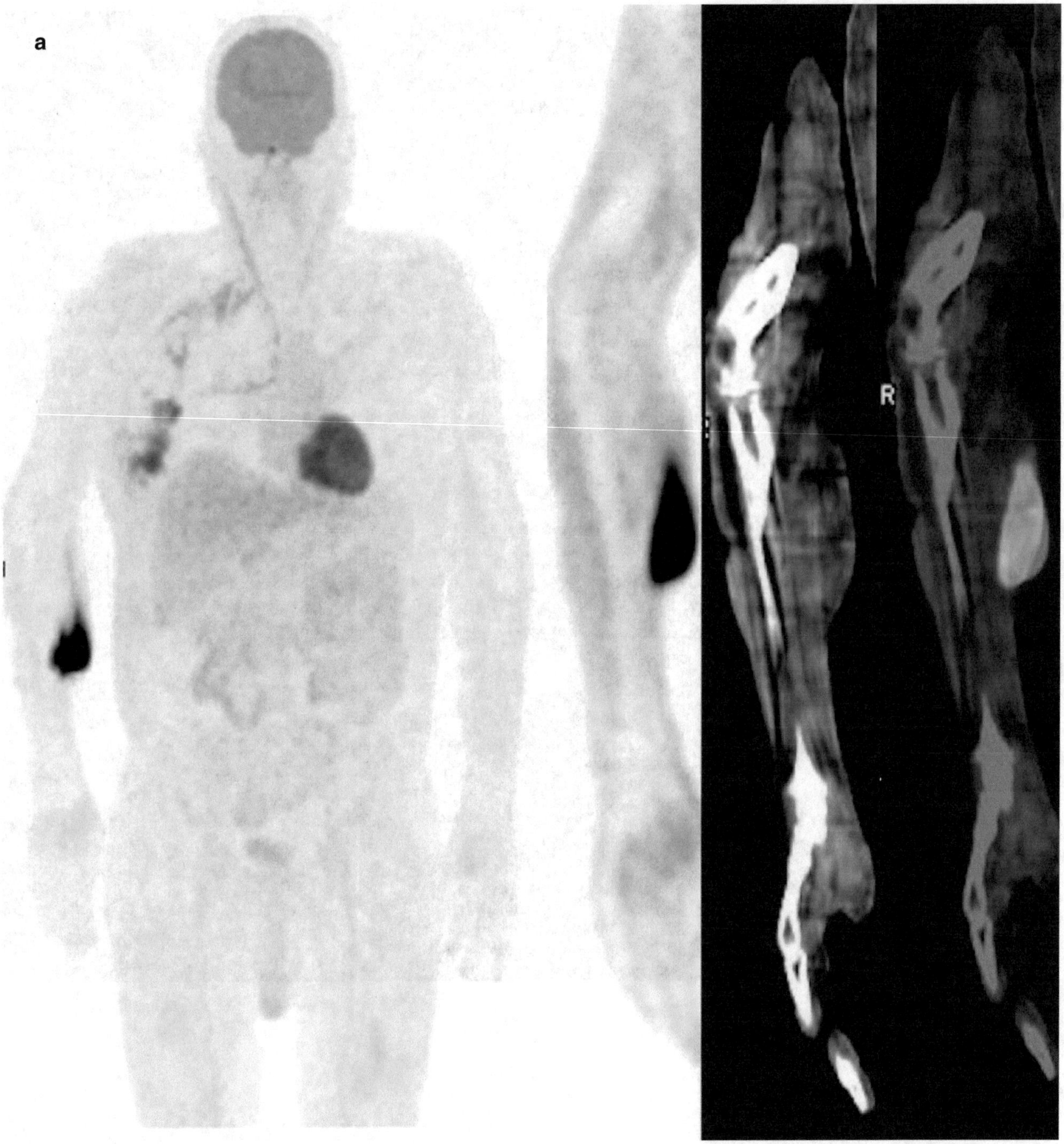

Fig. 7.31 (**a**) MIP image of [18F]FDG PET/CT (left panel) shows markedly increased tracer uptake in the right forearm; an ill-defined area with moderately increased [18F]FDG uptake is observed also in the right hemithorax. The right panel displays magnified coronal sections of right arm and forearm (from left to right: PET component, CT component, fused PET/CT image), clearly showing accumulation of [18F] FDG limited to the site of the arterovenous fistula. (**b**) Upper and lower panels display the transaxial and coronal sections, respectively, showing moderately increased [18F]FDG uptake at the peripheral edge of the posttraumatic chronic hematoma in the right chest wall, externally of the ribcage (from left to right: PET component, CT component, fused PET/CT image). The transaxial CT section also shows bilateral pleural effusion at the bases of lungs

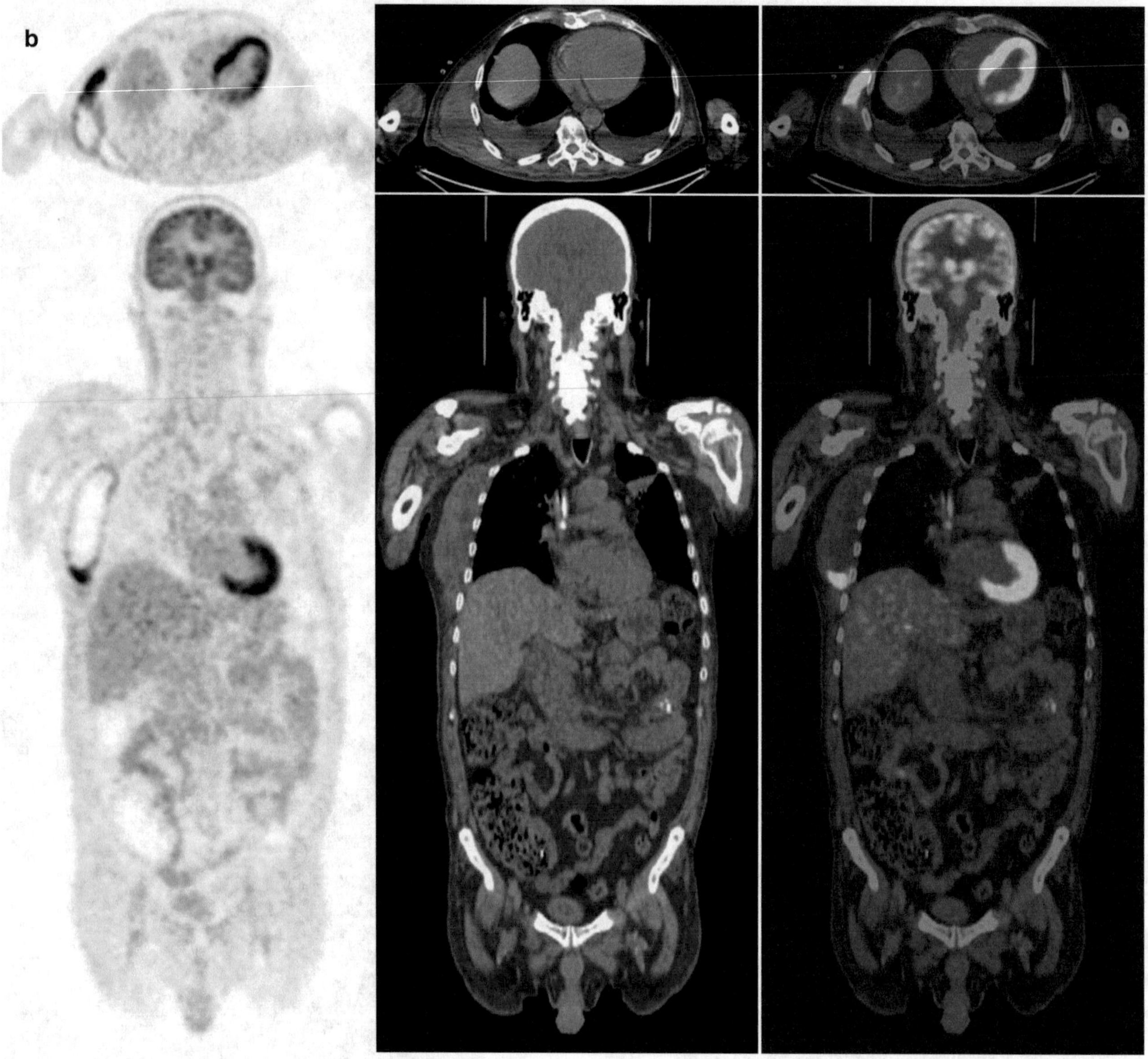

Fig. 7.31 (continued)

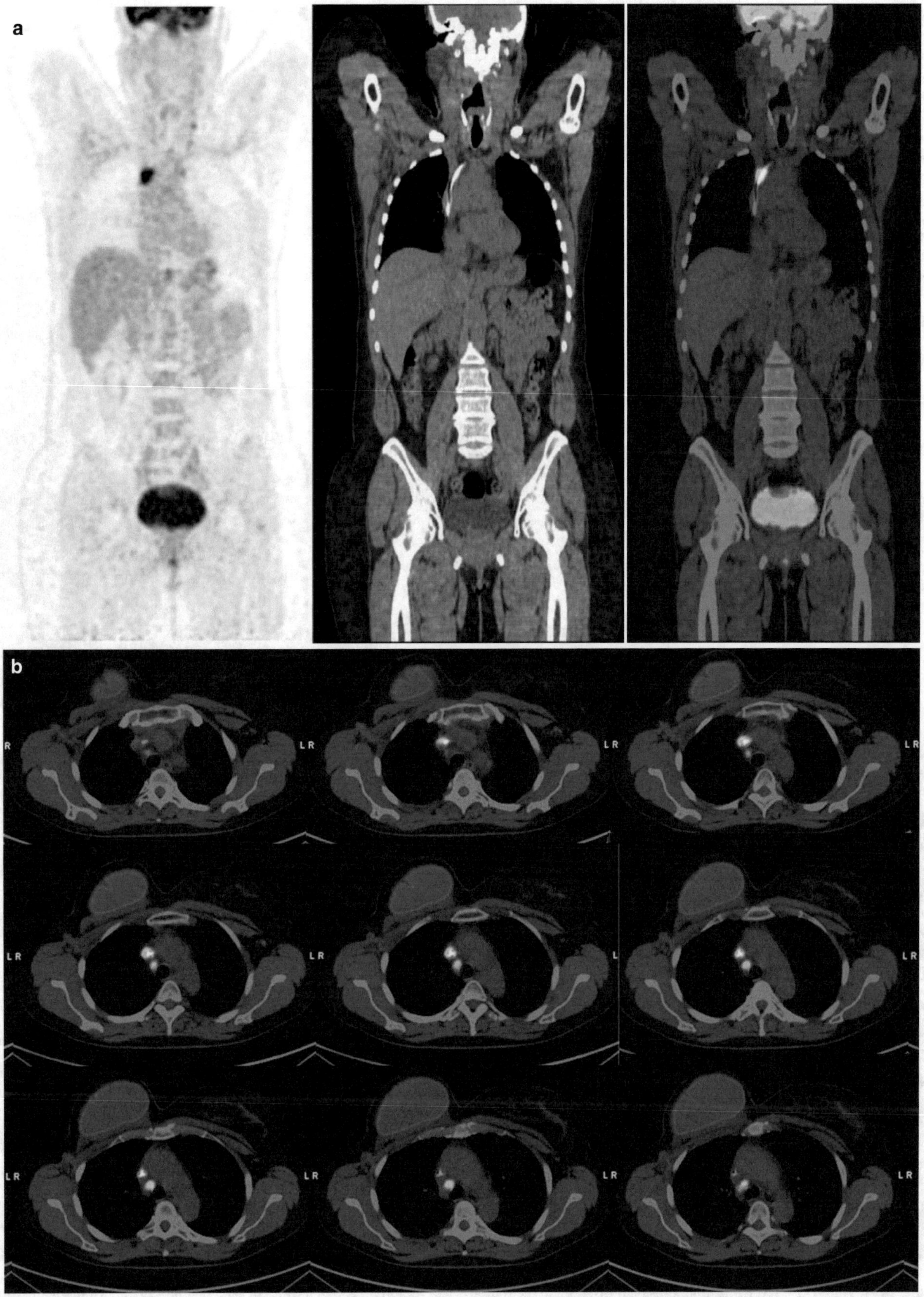

Fig. 7.32 Baseline [^{18}F]FDG PET/CT imaging. (**a**) Coronal sections of the [^{18}F]FDG PET/CT scan (from left to right: PET component, CT component, fused PET/CT image) show markedly increased tracer uptake along the intra-thoracic portion of the Port-a-Cath system. (**b**) Transaxial fused PETC/CT images at various levels confirm increased [^{18}F]FDG uptake along the intra-thoracic portion of the Port-a-Cath system, associated with increased tracer uptake in mediastinal lymph nodes

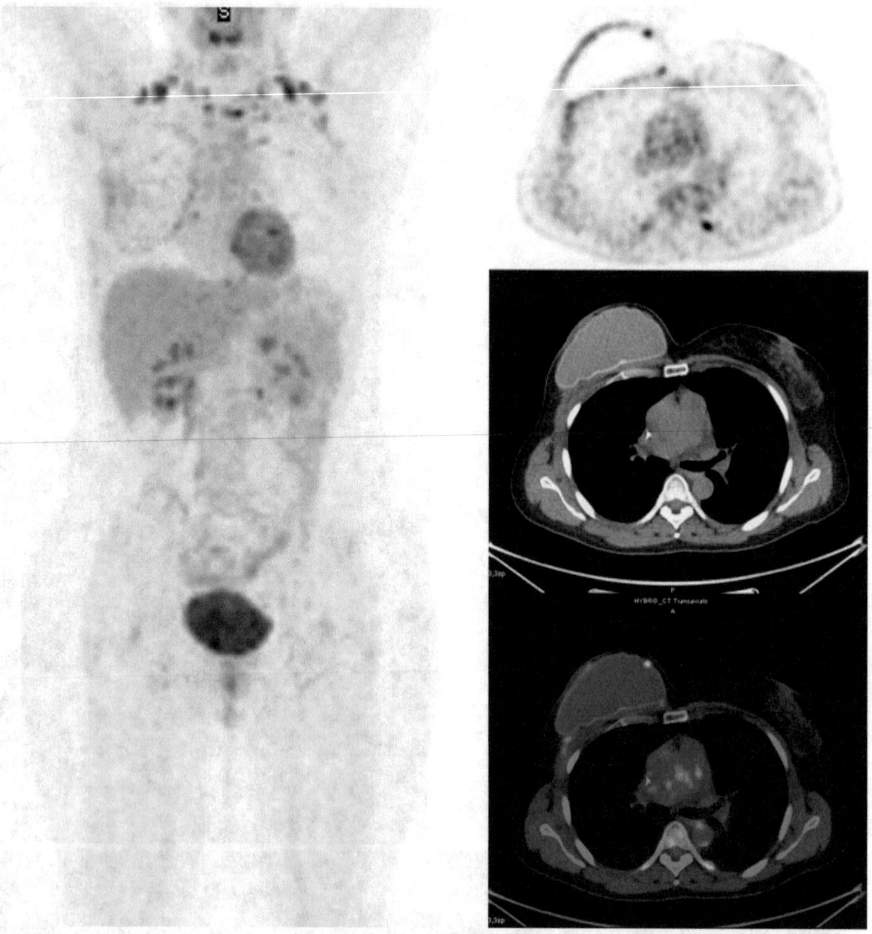

Fig. 7.33 Follow-up [^{18}F] FDG PET/CT scan acquired after antimicrobial therapy (MIP image in left panel, transaxial PET, CT, and fused PET/CT images in right panel). Disappearance of the previously detected areas of increased tracer uptake associated with the Port-a-Cath system. In this scan, it is possible to better identify a rim of mildly increased [^{18}F] FDG uptake at the periphery of the augmentation breast implant

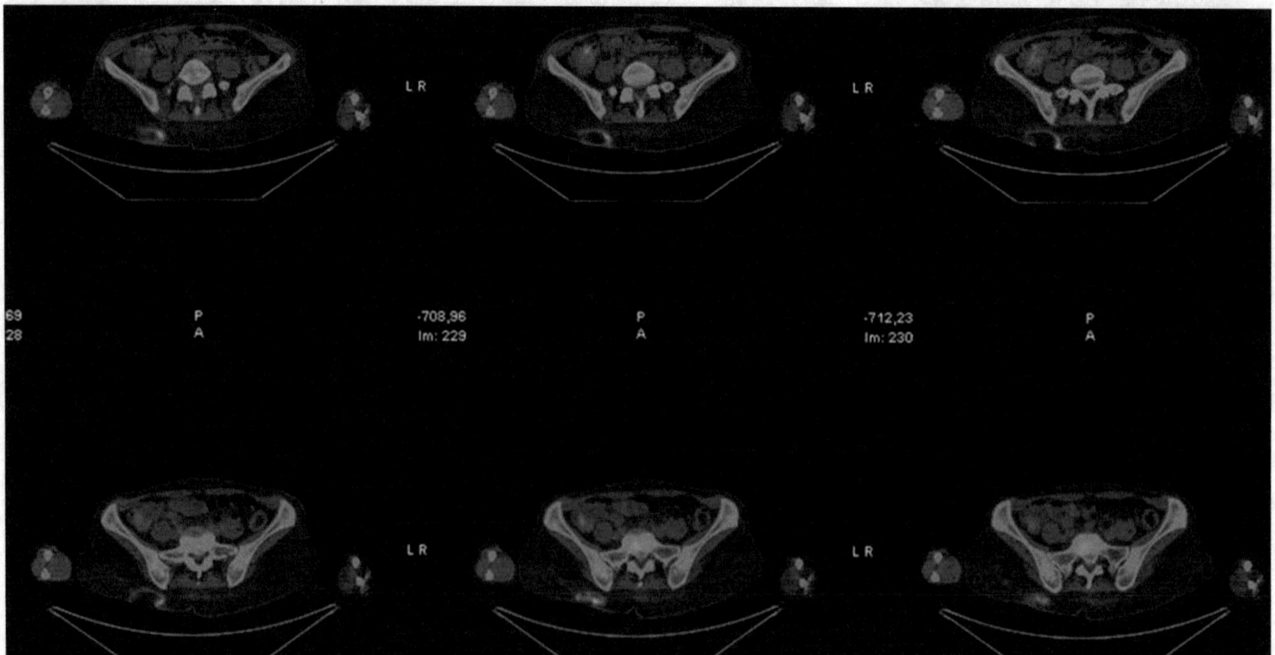

Fig. 7.34 [^{18}F]FDG PET/CT imaging. Tansaxial fused sections at different levels of the pelvis, clearly showing markedly increased [^{18}F] FDG uptake corresponding to the subcutaneous pocket in the right gluteal region, that was the site of the generator pocket of the neurostimulator that been implanted to treat urgence incontinence

References

1. Guggenbichler JP, Assadian O, Boeswald M, Kramer A. Incidence and clinical implication of nosocomial infections associated with implantable biomaterials—catheters, ventilator-associated pneumonia, urinary tract infections. GMS Krankenhhyg Interdiszip. 2011;6(1):Doc18.
2. Vincent JL. Nosocomial infections in adult intensive-care units. Lancet. 2003;361(9374):2068–77.
3. System NNIS. National Nosocomial Infections Surveillance (NNIS) system report, data summary from January 1992 to June 2002, issued August 2002. Am J Infect Control. 2002;30(8):458–75.
4. Safdar N, Crnich CJ, Maki DG. Nosocomial infections in the intensive care unit associated with invasive medical devices. Curr Infect Dis Rep. 2001;3(6):487–95.
5. SD E, PE C. The virulence of Staphylococcus pyogenes for man; a study of the problems of wound infection. Br J Exp Pathol. 1957;38(6):573–86.
6. Darouiche RO. Device-associated infections: a macroproblem that starts with microadherence. Clin Infect Dis. 2001;33(9):1567–72.
7. Maki DG, Stolz SM, Wheeler S, Mermel LA. Prevention of central venous catheter-related bloodstream infection by use of an antiseptic-impregnated catheter. A randomized, controlled trial. Ann Intern Med. 1997;127(4):257–66.
8. Pittet D, Tarara D, Wenzel RP. Nosocomial bloodstream infection in critically ill patients. Excess length of stay, extra costs, and attributable mortality. JAMA. 1994;271(20):1598–601.
9. Habib G, Erba PA, Iung B, Donal E, Cosyns B, Laroche C, et al. Clinical presentation, aetiology and outcome of infective endocarditis. Results of the ESC-EORP EURO-ENDO (European infective endocarditis) registry: a prospective cohort study. Eur Heart J. 2019;40(39):3222–32.
10. Cruse PJ, Foord R. The epidemiology of wound infection. A 10-year prospective study of 62,939 wounds. Surg Clin North Am. 1980;60(1):27–40.
11. Randrup E, Wilson S, Mobley D, Suarez G, Mekras G, Baum N. Clinical experience with Mentor Alpha I inflatable penile prosthesis. Report on 333 cases. Urology. 1993;42(3):305–8.
12. Al-Khatib SM, Greiner MA, Peterson ED, Hernandez AF, Schulman KA, Curtis LH. Patient and implanting physician factors associated with mortality and complications after implantable cardioverter-defibrillator implantation, 2002-2005. Circ Arrhythm Electrophysiol. 2008;1(4):240–9.
13. Wilhelm MJ, Schmid C, Hammel D, Kerber S, Loick HM, Herrmann M, et al. Cardiac pacemaker infection: surgical management with and without extracorporeal circulation. Ann Thorac Surg. 1997;64(6):1707–12.
14. Barrack RL, Harris WH. The value of aspiration of the hip joint before revision total hip arthroplasty. J Bone Joint Surg Am. 1993;75(1):66–76.
15. Stoodley P, Conti SF, DeMeo PJ, Nistico L, Melton-Kreft R, Johnson S, et al. Characterization of a mixed MRSA/MRSE biofilm in an explanted total ankle arthroplasty. FEMS Immunol Med Microbiol. 2011;62(1):66–74.
16. Stewart PS, Bjarnsholt T. Risk factors for chronic biofilm-related infection associated with implanted medical devices. Clin Microbiol Infect. 2020;26(8):1034–8.
17. Lorente L, Henry C, Martín MM, Jiménez A, Mora ML. Central venous catheter-related infection in a prospective and observational study of 2,595 catheters. Crit Care. 2005;9(6):R631–5.
18. Locci R, Peters G, Pulverer G. Microbial colonization of prosthetic devices. IV. Scanning electron microscopy of intravenous catheters invaded by yeasts. Zentralbl Bakteriol Mikrobiol Hyg B. 1981;173(6):419–24.
19. Chambless JD, Hunt SM, Stewart PS. A three-dimensional computer model of four hypothetical mechanisms protecting biofilms from antimicrobials. Appl Environ Microbiol. 2006;72(3):2005–13.
20. Habash M, Reid G. Microbial biofilms: their development and significance for medical device-related infections. J Clin Pharmacol. 1999;39(9):887–98.
21. Denstedt JD, Wollin TA, Reid G. Biomaterials used in urology: current issues of biocompatibility, infection, and encrustation. J Endourol. 1998;12(6):493–500.
22. Watnick P, Kolter R. Biofilm, city of microbes. J Bacteriol. 2000;182(10):2675–9.
23. Hall-Stoodley L, Costerton JW, Stoodley P. Bacterial biofilms: from the natural environment to infectious diseases. Nat Rev Microbiol. 2004;2(2):95–108.
24. Yang L, Liu Y, Wu H, Song Z, Høiby N, Molin S, et al. Combating biofilms. FEMS Immunol Med Microbiol. 2012;65(2):146–57.
25. Appelgren P, Ransjö U, Bindslev L, Espersen F, Larm O. Surface heparinization of central venous catheters reduces microbial colonization in vitro and in vivo: results from a prospective, randomized trial. Crit Care Med. 1996;24(9):1482–9.
26. Schembri MA, Klemm P. Biofilm formation in a hydrodynamic environment by novel fimh variants and ramifications for virulence. Infect Immun. 2001;69(3):1322–8.
27. Thomas WE, Trintchina E, Forero M, Vogel V, Sokurenko EV. Bacterial adhesion to target cells enhanced by shear force. Cell. 2002;109(7):913–23.
28. Donlan RM. Biofilm formation: a clinically relevant microbiological process. Clin Infect Dis. 2001;33(8):1387–92.
29. Costerton JW, Stewart PS, Greenberg EP. Bacterial biofilms: a common cause of persistent infections. Science. 1999;284(5418):1318–22.
30. Mermel LA, Allon M, Bouza E, Craven DE, Flynn P, O'Grady NP, et al. Clinical practice guidelines for the diagnosis and management of intravascular catheter-related infection: 2009 update by the Infectious Diseases Society of America. Clin Infect Dis. 2009;49(1):1–45.
31. Díaz ML, Villanueva A, Herraiz MJ, Noguera JJ, Alonso-Burgos A, Bastarrika G, et al. Computed tomographic appearance of chest ports and catheters: a pictorial review for noninterventional radiologists. Curr Probl Diagn Radiol. 2009;38(3):99–110.
32. Garner JS, Jarvis WR, Emori TG, Horan TC, Hughes JM. CDC definitions for nosocomial infections, 1988. Am J Infect Control. 1988;16(3):128–40.
33. Schiffer CA, Mangu PB, Wade JC, Camp-Sorrell D, Cope DG, El-Rayes BF, et al. Central venous catheter care for the patient with cancer: American Society of Clinical Oncology clinical practice guideline. J Clin Oncol. 2013;31(10):1357–70.
34. Chopra V, Anand S, Krein SL, Chenoweth C, Saint S. Bloodstream infection, venous thrombosis, and peripherally inserted central catheters: reappraising the evidence. Am J Med. 2012;125(8):733–41.
35. McLaws ML, Burrell AR. Zero risk for central line-associated bloodstream infection: are we there yet? Crit Care Med. 2012;40(2):388–93.
36. van de Wetering MD, van Woensel JB. Prophylactic antibiotics for preventing early central venous catheter Gram positive infections in oncology patients. Cochrane Database Syst Rev. 2007(1):CD003295.
37. Gilbert RE, Harden M. Effectiveness of impregnated central venous catheters for catheter related blood stream infection: a systematic review. Curr Opin Infect Dis. 2008;21(3):235–45.
38. Imataki O, Tamai Y, Watanabe M, Abe Y, Kawakami K. Central venous catheter-related thrombosis with infection in cancer patients-2 cases. Gan To Kagaku Ryoho. 2006;33(9):1353–6.

39. Borchardt RA, Raad I. Bloodstream infections: the risks and benefits of intravascular catheters. JAAPA. 2012;25(8):21–2.
40. Smit J, Rieg SR, Wendel AF, Kern WV, Seifert H, Schønheyder HC, et al. Onset of symptoms, diagnostic confirmation, and occurrence of multiple infective foci in patients with Staphylococcus aureus bloodstream infection: a look into the order of events and potential clinical implications. Infection. 2018;46(5):651–8.
41. Linnemann B. Management of complications related to central venous catheters in cancer patients: an update. Semin Thromb Hemost. 2014;40(3):382–94.
42. Wakabayashi H, Otani T, Yachida S, Okano K, Izuishi K, Suzuki Y. Central venous catheter-related infection diagnosed by CT. Lancet. 2006;368(9545):1466.
43. Cook RJ, Ashton RW, Aughenbaugh GL, Ryu JH. Septic pulmonary embolism: presenting features and clinical course of 14 patients. Chest. 2005;128(1):162–6.
44. Picardi M, Pagliuca S, Chiurazzi F, Iula D, Catania M, Rossano F, et al. Early ultrasonographic finding of septic thrombophlebitis is the main indicator of central venous catheter removal to reduce infection-related mortality in neutropenic patients with bloodstream infection. Ann Oncol. 2012;23(8):2122–8.
45. Gutfilen B, Lopes de Souza SA, Martins FP, Cardoso LR, Pinheiro Pessoa MC, Fonseca LM. Use of ^{99m}Tc-mononuclear leukocyte scintigraphy in nosocomial fever. Acta Radiol. 2006;47(7):699–704.
46. Lai CH, Chi CY, Chen HP, Lai CJ, Fung CP, Liu CY. Port-A catheter-associated Nocardia bacteremia detected by gallium inflammation scan: a case report and literature review. Scand J Infect Dis. 2004;36(10):775–7.
47. Miller JH. Detection of deep venous thrombophlebitis by gallium 67 scintigraphy. Radiology. 1981;140(1):183–6.
48. Chiu JS, Tzeng JE, Wang YF. Infection hunter: gallium scintigraphy for hemodialysis access graft infection. Kidney Int. 2006;69(8):1290.
49. Sullivan SJ, Quadri SM, Cunha BA. Hickman catheter Staphylococcus aureus bacteremia diagnosed by indium-111 scan. Heart Lung. 1992;21(5):505–6.
50. Bhargava P, Kumar R, Zhuang H, Charron M, Alavi A. Catheter-related focal FDG activity on whole body PET imaging. Clin Nucl Med. 2004;29(4):238–42.
51. Mahfouz T, Miceli MH, Saghafifar F, Stroud S, Jones-Jackson L, Walker R, et al. ^{18}F-fluorodeoxyglucose positron emission tomography contributes to the diagnosis and management of infections in patients with multiple myeloma: a study of 165 infectious episodes. J Clin Oncol. 2005;23(31):7857–63.
52. Miceli MH, Jones Jackson LB, Walker RC, Talamo G, Barlogie B, Anaissie EJ. Diagnosis of infection of implantable central venous catheters by [^{18}F]fluorodeoxyglucose positron emission tomography. Nucl Med Commun. 2004;25(8):813–8.
53. Vos FJ, Donnelly JP, Oyen WJ, Kullberg BJ, Bleeker-Rovers CP, Blijlevens NM. ^{18}F-FDG PET/CT for diagnosing infectious complications in patients with severe neutropenia after intensive chemotherapy for haematological malignancy or stem cell transplantation. Eur J Nucl Med Mol Imaging. 2012;39(1):120–8.
54. O'Horo JC, Sampathkumar P. Infections in neurocritical care. Neurocrit Care. 2017;27(3):458–67.
55. Ramanan M, Lipman J, Shorr A, Shankar A. A meta-analysis of ventriculostomy-associated cerebrospinal fluid infections. BMC Infect Dis. 2015;15:3.
56. van de Beek D, Drake JM, Tunkel AR. Nosocomial bacterial meningitis. N Engl J Med. 2010;362(2):146–54.
57. Berger C, Schwarz S, Schaebitz WR, Aschoff A, Schwab S. Serum procalcitonin in cerebral ventriculitis. Crit Care Med. 2002;30(8):1778–81.
58. Martínez R, Gaul C, Buchfelder M, Erbguth F, Tschaikowsky K. Serum procalcitonin monitoring for differential diagnosis of ventriculitis in adult intensive care patients. Intensive Care Med. 2002;28(2):208–10.
59. Fam MD, Zeineddine HA, Eliyas JK, Stadnik A, Jesselson M, McBee N, et al. CSF inflammatory response after intraventricular hemorrhage. Neurology. 2017;89(15):1553–60.
60. Walti LN, Conen A, Coward J, Jost GF, Trampuz A. Characteristics of infections associated with external ventricular drains of cerebrospinal fluid. J Infect. 2013;66(5):424–31.
61. Huy NT, Thao NT, Diep DT, Kikuchi M, Zamora J, Hirayama K. Cerebrospinal fluid lactate concentration to distinguish bacterial from aseptic meningitis: a systemic review and meta-analysis. Crit Care. 2010;14(6):R240.
62. Jamjoom AAB, Joannides AJ, Poon MT, Chari A, Zaben M, Abdulla MAH, et al. Prospective, multicentre study of external ventricular drainage-related infections in the UK and Ireland. J Neurol Neurosurg Psychiatry. 2018;89(2):120–6.
63. Seidelman J, Lewis SS. Neurosurgical device-related infections. Infect Dis Clin N Am. 2018;32(4):861–76.
64. Martin RM, Zimmermann LL, Huynh M, Polage CR. Diagnostic approach to health care- and device-associated central nervous system infections. J Clin Microbiol. 2018;56(11):pii:e00861–18
65. Sader E, Moore J, Cervantes-Arslanian AM. Neurosurgical infections. Semin Neurol. 2019;39(4):507–14.
66. O'Keeffe AB, Lawrence T, Bojanic S. Oxford craniotomy infections database: a cost analysis of craniotomy infection. Br J Neurosurg. 2012;26(2):265–9.
67. Delgado-López PD, Martín-Velasco V, Castilla-Díez JM, Galacho-Harriero AM, Rodríguez-Salazar A. Preservation of bone flap after craniotomy infection. Neurocirugia (Astur). 2009;20(2): 124–31.
68. Mustroph CM, Malcolm JG, Rindler RS, Chu JK, Grossberg JA, Pradilla G, et al. Cranioplasty infection and resorption are associated with the presence of a ventriculoperitoneal shunt: a systematic review and meta-analysis. World Neurosurg. 2017;103:686–93.
69. Cheah PP, Rosman AK, Cheang CK, Idris B. Autologous cranioplasty post-pperative surgical site infection: does it matter if the bone flaps were stored and handled differently? Malays J Med Sci. 2017;24(6):68–74.
70. Ho AL, Cannon JGD, Mohole J, Pendharkar AV, Sussman ES, Li G, et al. Topical vancomycin surgical prophylaxis in pediatric open craniotomies: an institutional experience. J Neurosurg Pediatr. 2018;22(6):710–5.
71. Ravikumar V, Ho AL, Pendhakar AV, Sussman ES, Kwong-Hon Chow K, Li G. The use of vancomycin powder for surgical prophylaxis following craniotomy. Neurosurgery. 2017;80(5):754–8.
72. Vinchon M, Dhellemmes P. Cerebrospinal fluid shunt infection: risk factors and long-term follow-up. Childs Nerv Syst. 2006;22(7):692–7.
73. Kulkarni AV, Drake JM, Lamberti-Pasculli M. Cerebrospinal fluid shunt infection: a prospective study of risk factors. J Neurosurg. 2001;94(2):195–201.
74. Conen A, Walti LN, Merlo A, Fluckiger U, Battegay M, Trampuz A. Characteristics and treatment outcome of cerebrospinal fluid shunt-associated infections in adults: a retrospective analysis over an 11-year period. Clin Infect Dis. 2008;47(1):73–82.
75. Tunkel AR, Hasbun R, Bhimraj A, Byers K, Kaplan SL, Scheld WM, et al. 2017 Infectious Diseases Society of America's clinical practice guidelines for healthcare-associated ventriculitis and meningitis. Clin Infect Dis. 2017;64(6):e34–65.
76. Stenehjem E, Armstrong WS. Central nervous system device infections. Infect Dis Clin N Am. 2012;26(1):89–110.
77. Stoodley P, Braxton EE, Nistico L, Hall-Stoodley L, Johnson S, Quigley M, et al. Direct demonstration of Staphylococcus biofilm in an external ventricular drain in a patient with a history of recurrent ventriculoperitoneal shunt failure. Pediatr Neurosurg. 2010;46(2):127–32.

78. Medina M, Viglietti AL, Gozzoli L, Lucano A, Ravasi L, Lucignani G, et al. Indium-111 labelled white blood cell scintigraphy in cranial and spinal septic lesions. Eur J Nucl Med. 2000;27(10):1473–80.
79. Liberatore M, Drudi FM, Tarantino R, Prosperi D, Fiore V, Missori P, et al. Tc-99m exametazime-labeled leukocyte scans in the study of infections in skull neurosurgery. Clin Nucl Med. 2003;28(12):971–4.
80. Wan DQ, Joseph UA, Barron BJ, Caram P, Nguyen AP. Ventriculoperitoneal shunt catheter and cerebral spinal fluid infection initially detected by FDG PET/CT scan. Clin Nucl Med. 2009;34(7):464–5.
81. Rehman T, Chohan MO, Yonas H. Diagnosis of ventriculoperitoneal shunt infection using [F-18]-FDG PET: a case report. J Neurosurg Sci. 2011;55(2):161–3.
82. Awan NR, Lozano A, Hamani C. Deep brain stimulation: current and future perspectives. Neurosurg Focus. 2009;27(1):E2.
83. Abode-Iyamah KO, Chiang HY, Woodroffe RW, Park B, Jareczek FJ, Nagahama Y, et al. Deep brain stimulation hardware-related infections: 10-year experience at a single institution. J Neurosurg. 2018:1–10.
84. Fenoy AJ, Simpson RK. Management of device-related wound complications in deep brain stimulation surgery. J Neurosurg. 2012;116(6):1324–32.
85. Hyam JA, de Pennington N, Joint C, Green AL, Owen SL, Pereira EA, et al. Maintained deep brain stimulation for severe dystonia despite infection by using externalized electrodes and an extracorporeal pulse generator. J Neurosurg. 2010;113(3):630–3.
86. Real R, Linhares P, Fernandes H, Rosas MJ, Gago MF, Pereira J, et al. Role of Tc-Sulesomab immunoscintigraphy in the management of infection following deep brain stimulation surgery. Neurol Res Int. 2011;2011:817951.
87. Bernstein JE, Kashyap S, Ray K, Ananda A. Infections in deep brain stimulator surgery. Cureus. 2019;11(8):e5440.
88. Fily F, Haegelen C, Tattevin P, Buffet-Bataillon S, Revest M, Cady A, et al. Deep brain stimulation hardware-related infections: a report of 12 cases and review of the literature. Clin Infect Dis. 2011;52(8):1020–3.
89. Kumar K, Hunter G, Demeria D. Spinal cord stimulation in treatment of chronic benign pain: challenges in treatment planning and present status, a 22-year experience. Neurosurgery. 2006;58(3):481–96; discussion -96
90. Follett KA, Boortz-Marx RL, Drake JM, DuPen S, Schneider SJ, Turner MS, et al. Prevention and management of intrathecal drug delivery and spinal cord stimulation system infections. Anesthesiology. 2004;100(6):1582–94.
91. Ghosh D, Mainali G, Khera J, Luciano M. Complications of intrathecal baclofen pumps in children: experience from a tertiary care center. Pediatr Neurosurg. 2013;49(3):138–44.
92. Montague DK. Penile prosthesis implantation in the era of medical treatment for erectile dysfunction. Urol Clin North Am. 2011;38(2):217–25.
93. Carson CC, Robertson CN. Late hematogenous infection of penile prostheses. J Urol. 1988;139(1):50–2.
94. Mulhall John P, Ahmed A, Branch J, Parker M. Serial assessment of efficacy and satisfaction profiles following penile prosthesis surgery. J Urol. 2003;169(4):1429–33.
95. McClellan DS, Masih BK. Gangrene of the penis as a complication of penile prosthesis. J Urol. 1985;133(5):862–3.
96. Roberts JA, Fussell EN, Lewis RW. Bacterial adherence to penile prosthesis. Int J Impot Res. 1989;1:167–78.
97. Fishman Irving J, Scott FB, Selim Ashraf M. Rescue procedure: an alternative to complete removal for treatment of infected penile prosthesis. J Urol. 1987;137(6):202A-A.
98. Montague DK, Angermeier KW, Lakin MM. Penile prosthesis infections. Int J Impot Res. 2001;13(6):326–8.
99. Gross MS, Reinstatler L, Henry GD, Honig SC, Stahl PJ, Burnett AL, et al. Multicenter investigation of fungal infections of inflatable penile prostheses. J Sex Med. 2019;16(7):1100–5.
100. Jarow JP. Risk factors for penile prosthetic infection. J Urol. 1996;156(2 Pt 1):402–4.
101. Parsons CL, Stein PC, Dobke MK, Virden CP, Frank DH. Diagnosis and therapy of subclinically infected prostheses. Surg Gynecol Obstet. 1993;177(5):504–6.
102. Chimento GF, Finger S, Barrack RL. Gram stain detection of infection during revision arthroplasty. J Bone Joint Surg Br. 1996;78(5):838–9.
103. Henry GD, Carson CC, Wilson SK, Wiygul J, Tornehl C, Cleves MA, et al. Revision washout decreases implant capsule tissue culture positivity: a multicenter study. J Urol. 2008;179(1):186–90; discussion 90
104. Hartman RP, Kawashima A, Takahashi N, LeRoy AJ, King BF. Inflatable penile prosthesis (IPP): diagnosis of complications. Abdom Radiol (NY). 2016;41(6):1187–96.
105. Moncada I, Jara J, Cabello R, Monzo JI, Hernández C. Radiological assessment of penile prosthesis: the role of magnetic resonance imaging. World J Urol. 2004;22(5):371–7.
106. Better N, Ahn CS, Drum DE, Tow DE. Identification of penile prosthetic infection on 67gallium scan. J Urol. 1994;152(2 Pt 1):475–6.
107. Achong D, Zloty M. In-111 WBC scintigraphy for evaluation of the painful penile prosthesis. J Nucl Med. 2008;49(supplement 1):266P-P.
108. Spear SL, Seruya M. Management of the infected or exposed breast prosthesis: a single surgeon's 15-year experience with 69 patients. Plast Reconstr Surg. 2010;125(4):1074–84.
109. Pittet B, Montandon D, Pittet D. Infection in breast implants. Lancet Infect Dis. 2005;5(2):94–106.
110. De Cholnoky T. Augmentation mammaplasty. Survey of complications in 10,941 patients by 265 surgeons. Plast Reconstr Surg. 1970;45(6):573–7.
111. Ahn CY, Ko CY, Wagar EA, Wong RS, Shaw WW. Microbial evaluation: 139 implants removed from symptomatic patients. Plast Reconstr Surg. 1996;98(7):1225–9.
112. Macadam SA, Mehling BM, Fanning A, Dufton JA, Kowalewska-Grochowska KT, Lennox P, et al. Nontuberculous mycobacterial breast implant infections. Plast Reconstr Surg. 2007;119(1):337–44.
113. Dessy LA, Corrias F, Marchetti F, Marcasciano M, Armenti AF, Mazzocchi M, et al. Implant infection after augmentation mammaplasty: a review of the literature and report of a multidrug-resistant Candida albicans infection. Aesthet Plast Surg. 2012;36(1):153–9.
114. Walsh R, Kliewer MA, Sullivan DC, Hertzberg B, Paulson EK, Soo MS, et al. Periprosthetic mycobacterial infection. CT and mammographic findings. Clin Imaging. 1995;19(3):193–6.
115. van Wingerden JJ, van Staden MM. Ultrasound mammography in prosthesis-related breast augmentation complications. Ann Plast Surg. 1989;22(1):32–5.
116. Khedher NB, David J, Trop I, Drouin S, Peloquin L, Lalonde L. Imaging findings of breast augmentation with injected hydrophilic polyacrylamide gel: patient reports and literature review. Eur J Radiol. 2011;78(1):104–11.
117. Lee CJ, Kim SG, Kim L, Choi MS, Lee SI. Unfavorable findings following breast augmentation using injected polyacrylamide hydrogel. Plast Reconstr Surg. 2004;114(7):1967–8.
118. Lui CY, Ho CM, Iu PP, Cheung WY, Lam HS, Cheng MS, et al. Evaluation of MRI findings after polyacrylamide gel injection for breast augmentation. AJR Am J Roentgenol. 2008;191(3):677–88.
119. Leslie K, Buscombe J, Davenport A. Implant infection in a transsexual with renal failure. Nephrol Dial Transplant. 2000;15(3):436–7.

120. Ellenberger P, Graham WP, Manders EK, Basarab RM. Labeled leukocyte scans for detection of retained polyurethane foam. Plast Reconstr Surg. 1986;77(1):77–9.
121. Chen CJ, Lee BF, Yao WJ, Wu PS, Chen WC, Peng SL, et al. A false positive F-FDG PET/CT scan caused by breast silicone injection. Korean J Radiol. 2009;10(2):194–6.
122. Bakheet SM, Powe J, Kandil A, Ezzat A, Rostom A, Amartey J. F-18 FDG uptake in breast infection and inflammation. Clin Nucl Med. 2000;25(2):100–3.
123. Adejolu M, Huo L, Rohren E, Santiago L, Yang WT. False-positive lesions mimicking breast cancer on FDG PET and PET/CT. AJR Am J Roentgenol. 2012;198(3):W304–14.
124. Lim HS, Yoon W, Chung TW, Kim JK, Park JG, Kang HK, et al. FDG PET/CT for the detection and evaluation of breast diseases: usefulness and limitations. Radiographics. 2007;27(Suppl 1):S197–213.
125. Sappington JM, Arriaga MA. Otology, neurotology, and skull base surgery: clinical reference guide: Theodore R. McRackan and Derald E. Brackmann; San Diego, CA: Plural Publishing, 2015. Otol Neurotol. 2016;37(5)
126. Yu KC, Hegarty JL, Gantz BJ, Lalwani AK. Conservative management of infections in cochlear implant recipients. Otolaryngol Head Neck Surg. 2001;125(1):66–70.
127. Tambyraja RR, Gutman MA, Megerian CA. Cochlear implant complications: utility of federal database in systematic analysis. Arch Otolaryngol Head Neck Surg. 2005;131(3):245–50.
128. Hirsch BE, Blikas A, Whitaker M. Antibiotic prophylaxis in cochlear implant surgery. Laryngoscope. 2007;117(5):864–7.
129. Rubin Grandis J, Branstetter BF, Yu VL. The changing face of malignant (necrotising) external otitis: clinical, radiological, and anatomic correlations. Lancet Infect Dis. 2004;4(1):34–9.
130. de Miguel-Martínez I, Ramos-Macías A, Borkoski Barreiro S. Efficacy of heptavalent pneumococcal conjugate vaccine in children with cochlear implant. Acta Otorrinolaringol Esp. 2008;59(1):2–5.
131. Rubin LG, Papsin B, et al. Cochlear implants in children: surgical site infections and prevention and treatment of acute otitis media and meningitis. Pediatrics. 2010;126(2):381–91.
132. Hall-Stoodley L, Hu FZ, Gieseke A, Nistico L, Nguyen D, Hayes J, et al. Direct detection of bacterial biofilms on the middle-ear mucosa of children with chronic otitis media. JAMA. 2006;296(2):202–11.
133. Shpizner BA, Holliday RA, Roland JT, Cohen NL, Waltzman SB, Shapiro WH. Postoperative imaging of the multichannel cochlear implant. AJNR Am J Neuroradiol. 1995;16(7):1517–24.
134. Hoep LS, Merkus P, van Schie A, Rinkel RN, Smit CF. The value of nuclear scans in cochlear implant infections. Eur Arch Otorhinolaryngol. 2006;263(10):895–9.

Nuclear Medicine Imaging of Infections and Inflammation of Central Nervous System and of the Head and Neck Structures

8

Alberto Signore, Tiziana Lanzolla, and Chiara Lauri

Contents

Learning Objectives

- To learn the most frequent intra- and extracranial infections
- To understand the role of nuclear medicine imaging in these patients
- To show several clinical cases and pictures diagnostic images to help physicians to correctly acquire and interpret nuclear medicine images

A. Signore (✉)
Department of Medical-Surgical Sciences and of Translational Medicine, Sapienza University of Rome, Roma, Italy

Nuclear Medicine Unit, AOU Sant'Andrea, Rome, Italy
e-mail: alberto.signore@uniroma1.it

C. Lauri
Department of Medical-Surgical Sciences and of Translational Medicine, Sapienza University of Rome, Rome, Italy

Nuclear Medicine Unit, AOU Sant'Andrea, Rome, Italy

T. Lanzolla
Nuclear Medicine Unit, AOU Sant'Andrea, Rome, Italy

8.1 Introduction

Infections of the central nervous system (CNS) and in the head and neck region (H&N) are frequent and often difficult to diagnose, in particular due their variable aetiology and poor/nonspecific symptoms. X-ray computerized tomography (CT) and magnetic resonance imaging (MRI) are always the first-line imaging modalities and can be very helpful in the presence of typical signs of infection and related inflammation. However, these modalities lack in sensitivity when post-therapy evaluation is required, in case of suspicion of a relapse, or when an 'interim' evaluation is required, in order to decide whether to discontinue or continue antibiotic therapy. In these cases, radionuclide imaging can be of great help and even more helpful if a pre-therapy scan is available. In the above conditions, the Nuclear Medicine modalities include scintigraphy with radiolabelled autologous white blood cells (WBC, particularly useful for malignant otitis and brain abscesses) and positron emission tomography

E. Lazzeri et al. (eds.), *Radionuclide Imaging of Infection and Inflammation*, https://doi.org/10.1007/978-3-030-62175-9_8

(PET) with the glucose analogue [^{18}F]fluoro-2-deoxyglucose ([^{18}F]FDG).

8.2 CNS Infections

Enclosed as it is in the cranial cavity and spinal canal, the CNS is efficiently protected from the risks and dangers of the outside environment. A particular and unique mode of defence is the biological blood–brain barrier (BBB) and the barrier between blood and the cerebrospinal fluid (CSF) that prevent the passage from blood to the nervous tissue of microorganisms and microbial toxins, but also of antibodies, complement and numerous chemotherapeutic drugs as well as radiopharmaceuticals.

The blood–CSF barrier is the consequence of the structure of capillaries of the choroid plexus; although it has a less dense basement membrane and less fenestrated endothelium than the BBB, the role of this barrier is conferred by the limited access to the highly vascularized villi, of epithelial cells, which are in direct continuation with the ependymal cells lining the walls of the ventricles. The permeability of these barriers varies throughout life (it is lower during neonatal age) and is reduced in some physiological conditions (menstruation, pregnancy) or pathological conditions (infections, stroke, cancer, poisoning).

The CNS can be reached by microorganisms through various routes, because:

- Isolation is not anatomically perfect; birth defects may allow the penetration into the CNS of microorganisms from proximal anatomical sites.
- Anatomical isolation is reduced after an injury, surgical interventions, after placing catheters or probes, and in all conditions that potentially allow the penetration of microorganisms.
- Microorganisms can reach the CNS from sites of contiguous infection, either by direct extension of the process or indirectly via the venous blood or following the course of nerves.
- From remote locations, microorganisms can reach the CSF via the blood and nerve tissue.
- Macrophages can be a vehicle to carry microorganisms from blood to CNS.
- Viruses typically arrive into the CNS via the nervous system, along the course of cranial or spinal nerves.
- The CNS can be reached by microorganisms also from the nasal mucosa along the olfactory nerve.

Despite the significant advances of radiological techniques occurred in recent years, particularly MRI and functional MRI (fMRI), there are situations in which the morphological pattern is not sufficient to characterize the lesion, particularly after surgery, radiotherapy, or in the presence of fibrotic tissue and after antibiotic treatment.

The most common infections of the CNS are abscess and encephalitis [1–3]. Brain abscess is defined as purulence and inflammation in one or more localized regions within the brain parenchyma. Direct spread of infection from a site contiguous to the CNS (sinusitis, otitis and dental abscesses) remains the most common route of infection, comprising about 50% of brain abscess cases, while rarely results from meningitis. The proportion of cases of brain abscess in which no primary focus of infection can be identified ranges from 10% to over 60% (Fig. 8.1).

Experimental studies demonstrated that the development of a brain abscess evolves from an early cerebritis stage (neutrophil accumulation, oedema and some tissue necrosis); subsequently, the area of cerebritis expands, a necrotic centre and a capsule develop, which is vascularized (so that ring enhancement on contrast CT imaging is evident); depending on the host immune response, there is a destruction of some surrounding healthy brain tissue in an attempt to sequester the infection.

Early findings on the CT scan are not specific; CT scanning with contrast during early cerebritis may show only oedema—an area of hypodensity—which may or may not enhance after contrast administration. The oedema pattern and moderate mass effect cannot be differentiated from tumour or stroke in some patients. MRI findings in patients with cerebritis may resemble findings in stroke, while findings in the infarcts that result from vasculitis and cerebritis may resemble those of embolic strokes. In an early stage, when cell damage and necrosis occur but before the formation of pus and a significant amount of leukocytes, scintigraphy with autologous labelled WBCs would be negative; however, even in the absence of a clear capsule on CT, a focal accumulation of labelled WBCs indicates that antibiotic therapy should begin while the process is still at the encephalitic stage when complete resolution by medical treatment alone may be achieved.

The main problem of clinical and imaging diagnosis remains, however the differential diagnosis of CT hypodense intracerebral cystic lesions, still solved only in part despite the great technical advances and the diagnostic accuracy of CT and MRI. Differentiating between brain abscesses and cystic brain tumours (such as high-grade gliomas and metastases) may be difficult even with conventional MRI, particularly in the absence of concurrent specific clinical signs of infection. In the differential diagnosis from malignant cystic tumours, the diagnosis of cerebral abscesses is of key importance both in the decision to operate and in planning of the surgical approach; in the presence of an abscess, the best approach is aspiration and biopsy, performed best using a CT-guided computer-assisted technique or with the aid of an external frame, which, with the aid of CT data, directs the placement of the aspiration needle. The operation should be

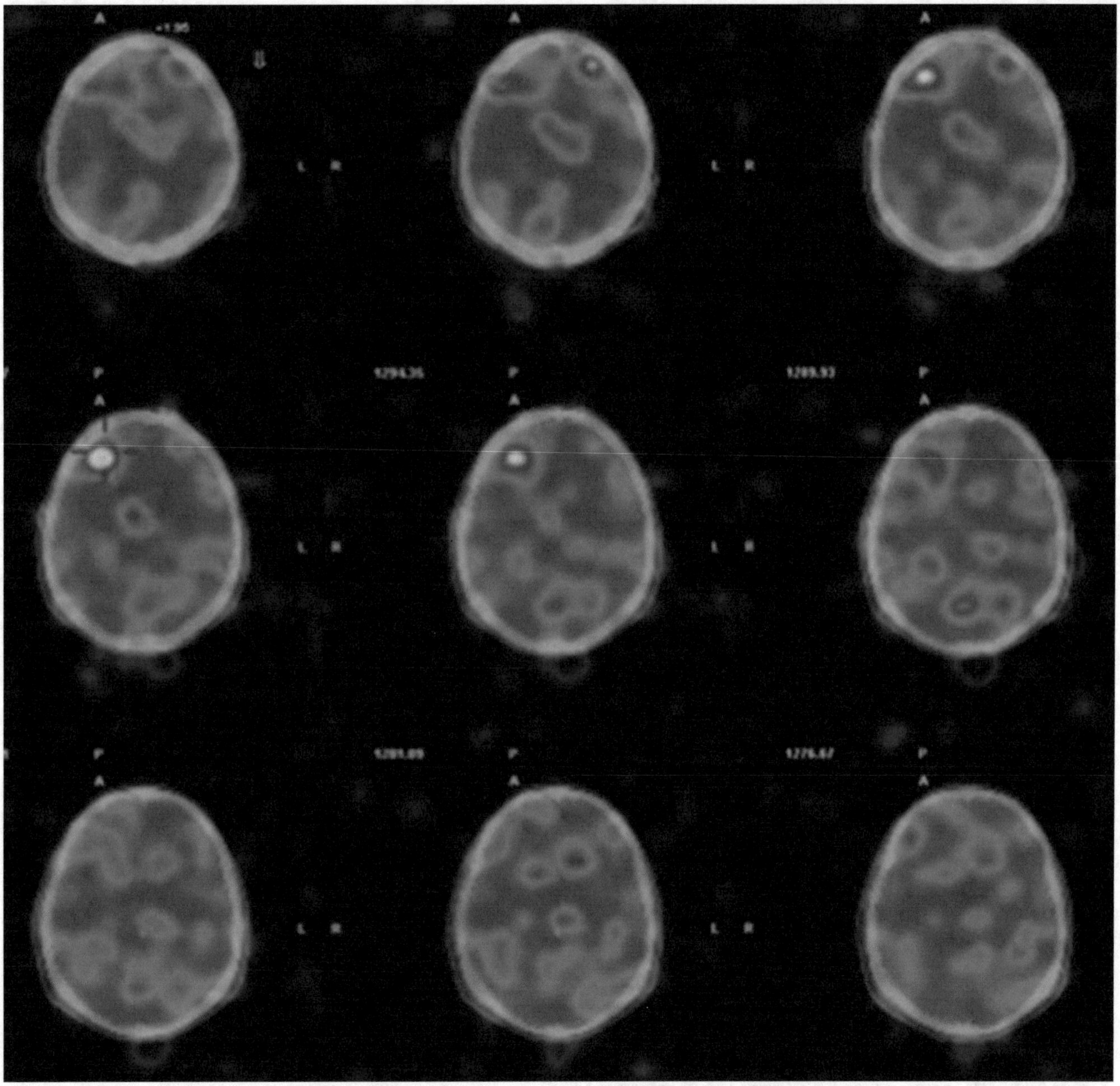

Fig. 8.1 A 44-year-old man who in a road accident occurred in 2011 suffered a fracture of the left frontal-ethmoid-orbit, of C7-T1 and of the spinal process of C6; the lesions were surgically treated with stabilization. The subsequent course was complicated with liquor fistula and infection due to *Candida albicans* and *Streptococcus epidermidis*, which required intensive antibiotic treatment. The patient was readmitted to the hospital in February and April 2012, due to recurrent meningitis with associated fever and laboratory findings of infection. The liquor culture identified *Candida albicans* infection. A WBC scan was performed in order to exclude infection in the cervical region due to stabilization and/or in the brain. SPECT/CT with ^{111}In-oxine-WBC showed a brain abscess in the right frontal lobe, as well as abnormal accumulation of radiolabelled WBS in the left frontal bone. The SPECT/CT images provided better diagnostic information than planar images (not shown here)

planned and conducted in such a way as to prevent the dissemination of purulent material.

When assessing patients in the period of post-operative/post-antibiotic treatment, WBC scintigraphy, with both ^{111}In-oxine and ^{99m}Tc-HMPAO, should be considered in order to verify if complete resolution of the problem by surgical/medical means has been achieved (Fig. 8.2).

Although the radiolabelled WBC scan cannot discriminate between a cerebral abscess and an abscess in a metastatic tumour, its main advantage is the possibility to identify primary or concomitant abscesses in other body regions, a finding that would have obvious diagnostic and therapeutic implications. Therefore, it is always advisable to perform a whole-body scan along with the brain scan.

Frequent diagnostic issues in neurosurgical patients involve the presence of infection along the extracranial path of implanted shunts, the differentiation between sepsis of the skin flap, hematoma and CSF collection. In this regard, it

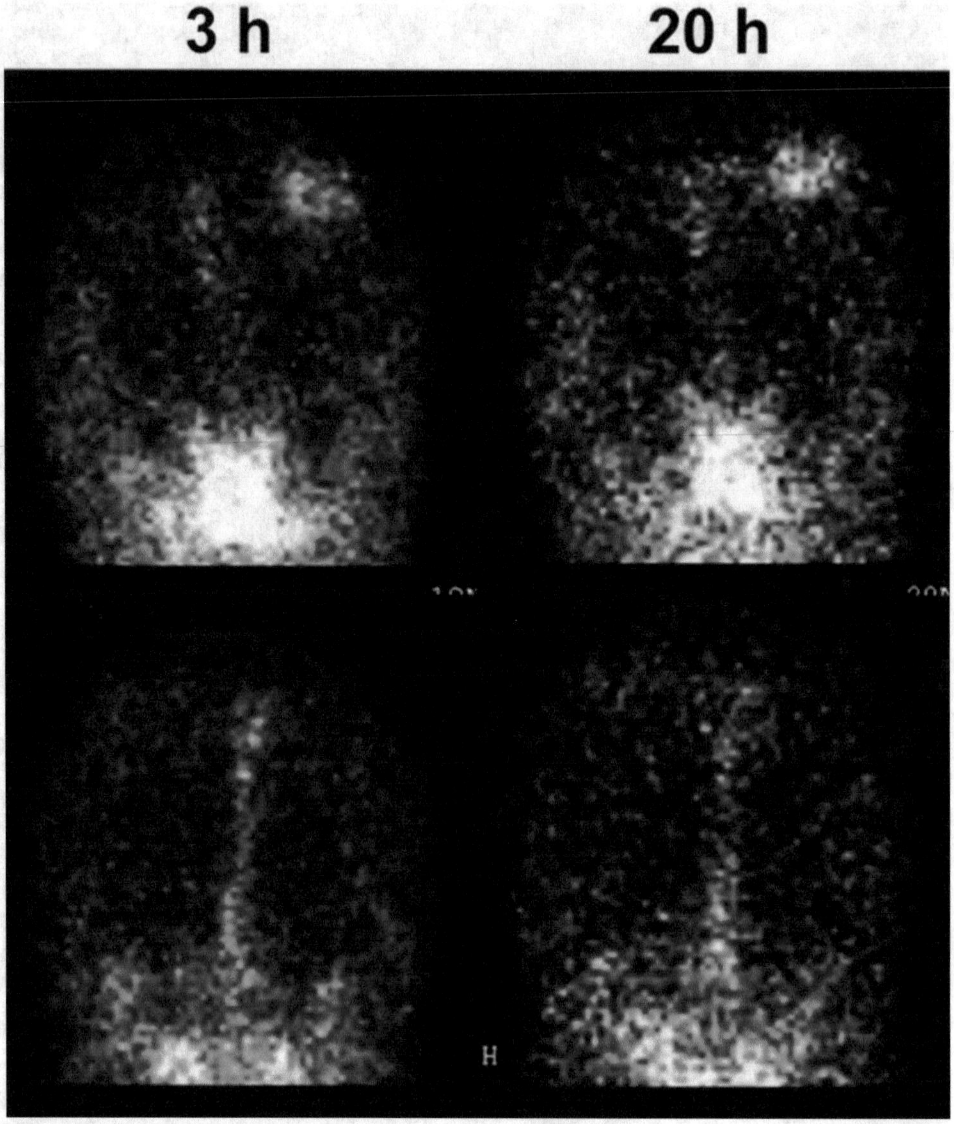

Fig. 8.2 Planar anterior (upper row) and posterior (lower row) views acquired 3 h and 20 h (left and right columns, respectively) after i.v. infusion of ^{99m}Tc-HMPAO-WBC in a 53-year-old woman with congenital hydrocephalus who had been submitted to multiple surgeries for ventricle-peritoneal derivation and who subsequently presented with a fistula in the left frontal region. CT showed thickening of the frontal bone and subcutaneous tissues near to left frontal surgical scar. The anterior images acquired up to 20 h post-injection show a clear accumulation of activity with time, indicating osteomyelitis

should be noted that, in patients previously submitted to spinal surgery with implantation of a titanium prosthesis, both X-rays and MRI imaging may be difficult to interpret due to the presence of artefacts.

Nuclear medicine techniques used to investigate intracranial and extracranial infections include scintigraphy with ^{111}In-oxine-WBC or, preferably, ^{99m}Tc-HMPAO-WBC for imaging based on single-photon emission.

The use of [^{18}F]FDG PET/CT in patients with cranial lesions is in general limited to the search for the primary tumour in cases of suspected secondary infection of tumour lesions of the brain, or in patients with HIV infection [4–6]. In these cases, the differential diagnosis involves malignant lesions (usually lymphoma) and benign infected lesions (toxoplasmosis, syphilis, multifocal progressive leuko-encephalopathy) [7–16]. Usually higher SUV values are observed in malignant lesions than in benign infected lesions, especially in toxoplasma lesions.

Key Learning Points

- Nuclear medicine imaging can be useful for differential diagnosis and for follow-up after therapy.
- Several radiopharmaceuticals have been described to investigate inflammatory encephalitis and multiple sclerosis but are not routinely used since MR imaging is the investigation of choice.
- Radiolabelled WBC scintigraphy is a very accurate modality to investigate cranial abscesses.
- Therapy follow-up with radiolabelled WBC scintigraphy is extremely useful, particularly if a pre-therapy scan is available for comparison.

8.3 Otitis and Sinusitis

The most frequent extracranial infections are otitis and sinusitis (Fig. 8.3). Infections of cochlear implants (CI) are also frequent (1.7–16.6%) related to the biofilm covering the devices, to the spread of microorganisms into the inner ear during surgery, or to bacteraemia [17–19]. CI infections include cutaneous necrosis and surgical wound dehiscence (early or late after surgery), otitis, cerebritis and meningitis. The diagnostic of CI-related infections is essentially clinical. CT is the radiological technique of choice for detecting collections beneath the receiver/stimulator, even though metallic artefacts can interfere with image interpretation. Nuclear medicine imaging techniques have a limited role for diagnosing CI infections, especially in the acute forms. However, bone scintigraphy with ^{99m}Tc-diphosphonates as well as [^{18}F]FDG-PET can be valuable tools in case of a late low-grade CI-related infection. In fact, in case of chronic osteomyelitis of the petrosal bone, where the minimal signs of infection are often undetectable with radiologic imaging, nuclear medicine techniques can reveal the presence of abnormal radiopharmaceutical uptake [20].

Malignant otitis externa (MOE) is an infection of the external auditory canal that can spread to the mastoid process and to the skull base; the most common presenting symptoms are otalgia, associated with temporal and occipital headache. The diagnosis of necrotizing, or 'malignant', otitis externa is typically based on the clinical presentation of a severe otitis externa, often in diabetic or immunocompromised patients, with associated skull base soft tissue infection and osteomyelitis, as visualized on MRI or CT imaging. Once clinical parameters and laboratory markers are normalized, the otolaryngologist faces the problem of how to determine if treatment has been adequate and can be discontinued with minimal risk of recurrence. As soft tissue involvement is expected to have resolved, a possible persistence of internal osteomyelitis must be excluded. Nuclear medicine imaging can help define the extent of infection or its eradication. Three-phase bone scintigraphy with ^{99m}Tc-hydroxymethylene-diphosphonate (^{99m}Tc-HDP) or ^{99m}Tc-methylenediphosphonate (^{99m}Tc-MDP) has traditionally been used for the initial diagnosis of osteomyelitis, by identifying sites of increased osteoblast activity. Although sensitive for osteomyelitis, this scan is unable to differentiate between active infection and bone re-modelling. By contrast, ^{99m}Tc-HMPAO-WBC scintigraphy is able to identify residual neutrophil-mediated inflammation and therefore is the best modality for follow-up after treatment [21].

Key Learning Points

- Nuclear medicine imaging is particularly useful in diagnosis and follow-up of malignant otitis.
- Radiolabelled WBC scintigraphy is the most accurate modality for therapy follow-up in patients with MOE.

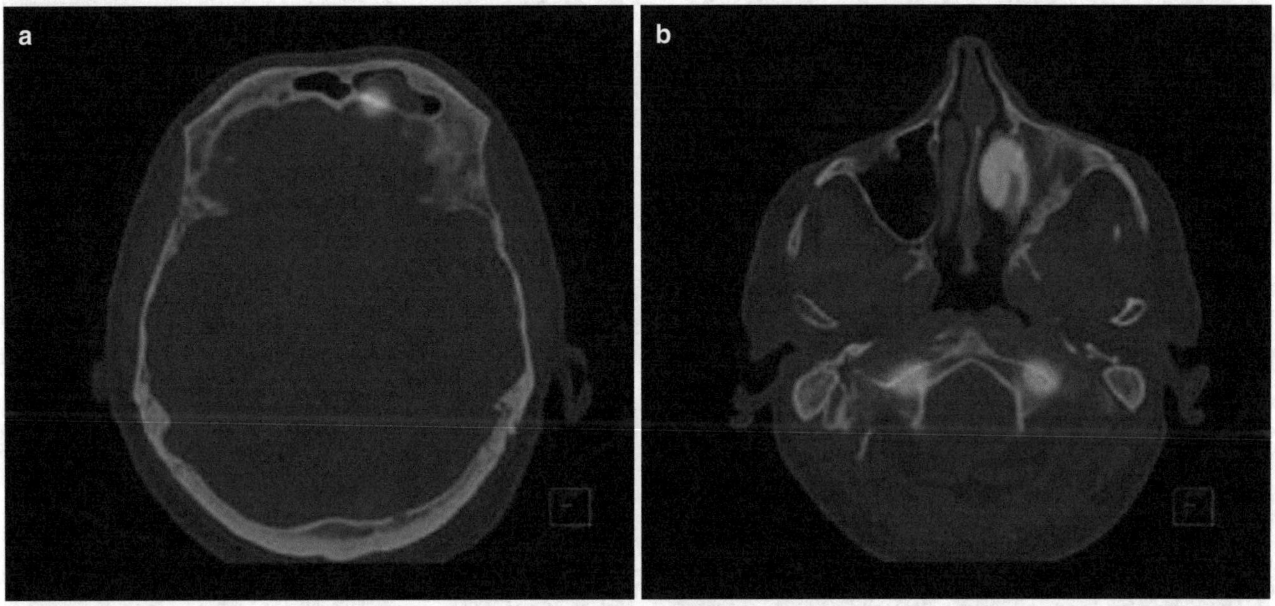

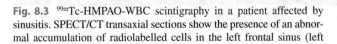

Fig. 8.3 ^{99m}Tc-HMPAO-WBC scintigraphy in a patient affected by sinusitis. SPECT/CT transaxial sections show the presence of an abnormal accumulation of radiolabelled cells in the left frontal sinus (left images) and left nasal turbinate (right images). In head and neck infections, SPECT/CT images help to correctly define the anatomical site of infection and its extent to nearby structures

8.4 Infections Associated with Dermal Fillers

In recent years, we are facing an increasing rate of soft tissue infections of the face, peri-orbital or labial and zygomatic as a complication of dermal filler injection for cosmetic reasons. In these cases, it is extremely important to distinguish sterile inflammation from infection, because different therapy and outcome are different in these two conditions (Fig. 8.4). Ultrasound and MRI do not have sufficient accuracy to distinguish between these two conditions, although they might be important for the identification of the material used as filler, which is also important for therapeutic and prognostic reasons and is often not known by the patient [22–27].

Key Learning Points

- Nuclear medicine imaging can help in detecting infection associated with dermal filler injection.
- Radiolabelled WBC scintigraphy has higher diagnostic accuracy than ultrasound and MRI.
- Ultrasound is mandatory to identify the nature of the filler used.

8.5 Dental Abscesses

Dental abscesses are also frequently observed and can be the port of entry for other infections [28]. Osteo-integrated dental implants may be subject to mobilization or infections. Bone scintigraphy with SPECT (or preferably SPECT/CT) acquisitions can be used to detect infections of the jaw associated with bone-integrated implants, allowing an exact localization of areas with complicated healing. Radiolabelled leukocytes scintigraphy may be useful in the evaluation of dental implant infection when osteomyelitis is suspected [29–31]. The diagnosis of dental abscesses can also be an incidental finding during radiolabelled WBC scintigraphy performed in search for other primary sites of infection or in case of fever of unknown origin (Fig. 8.5). Currently, few data are available about the role of [^{18}F]FDG-PET/CT in the evaluation of dental implant infections, particularly if associated with osteomyelitis; whereas, the role of this imaging technique is being tested in larger series of patients with other oral cavity disease, such as periodontal disease and apical periodontitis.

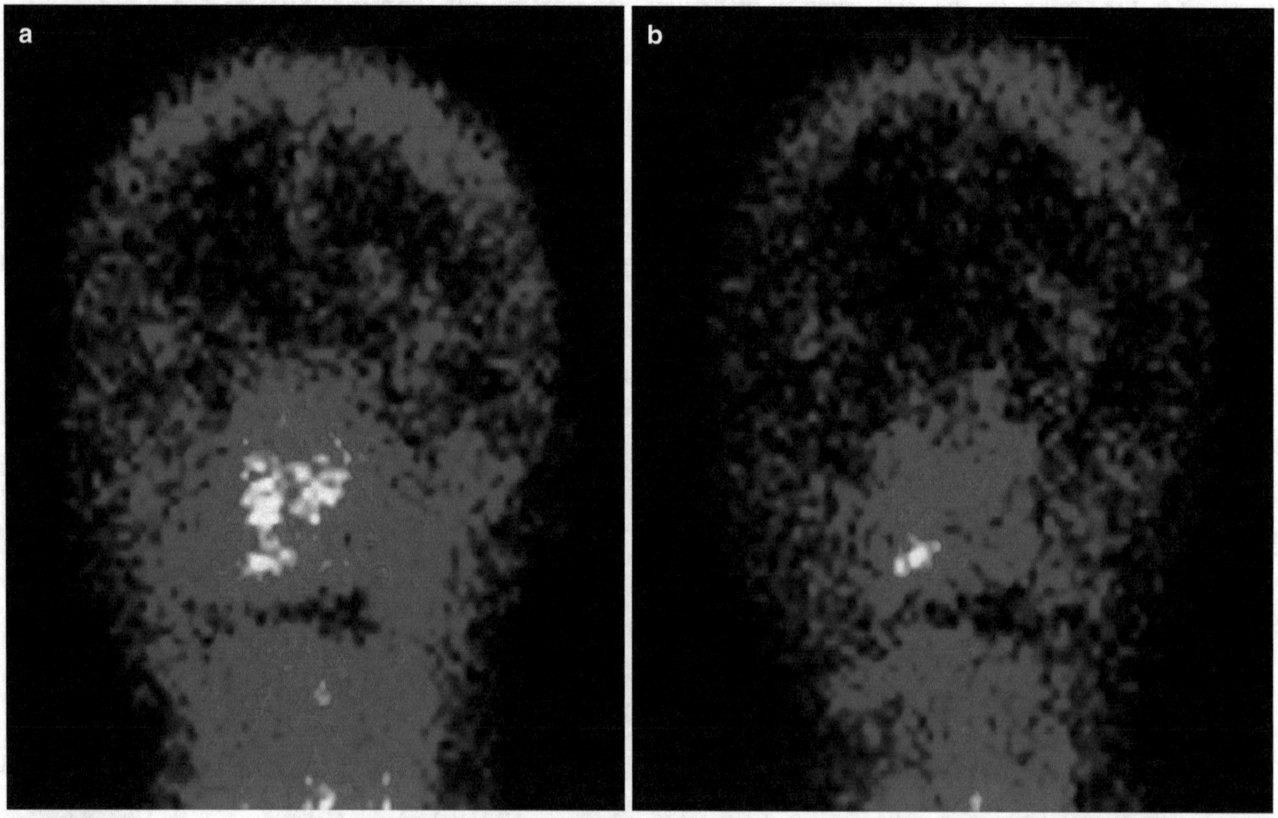

Fig. 8.4 Planar anterior and posterior views of the head of a patient with suspected infection of a labial silicon dermal filler. Images were acquired 3 h and 20 h after i.v. infusion of 22 mCi of ^{99m}Tc-HMPAO-WBC. An increase of activity and size between the 3-h scan and the 20-h scan in the right upper lip is clearly observed, indicating infection. The patient had a positive swab and underwent antibiotic therapy before surgical removal of the filler

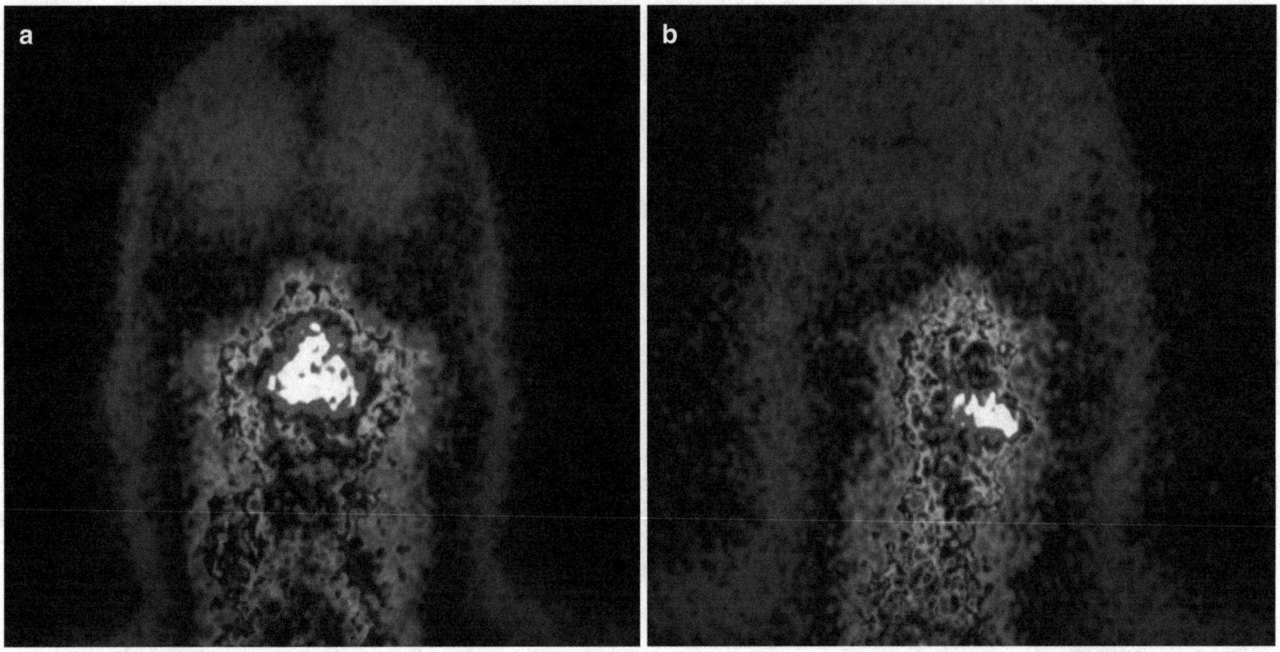

Fig. 8.5 Planar anterior images of the head and neck in a 68-year-old patient with FUO and high probability of infection. Images were acquired 3 h (**a**) and 20 h (**b**) after i.v. administration of 16 mCi of ^{99m}Tc-HMPAO-WBC. Total body images were also acquired, but did not show any additional site of abnormal accumulation of the labelled cells. Abnormal accumulation of labelled cells was observed at the left upper jaw, increasing with time between the 3-h scan and the 20-h scan. The patient had an infection associated to a dental implant

Key Learning Points

- Nuclear medicine imaging is useful to detect infections associated with dental implants.
- Radiolabelled WBC scintigraphy and [^{18}F]FDG PET have been proposed with a good diagnostic accuracy, although few reports have so far been published.

8.6 Thyroiditis and Exophthalmos

8.6.1 Acute and Subacute Thyroiditis

The term 'thyroiditis' includes a heterogeneous group of inflammatory disorders with different presentation, aetiology and clinical course. Acute thyroiditis is extremely rare and has a bacterial origin (most often *Streptococcus pyogenes*, *Staphylococcus aureus*, *Pneumococcus pneumoniae*); it has an acute clinical presentation with neck pain, dysphagia, dysphonia and fever.

Subacute thyroiditis includes granulomatous thyroiditis (or De Quervain's thyroiditis) and the silent form. A transient hyperthyroidism may occasionally be observed, caused by the efflux of thyroid hormones from damaged thyroid cell or follicles. *Restitutio ad integrum* is usually observed in the acute forms after antibiotic therapy, while some patients with subacute thyroiditis develop hypothyroidism.

The diagnostic accuracy of radionuclide imaging in acute/subacute thyroiditis is extremely variable and depends on the phase of the disease (Fig. 8.6).

The chronic form of thyroiditis is called Hashimoto's thyroiditis and is characterized by a diffused lymphocytic infiltration of the gland and release of several cell antigens that induce the production of several autoantibodies (most frequently antibodies against thyroglobulin and against thyroid peroxidase).

8.6.2 Graves' Disease and Autoimmune Exophthalmos

Graves' disease, also known as diffused toxic goitre, is a disease characterized by hyperthyroidism, diffusively enlarged thyroid and in some patients exophthalmopathy. It is an autoimmune disorder caused by the presence of antibodies against the TSH receptor that, upon binding, stimulate rather than inactivate the gland; these antibodies are involved also in the activation of retro-orbital fibroblasts.

Thyroid scintigraphy with ^{99m}Tc-pertechnetate or radioiodide helps in the differential diagnosis between Graves' hyperthyroidism and the other causes of thyrotoxicosis.

Mixoedema, a rare complication that occurs in about 1–5% of patient with Graves' disease, is an infiltrative dermopathy that presents as a waxy, discoloured induration of the skin of the 'pretibial area', spreading to the dorsum of the feet. Mixoedema is mainly due to a fibroblast activation and

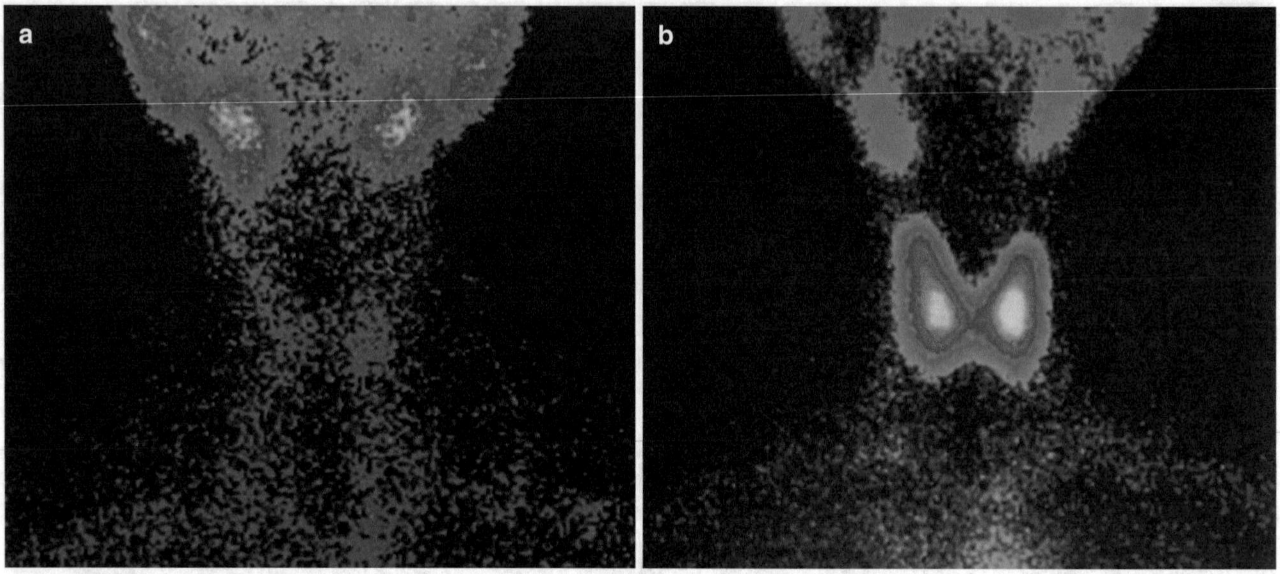

Fig. 8.6 ^{99m}Tc-perthecnetate thyroid scintigraphy in a 24-year-old woman with hyperthyroidism characterized by early appearance of tachycardia. (**a**) The scan at initial presentation shows no activity in the thyroid parenchyma, indicating acute/subacute thyroiditis. (**b**) The follow-up scan performed in the same patient after 2 months of therapy (anti-inflammatory drugs and beta-blockers) shows complete recovery of thyroid function

lymphocyte infiltration that causes an increased deposition of connective tissue components such as glycosaminoglycan, hyaluronic acid and others mucopolysaccharides, which results in osmotic oedema and fluid retention. The diagnosis is almost exclusively based on clinical ground.

Radionuclide-based evaluation of Graves' exophthalmos has been investigated with radiolabelled somatostatin analogues (for somatostatin radioreceptor scintigraphy, or SRS) and with radiolabelled interleukin-2 (IL2). In particular, radiolabelled IL2, by targeting activated lymphocytes, can highlight the presence of an active retro-bulbar lymphocytic infiltration of the eye muscles, an information that is very useful for therapy decision-making and follow-up [32].

On the other hand, SRS has been successfully used in Graves' exophthalmopathy because the accumulation of this radiopharmaceutical in the eye muscles mirrors the activity state of the disease and provides a rationale for treatments with unlabelled long-acting somatostatin analogues or with anti-TNF monoclonal antibodies (Fig. 8.7) [33, 34].

Key Learning Points

- Nuclear medicine plays a leading role in cases of suspected thyroiditis, to assess both the extent and the evolution of the inflammatory process, particularly in forms associated with transient thyrotoxicosis.
- When thyroiditis is suspected, thyroid scintigraphy with ^{99m}Tc-perthecnetate or with radioiodide should always be considered in the diagnostic work-up, together with the measurement of the radioiodide thyroid uptake.
- Scintigraphy with radiolabelled somatostatin analogues has shown to be very useful to quantify retro-bulbar inflammation in patients with exophthalmous and for detecting associated diseases (rheumatic and of salivary glands).

8.7 Other Neck Infections

A few sporadic reports have been published on the role of nuclear medicine imaging (based on radiolabelled WBC scintigraphy) in patients with head and neck infections, such as infected brachial cysts, salivary gland infections and other similar conditions (Fig. 8.8) [35, 36]. The first-line imaging modalities in these conditions currently include contrast enhanced MRI, CT and/or ultrasound, which are often sufficient for an accurate diagnosis.

Acknowledgments The current chapter is a revision of the original chapter written by Alberto Signore and Alberto Biggi in the previous edition of the book.

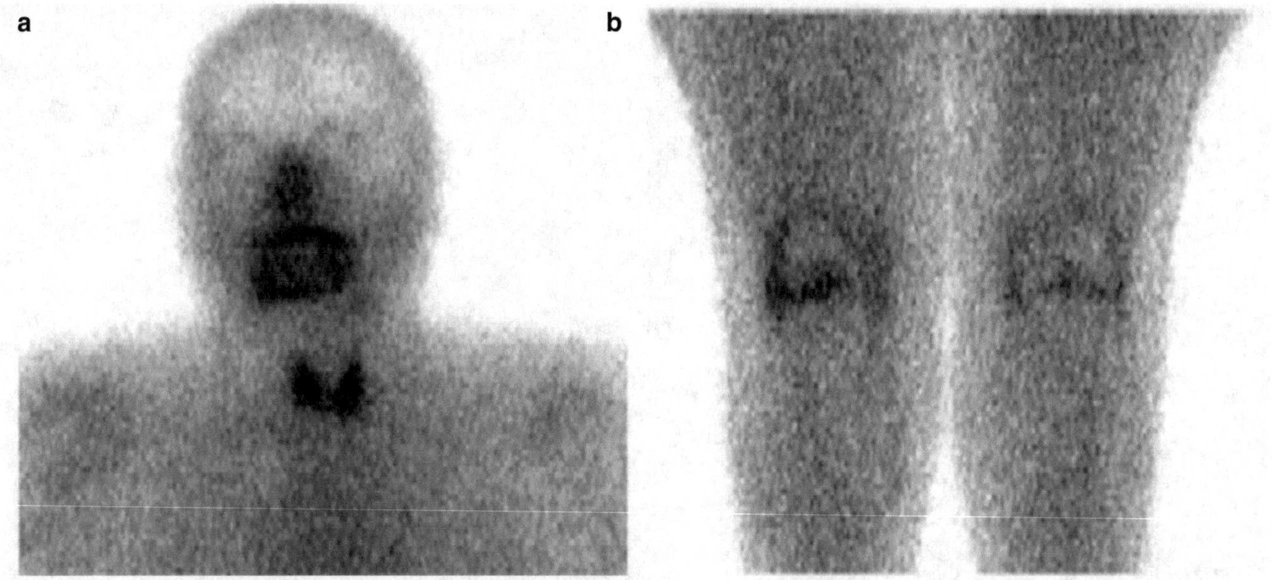

Fig. 8.7 Scintigraphy acquired 3 h after the i.v. administration of 10 mCi of ^{99m}Tc-HYNYC-TOC (a somatostatin analogue) in a patient with rheumatoid arthritis associated with Sjogren's syndrome and autoimmune thyroiditis, with the purpose of visualizing the expression of somatostatin receptors in inflamed tissues. This radiopharmaceutical is important for therapy decision-making, as it has been reported that patients with a positive scan may respond to therapy with unlabelled somatostatin analogues

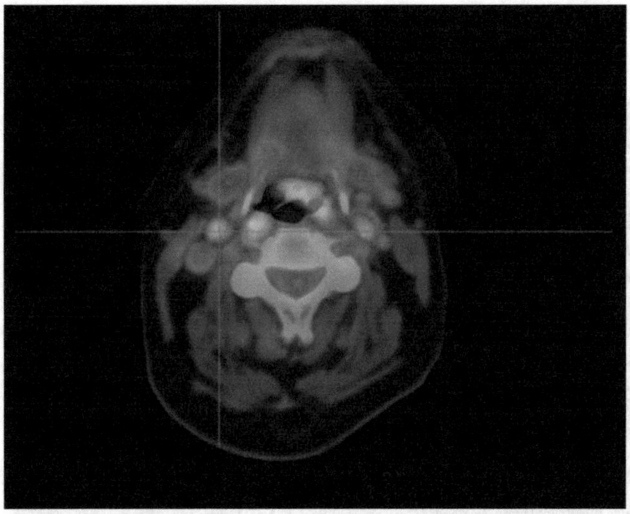

Fig. 8.8 [^{18}F]FDG PET/CT in a patients with carotid atherosclerotic plaque: the fused transaxial section shows [^{18}F]FDG uptake in the internal carotid artery. According to recent reports, carotid plaques are often characterized by increased [^{18}F]FDG uptake, due to the presence of macrophages in the lesion that indicates an inflammatory reaction within the plaque; this finding is not specific for infection

Clinical Cases

Case 8.1

Alberto Signore

Woman, 54 years old. 2011: Large dermoid lesion in the posterior fossa treated with surgery and requiring subsequent ventriculoperitoneal shunt surgery. Approximately 1 year later, worsening ataxia and dysarthria and appearance of intense vomiting and paralysis of the VII cranial nerve. The neurologic examination results were abnormal, but the CT scan performed in the Emergency Department showed only a mild increase of ventricular spaces. Hematological values as well as inflammatory parameters such as CRP (<5 mg/dL) and ESR (16 mm/h) were normal. MRI with gadolinium (04.06.2012) was requested, because of clinical suspicions of brain lesion, demonstrating the mass in the posterior fossa suspected for abscess (Figs. 8.9, 8.10 and 8.11).

Suspected Site of Infection

Brain abscess.

Radiopharmaceutical Activity

330 MBq of ^{99m}Tc-HMPAO-leukocytes.

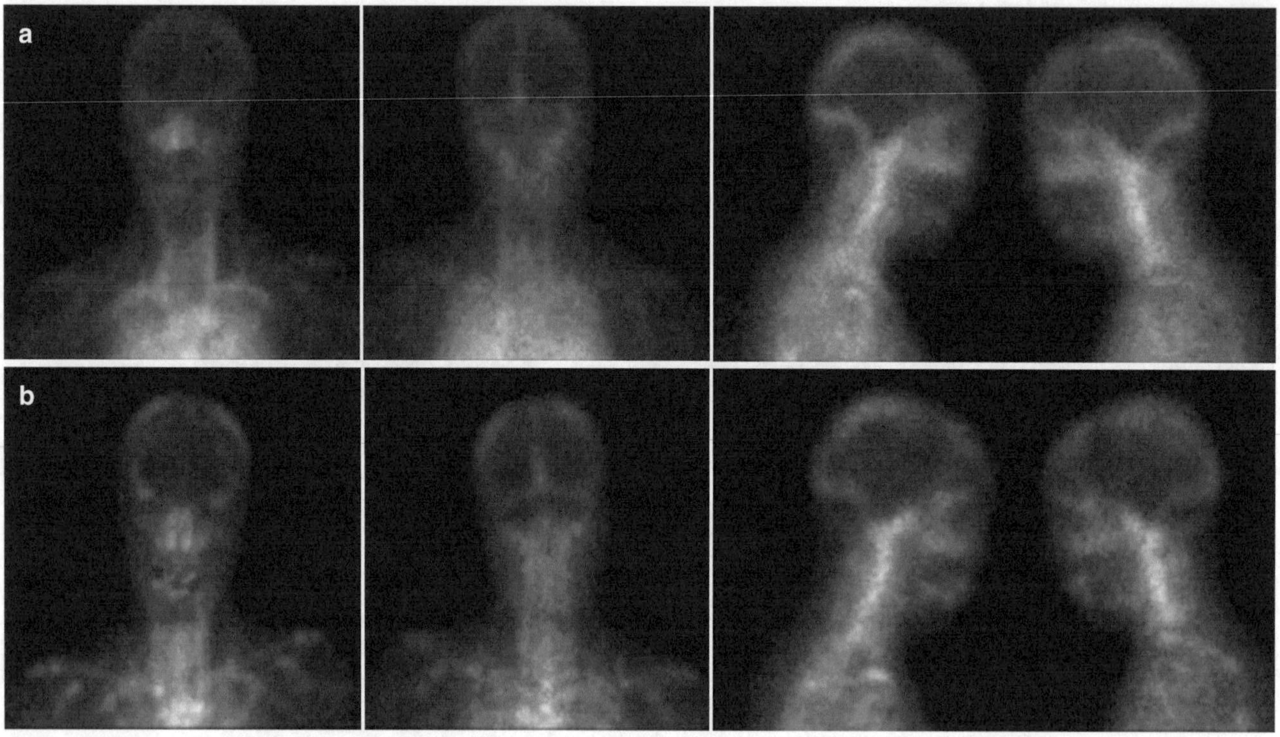

Fig. 8.9 Early (**a**) and delayed (**b**) spot images in anterior (left), posterior (middle), and lateral (right) views of the head and neck region. No areas of abnormal radioactivity accumulation are evident

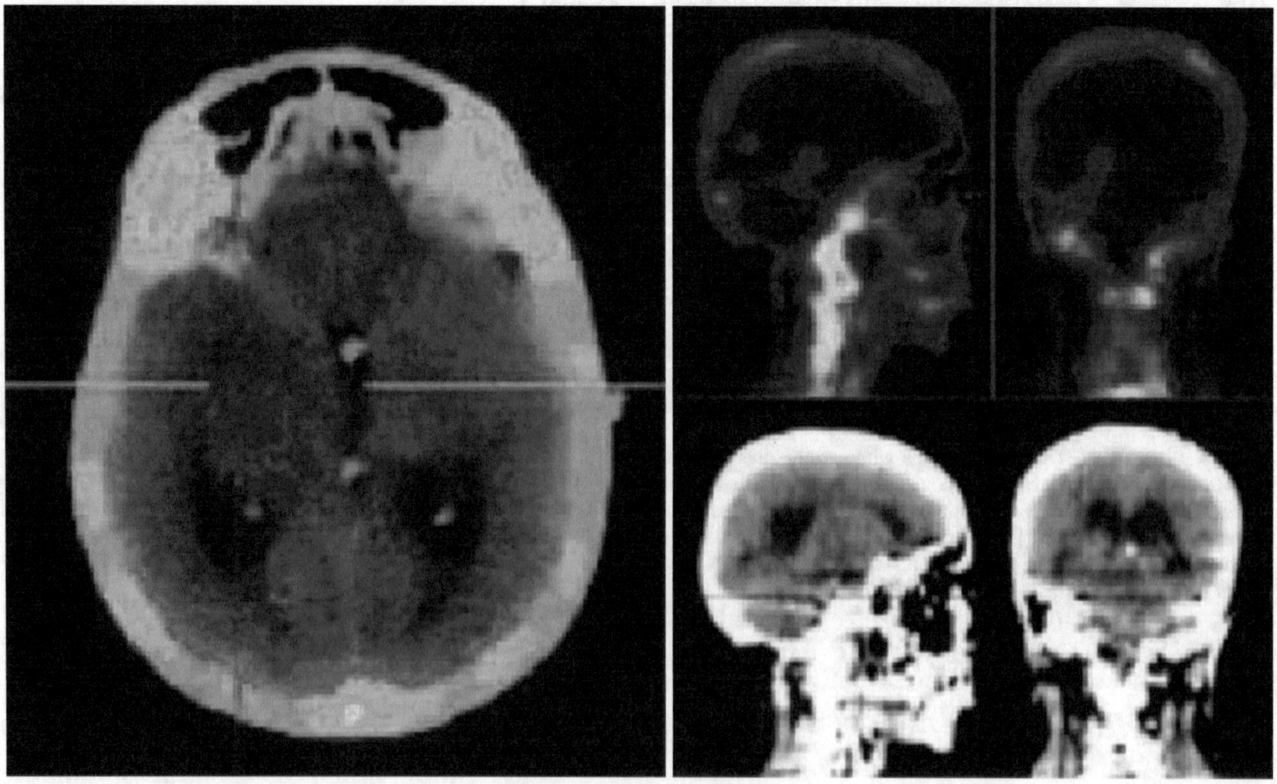

Fig. 8.10 No pathologic uptake is shown by ^{99m}Tc-HMPAO-leukocyte SPECT/CT images (5 h) (transaxial fused image, left; sagittal and coronal fused images, upper right; sagittal and coronal CT images, bottom right), particularly at the site of the brain lesion

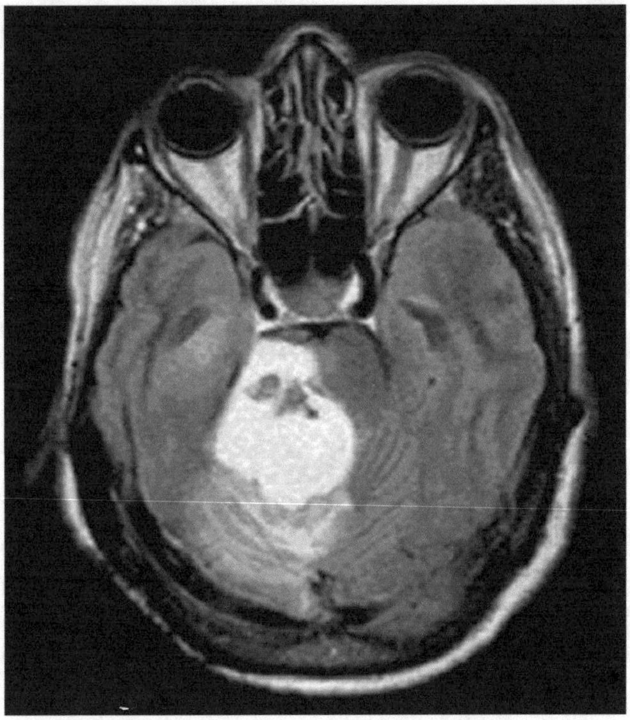

Fig. 8.11 MRI with gadolinium (transaxial section) showed a large right brain lesion

Imaging

Whole-body scan 30 min p.i. and planar spot antero-posterior and lateral images 4 and 24 h p.i. (Fig. 8.9) and SPECT/CT 24 h p.i. (Fig. 8.10).

Conclusion/Teaching Point

This is an example of the usefulness of ^{99m}Tc-HMPAO-WBC scintigraphy in the differential diagnosis between infectious and noninfectious lesions. MRI findings suggested an abscess because of the presence of liquid areas in the brain lesion. Based on the ^{99m}Tc-HMPAO-WBC scintigraphy results, a new craniotomy was performed (about one month after onset of symptoms) and the lesion at the posterior fossa was surgically removed. Histology indicated a dermoid cyst, consistent with the scintigraphy results.

Case 8.2

Alberto Signore

A 72-year-old man presented with a history of worsening right-sided otalgia, aural discharge, and hearing loss, associated with a right-sided facial weakness. This was assumed to be secondary to malignant external otitis. In August 2008, diagnosis of malignant external otitis with osteomyelitis of the right temporal bone was made. In September 2008, right tympanoplasty was carried out with decompression of the facial nerve. In 2009, ^{99m}Tc-HMPAO-WBC scintigraphy and three-phase bone scintigraphy were performed to confirm the absence of infection. Following positivity of both scans, the patient was treated with antibiotic therapy for 3 months. In 2010, a repeat three-phase bone scintigraphy showed the persistence of an inflammatory process in the temporal bone, mastoid region, and the right external auditory meatus. The patient started new treatment with antibiotics and was followed up clinically. In 2012, a new scan with ^{99m}Tc-HMPAO-WBC showed disappearance of infection.

Suspected Site of Infection

Right temporal bone osteomyelitis

Radiopharmaceutical Activity

A standard protocol was used to label autologous leukocytes with ^{99m}Tc-HMPAO (680 MBq) ^{99m}Tc-HDP bone scan: 740 MBq.

Imaging

^{99m}Tc-HMPAO-WBC scintigraphy: planar and SPECT images of the head were acquired at 30 min, 3 h, and 20 h p.i. (Fig. 8.12). Bone scan was performed after intravenous administration, acquisitions were dynamic for the first minute and then a planar blood-pool image was taken at 5 min, followed by a total body acquisition after 2 h, in particular of the skull (data not shown).

Conclusion/Teaching Point

The WBC scan in this case is more specific than the three-phase bone scan and should be used (possibly also with SPECT/CT acquisitions) to follow-up the efficacy of therapy.

Case 8.3

Alberto Biggi*

Male, age 53 years. Neurosurgical procedure at age of 14 years due to III ventricle pseudo-tumor (colloidal cyst) with apposition of ventricular-peritoneal shunt. October 2007, March and July 2009: admitted to neurology due to episodes of cerebritis associated with partial seizure crisis. February 2011: acute onset of high temperature associated with generalized seizure crisis. The liquor sample was negative.

* Dr. Alberto Biggi died prematurely on October 29, 2019.

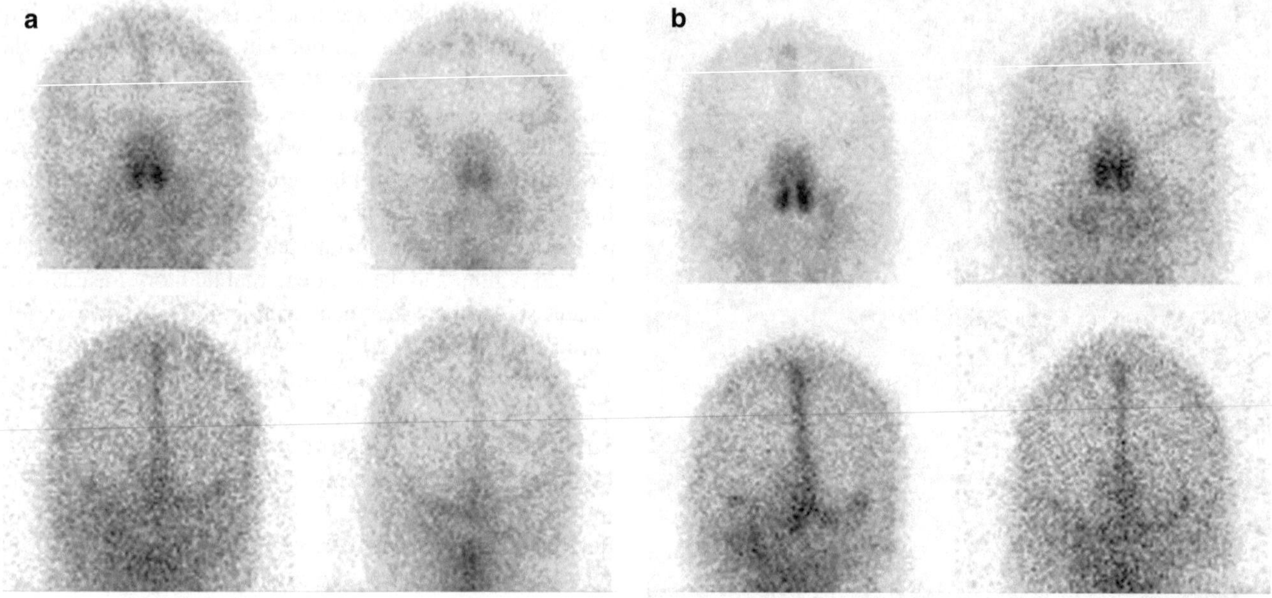

Fig. 8.12 ^{99m}Tc-HMPAO-WBC scintigraphy in external malignant otitis at the end of therapy. The images show anterior (top) and posterior (bottom) acquisitions obtained 3 h (left part in both panels) and 20 h (right part in both panels) after administration of cells. (**a**) Scan performed after treatment in 2009 and (**b**) after treatment in 2012

MRI, February 14, 2011: 2 cm area close to the anterior horn of the right lateral ventricle and a second area close to the "corpus callosum."

^{111}In-oxine-WBC, February 15, 2011: two focal areas of radiolabelled WBC accumulation near the anterior horn of the right lateral ventricle and in the parietal posterior region close to the posterior extremity of the shunt.

The patient started with antibiotic therapy. The first follow-up WBC scan in March 2011 demonstrated the progressive reduction of the focal uptake compared to the baseline study, with complete disappearance in the subsequent scan performed in May 2011.

Suspected Site of Infection

Brain.

Radiopharmaceutical Activity

^{111}In-oxine-WBC: February 2011, injected activity 20 MBq. March–May 2011: injected activity 20 MBq.

Imaging

Planar imaging acquisition after 4 h and after 24 h. SPECT/CT images of the head after 24 h. Static planar spot images (10 min/image; 128 × 128 matrix). SPECT/CT images of the abdomen: dual head SPET, matrix size 64 × 64, 35 s/step, 360° rotation, 5 mm/slice; low dose CT: slice thickness, 5 mm (Fig. 8.13).

Conclusion/Teaching Point

Late images after 24 h are necessary to confirm/exclude brain infection. SPECT/CT images are definitely superior to planar images in the identification and localization of the lesions. SPECT ^{111}In-oxine-WBC imaging of the brain represent the best approach to confirm the resolution of a brain septic process.

Case 8.4

Annibale Versari

An 80-year-old woman presented complaining of severe, constant pain in the right orbital region and blindness in the right eye. Horton arteritis was suspected, and the patient was referred for [^{18}F]FDG PET/CT (Fig. 8.14).

Biopsy of the abnormal intracranial tissue exhibiting increased [^{18}F]FDG uptake and altered MR signal yielded an histological pattern consistent with aspergillus infection, which was confirmed by subsequent microbiological tests. The patient is now undergoing antifungal therapy, and a follow-up PET/CT scan with [^{18}F]FDG is planned after an adequate period of treatment, to assess the efficacy of therapy both on the intracranial lesion and on the chest lesion.

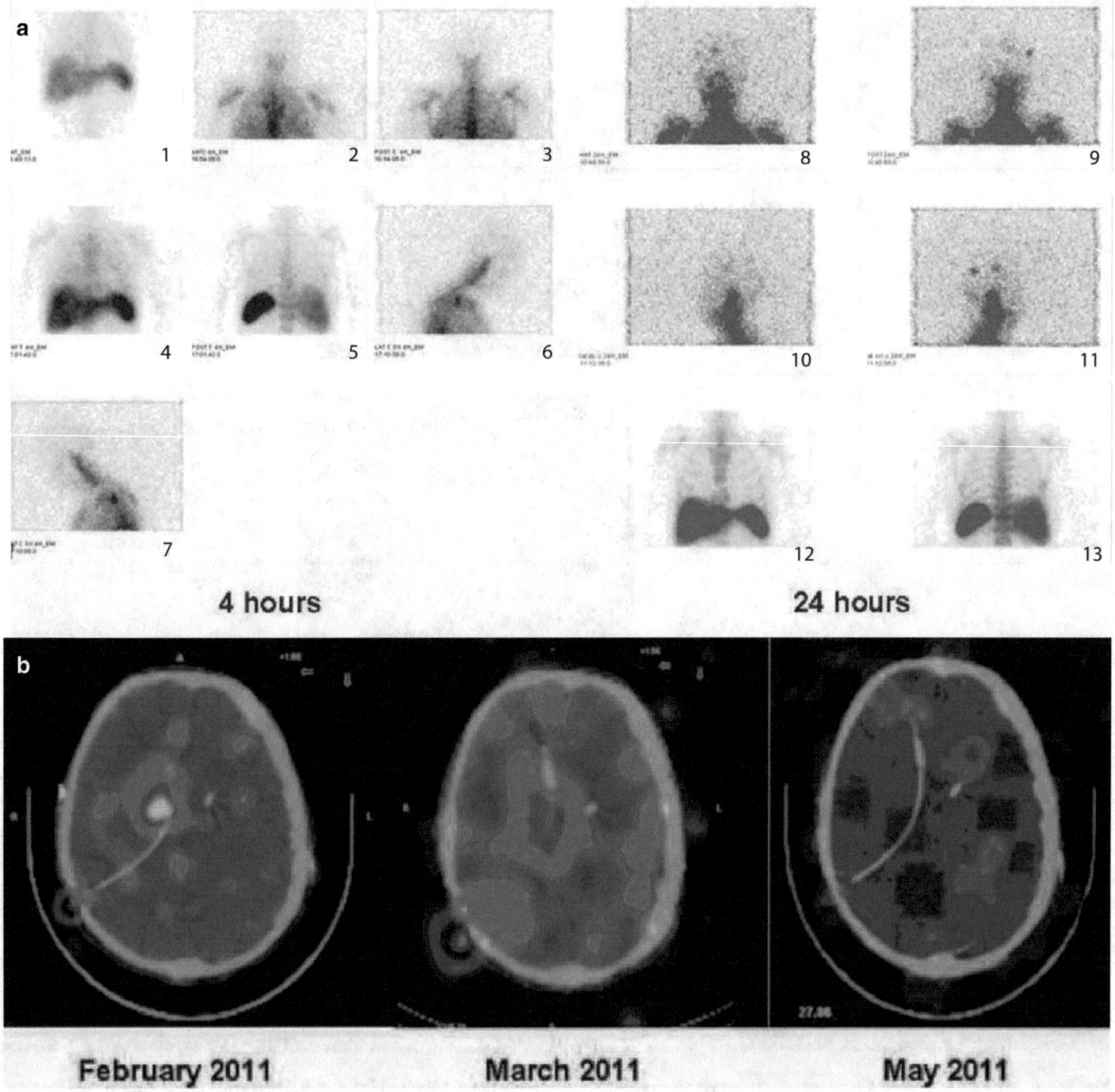

Fig. 8.13 ^{111}in-oxine-WBC: (**a**) Planar images acquired after 4 h and 24 h: normal biodistribution of the labelled WBCs in lung/liver; two focal areas of radiolabelled WBC accumulation near to the anterior horn of the right lateral ventricle and in the parietal posterior region close to the posterior extremity of the shunt. 4 h: *1* posterior of head, *2* anterior of head, *3* anterior of abdomen, *4* anterior of chest, *5* posterior of chest, *6* and *7* lateral of head. 24 h: *8* anterior of head, *9* posterior of head, *10* and *11* lateral of head, *12* anterior of chest, *13* posterior of chest. (**b**) SPECT/CT transaxial image confirms the presence of focal area of uptake and precisely locates the spot

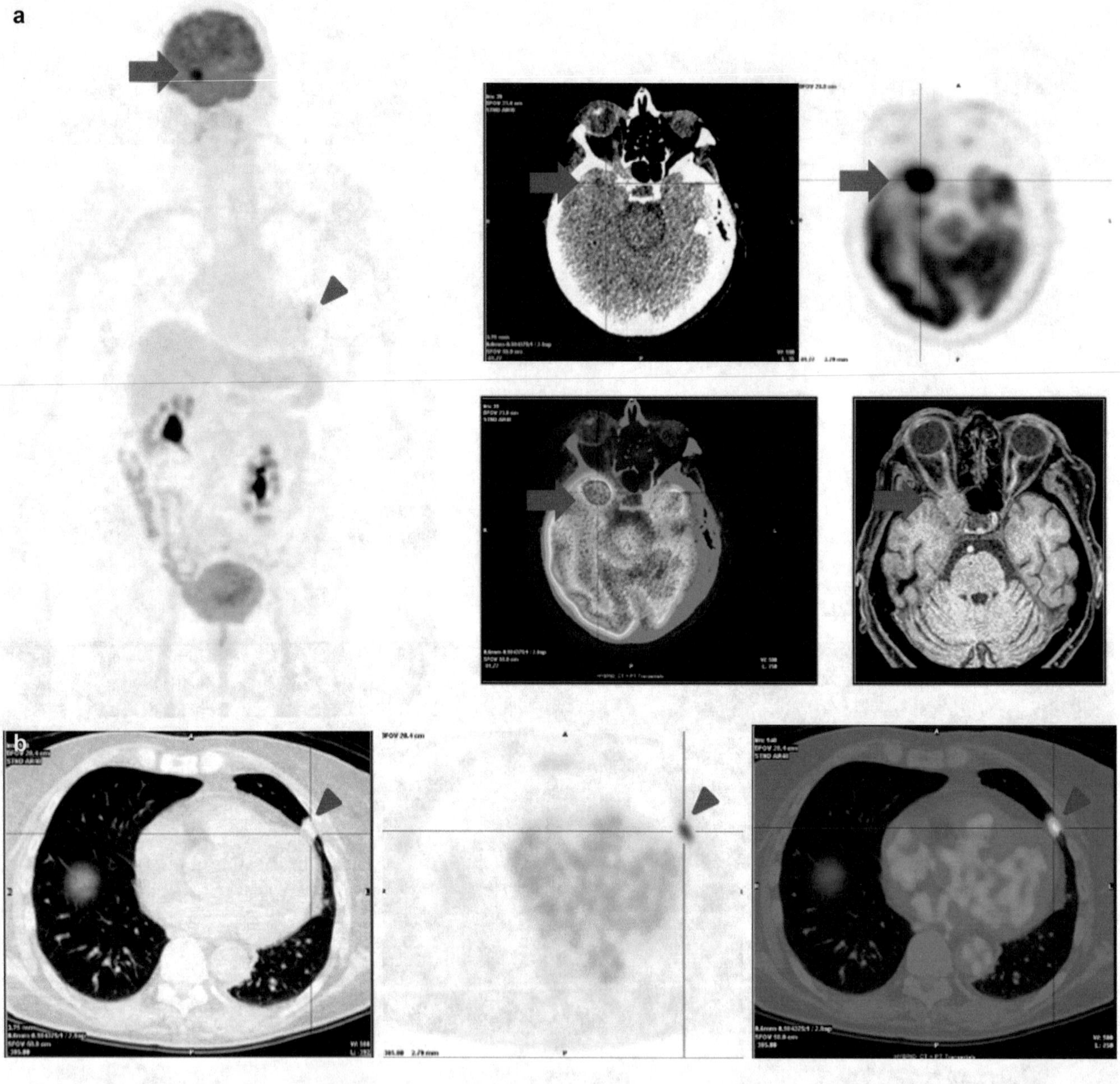

Fig. 8.14 (**a**) The MIP image (shown in left panel) demonstrates a focus of intense [^{18}F]FDG uptake within the brain (indicated by red arrow, with SUV_{max}=16). The axial sections shown in the right panel (CT component in the upper left corner, PET component in the upper right corner, fused PET/CT image in the lower left corner) localize more precisely this focus of increased tracer uptake anteriorly of the right temporal lobe, with apparent extension to the adjacent upper orbital fissure and sphenoid (small wing and body). The MRI image shown in the lower right corner of the right panel visualizes abnormal tissue mainly located in the anterior portion of the cavernous sinus and extended through the upper and lower orbital fissure in the region of the orbital apex, with involvement of the endo-orbital adipose tissue and circumferential compression of the apical portion of the optic nerve; (**b**) Axial sections of CT component (left panel), PET component (central panel) and fused PET/CT (right panel) localize the focus of moderately increased [^{18}F]FDG uptake in the left chest, as a parenchymal lung nodule in the left lingula (indicated by red arrowheads, with a SUV_{max}= 6)

References

1. Liberatore M, Drudi FM, Tarantino R, Prosperi D, Fiore V, Missori P, Venditti M, Delfini R. Tc-99m exametazime-labeled leukocyte scans in the study of infections in skull neurosurgery. Clin Nucl Med. 2003;28:971–4.
2. Medina M, Viglietti AL, Gozzoli L, Lucano A, Ravasi L, Lucignani G, Camuzzini G. Indium-111 labelled white blood cell scintigraphy in cranial and spinal septic lesions. Eur J Nucl Med. 2000;27:1473–80.
3. Braga FJ, Maes A, Vanteenkiste P, Flamen P, Peetermans W, Mortelmans L. Neural tuberculosis detected by F-18 FDG positron emission tomography. Clin Nucl Med. 2001;26:706.
4. Heald AE, Hoffman JM, Bartlett JA, Waskin HA. Differentiation of central nervous system lesions in AIDS patients using positron emission tomography (PET). Int J STD AIDS. 1996;7:337–46.

5. Villringer K, Jäger H, Dichgans M, Ziegler S, Poppinger J, Herz M, Kruschke C, Minoshima S, Pfister HW, Schwaiger M. Differential diagnosis of CNS lesions in AIDS patients by FDG-PET. J Comput Assist Tomogr. 1995;19:532–6.
6. Hoffman JM, Waskin HA, Schifter T, Hanson MW, Gray L, Rosenfeld S, Coleman RE. FDG-PET in differentiating lymphoma from nonmalignant central nervous system lesions in patients with AIDS. J Nucl Med. 1993;34:567–75.
7. Yilmaz K, Yilmaz M, Mete A, Celen Z. A correlative study of FDG PET, MRI/CT, electroencephalography, and clinical features in subacute sclerosing panencephalitis. Clin Nucl Med. 2010;35:675–81.
8. Wang HC, Zhao J, Zuo CT, Zhang ZW, Xue FP, Liu P, Hua FC, Tan HB, Guan YH. Encephalitis depicted by a combination of C-11 acetate and F-18 FDG PET/CT. Clin Nucl Med. 2009;34:952–4.
9. Dimitrakopoulou-Strauss A, Wilmsmeyer M, König S, Schubert S, Neff KW, Haberkorn U, Strauss LG. ^{18}F-FDG PET in a 10-year-old female patient with subacute sclerosing panencephalitis. Eur J Nucl Med Mol Imaging. 2006;33:1100–1.
10. Hsieh HJ, Lin SH, Chu YK, Chang CP, Wang SJ. F-18 FDG and F-18 FDOPA PET brain imaging in subacute sclerosing panencephalitis. Clin Nucl Med. 2005;30:519–20.
11. Lee BY, Newberg AB, Liebeskind DS, Kung J, Alavi A. FDG-PET findings in patients with suspected encephalitis. Clin Nucl Med. 2004;29:620–5.
12. Kassubek J, Juengling FD, Nitzsche EU, Lücking CH. Limbic encephalitis investigated by ^{18}FDG-PET and 3D MRI. J Neuroimaging. 2001;11:55–9.
13. Provenzale JM, Barboriak DP, Coleman RE. Limbic encephalitis: comparison of FDG PET and MR imaging findings. AJR Am J Roentgenol. 1998;170:1659–60.
14. Pichler R, Ciovica I, Rachinger J, Weiss S, Aichner FT. Multitracer study in Heidenhain variant of Creutzfeldt-Jakob disease: mismatch pattern of cerebral hypometabolism and perfusion imaging. Neuro Endocrinol Lett. 2008;29:67–8.
15. Engler H, Lundberg PO, Ekbom K, Nennesmo I, Nilsson A, Bergström M, Tsukada H, Hartvig P, Långström B. Multitracer study with positron emission tomography in Creutzfeldt-Jakob disease. Eur J Nucl Med Mol Imaging. 2003;30:85–95.
16. Henkel K, Zerr I, Hertel A, Gratz KF, Schröter A, Tschampa HJ, Bihl H, Büll U, Grünwald F, Drzezga A, Spitz J, Poser S. Positron emission tomography with [^{18}F]FDG in the diagnosis of Creutzfeldt-Jakob disease (CJD). J Neurol. 2002;249:699–705.
17. Tambyraja RR, Gutman MA, Megerian C. Cochlear implant complications: utility of federal database in systematic analysis. Arch Otolaryngol Head Neck Surg. 2005;131:245–50.
18. Yu KC, Hegarty J, Gantz B, Lalwani A. Conservative management of infections in cochlear implant recipients. Otolaryngol Head Neck Surg. 2001;125:66–70.
19. Antonelli PJ, Lee JC, Burne RA. Bacterial biofilms may contribute to persistent cochlear implant infection. Otol Neurotol. 2004;25:953–7.
20. Hoep LS, Merkus P, van Schie A, Rinkel RN, Smit CF. The value of nuclear scans in cochlear implant infections. Eur Arch Otorhinolaryngol. 2006;263:895–9.
21. Courson AM, Vikram HR, Barrs DM. What are the criteria for terminating treatment for necrotizing (malignant) otitis externa? Laryngoscope. 2014;124:361–2.
22. Di Girolamo M, Mattei M, Signore A, Grippaudo FR. MRI in the evaluation of facial dermal fillers in normal and complicated cases. Eur Radiol. 2015;25:1431–42.
23. Grippaudo FR, Di Girolamo M, Mattei M, Pucci E, Grippaudo C. Diagnosis and management of dermal filler complications in the perioral region. J Cosmet Laser Ther. 2014;16:246–52.
24. Grippaudo FR, Pacilio M, Di Girolamo M, Dierckx RA, Signore A. Radiolabelled white blood cell scintigraphy in the work-up of dermal filler complications. Eur J Nucl Med Mol Imaging. 2013;40:418–25.
25. Faundez E, Vega N, Vera E, Vega P, Sepulveda D, Wortsman X. Clinical and color Doppler ultrasound evaluation of polyacrylamide injection in HIV patients with severe facial lipoatrophy secondary to antiretroviral therapy. Skin Res Technol. 2017;23:243–8.
26. Tal S, Maresky HS, Bryan T, Ziv E, Klein D, Persitz A, Heller L. MRI in detecting facial cosmetic injectable fillers. Head Face Med. 2016;12(1):27.
27. Ginat DT, Schatz CJ. Imaging features of midface injectable fillers and associated complications. AJNR Am J Neuroradiol. 2013;34:1488–95.
28. Kao CH, Wang SJ. Spread of infectious complications of odontogenic abscess detected by Technetium-99m-HMPAO-labeled WBC scan of occult sepsis in the intensive care unit. J Nucl Med. 1992;33:254–5.
29. Schliephake H, Berding G. Evaluation of bone healing in patients with bone grafts and endosseous implants using single photon emission tomography (SPECT). Clin Oral Implants Res. 1998;9:34–42.
30. Concia E, Prandini N, Massari L, Ghisellini F, Consoli V, Menichetti F, Lazzeri E. Osteomyelitis: clinical update for practical guidelines. Nucl Med Commun. 2006;27:645–60.
31. Bruni C, Padovano F, Travascio L, Schillaci O, Simonetti G. Usefulness of hybrid SPECT/CT for the ^{99m}Tc-HMPAO-labeled leukocyte scintigraphy in a case of cranial osteomyelitis. Braz J Infect Dis. 2008;12:558–60.
32. Pacilio M, Lauri C, Prosperi D, Petitti A, Signore A. New SPECT and PET radiopharmaceuticals for imaging inflammatory diseases: a meta-analysis of the last 10 Years. Semin Nucl Med. 2018;48:261–76.
33. Sun H, Jiang XF, Wang S, Chen HY, Sun J, Li PY, Ning G, Zhao YJ. ^{99m}Tc-HYNIC-TOC scintigraphy in evaluation of active Graves' ophthalmopathy (GO). Endocrine. 2007;31:305–10.
34. Colao A1, Pivonello R, Lastoria S, Faggiano A, Ferone D, Lombardi G, Fenzi G. Clinical implications of somatostatin-receptor scintigraphy in ophthalmic Graves' disease. Eur J Endocrinol. 2000;143(Suppl 1):S35–42.
35. Chisin R, Noyek AM, Israel O, Witterick IJ, Front D, Kirsh JC. Contribution of nuclear medicine to the diagnosis and management of extracranial head and neck diseases (excluding thyroid and parathyroid). Isr J Med Sci. 1992;28:254–61.
36. Epstein JS, Ganz WI, Lizak M, Grobman L, Goodwin WJ, Dewanjee MK. Indium 111-labelled leukocyte scintigraphy in evaluating head and neck infections. Ann Otol Rhinol Laryngol. 1992;101:961–8.

Infective Endocarditis and Cardiovascular Implantable Electronic Device Infection

9

Martina Sollini, Francesco Bandera, Francesco Bartoli, Roberta Zanca, Elena Lazzeri, and Paola Anna Erba

Contents

M. Sollini
Department of Biomedical Sciences, Humanitas University, Pieve Emanuele, Italy

Humanitas Clinical and Research Center - IRCCS, Rozzano, Italy

F. Bandera
Department of Biomedical Sciences for Health, University of Milan, Milan, Italy

Cardiology University Department, Heart Failure Unit, IRCCS Policlinico San Donato, San Donato Milanese, Milan, Italy

F. Bartoli · R. Zanca
Department of Translational Research and Advanced Technologies in Medicine and Surgery, Regional Center of Nuclear Medicine, University of Pisa, Pisa, Italy

E. Lazzeri
Regional Center of Nuclear Medicine, University Hospital of Pisa, Pisa, Italy

P. A. Erba (✉)
Department of Translational Research and Advanced Technologies in Medicine and Surgery, Regional Center of Nuclear Medicine, University of Pisa, Pisa, Italy

Regional Center of Nuclear Medicine, University Hospital of Pisa, Pisa, Italy
e-mail: paola.erba@unipi.it

E. Lazzeri et al. (eds.), *Radionuclide Imaging of Infection and Inflammation*, https://doi.org/10.1007/978-3-030-62175-9_9

Learning Objectives

- To learn the epidemiology of IE and CIED-related infections
- To understand the pathophysiology, clinical presentation, and management of patients with IE and CIED-related infections
- To understand the roadmap of the diagnostic algorithm of IE and CIED-related infections
- To understand the requirements of an imaging procedure to be used in the diagnostic algorithm of IE and CIED-related infections
- To learn the benefits of each imaging technique in patients with IE and CIED-related infections
- To understand the limitations of each imaging technique in patients with IE and CIED-related infections
- To learn the main protocols for scintigraphy with labeled autologous leukocytes (including SPECT/CT imaging) and for [^{18}F]FDG PET/CT imaging in patients with IE and CIED-related infections
- To recognize pitfalls and sources of uncertainty for labeled leukocyte SPECT/CT and [^{18}F]FDG PET/CT imaging in patients with IE and CIED-related infections
- To understand the diagnostic strategy addressing specific clinical issues in patients with IE and CIED-related infections
- To understand the rationale of implementing and operating ready for the clinical discussion within a cardiovascular multidisciplinary team for clinical discussion of patients with suspected IE and CIED-related infections

9.1 Cardiovascular Infections

Cardiovascular infections have been recognized as a significant cause of cardiac diseases for many decades. The spectrum of microorganisms causing cardiovascular infections is very broad and includes all classes of microbes. Infection can involve various components of the native structure of the heart—pericardium, muscle, endocardium, valves, autonomic nerves, and the vessels—as well as implanted devices such as valve prosthesis (all types of prosthetic valves, annuloplasty rings, intracardiac patches, and shunts), cardiovascular implantable electronic devices (CIED), left ventricular assist device (LVAD), catheters, and vascular graft. In this chapter, we focus on IE and CIED infections.

Due to important technological advances and longevity, the use of implantable devices and surgical biomaterials in medicine has increased significantly during the last decades and is expected to increase further over the next years. As a consequence, an increased number of complications associated with implanted medical devices are foreseen. Healthcare-associated infections represent the most common noncardiac complication after cardiac surgery and device implants, affecting about 1.7 million patients each year, and are associated with nearly 100,000 deaths in the USA [1, 2]. Infections associated with cardiovascular implants are of particular concern, since patients undergoing cardiac surgery are becoming progressively older and have many comorbidities. In fact, their infection risk [3, 4] is nearly 5% in the first 2 months following cardiac surgery, with a tenfold higher risk for mortality [5].

The severity of cardiovascular infection depends on the involved microorganism and on maturity of the biofilm (a community of adherent microorganisms embedded within a self-produced matrix of extracellular polymeric substances) that develops on the device [6, 7], on the location and type of the biomaterial, and on the host defense status. A common key characteristic of cardiovascular infections is that matrix-embedded bacterial communities tolerate efficiently antibiotics and host phagocytic defenses. Therefore, often the only opportunity to efficaciously eradicate the infection is surgical treatment, including sometimes removal of the infected device.

Key Learning Points

- Cardiovascular infections can involve native structure of the heart as well as implanted devices.
- The use of implantable devices and surgical biomaterials in medicine has increased significantly.
- Healthcare-associated infections represent the most common noncardiac complication after cardiac surgery and device implants.
- The severity of cardiovascular infection depends on the involved microorganism and maturity of the biofilm on the device, on the location and type of the biomaterial, and on the host defense status.
- Surgery is often required to eradicate the infection, including sometimes removal of the infected device.

9.2 Infective Endocarditis

9.2.1 General Introduction

Infective endocarditis (IE), an infection of the endocardial surface of the heart [8], represents a complex and potentially deadly disease, associated with cardiac-located infection and often with multi-organ complications. The incidence of IE, which remains along with prognosis unchanged (or even increased) despite improvements in diagnostic and therapeutic strategies, varies from one country to another, within a range of 3–10 episodes/100,000 people per year [9]. There are numerous reasons for such persistently poor prognosis, including an increasing proportion of older patients with more severe disease, changing epidemiological profiles, and greater numbers of patients with prosthetic valve or device-related infection [9, 10].

Recent data from the EURO-ENDO registry [11], which provides a unique opportunity to assess the current characteristics of IE in Europe (including clinical presentation, microbiology, complications, management, and prognosis), show that IE more frequently affects men around 60 years of age and still presents an unacceptably poor prognosis, with a mortality of about 17.1% which is consistent with the 18% mortality observed in the ICE cohort [12], but higher than the 12.6% mortality observed in the Euro Heart survey [13]. The in-hospital mortality rate is associated with known risk factors, including prosthetic valve infective endocarditis (PVIE), age, comorbidities, *Staphylococcus aureus* infection, congestive heart failure, cerebral complications, perivalvular lesions, and vegetation length. The major cause of death was heart failure. Interestingly, mortality was particularly high in EURO-ENDO [11], when surgery was indicated but not performed, thus emphasizing the crucial role of an aggressive surgical strategy in these patients. Although the exact reason to contraindicate surgery in 58.2% of patients with a theoretical surgical indication is unknown, it is probably related to a combination of several parameters (age, frailty, left ventricular dysfunction, and multiple surgeries).

IE can be classified according to the site of the infection (left-sided native valve, prosthetic valve, right-sided), the pathogenesis of infection (nosocomial, community-acquired, etc.), or according to the responsible microorganism [14]. The epidemiological profile of IE has changed in recent decades, with important differences between countries and increasing numbers of staphylococcal and nosocomial cases [15]. The main etiology was in the past typically represented by *Streptococcus sporigenous* infection, but has recently changed to *Staphylococcus sporigenous* [16, 17]. Predisposing conditions, such as rheumatic and congenital disease or syphilis, are nowadays less frequent than prolapsed mitral valve, mitral and aortic valve calcifications, prosthetic valves and devices, and intravenous drug abuse [17–19]. Finally, the population of patients has also changed, younger patients being increasingly more frequently affected than in the past [20, 21]. PVIE, device-related IE (CDRIE), nosocomial, staphylococcal, and enterococcal IE are currently the more frequent IE variants [11].

9.2.2 Clinical Presentation and Diagnosis of IE

IE may present as an acute, rapidly progressive infection, but also as a subacute or chronic disease with low-grade fever and nonspecific symptoms that may thwart or confuse initial assessment. Therefore, patients may refer initially to a variety of specialists who may consider a range of alternative diagnoses. The diagnosis of IE is essentially clinical [15, 22] and should be suspected in all patients presenting with fever of unknown origin, particularly when fever (up to 90% of cases) is associated with cardiac signs, laboratory signs of infection, anemia, and microscopic hematuria; embolic manifestations are also frequently present (brain, lung, or spleen, in about 30% of cases) [23, 24]. The main cardiac signs include heart murmur (up to 85% of cases) and progressive heart failure; systemic signs, typically represented by spleen enlargement, glomerulonephritis, and peripheral stigmata, are observed when IE remains undiagnosed for a long time [15]. Vascular and immunological phenomena, such as splinter hemorrhages and/or Roth's spots (retinal hemorrhages), are common. However, clinical presentation is frequently atypical in elderly or immunocompromised patients [22].

EURO-ENDO [11] confirms the high risk of embolic events in IE, that in general occur in up to 40% of patients with IE (with a high burden of cerebral manifestations [22, 23]) and are associated with increased morbidity and mortality [25]. The risk of new embolic events (i.e., after initiation of antibiotic therapy) is only 6–21% [26], yet embolism was already present on admission in 25.2% patients in the EURO-ENDO registry, and the rate of new embolic events occurring during hospitalization was very high (20.5%). For reference, embolic events were observed in 23% in the ICE cohort [12], and embolism was the reason for surgery in 18% of the Euro Heart survey [13]. Factors associated with embolic events were similar to previous studies, with a major role of staphylococcal infection, vegetation presence, and size. Tricuspid, pulmonary, and aortic IE was associated with the highest risk of embolism.

9.2.3 Diagnosis and Prognostic Stratification of IE

New strategies have been developed to improve diagnosis and prognosis. The ESC Guidelines on the management of

IE were published in 2015 and provided new insights into the diagnostic and therapeutic management of these patients [27]. Although echocardiography (ECHO) is the main diagnostic imaging technique used in IE, other noninvasive imaging techniques have received increasing attention, including multislice computed tomography (MSCT), magnetic resonance imaging (MRI), and nuclear imaging ([^{18}F]FDG PET/CT and leucocyte scintigraphy) [28–32].

Two main diagnostic challenges must be taken into account when facing a patient with IE or CDI suspicion. First, confirming local involvement at the cardiac/device level and, second, detecting distant lesions related to the infectious process. Each technique has its diagnostic pros and cons when trying to solve these two issues (Table 9.1). In this regard, clinical discussion within the endocarditis team is in our experience the best way to overcome limitations of the imaging techniques, thus optimizing the imaging results for the subsequent patients' management.

Table 9.1 The ESC 2015 modified criteria for the diagnosis of IE, with modifications in italics-bold (modified from ref. 31)

Major criteria

1. Blood cultures positive for IE.
   - (a) Typical microorganisms consistent with IE from two separate blood cultures:
     - Viridans streptococci, *Streptococcus gallolyticus* (*Streptococcus bovis*), HACEK group, *Staphylococcus aureus*.
     - Community-acquired enterococci, in the absence of a primary focus.
   - (b) Microorganisms consistent with IE from persistently positive blood cultures:
     - ≥2 positive blood cultures of blood samples drawn >12 h apart
     - All of three or a majority of ≥4 separate cultures of blood (with first and last samples drawn ≥1 h apart).
   - (c) Single positive blood culture for *Coxiella burnetii* or phase I IgG antibody titer >1:800
2. Imaging positive for IE.
   - (a) Echocardiogram positive for IE:
     - Vegetation.
     - Abscess, pseudoaneurysm, intracardiac fistula.
     - Valvular perforation or aneurysm.
     - New partial dehiscence of prosthetic valve.
   - (b) ***Abnormal activity around the site of prosthetic valve implantation detected by [^{18}F]FDG PET/CT (only if the prosthesis was implanted >3 months previously) or by radiolabeled leucocyte SPECT/CT.***
   - (c) ***Definite paravalvular lesions by cardiac CT.***

Minor criteria

1. Predisposition such as predisposing heart condition or injection drug use.
2. Fever defined as temperature > 38 °C.
3. Vascular phenomena (***including those detected only by imaging***): major arterial emboli, septic pulmonary infarcts, infectious (mycotic) aneurysm, intracranial hemorrhage, conjunctival hemorrhages, and Janeway's lesions.
4. Immunological phenomena: glomerulonephritis, Osler's nodes, Roth's spots, and rheumatoid factor.
5. Microbiological evidence: positive blood culture but does not meet a major criterion as noted above or serological evidence of active infection with organism consistent with IE.

Key Learning Points

- IE can be a deadly disease.
- Poor prognosis is due to an increasing proportion of older patients with more severe disease, changing epidemiological profiles, and greater number of patients with prosthetic valve or device-related infection.
- IE more frequently affects men around 60 years of age.
- The main etiology is *Staphylococcus sporigenous.*
- The most frequent predisposing conditions are prolapsed mitral valve, mitral and aortic valve calcifications, prosthetic valves and devices, and intravenous drug abuse.
- PVIE, CDRIE, nosocomial, staphylococcal, and enterococcal IE are currently the more frequent IE variants.
- IE may present as an acute, rapidly progressive infection, but also as a subacute or chronic disease with low-grade fever and nonspecific symptoms.
- The main cardiac signs include heart murmur and progressive heart failure.
- Systemic signs such as spleen enlargement, glomerulonephritis, and peripheral stigmata are observed when IE remains undiagnosed for a long time.
- Clinical presentation is frequently atypical in elderly or immunocompromised patients.
- Embolic events occur in up to 40% of patients with IE and are associated with increased morbidity and mortality.
- Factors associated with embolic events are staphylococcal infection, presence of vegetation, and size.
- Tricuspid, pulmonary, and aortic IE are associated with the highest risk of embolism.
- ECHO is the main diagnostic imaging technique used in IE.
- ECHO, MSCT, PET/CT, and labeled leucocyte imaging are complementary tools in the diagnostic algorithm of IE.

9.2.4 Diagnosis of IE: From the Duke Criteria to the 2015 ESC Criteria

According to the modified Duke criteria, microbiological tests for germ characterization along with positive echocardiographic findings are necessary to establish the diagnosis of IE according to the "definite," "possibly," or "rejected" categories [33, 34]. Overall, the Duke criteria have 80% sensitivity [35]. However, 24% of the patients with pathologically proven endocarditis may be misclassified as "possible" according to these criteria [34]. The main reasons for misclassification using the Duke criteria are represented by either a negative blood culture or failure to demonstrate an endocardial vegetation at ECHO.

Negative blood cultures occur in 2.5–31% of patients with IE, more commonly because of prior antibiotic therapy [36, 37]. A negative blood culture results in delayed diagnosis and has therefore a negative impact on the outcome of the patients [38].

Both transthoracic echocardiography (TTE) and transesophageal echocardiography (TEE or TOE) are used for detecting endocardial vegetations. The three major echocardiographic findings for the diagnosis of IE are the presence of vegetation, abscess, or a new dehiscence of a prosthetic valve [8]. TEE is especially useful for evaluating patients with suspected prosthetic valve endocarditis [39] and is also superior to TTE for detecting mechanical complications such as valve perforation and chordal rupture [40]. A negative TOE has a very high negative predictive value for IE (86–97%) [41]. Overall, the sensitivity of TTE and TOE for the diagnosis of vegetations is 70% and 96%, respectively, in native-valve endocarditis (NVE) and 50% and 92%, respectively, in prosthetic-valve endocarditis (PVE). For abscess detection, sensitivity of TTE is about 50%, compared with 90% for TOE (with specificity >90% for both modalities) [42]. At ECHO, the detection of lesions in patients with prosthetic valves is more difficult than in patients with native valves, and normal or inconclusive results have been reported in up to 30% of cases. False-positive results can also occur.

Therefore, in the latest update of the European Society of Cardiology (ESC) guideline for the management of IE, multimodality imaging has been integrated in the diagnostic algorithm of IE [11] (Table 9.1 and Fig. 9.1). Along with blood cultures and ECHO, which remains the first imaging test that plays a central role in both the diagnosis and the subsequent clinical management of patients with IE, other imaging techniques were introduced. Cardiac/whole-body CT scan, cerebral MRI, [^{18}F]FDG PET/CT, and radiolabeled leucocyte SPECT/CT are in a pivotal position of the diagnostic work-up, since they have been demonstrated to contribute to reach an early and accurate diagnosis [11]. The value of cardiac CT has also been emphasized in the American Heart Association (AHA)/American College of Cardiology (ACC) guidelines [43]. According to the "ESC 2015 modified diagnostic criteria," the echocardiographic findings that are considered major criteria for the diagnosis of IE remained unchanged. However, in case of PVE, three additional imaging-based findings are now included as either major or minor criteria, as follows: (1) the identification of paravalvular lesions by cardiac CT should be considered as a major criterion; (2) when suspecting PVE, abnormal uptake by [^{18}F]FDG PET/CT or labeled leucocyte SPECT/CT should be considered as a major criterion; (3) the identification by

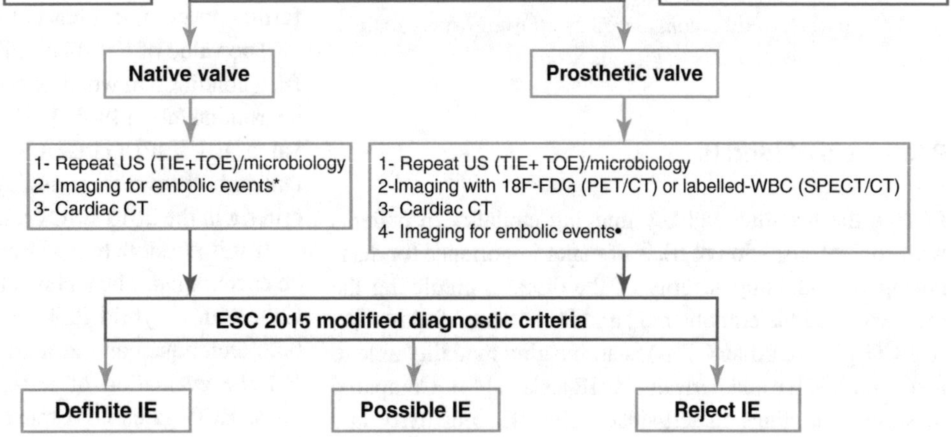

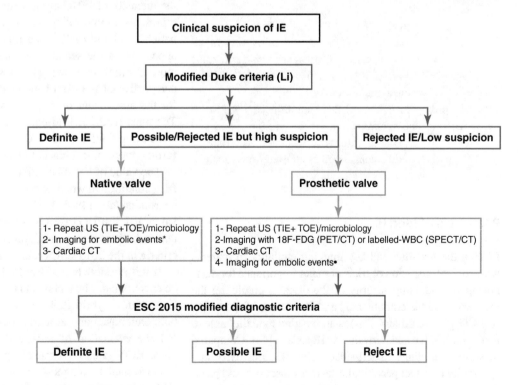

Fig. 9.1 Diagrammatic block flowchart showing the diagnostic path initiated by the clinical suspicion of IE. *TTE*, *TOE*, *ESC* European Society of Cardiology, *US* ultrasound examination [reproduced with permission from ref. 31]

imaging of recent embolic events or infectious aneurysms (silent events) should be considered as a minor criterion.

Key Learning Points

- The modified Duke criteria rely on microbiological and echocardiographic findings to establish the diagnosis of IE as "definite," "possibly," or "rejected."
- Overall, the Duke criteria have 80% sensitivity.
- The main reasons for misclassification using the Duke criteria are represented by either negative blood culture or ECHO.
- Negative blood cultures occur in 2.5–31% of patients with IE.
- The three major echocardiographic findings for the diagnosis of IE are the presence of vegetation, abscess, or a new dehiscence of a prosthetic valve.
- Overall, the sensitivity of TTE and TEE for detecting vegetations is 70% and 96%, respectively, in NVE and 50% and 92%, respectively, in PVE.
- In patients with native valves, normal or inconclusive results have been reported in up to 30% of cases; false-positive results can also occur.
- In the latest update of the ESC Guideline for the management of IE, multimodality imaging has been integrated in the diagnostic algorithm of IE.
- CT scan, cerebral MRI, [18F]FDG PET/CT, and radiolabeled leucocyte SPECT/CT are pivotal diagnostic work-up.
- According to the "ESC 2015 modified diagnostic criteria," in case of PVE the identification of paravalvular lesions by cardiac CT and abnormal uptake by [18F]FDG PET/CT or leucocyte SPECT/CT should be considered as a major criterion.
- According to the "ESC 2015 modified diagnostic criteria," the identification by imaging of recent embolic events or infectious aneurysms (silent events) should be considered as a minor criterion.

9.2.5 Left-Sided IE

ECHO, the first-line and key imaging modality in patients with clinical suspicion of IE, is of major importance for diagnosing IE, assessing severity of the disease, predicting the prognosis and the embolic risk, and for patients' follow-up.

ECG-gated cardiac CT(A) is an imaging modality able to assess both valve and perivalvular IE lesions [44]. Compared to surgical findings in left-sided valve IE, sensitivity and specificity to detect perivalvular lesions (abscesses and pseudoaneurysms) are very high (>95%) [44], especially in the aortic localization [45]. Detection of valve lesions as vegetations, leaflet thickening, valve perforation, or valve aneurysm is also possible [44]. Excellent correlation with operative findings has been reported, with 96% sensitivity and 97% specificity of CT, considering surgery as the reference standard in the "per valve" analysis [45], as well as excellent interobserver agreement. Nonetheless, it should be considered that data on the value of cardiac CT(A) in IE are relatively scarce, including few patients in highly experienced centers; therefore, this experience might not be valid for all centers managing patients with IE. Cardiac CT(A) also allows a noninvasive coronary angiography to be obtained preoperatively in patients with surgical indication, in whom conventional invasive angiography could be contraindicated. The main relative limitations of CT are the high radiation exposure and the risk of nephrotoxicity associated with the use of iodinated contrast medium. However, the potential advantages of CT to provide relevant diagnostic information overcome these limitations.

Sensitivity of SPECT/CT with labeled leucocytes (WBC) has been reported to range between 64% and 90%, associated with 36% and 100% specificity, 85% and 100% positive, and 47% and 81% negative predictive values [30, 46]. In case of abscess, WBC SPECT/CT has been reported to have 83–100% sensitivity, 78–87% specificity, 43–71% positive, and 93–100% negative predictive values [47], even in the early post-intervention phase [30, 47]. Compared to [18F]FDG PET/CT, WBC SPECT/CT has an excellent positive predictive value for the detection of perivalvular infection and abscesses in patients with suspected PVE. In addition, the intensity of WBC accumulation in the perivalvular area represents an interesting marker of local infectious activity: patients with mild activity accumulation on the first scan disappearing on the second imaging evaluation seem to have more favorable outcome [47]. This opens the very interesting perspective of the use of molecular multimodality imaging for the assessment of response to antimicrobial treatment. The most recent hybrid equipment allows to perform CTA also during a WBC SPECT/CT scan. However, this potential further development has not been yet evaluated.

The value of [18F]FDG PET/CT is limited in native valve IE, a condition in which sensitivity is too poor to recommend its routine use [48–50]. However, in patients with native valve IE, [18F]FDG PET/CT is useful for the detection of distant embolic events, a condition currently considered a minor criteria in the 2015 ESC criteria (see further below).

If it is possible to perform PET/CTA, its use must always be encouraged. The technical requisites for performing PET/CTA with a hybrid PET/CT scanner are cardiac gating for both techniques and at least a 64-detector row CT scanner. For the evaluation of left-sided prosthetic IE, an arterial phase ECG-gated CTA must be performed. When PET/CTA is performed to diagnose device infection, a prospective, ECG-gated, venous phase CTA sequence is recommended to evaluate local soft tissue changes, lead vegetations, and venous thrombosis of the vascular accesses [51].

The advantage of ECG-gated [18F]FDG PET/CTA is the identification of a larger number of anatomic lesions than non-gated [18F]FDG PET/CT, the reduction of doubtful studies on non-gated [18F]FDG PET/CT [51, 52] and in specific clinical situations such as patients with aortic grafts, patients with congenital heart diseases who have a complex anatomy, as their surgical treatment often requires implantation of a large amount of prosthetic material.

On the other hand, in case of prosthetic material, [18F]FDG PET/CT and WBC SPECT/CT imaging are very useful. Abnormal activity around the site of prosthetic valve implantation detected by [18F]FDG PET/CT or labeled leukocytes SPECT/CT is considered a major criteria. If PET/CT acquisition is combined with a cardiac CT (PET/CTA), the metabolic findings provided by the [18F]FDG uptake distribution and intensity might be added to the anatomic findings already described for cardiac CTA within a single imaging procedure. In a recent systematic review on the assessment of PVE, [18F]FDG PET/CT sensitivity and specificity have been reported to range between 73–100% and 71–100%, respectively, with 67–100% positive and 50–100% negative predictive values (PPV and NPV, respectively). Adding [18F]FDG PET/CT to the modified Duke criteria increased sensitivity for a definite IE from 52–70% to 91–97% [53] by reducing the number of possible PVE cases. This finding has been confirmed in several series [28, 46, 51, 54–57].

[18F]FDG PET/CT has been reported to have similar sensitivities as ECHO for vegetations, perivalvular sequelae, and prosthetic valve dehiscence [28]. When [18F]FDG PET/CT is combined with CT-angiography ([18F]FDG PET/CTA), sensitivity and specificity for IE increased to 91%, with 93% PPV and 88% NPV [51, 58]. In association with the Duke criteria, [18F]FDG PET/CTA allowed reclassification of 90% of the cases initially classified as "possible" IE and provided a more conclusive diagnosis (definite/reject) in 95% of the patients. This combined multimodality procedure should be considered in all the patients in whom ECHO presents significant limitations. In fact, its ability to provide relevant information on the local extent of the disease such as the presence of pseudo-aneurysms, fistulas, thrombosis and coronary involvement, are significant for subsequent clinical and surgical decision-making.

Key Learning Points

- ECHO is the first-line and key imaging modality when suspecting IE.
- ECHO is of major importance for diagnosing of IE, assessing the severity of the disease, predicting prognosis and embolic risk, and for patients' follow-up.
- ECG-gated cardiac CT(A) is able to assess both valve and perivalvular IE lesions.
- CT(A) has excellent correlation with operative findings, with 96% sensitivity and 97% specificity in comparison with surgery in the "per valve" analysis, as well as excellent interobserver agreement.
- Data on the value of cardiac CT(A) in IE are relatively scarce, including few patients in highly experienced centers.
- The main relative limitations of CT are its high radiation exposure and the risk of nephrotoxicity associated with the use of iodinated contrast.
- Sensitivity of WBC SPECT/CT ranges between 64–90%, with 36–100% specificity, 85–100% positive, and 47–81% negative predictive values.
- WBC SPECT/CT has excellent positive predictive value for the detection of perivalvular infection and abscesses in patients with suspected PVE.
- The intensity of WBC accumulation in the perivalvular area constitutes an interesting marker of local infectious activity.
- The value of [18F]FDG PET/CT is limited in native valve IE and its use is mainly related to the detection of distant embolic events.
- If it is possible to obtain PET/CTA, its use must always be encouraged.
- The advantage of [18F]FDG PET/CTA is the identification of a larger number of anatomic lesions than non-gated [[18F]FDG PET/CT, and the reduction of doubtful studies on non-gated [18F]FDG PET/CT.
- In case of prosthetic material, [18F]FDG PET/CT and WBC imaging are very useful.
- In patients with PVE, [18F]FDG PET/CT sensitivity and specificity range between 73–100% and 71–100%, respectively, with a 67–100% PPV and 50–100% NPV, respectively.
- Adding [18F]FDG PET/CT to the modified Duke criteria increased sensitivity for a definite IE from 52–70% to 91–97%, by reducing the number of possible PVE cases.
- [18F]FDG PET/CTA has 91% sensitivity and 93% specificity, with 93% PPV and 88% NPV.
- When associated with Duke criteria, [18F]FDG PET/CTA allowed reclassification of 90% of the cases initially classified as "possible" IE and provided a more conclusive diagnosis (definite/reject) in 95% of the patients.

9.2.6 Right-Sided IE

Involvement of the right heart is usually easy to detect using TTE because of the anterior location of the tricuspid valve and usually large vegetations [59], although the right heart has many echocardiographically anomalous anatomic facets that may be difficult to distinguish from vegetations [60]. Eustachian and pulmonary valves should always be assessed. TEE is more sensitive in the detection of pulmonary vegetations [61], associated left-sided involvement, central intravenous catheters and devices, prosthetic valve endocarditis, foreign bodies, unusual locations of right-side IE, and complications (e.g., perivalvular abscesses) after failure to respond to therapy [62]. TTE better defines the presence of prognostic features such as pericardial effusion, ventricular dysfunction, and increased pulmonary arterial pressure. TEE is superior to TTE in the detection and sizing of vegetations [63] and allows visualization of lead vegetations in the right atrium-superior vena cava area and in other regions less well visualized by TTE.

CTA, [^{18}F]FDG PET/CT(A) (or [^{18}F]FDG PET/CT), and WBC SPECT/CT might be used in all the cases when right-sided IE (particularly PVE) is suspected. Contrast-enhanced CT may reveal pulmonary embolism, infarcts, and abscesses. Ventilation-perfusion scintigraphy may be an alternative to CT in order to screen patients for septic pulmonary embolism [64], although [^{18}F]FDG PET/CT(A) and WBC SPECT/CT have largely replaced ventilation-perfusion scintigraphy, since they allow simultaneous assessment of right- and left-side valves, of sites of distant embolisms, and of potential portal of entry (POE) of the infection [32].

Key Learning Points

- Right heart involvement is usually easy to detect using TTE because of the anterior location of the tricuspid valve and usually large vegetations.
- TEE is more sensitive in the detection of pulmonary vegetations, associated left-sided involvement, central intravenous catheters and devices, prosthetic valve endocarditis, foreign bodies, unusual locations of right-sided IE, and of the associated complications.
- TTE better evaluates prognostic features such as pericardial effusion, ventricular dysfunction, and pulmonary arterial pressure.
- TEE is superior to TTE in the detection and sizing of vegetations.
- CTA, [^{18}F]FDG PET/CT(A) (or [^{18}F]FDG PET/CT), and WBC SPECT/CT might be used in all the cases when right-sided IE (particularly PVE) is suspected.
- Contrast-enhanced CT may reveal pulmonary embolism, infarcts and abscesses.
- Ventilation-perfusion scintigraphy may be an alternative to CT in order to screen for septic pulmonary embolism.
- [^{18}F]FDG PET/CT(A) and WBC SPECT/CT have largely replaced ventilation-perfusion scintigraphy, since they allow simultaneous assessment of right and left side valves, sites of distant embolisms, and potential portals of entry for the infection.

9.2.7 Embolic Burden in IE

Extracardiac manifestations of IE (both NVE and PVE) are reported in 30–80% of patients. The most frequent events are embolic stroke or septic embolization to bone, spleen, or kidneys [84], although only some of these are symptomatic [10, 65]. The majority of embolisms take place within the first 14 days after treatment initiation [66], they can appear as the initial symptom leading to the diagnosis and are frequently recurrent [66]. Localization of the emboli and their cerebral/extracerebral proportion vary according to the studies, in particular according to the frequency and modalities of imaging, and the proportion of right-sided and left-sided IE.

The search for asymptomatic embolic events through systematic extracardiac imaging has become very important, due to the fact that the detection of asymptomatic embolic events is now considered a minor Duke criterion in the 2015 ESC criteria [11]. This represents another main difference between the ESC and the American Heart Association (AHA) recommendations, in which only symptomatic extracardiac localizations of IE are considered as Duke classification minor criteria [43].

The panel of imaging modalities used routinely to evaluate patients with extracardiac infective processes includes dental radiography, abdominal ultrasound, CT scan of the brain, whole-body CT or MRI scan. The CT scan (including the brain) has long been considered the main imaging technique for the diagnosis of embolic events in IE patients; MRI is a valuable alternative in case of cerebral embolism, with the advantage of a higher sensitivity in detecting recent ischemic lesions, and small ischemic or hemorrhagic lesions, without the use of iodine contrast. A noticeable advantage of [^{18}F]FDG PET/CT and WBC SPECT/CT is the possibility to perform the extracardiac work-up within a single imaging procedure, thus revealing the concomitant presence of extracardiac infection sites as the consequence of septic embolism, as well as primary infective processes. ECHO is also useful for predicting embolic events. Among the several factors that have been associated with an increased risk of embolism [67] (age, diabetes, atrial fibrillation, embolism before antibiotics, vegetation length, and *Staphylococcus aureus* infection [10]), size and mobility of the vegetations are the most potent predictors of new embolic event in patients with IE [23, 25, 66, 68, 69]. A recent study found that the risk of neurological complications was particularly high in patients with very large vegetations (>30 mm length) [70]. The 2015 ESC guidelines recommend urgent surgical therapy in case of large (>10 mm) vegetation following one or more embolic episodes, and when the large vegetation is associated with other predictors of complicated course [27].

Key Learning Points

- Extracardiac manifestations are reported in 30–80% of IE patients.
- The most frequent events are embolic stroke or septic embolization to bone, spleen, or kidneys, although only some of these are symptomatic.
- The majority of embolisms take place within the first 14 days after initiation of treatment.
- The search for asymptomatic embolic events through systematic extracardiac imaging has become very important, because the detection of asymptomatic embolic events is now considered a minor Duke criterion in the 2015 ESC criteria.
- A panel of imaging modalities is used routinely to evaluate patients with extracardiac infective processes.
- CT (including the brain) has long been considered the main imaging technique for the diagnosis of embolic events in IE patients.
- MRI is a valuable alternative in case of cerebral embolism, with higher sensitivity in detecting recent ischemic lesions and small ischemic or hemorrhagic lesions, without the use of iodine contrast.
- A noticeable advantage of [^{18}F]FDG PET/CT and WBC SPECT/CT is the possibility to perform the extracardiac work-up within a single imaging procedure.
- ECHO is also useful for predicting embolic events.
- Among the several factors that have been associated with an increased risk of embolism, size and mobility of the vegetations are the most potent predictors of new embolic event in patients with IE.

9.3 Cardiovascular Implantable Electronic Devices

Implantation of cardiovascular electronic devices (CIED), such as permanent pacemakers, implantable cardioverter/defibrillator, or cardiac resynchronization therapy devices with or without defibrillators, has increased significantly over the last decade, due to growing evidence of improved quality of life and prolonged survival among certain groups of patients [71–73]. The number of devices that are implanted is estimated to exceed one million per year [74]. At least 2% of patients over the age of 65 years have a CIED. Simultaneously with the rise in device implants, the rate of infectious complications is also increasing by an estimated 5% per year [75], reaching an incidence of 1.4 per 1000 device-years [76]. This dramatic increase in the rate of device infections corresponded to an increase in the prevalence of major comorbidities, including renal failure, heart failure, respiratory failure, and diabetes mellitus in CIED recipients [77]. In addition to morbidity for patients, CIED infection has been linked to increase in-hospital mortality, by more than twofold [78, 79], and higher rates of readmission up to 3 years following device implantation [79–81]. CIED infections are estimated to cost over US $500 million per year worldwide [80, 81].

CIED infections occur via two major mechanisms. The most common is contamination of leads and/or pulse generator during implantation or subsequent manipulation [82]. Device erosion late after interventions may either be due to, or result in pocket infection. In either case, contamination and subsequent bacterial colonization result in pocket infection, which can spread along the intravascular parts of the leads and progress to systemic infection. The second mechanism is a bloodstream infection [83]. Direct lead seeding can occur during bacteremia caused by a distant infectious focus, such as a local septic thrombophlebitis, osteomyelitis, pneumonia, surgical site infection, contaminated vascular catheters or bacterial entry via the skin, mouth, gastrointestinal, or urinary tract. The patient's own skin flora can be introduced into the wound at the time of skin incision and thereby contaminate the device. Contamination may also occur before implantation via the air in the operating room (both host and staff) or via the hands of anyone handling the device. From a pathophysiological standpoint, device-related factors which favor the infections are those affecting bacterial adherence to the generator or lead, and the biofilm formation on these surfaces. Bacterial adherence is facilitated by irregular and hydrophobic surfaces [84]. Staphylococci are the main etiological agents (60–80%), and *Staphylococcus aureus* is the most common cause of bacteremia and early pocket infections. Altogether, methicillin-resistant staphylococci were isolated in 33.8%of CIED infections (49.4% of all staphylococcal infections) [85], their frequency varying by country, and even by hospital. Over the past decade, the rates of methicillin resistance seem to be greater than those reported earlier [16], while Gram-negative bacteria were isolated in 8.9%. Gram-negative bacilli represent 5–10% of the cases, and cultures are negative in another 10% of the cases. Infection from fungi or mycobacteria is rare. CIED-related infection may occur either as a surgical site infection within 1 year after implantation [86] or as late-onset leading to endocarditis [87].

Risk factors for CIED infection can be classified as patient-related, procedure-related, and device-related factors. These risk factors may be modifiable or non-modifiable. Identification of modifiable risk factors is important because they may allow for preventive measures to reduce the risk. Considering that CIED infections occur in the presence of multiple host and procedure-related factors, risk scores have been developed to identify patients at low and high risk. Scoring systems could play a role in better identifying patients at risk than individual factors, especially considering the inconsistency of the reported factors in various studies. However, despite the potential practical use of such risk scores, they are currently not recommended for clinical use because the evidence behind them remains weak.

Key Learning Points

- At least 2% of patients over the age of 65 years have a CIED.
- The rate of infectious complications is increasing by an estimated 5% per year.
- The most common pathogenetic mechanism of CIED infections is contamination of leads and/or pulse generator during implantation or subsequent manipulation.
- The second mechanism is a bloodstream infection.
- Bacterial adherence is facilitated by irregular and hydrophobic surfaces.
- Staphylococci are the main etiological agents, *Staphylococcus aureus* being the most common cause of bacteremia and early pocket infections.
- Gram-negative bacteria are isolated in 8.9% of the cases.
- CIED-related infection may occur either as a surgical site infection within 1 year after implantation or as late-onset leading to endocarditis.
- Risk factors for CIED infection are classified as patient-related, procedure-related, and device-related factors.
- Risk scores developed to identify patients at low and high risk have not yet been sufficiently validated for routine clinical use.

9.3.1 Clinical Classification and Management of CIED Infections

From a clinical perspective, it is very important to distinguish among different entities, which require different treatment management. Indeed, a superficial incisional infection should be distinguished from a pocket infection, as it involves only the skin and the subcutaneous tissue without communication with the pocket (and hence does not require extraction of the CIED system) [88, 89]. Pocket infection is defined as an infection limited to the generator pocket. It is clinically associated with local signs of inflammation that may be mild and characterized by erythema, warmth, and fluctuation [83]. Deformation of the pocket, adherence, or imminent risk of erosion are often signs of low-grade, indolent infection. Symptoms and signs of an infected surgical wound may fluctuate and although it can be difficult to recognize initially it is not recommended to take a sample of pocket material. Once a wound dehiscence occurs, a purulent drainage or a sinus is established, and a pocket infection is clearly present. If the generator or proximal leads are exposed, the device should be considered infected, irrespective of the results of microbiology. Material from the pocket may be used for culture, recognizing the potential for contamination. Pocket infections may be associated with lead infections and CIED systemic infections and/or IE.

When systemic infection and IE complicate a CIED infection without local infection, the diagnosis may be more challenging since symptoms may be nonspecific (fever, chills, night sweats), and a long period may elapse between CIED implantation and symptom onset. C-reactive protein (CRP) may be helpful although nonspecific and procalcitonin (PCT) test may be of value, especially if positive (>0.05) due to the high specificity for pocket infection compared to no infection and in case of embolic phenomena and *Staphylococcus aureus* endocarditis [92, 93]. In many cases, local and systemic symptoms coexist, but a systemic infection can also occur not associated with any local symptoms, as observed more frequently in late-onset infections. Patients with CIED infection may present with embolic involvement of the lungs and pleural space, frequently misdiagnosed as pulmonary infections [90, 91]. CIED infections may also be revealed by other distant foci, such as vertebral osteomyelitis and discitis. In a recent international cohort, 10% of 2781 episodes of IE were represented by device-related endocarditis [12]. When endocarditis is present, it is right-sided with involvement of the tricuspid valve or the mural endocardium. Although the mitral and/or aortic valves are involved only in exceptional cases, in such instance systemic embolism, stroke, congestive heart failure, and metastatic infections are more frequent and have a more severe prognosis.

The key issue for successful treatment of definite CIED infections is complete removal of all parts of the system and transvenous hardware, including the device and all leads [94, 95]. This treatment concept applies to systemic as well as localized CIED pocket infections [96]. Patients with cardiac implantable electronic device with superficial wound infections early after implantation, device exchange, or revision surgery should not undergo device and lead removal. Superficial infections are confined to the skin and the subcutaneous tissue without involvement of any parts of the CIED system. Distinguishing between a superficial and a pocket infection can be a clinical challenge. Therefore, it is important to closely watch patients who are under suspicion of having a superficial infection. In such patients, an oral antibiotic therapy (7–10 days) is reasonable [78].

Key Learning Points

- Superficial incisional infection involves only the skin and the subcutaneous tissue, without communication with the pocket.
- Superficial incisional infection does not require extraction of the CIED system.
- Pocket infection is an infection limited to the generator pocket, clinically associated with local signs of inflammation that may be mild and characterized by erythema, warmth, and fluctuation.
- Material from the pocket may be used for culture, recognizing the potential for contamination.
- Pocket infections may be associated with lead infections and CIED systemic infections and/or IE.
- When systemic infection and IE complicates a CIED infection without local infection, the diagnosis may be more challenging.
- Patients with CIED infection may present with embolic involvement of the lungs and pleural space, vertebral osteomyelitis, and discitis.
- Serum CRP is helpful, although nonspecific, and the PCT test may be of value, especially if positive.
- When endocarditis is present, it is right-sided with involvement of the tricuspid valve or the mural endocardium.
- The mitral and/or aortic valves are involved only in exceptional cases.
- The key issue for successful treatment of definite CIED infections is complete removal of all parts of the system and transvenous hardware, including the device and all leads.
- This treatment concept applies to systemic as well as to localized CIED pocket infections.

9.3.2 Diagnosis of CIED Infections

There is no standardized diagnostic tool for CIED endocarditis. The modified Duke criteria [26] and the ESC 2015 criteria [27] have generally been employed for the diagnosis. However, none represents a validated and standardized tool for diagnosis in this specific setting. Very recently, additional criteria merging of the modified Duke criteria with the ESC 2015 criteria, known as the 2019 International CIED Infection Criteria, have been established [97] (Fig. 9.2).

9.3.3 Microbiology of CIED Infections

Identification of the microorganisms causing a CIED infection is pivotal for effective antibiotic therapy. Therefore, every effort should be made to obtain cultures prior to the starting antibiotic therapy. Blood cultures should be repeated in patients with CIED and fever without clear signs of local infections and IE. Every positive blood culture should be carefully evaluated and prompt active exclusion of CIED infection with other diagnostic techniques [97]. In case of negative blood cultures, increased incubation time (10–14 days) and the use of biomolecular methods (DNA amplification and/or gene sequencing) to detect fastidious or atypical pathogens [98] may be considered. Swabs collected from the chronic draining sinus or fistula for culture are discouraged, whereas tissue or fluid collected from the pocket via an adjacent intact portion of the skin (via a sterile needle or syringe) is encouraged in order to avoid passing through the sinus to identify the bacterial strain. During a CIED extraction procedure, distal and proximal lead fragments, lead vegetation (if present), and generator pocket tissue should be sent for culture.

9.3.4 Imaging of CIED Infections

ECHO should be the first-line imaging tool to assess patients with CIED, in order to identify lead vegetations and valvular involvement [27]. TTE and TEE are both recommended in case of suspected CIED infections. While TTE better defines pericardial effusion, ventricular dysfunction, and pulmonary vascular pressure, TEE is superior for the detection and sizing of vegetations [63], especially in the right atrium-superior vena cava area and in regions less well visualized by TTE. In the absence of typical vegetations of measurable size, both TTE and TEE may be false negative in CIED-related IE. Lead masses in asymptomatic CIED carriers may be observed on TTE/TEE and do not predict CIED-related IE over long-term follow-up [99, 100]. Therefore, once a lead mass is identified, careful clinical assessment to rule out

Fig. 9.2 - Recommendations for the diagnosis of CIED infections and/or IE: the Novel 2019 International CIED Infection Criteria, obtained merging the modified Duke, the ESC 2015 Guidelines criteria, and adding specific points for to CIED-related infection criteria (in green). *CIED* cardiac implantable electronic device, *CT* computerized tomography, *E* expert opinion, *ICE* intracardiac echocardiography, *IE*, *M* meta-analysis, *O* observational studies, *R* randomized trials, *SPECT* single-photon emission tomography, *WBC* white blood cells [modified from ref. 97]

Consensus statement	Statement class	Scientific evidence coding
TTE is recommended as the first-line imaging modality in patients with suspected CIED-related IE	♥	O
A chest X-ray should be performed in all patients with suspected CIED infection	♥	E
TEE is recommended in suspected CIED infection with positive or negative blood cultures, independent of TTE results before an extraction, to evaluate CIED infection and IE	♥	O
Repeat TTE and/or TEE within 5–7 days is recommended in case of initially negative examination when clinical suspicion of CIED-related IE remains high	♥	O
TEE should be performed in CIED patients with *S. aureus* bacteraemia	♥	O
ICE may be considered if suspected CIED-related IE, with positive blood cultures and negative TTE and TEE results	♡	O, E
[^{18}F]FDG PET/CT scanning or radiolabelled WBC scintigraphy or contrast enhanced CT are recommended if suspected CIED-related IE, positive blood cultures, and negative echocardiography (attention in imaging interpretation early after device implant)	♥	O, M
[^{18}F]FDG PET/CT should be performed in case of *S. aureus* bacteremia in CIED patients	♥	O, E
[^{18}F]FDG PET/CT, radiolabelled WBC scintigraphy and/or contrast enhanced CT is recommended for identification of unexpected embolic localizations (i.e. lung embolism) and metastatic infections	♥	O, M
The identification of the infection portal of entry may be considered by [^{18}F]FDG PET/CT and WBC imaging in order to prevent IE relapse	♡	O, E
Pulmonary CT angiography is recommended in patients with recurrent pneumonia	♥	O, E
In patients with CIED infection treated with percutaneous lead extraction, TTE/TEE before hospital discharge are recommended to detect presence of retained segments of pacemaker lead, and to assess tricuspid valve function, RV function, and pulmonary hypertension	♥	O
In case of persistent sepsis after device extraction: - TEE is recommended to identify residual insulation material and local complications - [^{18}F]FDG PET/CT, radiolabelled WBC scintigraphy and/or contrast enhanced CT for better assessment of local extension of the infection and whole body assessment	♥	O, M
A multidisciplinary team (the Endocarditis Team) is recommended for evaluation of imaging results	♥	E

either infection or non-bacterial lead-thrombotic endocarditis is needed, including serial TTE/TEE or additional imaging tests.

Intracardiac echocardiography (ICE) is effective and has high sensitivity for the detection of vegetations in cardiac devices [101, 102]. Therefore, a vegetation seen with ICE may be considered a major criterion for diagnosis. Recently, transvenous biopsy, guided by TEE, has been shown to be useful to distinguish vegetation from thrombus [103].

In patients with CIED infections treated with percutaneous lead extraction, a TTE before hospital discharge is recommended to detect retained segments of the pacemaker lead and to assess tricuspid valve function, right ventricular function, and pulmonary hypertension. A TEE (and additional imaging tests) should be considered after percutaneous lead extraction, in order to detect infected material, ghosts [104], and potential tricuspid valve complications, particularly in patients with persistent sepsis after extraction. It is important to consider that a normal ECHO does not rule out CIED-related IE.

Some radiographic and CT findings (i.e., presence of fluid density between the heart and the device) [105] may suggest the presence of infection; however, these findings can be observed also in the postoperative or inflammatory changes that are noninfectious. Furthermore, the absence of crumpling of patches in plain X-ray or fluid around the heart in the CT scan does not exclude the possibility of underlying infection at these sites.

Different nuclear medicine imaging techniques have been employed to evaluate patients with suspected or ascertained CIED infection. In particular ^{67}Ga-citrate scintigraphy has been successfully employed in a small series of patients with CIED infection [106]. The role of scintigraphy with ^{111}In-oxine-leukocytes or ^{99m}Tc-HMPAO-leukocytes has also been tested in this clinical setting, demonstrating that this technique helps in some cases to define the presence of CIED infection and to evaluate its extent [107, 108], Additionally ^{99m}Tc-HMPAO-leukocyte SPECT/CT allows the detection of additional unsuspected extracardiac sites of infection in up to 23% of patients with device-related sepsis [109], although with some limitations in the case of small CNS embolism. Similar results have been published in one case of lead-associated infection using SPECT/CT with ^{99m}Tc-sulesomab [110].

[^{18}F]FDG PET/CT is also promising for identifying CIED infections [111], particularly when the examination is performed to rule out device involvement during infection [112] and to define the embolic burden [111, 113–115]. Recently, the performance of [^{18}F]FDG PET/CT in CIED infections has been reported to improve when adopting ad hoc developed diagnostic criteria [116]. Similarly to what has been described for PVE, WBC SPECT/CT and [^{18}F]FDG PET/CT can be used to confirm or exclude infection and to characterize the extension of the infectious process, including extracardiac work-up. The value of [^{18}F]FDG PET/CT in the diagnosis of CIED infection is confirmed by a large body of literature. The diagnosis of local infections is quite straightforward. A recent meta-analysis provides a pooled specificity and sensitivity in this subgroup of 93% (95% CI, 84–98%) and 98% (95% CI, 88–100%), respectively, and the area under the ROC curve was 0.98 for [^{18}F]FDG PET/CT [117, 118]. The largest study with labeled leukocyte scintigraphy ($n = 63$) reported a sensitivity of 94% and a specificity of 100% [89]. Using these imaging modalities, it is possible to distinguish between superficial and deep pocket infection, which necessitates removal of the generator rather than a medical treatment. Non-attenuation corrected images should be used for final interpretation of the images. Semi-quantitative parameters such as semi-quantitative ratio of maximum count rate of the pocket device over mean count rate of lung parenchyma [116] or normalization of SUV_{max} around the CIEDs to the mean hepatic blood pool ratio activity [119] might help in differentiated mild postoperative residual inflammation up to 2 months after device implantation versus infection. The diagnostic accuracy for lead infections is lower, with overall pooled sensitivity of 65% (95% CI, 53–76%), specificity of 88% (95% CI, 77–94%), and AUC of 0.861 [117]. Such a finding is mainly related to the small size of the vegetations along the leads, which are often under the spatial resolution of the system [111]. The [^{18}F]FDG PET/CT and WBC scintigraphy findings associated with Duke criteria also allowed reclassifying most of cases initially classified as "possible" IE [51], distinguishing infection limited to the pocket or leads from a more severe infection affecting the whole device [120], and identifying patients requiring device extraction [121].

In addition, also in the case of CIED infections, accurate evaluation of the whole-body imaging might detect septic embolisms and identify the possible infection portal of entry, impacting on the subsequent therapeutic management and reducing the risk of relapse [122]. Indeed, in CIED infection, the detection of lung embolism, considered as a major criterion of the Duke score, has shown to increase the diagnostic sensitivity [91].

Therefore, both imaging approaches, WBC SPECT/CT and [^{18}F]FDG PET/CT, can be suggested in patients with CIED infections as a guide to clinicians for choosing the most suitable treatment, i.e., conservative treatment (ESC class IIb recommendations) [27]. PET/CT imaging may also contribute to assess the mortality risk stratification after lead extraction. Patients with definite CIED infection without pocket involvement on [^{18}F]FDG PET/CT had unfavorable outcome, suggesting that the presence of an endovascular infection stemming from an unrecognized/distant site is associated with poor prognosis [123].

Contrast-enhanced CT combined with PET may prove useful in selected patients. The addition of contrast-enhanced CT to the standard [^{18}F]FDG PET/CT protocol resulted in a high rate of reclassifications from "possible" to "definite" IE, improving the overall diagnostic accuracy with or without the Duke criteria in a series of patients with suspected pulmonary embolism or CIED infections [51]. Cardiac CT angiography may also add important information on remote vascular complications, including mycotic aneurysm, arterial emboli, and septic pulmonary infarcts, which add to the diagnostic criteria and affect the overall treatment strategy. In addition, pulmonary CT angiography may be useful in patients with recurrent pneumonia [124]. A wider use of contrast-enhanced CT is limited by the deleterious impact of contrast agents on kidney function, particularly as the patients are exposed to nephrotoxic antibiotic therapy. An extensive description of the technical aspects and the interpretation criteria for multimodality imaging has recently been published [31].

Multidisciplinary team (the endocarditis team) evaluations of imaging results are recommended and have been

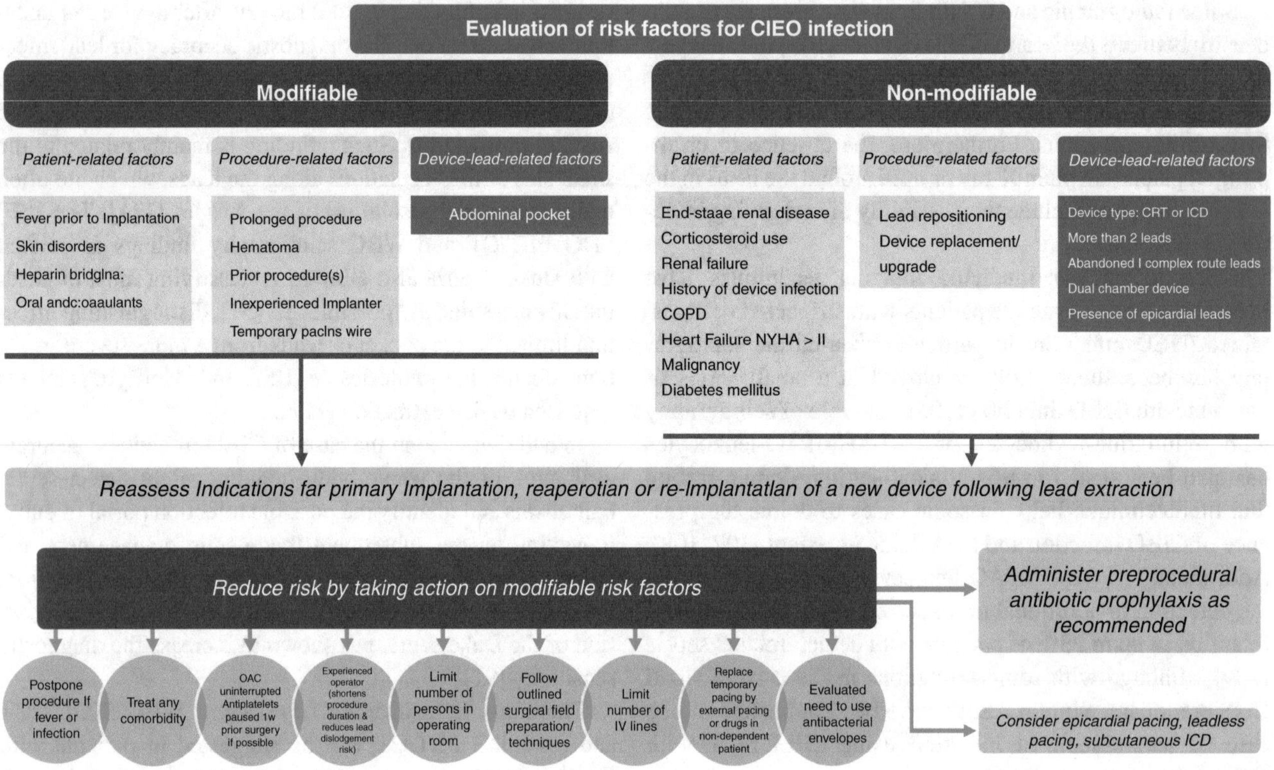

Fig. 9.3 Recommendations for the diagnosis of CIED-related infections based on imaging, developed by the European Heart Rhythm Association in consensus with other scientific societies. *IE*, *TTE*, *TOE*, *ICE* intracardiac echocardiography, *RV* right ventricular, *E* expert opinion, *M* meta-analysis, *O* observational studies, *R* randomized trials, green heart = recommended/indicated or "should do this"; yellow heart = May be used or recommended [reproduced with permission from ref. 97]

shown to significantly reduce the 1-year mortality from 18.5% to 8.2% [98]. Figure 9.3 shows the proposed diagnostic flowchart for the use of imaging in patients with suspected CIED infection.

Key Learning Points

- There is no standardized diagnostic tool for CIED-related endocarditis.
- The 2019 International CIED Infection Criteria have been recently proposed.
- Identification of the microorganisms causing a CIED infection is pivotal for effective antibiotic therapy.
- Blood cultures should be repeated in patients with CIED and fever without clear signs of local infections and IE.
- Every positive blood culture should be carefully evaluated and prompt active exclusion of CIED infection with other diagnostic techniques.
- Fastidious or atypical pathogens should also be considered.
- Swabs collected from the chronic draining sinus or fistula for culture are discouraged.
- Tissue or fluid collected from the pocket via an adjacent intact portion of the skin (via a sterile needle or syringe) is encouraged.
- During an extraction procedure, distal and proximal lead fragments, lead vegetation (if present), and generator pocket tissue should be sent for culture.
- ECHO should be the first imaging tool in the assessment of patients with CIED, in order to identify lead vegetations and valvular involvement.
- TTE and TEE are both recommended in case of suspected CIED-related infections.
- Lead masses in asymptomatic CIED carriers observed on TTE/TEE do not predict CIED-related IE over long-term follow-up.
- ICE is effective and highly sensitive for the detection of vegetations in cardiac devices.
- Any vegetation seen with ICE can be considered a major diagnostic criterion.

- In patients with CIED infections treated with percutaneous lead extraction, a TTE before hospital discharge is recommended.
- A TEE (and additional imaging tests) should be considered after percutaneous lead extraction, in order to detect infected material, ghosts, and potential tricuspid valve complications, particularly in patients with persistent sepsis after extraction.
- A normal echocardiography does not rule out CIED-related IE.
- Some radiographic and CT findings may suggest the presence of infection.
- Scintigraphy with ^{111}In-oxine-leukocytes or ^{99m}Tc-HMPAO-leukocytes has been tested to detect CIED-related infection.
- ^{99m}Tc-HMPAO-leukocyte SPECT/CT allows the detection of additional unsuspected extracardiac sites of infection in up to 23% of patients.
- The diagnostic performance of [^{18}F]FDG PET/CT in CIED infections has been reported to improve when adopting ad hoc developed diagnostic criteria.
- [^{18}F]FDG PET/CT might be used to confirm/exclude infection and characterize the extension of the infectious process, including extracardiac work-up.
- [^{18}F]FDG PET/CT has 93% specificity (95% CI, 84–98%) and 98% sensitivity (95% CI, 88–100%) for the diagnosis of local infections.
- The largest study with WBC scintigraphy reported 94% sensitivity and 100% specificity.
- Semi-quantitative parameters might help in distinguishing mild postoperative residual inflammation up to 2 months after device implantation versus infection.
- The diagnostic accuracy for lead infections is lower, with overall pooled sensitivity of 65% and specificity of 88%.
- [^{18}F]FDG PET/CT and WBC scan findings in association with Duke criteria also allowed reclassifying most of cases initially classified as "possible" IE, thus identifying patients requiring device extraction.
- Accurate evaluation of the whole body imaging can detect septic embolisms and identify possible infection portal of entry, impacting on the subsequent therapeutic management and reducing the risk of relapse.
- PET/CTA resulted in a high rate of reclassifications from "possible" to "definite" IE, thus improving the overall diagnostic accuracy.
- Cardiac CT angiography may also add important information on distant vascular complications including mycotic aneurysm, arterial emboli, and septic pulmonary infarcts.
- Pulmonary CT angiography may be useful in patients with recurrent pneumonia.
- A wider use of contrast-enhanced CT is limited by the deleterious impact of contrast agents on kidney function particularly as the patients are exposed to nephrotoxic antibiotic therapy.
- Multidisciplinary team (the endocarditis team) evaluations of imaging results are recommended and have been shown to significantly reduce the 1-year mortality.

9.4 Infections Associated with Left Ventricular Assist Devices

Implantable left ventricular assist devices (LVAD) constitute a major medical advance for end-stage heart failure in selected patients [125]. This treatment is currently used as a bridge-to-transplantation, a bridge-to-recovery, or as destination therapy as the last resort in patients with neither perspectives of recovery, nor of heart transplant. Implantable LVAD intended for long-term use rely on a percutaneous driveline, to carry electric signals and energy from the controller and batteries to the implanted pump. As with any other implantable foreign device, it is subject to LVAD-related infections. The presence of a driveline piercing the skin places the patient at continual risk of infection that can affect the exit site, the subcutaneous tunnel, the abdominal pocket (if present), and the implanted pump and that can disseminate through bloodstream infection. The transition from pulsatile to continuous-flow LVAD significantly improved the clinical outcome [126] and decreased the risk of infectious complications. Nonetheless, LVAD-related infections are still common with a prevalence that ranges from 23% to 58%, being associated with a high mortality rate (15–44%) [109]. The major sites of infection include the mediastinum drivelines and the device surface, identified as LVAD endocarditis [127]. The major pathogens involved in these emerging foreign device-related infectious diseases are—as it could be expected—the "big five": *Staphylococcus aureus*, Enterobacteriaceae, *Pseudomonas aeruginosa*, coagulase-negative Staphylococci, and *Corynebacterium sporigenous* [128]. The management of LVAD infections, due to the few data currently available in literature and the lack of specific guidelines, is poorly standardized and is mainly derived from the available recommendation of other CIEDs infections, prosthetic valves, or vascular prosthesis, although their characteristics differ significantly. The only available specific recommendation to assist therapeutic decisions (i.e., the use of antimicrobial treatment and surgery) in this challenging context, is based on observational studies and expert opinion [129].

9.4.1 Diagnostic Work-Up of Infections Associated with Left Ventricular Assist Devices

The use of CT as main diagnostic imaging in these patients relies on the possibility to detect the presence of edema as primary sign of infection, a finding that is often nonspecific. The usefulness of WBC SPECT/CT and [^{18}F]FDG PET/CT for the diagnosis of LVAD-related infection has been shown in small patient groups under routine clinical conditions. Molecular imaging allows precise anatomic localization and accurate assessment of the extent of a suspected infection [109], with 100% sensitivity and 94% specificity for [^{18}F]FDG PET/CT [130]. The use of the metabolic volume has recently been reported to be associated with increased diagnostic accuracy as compared to the SUV_{max} in a series of 48 patients. In particular, the NPV and sensitivity increased up to >95% by using the metabolic volume compared to 87.5% when using SUV_{max} [131].

Key Learning Points

- LVAD represents a major medical advance for end-stage heart failure in selected patients.
- LVAD-related infections are common, with a prevalence that ranges from 23% to 58%, being associated with a high mortality rate (15–44%).
- The major sites of infection include the mediastinum drivelines and device surface, identified as LVAD endocarditis.
- The major pathogens involved are *Staphylococcus aureus*, Enterobacteriaceae, *Pseudomonas aeruginosa*, coagulase-negative Staphylococci, and *Corynebacterium sporigenous*.
- The use of CT as main diagnostic imaging in these patients relies on the possibility to detect the presence of edema as primary sign of infection, a finding that is often nonspecific.
- The usefulness of WBS SPECT/CT and [^{18}F]FDG PET/CT for the diagnosis of LVAD-related infection has been shown in small patient groups under routine clinical conditions.
- Molecular imaging allows precise anatomic localization and accurate assessment of the extent of a suspected infection, with 100% sensitivity and 94% specificity for [^{18}F]FDG PET/CT.
- NPV and sensitivity increased up to >95% by using the metabolic volume, compared to 87.5% when using SUV_{max}.

9.5 Technical Considerations on Patient Preparation, Radiopharmaceutical Preparation, Acquisition Protocols, Post-acquisition Image Processing, and Image Reading/Interpretation

9.5.1 Labeled Leukocyte SPECT/CT

9.5.1.1 Patient Preparation

In case of cardiovascular infection, the procedure for labeled leukocyte scintigraphy is very similar to the one used for any other infection. No specific patient preparation is required, besides the standard preparation for WBC imaging. The general rules for the radiolabeling of WBC preparation are also applied. An important aspect of WBC imaging in cardiovascular infections is the image acquisition protocol that should include planar acquisitions at 30 min (early images), at 4–6 h (delayed images), and at 20–24 h (late images) after reinjection of the radiolabeled leukocytes (most frequently ^{99m}Tc-HMPAO-WBC in the current clinical practice) with a mandatory SPECT/CT acquisition as part of the standard imaging protocol. The importance of including a SPECT/CT acquisition is due to the failure of planar imaging alone to detect the site and the extension of infections in the cardiovascular system [30, 31]. Therefore, in this scenario, SPECT/CT images are used not only to confirm and localize findings at planar images consistent with infection (area or increased accumulation intensity or size over time) but also to increase the diagnostic accuracy. If semi-quantitative evaluation of WBC is used for the diagnosis, it is very important that both planar and SPECT/CT images are always acquired with a "time-corrected for isotope decay" modality. SPECT/CT images should cover the thorax in case of IE and the thorax-upper abdominal area in case of CIEDs and LVAD infections, ensuring that all components of the device are included in the field of view, considering all the possible generator positions (i.e., abdomen).

When interpreting WBC imaging, some important issues should be taken into consideration. Rarely, false-positive findings have been described for WBC imaging in IE and CIED infections, even in case of very early infections. On the other hand, false-negative scans have been observed in the presence of IE caused by some specific strains [30]. The same limitation must always be considered in case of CIED infections, in particular the presence of very small vegetation(s) along the electrocatheter. Embolisms at WBC imaging might appear either as area of increased uptake over time in the brain, lung and soft tissue or as cold spot when spleen embolism and spondylodiscitis occur. This latter appearance must be considered nonspecific for infectious embolisms, since it might be present in other benign or malignant conditions, such as in the case of vertebral crush or metastasis. Therefore, although these findings in patients with IE are highly suggestive for septic embolism, they should be confirmed by additional diagnostic imaging tests. Due to the limited spatial resolution, reduced sensitivity has been described in case of small embolism [132].

Key Learning Points

- In case of CVS infection, the WBC scan procedure is very similar to the one used for any other infection.
- No specific patient preparation is required besides the standard preparation for a WBC scan.
- The image acquisition protocol must include a SPECT/CT acquisition as part of the standard imaging protocol.
- SPECT/CT images are used not only to confirm and localize findings at planar images consistent with infection (area or increased accumulation intensity or size over time) but also to increase the diagnostic accuracy.
- False-positive findings have rarely been described for WBC imaging in IE and CIED infections, even in case of very early infections.
- False-negative scans have been observed for IE caused by some specific strains, in the presence of very small vegetation(s) along the electrocatheter.
- Embolisms at WBC imaging might appear either as area of increased uptake over time in the brain, lung, and soft tissue or as cold spot when spleen embolism and spondylodiscitis occur.
- Although these findings in patients with IE are highly suggestive for septic embolism, they should be confirmed by additional diagnostic imaging tests.
- Due to the limited spatial resolution, reduced sensitivity has been described in case of small embolism.

9.5.2 [^{18}F]FDG PET/CT

Performing an [^{18}F]FDG PET/CT for cardiovascular infections is more complex than a simple translation of the standard protocol used in oncology. Starting from patient's preparation, some specific aspects of the imaging protocol and imaging reading should be considered. An extensive review of the main critical technical issues is provided in the "Recommendation on nuclear and multi-modality imaging in IE and CIED Infections" released by the EANM [31]. Briefly, we will discuss here some crucial points for a correct imaging procedure.

Patient preparation is very important to reduce the physiological uptake of [^{18}F]FDG in the myocardium. This can be achieved by the application of a proper fat-enriched, low-carbohydrate diet followed by fasting. Additionally, intravenous heparin approximately 15 min prior to [^{18}F]FDG injection can be used [133]. There is a general agreement that high-fat, low-carbohydrate diet for at least two meals with a fast of at least 4 h is the minimum to obtain a suppression of physiologic myocardial utilization of glucose. Since there is no evidence demonstrating that a specific patient preparation technique is superior to another, each institution should continuously evaluate its image quality data to ensure that more than 80% of the scans achieve adequate suppression of physiological [^{18}F]FDG myocardial uptake. Efforts should be made to decrease blood glucose to the lowest possible level, although hyperglycemia does not represent an absolute contraindication for performing the study [134]. Indeed, in case of infection and inflammation neither diabetes nor hyperglycemia at the time of the study has been demonstrated to increase the PET/CT false-negative rate [135].

The [^{18}F]FDG activity recommended in the joint EANM/SNMMI guidelines on PET imaging in inflammation/infection is 2.5–5.0 MBq/kg (175–350 MBq in a 70 kg standard adult) [134]. Although antimicrobial treatment is expected to decrease the intensity of [^{18}F]FDG uptake [136], there is no evidence at this stage to routinely recommend treatment discontinuation before performing PET/CT. On the contrary, corticosteroid treatment should be discontinued or at least reduced to the lowest possible dosage in the 24 h preceding the examination [137].

Image acquisition generally starts after an uptake time of 45–60 min, the emission time/bed position depending on sensitivity of the scanner. The field of acquisition, as in oncology, generally includes from skull base to mid thighs (total body). Whole body images including the lower limbs are suggested to detect complications of IE, such as mycotic aneurysms that may require specific treatment by embolization to prevent rupture [138]. An additional separate bed position on the cardiac region is useful to record gated images. Diagnostic angio-CT (CTA) scan might also be performed, to maximize the diagnostic information provided by the examination. Although delayed imaging has been proposed to increase specificity in diagnosing infection of cardiovascular implants [139, 140], recent data suggest that in IE delayed images are more prone to false-positive results

[141]. Also in case of [^{18}F]FDG PET/CT, image reconstruction with and without attenuation correction is recommended to identify potential reconstruction artifacts. Metal artifact reduction techniques are useful to minimize overcorrection, even if they do not always recover completely PET image quality.

Metabolic activity is evaluated both qualitatively and quantitatively. A focal or heterogeneous [^{18}F]FDG uptake distribution on visual assessment generally correlates with an infectious process. The intensity of [^{18}F]FDG uptake can be measured as the maximum standardized uptake value (SUV_{max}) in the abnormal area. To overcome bias related to individual differences in [^{18}F]FDG metabolism, the ratio of the prosthetic material SUV_{max} to the mean SUV of the blood pool or the liver (SUV_{ratio} or target-to-background ratio) can be used [119]. Quantitative assessment supports visual information, but as there are many factors that may affect measurements, the values obtained should be considered only a guide and not conclusive data [31, 142].

Recent data suggest that quantification of [^{18}F]FDG uptake around prosthetic valves using a cut-off of ≥2.0 as SUV_{ratio} has a very high predictive value for PVE (100% sensitivity, 91% specificity) after proper standardization of the scanner (European Association of Nuclear Medicine Research Ltd. (EARL), accreditation program) [143]. If SUV is used, all the factors affecting its quantification should be carefully considered, including those related to patient preparation (glycaemia, concurrent treatment, etc.), time of uptake, and the use of radiological contrast.

Several physiological variants and pathological conditions that enter in the differential diagnosis with IE/CIED infection should be recognized to prevent misinterpretation of a positive scan. Therefore, specific training in the field should be always undertaken before implementing the technique in a new center on a daily basis.

A physiological variant that might represent a confounding factor while reading the images is the presence of increased metabolic activity along the posterior part of the heart, where lipomatous hypertrophy of the interatrial septum may appear as a fat-containing mass with increased [^{18}F]FDG uptake [144]. One of the major findings that should be recognized is the presence of faint and homogeneous [^{18}F]FDG uptake strictly limited to the valve annulus, very similar to the pattern observed in prosthetic vascular graft [145]. This pattern of uptake around the prosthetic valve is frequently visible and may have different causes, particularly early after surgery. It most likely results from the persistent host reaction against the biomaterial coating the sewing ring of prosthetic valve. A recent experience by Pizzi et al. suggests that the metabolic and anatomic patterns might help distinguishing between inflammation and infection in these patients [146]. In particular, a postoperative inflammatory response may result in nonspecific [^{18}F]FDG uptake in the immediate postoperative period [147]. In this regard, it is important to consider the prior use of surgical adhesives during PV implantation. In this regard, PET/CT is not recommended by guidelines until 3 months after surgery. However, Mathieu et al. have recently showed that the mean amount of [^{18}F]FDG uptake was not significantly different between patients scanned within 3 months [148]. This has been confirmed in a recent multicenter study on a large cohort of patients, where recent valve implantation was not a significant predictor of false-positive interpretation [143].

Focally increased [^{18}F]FDG uptake can be observed in many other conditions such as active thrombi [149], soft atherosclerotic plaques [150], vasculitis [151], primary cardiac tumors [152], cardiac metastasis [59], post-surgical inflammation [62], and foreign body reactions (such as BioGlue, a surgical adhesive used to repair the aortic root) [60], stitches [61], and in case of Libman–Sacks endocarditis [62]. Therefore, it is necessary to adopt accurate patient's selection and inclusion criteria as well as accurate imaging reading to maintain a high specificity for IE using [^{18}F]FDG. As already discussed, antimicrobial therapy and/or vegetation size could account for false-negative results on [^{18}F]FDG PET/CT.

Key Learning Points

- Performing [^{18}F]FDG PET/CT for cardiovascular infections is more complex than a simple translation of the standard protocol used in oncology.
- A high-fat, low-carbohydrate diet for at least two meals and fasting of at least 4 h is the minimum condition to suppress physiologic myocardial glucose utilization.
- IV heparin approximately 15 min prior to [^{18}F]FDG injection can be used.
- Blood glucose should be the lowest possible, although hyperglycemia does not constitute an absolute contraindication to the study.
- Although antimicrobial treatment is expected to decrease the intensity of [^{18}F]FDG uptake, there is no evidence to routinely recommend treatment discontinuation before performing PET/CT.
- Corticosteroid treatment should be discontinued, or at least reduced to the lowest possible dosage in the 24 h preceding the examination.
- The field of acquisition, as in oncology, generally includes from skull base to mid thighs (total body).

- Whole-body images including the lower limbs is suggested to detect complications of IE such as mycotic aneurysms that may require specific treatment by embolization to prevent rupture.
- A CTA scan might also be performed, to maximize the diagnostic information provided by the examination.
- Metabolic activity is evaluated both qualitatively and quantitatively.
- A focal or heterogeneous [^{18}F]FDG uptake distribution on visual assessment generally correlates with an infectious process.
- Quantitative assessment supports visual information, but there are many factors that may affect measurements.
- If SUV is used, all the factors affecting it should be carefully considered, including those related to patient preparation, time of uptake, and the use of contrast.
- Several physiological variants and pathological conditions that enter in the differential diagnosis with IE/CIED infection should be recognized to prevent misinterpretation of a positive scan.
- Faint and homogeneous [^{18}F]FDG uptake strictly limited to the valve annulus is frequently visible and may have different causes, particularly early after surgery.
- Metabolic and anatomic patterns help distinguishing between inflammation and infection in these patients.
- Causes of false-positive [^{18}F]FDG findings should be ruled out.

Clinical Cases

Case 9.1

Background

A 52-year-old man was hospitalized for deep vein thrombosis of the right lower limb presenting as acute compartment syndrome, and underwent emergency fasciotomy. This treatment failed, and right limb amputation had to be subsequently performed. About 3 years prior to this acute episode, the patient had been submitted to the replacement of the aortic valve and ascending aorta. After the amputation, he experienced raise of C-reactive protein (CRP) and fibrinogen (10.4 mg/dL and 648 mg/dL, respectively); pro-calcitonin was in the normal range, and blood cultures were negative. TTE did not show any abnormality. Despite negativity of blood cultures and TTE, empiric antimicrobial treatment was started based on the high clinical suspicious of infection, and TEE was planned, which showed mild aortic valve regurgitation. Since the patient presented one major and one minor criteria, he was classified as possible IE with persisting high suspicious of infection; as recommended by the latest ESC 2015 Guidelines, he was therefore referred for molecular imaging. [^{18}F]FDG PET/CT (Fig. 9.4) confirmed the suspicious of IE, showing high tracer uptake on the prosthetic aortic valve. Empiric antimicrobial treatment was continued and after 2 months, when both CRP and fibrinogen were in the normal range, he underwent a follow-up [^{18}F]FDG PET/CT scan (Fig. 9.5) during therapy. The 2-month follow-up scan confirmed the presence of prosthetic valve endocarditis and showed additional infection involving soft tissues of the right amputation stump.

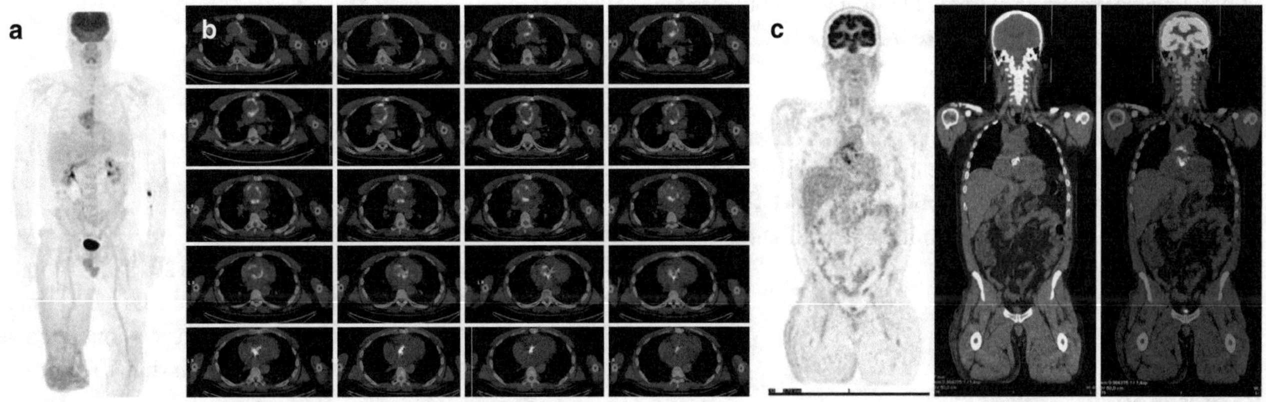

Fig. 9.4 [^{18}F]FDG PET/CT in a patient with prosthetic valve endocarditis. The MIP image (**a**) shows increased [^{18}F]FDG uptake in the mediastinum and at the right amputation stump. (**b**) Transaxial fused PET/CT sections. (**c**) Coronal sections (PET left; CT middle; fused PET/CT right). Intense [^{18}F]FDG uptake at the prosthetic valve is clearly detectable indicating IE. The moderate and diffuse tracer uptake at the right amputation stump suggests post-surgical inflammation

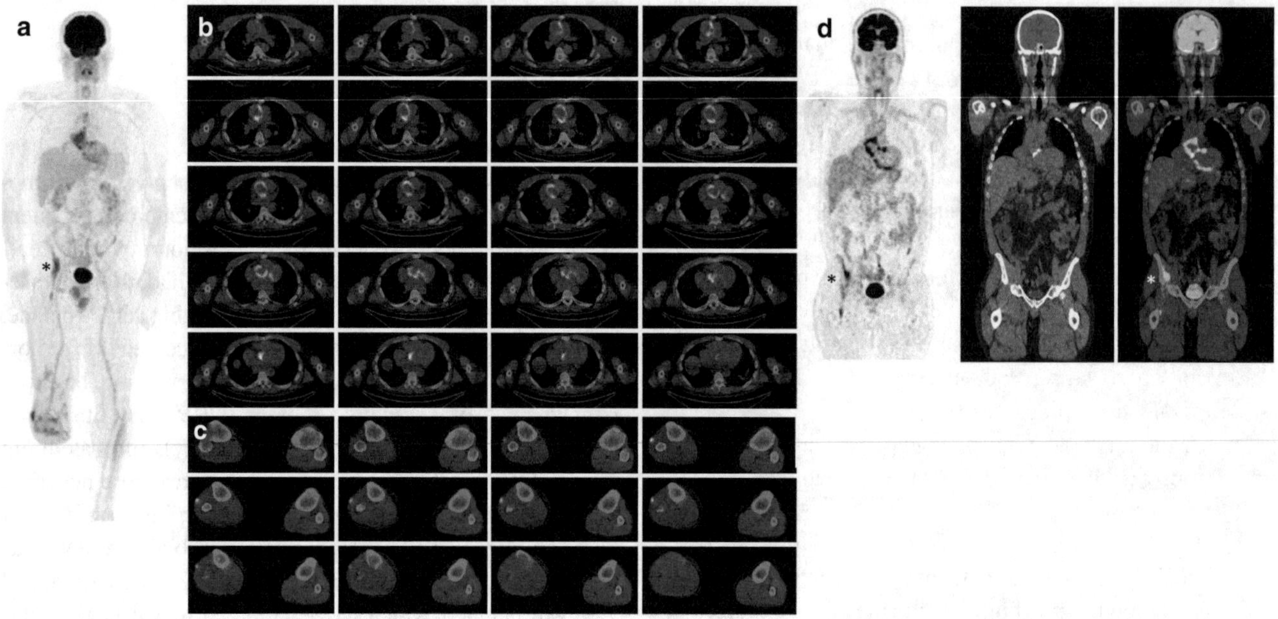

Fig. 9.5 Follow-up [^{18}F]FDG PET/CT scan in the same patient as in Fig. 9.4, with prosthetic valve endocarditis and infection of amputation stump. (**a**) The MIP image shows increased [^{18}F]FDG uptake in the mediastinum and in the lateral side of the right amputation stump. The transaxial fused PET/CT (**b**) and coronal (**c**) images (PET, left; CT, middle; fused, right) confirm intense [^{18}F]FDG uptake at the prosthetic valve, almost unchanged from the previous examination. The focal area of increased [^{18}F]FDG uptake in the lateral side of the right amputation stump suggests spread of infection to the soft tissues of the knee, as shown by axial fused images (**d**). The moderately increased tracer uptake at the right groin (indicated by "asterisk") is related to muscular uptake

Suspected Site of Infection
PVIE.

Radiopharmaceutical Activity
[^{18}F]FDG, 295 MBq.

Imaging
The acquisition included scout view (120 kV, 10 mA), whole-body CT scan (140 kV, 80 mA), and PET (3D, 3 min/FOV). Images were reconstructed with and without attenuation correction using the low-dose transmission CT scan.

Conclusion/Teaching Point
[^{18}F]FDG PET/CT identified the presence of IE, was helpful to monitor response to treatment, and identified an additional, unexpected site of infection. [^{18}F]FDG PET/CT is highly sensitive also during antimicrobial treatment.

Case 9.2

Background
A 60-year-old obese woman with aortic valve prosthesis went to the emergency department for chest pain and fever. IE was suspected due to the presence of fever associated to relevant cardiac risk factors (prosthetic valve). Blood cultures were positive for *Staphylococcus epidermidis*. TEE showed a doubtful image on the prosthetic valve, suspected for IE but inconclusive. [^{18}F]FDG PET/CT (Fig. 9.6) showed an area of focal tracer uptake at the aortic valve prosthesis, and a large lesion in the spleen characterized by a "hot" rim surrounding a "cold" core. Overall, these findings were suggestive for prosthetic valve endocarditis with splenic septic embolism.

Suspected Site of Infection
Prosthetic valve endocarditis.

Radiopharmaceutical Activity
[^{18}F]FDG, 347 MBq.

Imaging
The acquisition included scout view (120 kV, 10 mA), whole-body CT scan (140 kV, 80 mA), and PET (3D, 3 min/FOV). Images were reconstructed with and without attenuation correction using the low-dose transmission CT scan.

Conclusion/Teaching Point
[^{18}F]FDG PET/CT identified the presence of IE with associated splenic septic embolism.

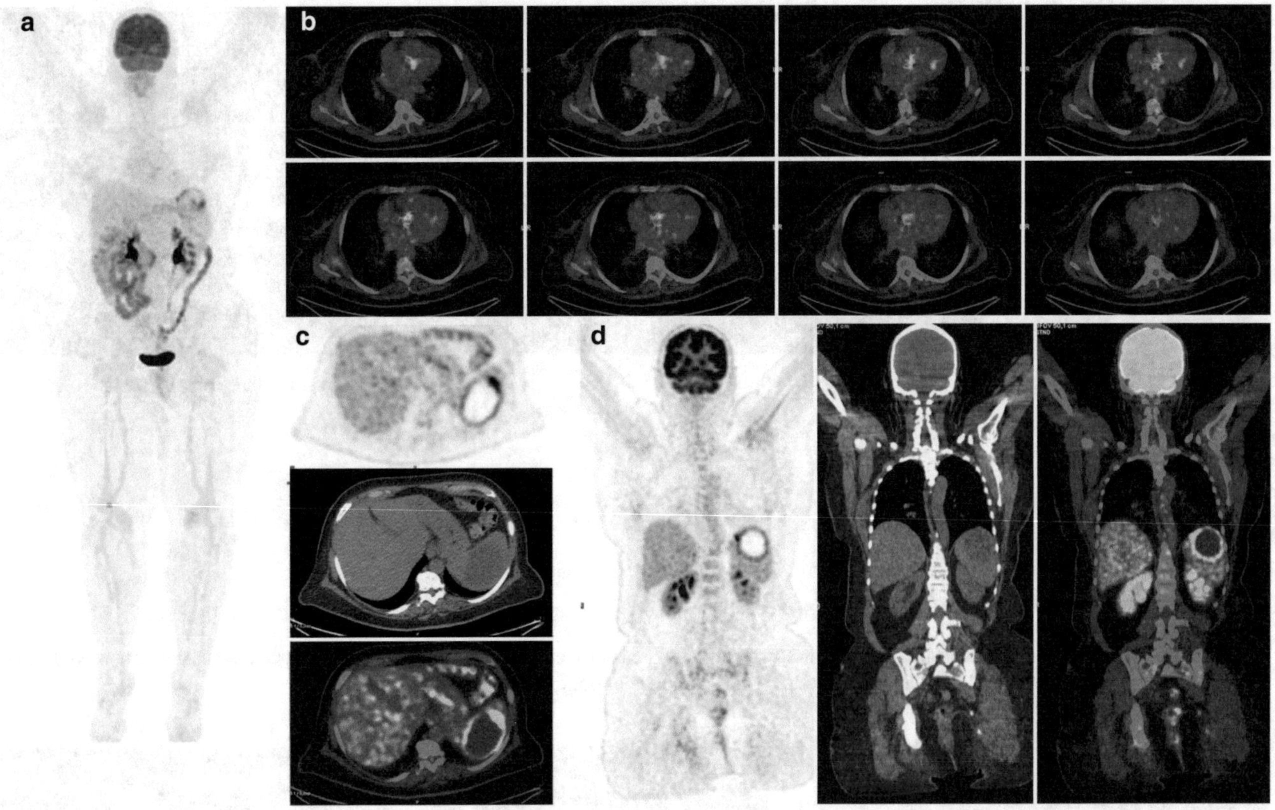

Fig. 9.6 The [^{18}F]FDG PET/CT MIP image (**a**) shows an area of mildly increased focal uptake in the cardiac region and a lesion in the spleen. Axial fused sections (**b**) confirm an area of focal uptake which involves the aortic valve prosthesis, indicating IE. (**c**) Axial (PET, upper; CT, middle; fused PET/CT, bottom) and (**d**) coronal (PET, left; CT, middle; fused PET/CT, right) sections show a large lesion in the spleen characterized by a "hot" rim surrounding "cold" core, suggesting septic embolism (abscess)

Case 9.3

Background

A 70-year-old woman with aortic and mitral valve prosthesis went to the emergency department for persistent fever unresponsive to antimicrobial treatment. Lab tests raised the suspicion of infection, with high C-reactive protein (38 mg/dL), and fibrinogen (521 mg/dL). Blood cultures were negative. TTE was negative. A doubtful image suspected for vegetation at the aortic valve was detected on TEE. Accordingly, the patient was referred for [^{18}F]FDG PET/CT (Fig. 9.7), which showed increased tracer uptake at both prosthetic valves. A ^{99m}Tc-HMPAO-labeled-WBC scintigraphy (Fig. 9.8) confirmed with the presence of IE involving both the aortic and the mitral prosthetic valves. Nonetheless, the disease burden identified by ^{99m}Tc-HMPAO-WBC scintigraphy was lower compared to [^{18}F]FDG PET/CT.

Suspected Site of Infection

Prosthetic valve endocarditis.

Radiopharmaceutical Activity

[^{18}F]FDG, 202 MBq; ^{99m}Tc-HMPAO-WBC, 740 MBq.

Imaging

The PET/CT acquisition included scout view (120 kV, 10 mA), whole-body CT scan (140 kV, 80 mA), and PET (3D, 3 min/FOV). Images were reconstructed with and without attenuation correction using the low-dose transmission CT scan.

^{99m}Tc-HMPAO-WBC scintigraphy: planar images of the thorax acquired at 30 min, 4 h and 20 h. SPECT/CT imaging of the thorax at 4 h and 20 h, with 3D reconstruction.

Conclusion/Teaching Point

Both [^{18}F]FDG PET/CT and ^{99m}Tc-HMPAO-WBC SPECT/CT allow identification of blood culture-negative prosthetic valve endocarditis. ^{99m}Tc-HMPAO-WBC scintigraphy requires SPECT/CT acquisition in suspected cardiovascular infection. As expected, ^{99m}Tc-HMPAO-WBC scintigraphy is more accurate than [^{18}F]FDG PET/CT for defining the infection burden.

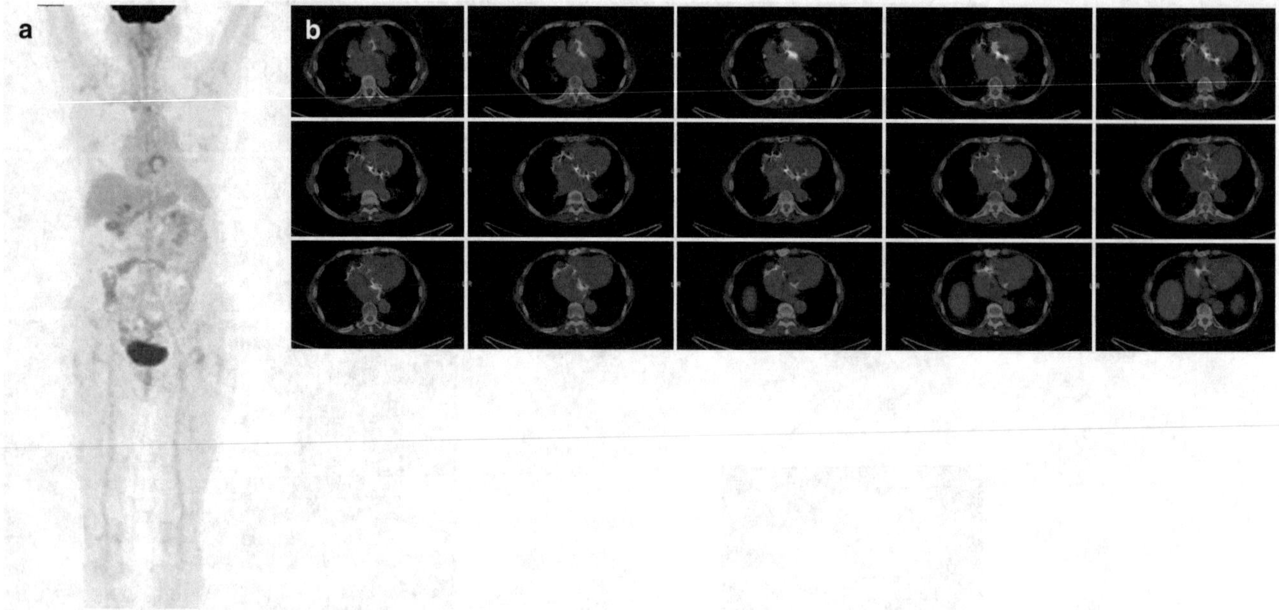

Fig. 9.7 The [^{18}F]FDG PET/CT MIP image (**a**) shows two ring-like areas of increased the tracer uptake in the cardiac region. Transaxial fused PET/CT sections (**b**) demonstrates involvement of both the aortic and the mitralic valve prosthesis

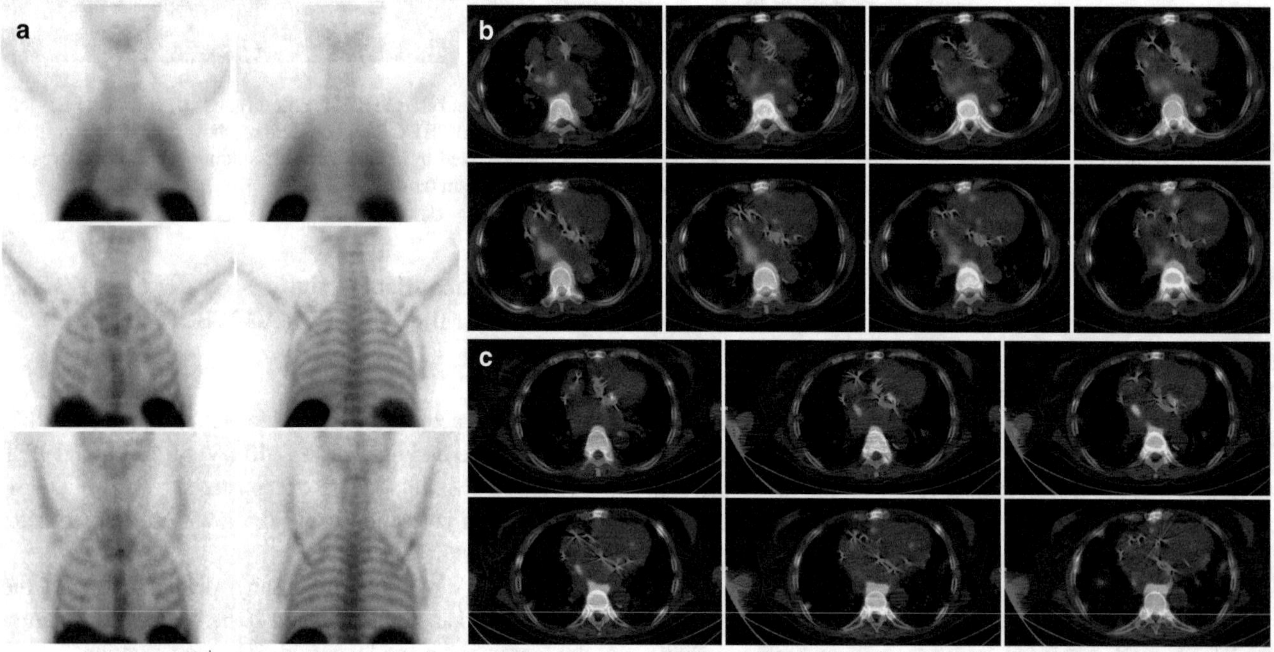

Fig. 9.8 (**a**) ^{99m}Tc-HMPAO-WBC planar images (anterior views in the left panels, posterior views in the right panels) of the thorax at 30 min, 4 h, and 20 h (from top to bottom), showing a mild time-dependent increase of radioactivity accumulation in the lower third of the sternum. Fused transaxial SPECT/CT sections acquired at 4 h (**b**) and at 20 h (**c**), showing increased WBC accumulation at both the aortic and the mitral valve prosthesis

Case 9.4

Background

An 81-year-old man had been submitted to ICD implant several years before being referred to the emergency department because of dyspnea and fever. Lab tests showed increased C-reactive protein (1.2 mg/dL, normal value <0.5 mg/dL) and erythrocyte sedimentation rate (85 mm/h, normal value <30 mm/h). Blood cultures were positive for *Staphylococcus aureus*, but both transthoracic and TEE

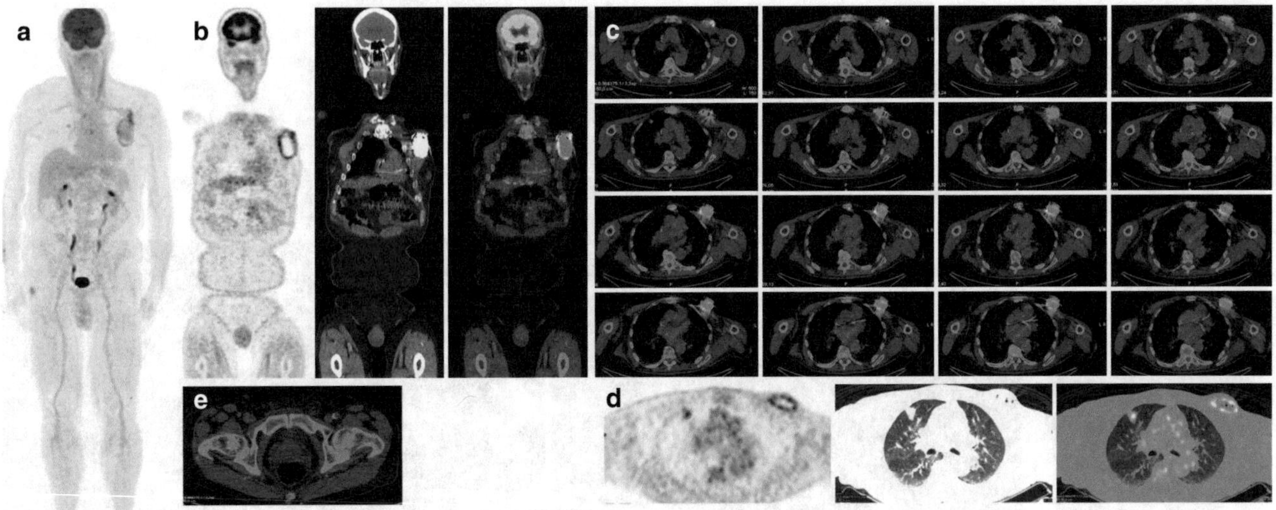

Fig. 9.9 The [18F]FDG PET/CT MIP image (**a**) shows increased tracer uptake in the upper region of the left hemithorax. (**b**) Coronal sections (PET, left; CT, middle; fused PET/CT, right) show intense and diffuse [18F]FDG uptake at the ICD pocket, in the left hemithorax. (**c**) Transaxial fused sections confirm the presence of ICD pocket infection, EC involvement and a hot spot in the upper lobe of right lung, classified as lung embolism; faint [18F]FDG uptake is detectable also in small bilateral axillary lymph nodes, as for nonspecific inflammation. (**d**) Selected transaxial sections (PET, left; CT, middle; fused PET/CT, right) showing in the same plane the pocket infection in the left hemithorax and the septic embolism in right lung. (**e**) The area of focal [18F]FDG uptake at the posterior right greater trochanter is due to nonspecific muscular uptake

excluded the presence of vegetation or any other signs of IE. Because of high clinical suspicion of ICD-related IE, the patient was referred for [18F]FDG PET/CT (Fig. 9.9), which showed high [18F]FDG uptake at the ICD generator pocket, along the EC, and in the right lung; this pattern was consistent with CIED infection with lung embolism. Small bilateral axillary lymph nodes exhibited faint, nonspecific tracer uptake.

Suspected Site of Infection

Cardiac device.

Radiopharmaceutical Activity

[18F]FDG, 291 MBq.

Imaging

The acquisition included scout view (120 kV, 10 mA), whole-body CT scan (140 kV, 80 mA), and PET (3D, 3 min/FOV). Images were reconstructed with and without attenuation correction using the low-dose transmission CT scan.

Conclusion/Teaching Point

[18F]FDG PET/CT identified the presence of ICD pocket infection, with associated septic lung embolism.

Case 9.5

Background

A 73-year-old man had been submitted ICD positioned for heart failure about 3 years before being referred to the emergency department for persistent fever unresponsive to antimicrobial treatment. Lab tests showed increased C-reactive protein (2.5 mg/dL, normal value <0.5 mg/dL), and erythrocyte sedimentation rate (96 mm/h, normal value <30 mm/h). Blood cultures were positive for *Streptococcus dysgalactiae*. TTE did not show any abnormality, while TEE was doubtful for a vegetation along the lead of ICD. Because of the high clinical suspicion for infection together with uncertain TEE findings, [18F]FDG PET/CT was performed (Fig. 9.10), which showed increased tracer uptake along the lead of ICD, thus confirming the doubtful TEE findings; in addition a focus of increased [18F]FDG uptake was noted in the soft tissues of the sacral region.

Suspected Site of Infection

Cardiac device.

Radiopharmaceutical Activity

[18F]FDG, 239 MBq.

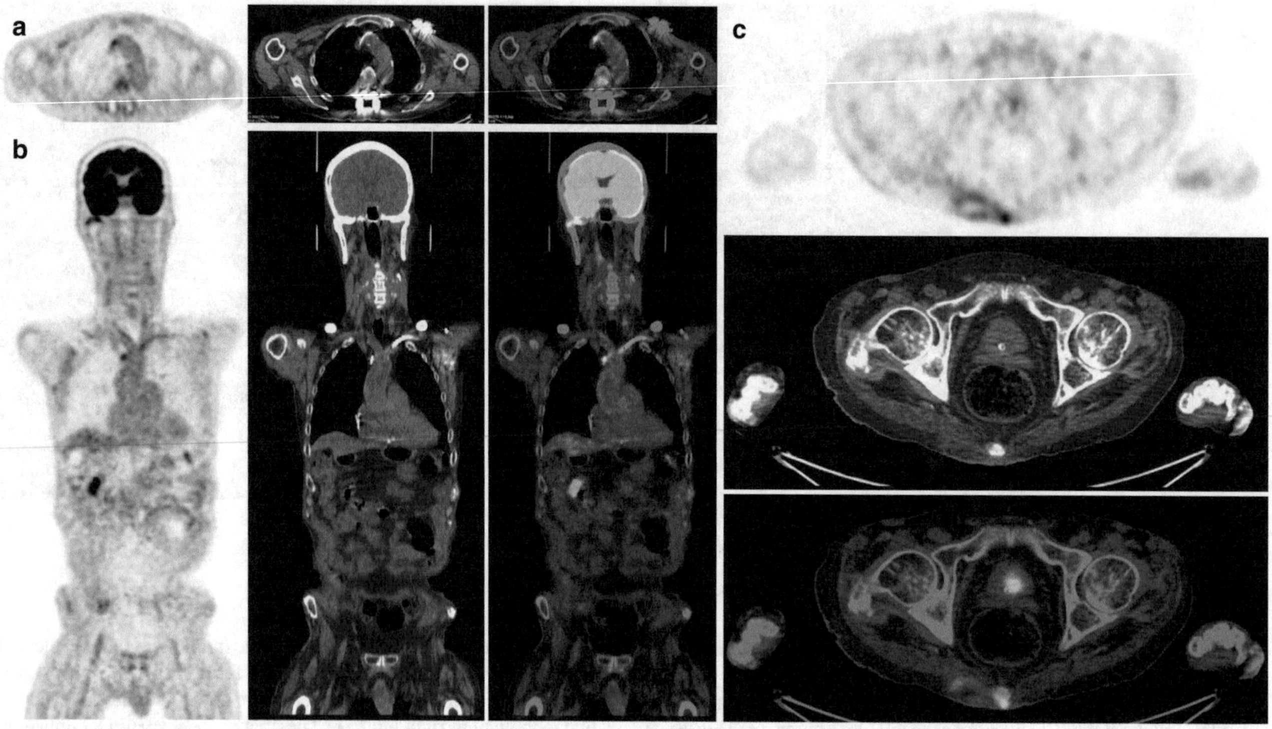

Fig. 9.10 [18F]FDG PET/CT in a patient with cardiac device infection. (**a**) Transaxial section on a selected plane (PET, left; CT, middle; fused PET/CT, right). (**b**) Coronal section on a selected plane (PET, left; CT, middle, fused PET/CT, right). The images show increased [18F]FDG uptake along the lead of the ICD, thus confirming the doubtful TEE findings as due to infection. (**c**) Transaxial sections on a selected plane (PET, top; CT, middle; fused PET/CT, bottom), demonstrating a focus of increased [18F]FDG uptake in the soft tissues of the sacral region

Imaging

The acquisition included scout view (120 kV, 10 mA), whole-body CT scan (140 kV, 80 mA), and PET (3D, 3 min/FOV). Images were reconstructed with and without attenuation correction using the low-dose transmission CT scan.

Conclusion/Teaching Point

[18F]FDG PET/CT identified ICD-related infection and also identified the probable portal of entry for bacteria.

Case 9.6

Background

A 74-year-old obese man with prior implantation of ICD went to the emergency department for dyspnea and persistent fever unresponsive to antimicrobial treatment. Lab tests indicated very high level of C-reactive protein (22 mg/dL) and mildly increased pro-calcitonin (1.8 ng/dL), but still in the range of sepsis uncertainty (0.5–2 ng/dL). Blood cultures were positive for *Staphylococcus aureus*. While TTE was negative, at TEE two faint vegetations were seen along the lead of ICD and at the tricuspid valve, respectively. [18F] FDG PET/CT was performed to confirm/exclude infection based on the high clinical suspicious (cardiac risk factors, lab tests, bacteremia, and suspected, even if uncertain, TEE findings). The PET/CT scan (Fig. 9.11) showed increased [18F]FDG uptake along the intracardiac portion of the lead of ICD and at the pericardium of the right atrium. In addition, lung embolisms were detected.

Suspected Site of Infection

Infection of device.

Radiopharmaceutical Activity

[18F]FDG, 367 MBq.

Imaging

The acquisition included scout view (120 kV, 10 mA), whole-body CT scan (140 kV, 80 mA), and PET (3D, 3 min/FOV). Images were reconstructed with and without attenuation correction using the low-dose transmission CT scan.

Conclusion/Teaching Point

[18F]FD-PET/CT identified the presence of ICD infection, associated with pericarditis and lung septic embolisms.

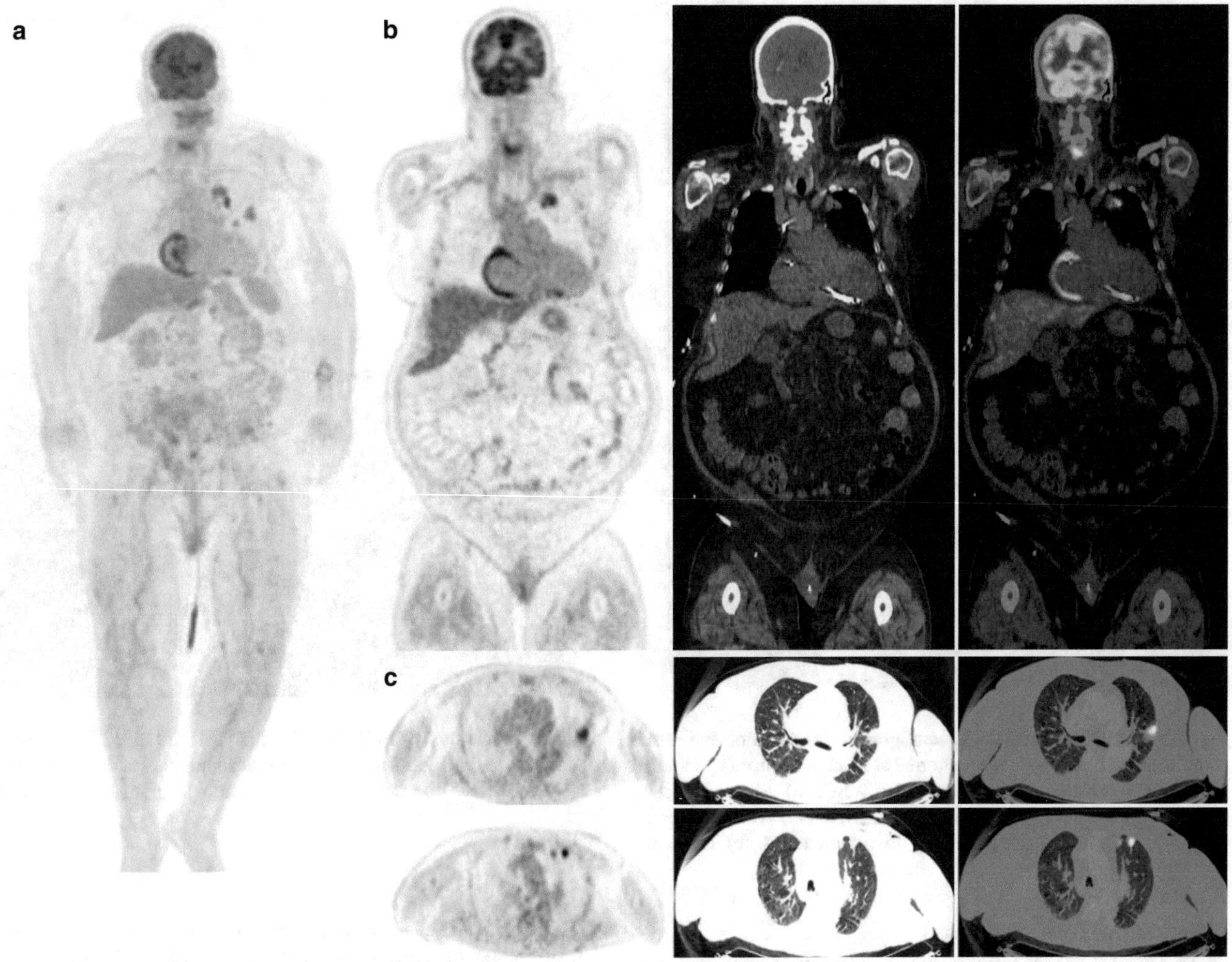

Fig. 9.11 (**a**) [^{18}F]FDG PET/CT MIP image. (**b**) Coronal sections (PET, left; CT, middle; fused PET/CT, right). The images show increased [^{18}F]FDG uptake at the intracardiac portion of the ICD lead, associated with intense and diffuse tracer uptake involving the pericardium of the right atrium. (**c**) Transaxial sections (PET, left; CT, middle; fused PET/CT, right), showing focal sites of [^{18}F]FDG uptake consistent with embolisms in the upper lobe of left lung

Case 9.7

Background

An 80-year-old man with ICD went to the emergency department for persistent fever unresponsive to antimicrobial treatment. Lab tests supported the clinical suspicion of infection, with increased C-reactive protein (14 mg/dL, normal value <0.5 mg/dL) and increased fibrinogen (486 mg/dL, normal range 150–400 mg/dL). Blood cultures were negative. TTE was negative. TEE identified a doubtful image suspected for vegetation along the lead. The patient underwent a ^{99m}Tc-HMPAO-WBC scintigraphy (Fig. 9.12), which identified device-related infection based on the presence of time-dependent radioactivity accumulation increase at the ICD pocket and along the intravascular portion of the ICD lead.

Suspected Site of Infection

Cardiac device.

Radiopharmaceutical Activity

^{99m}Tc-HMPAO-WBC, 740 MBq.

Imaging

Planar images of the thorax acquired at 30 min, 4 h, and 20 h. SPECT/CT imaging of the thorax at 4 h and 20 h, with 3D reconstruction.

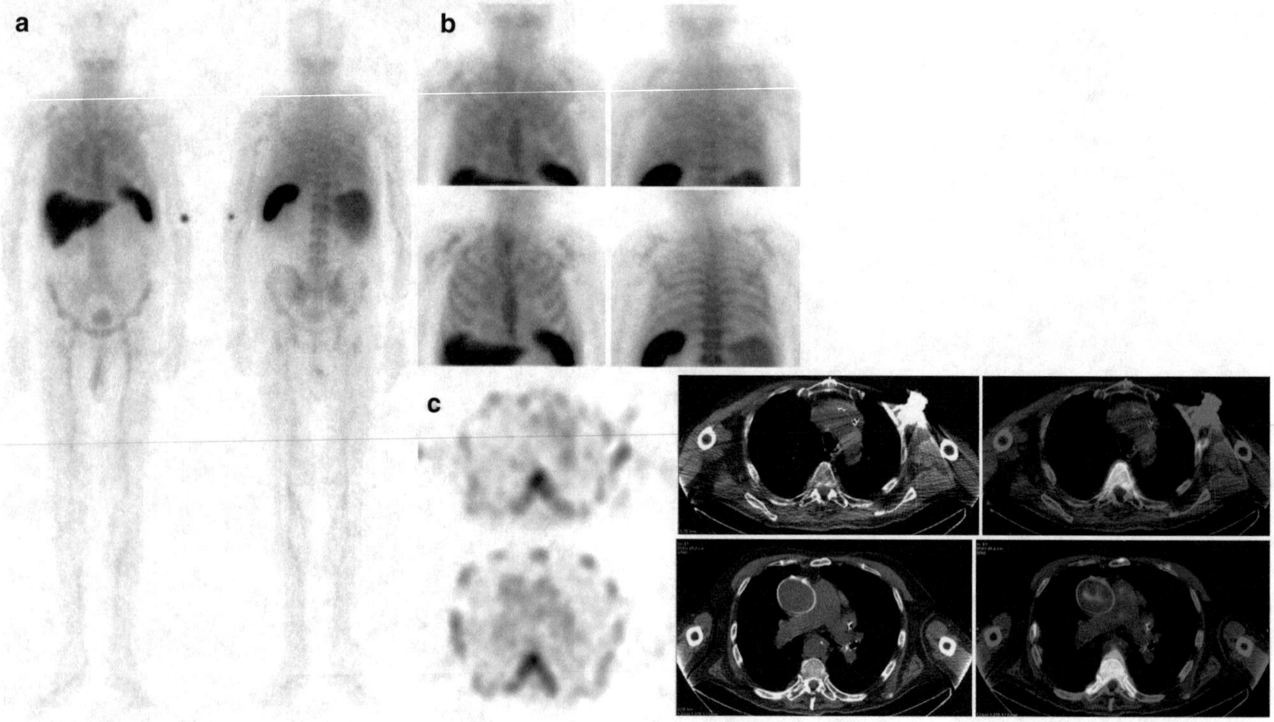

Fig. 9.12 ^{99m}Tc-HMPAO-WBC scintigraphy. (**a**) Anterior and posterior planar whole-body images acquired at 30 min, confirming a normal biodistribution pattern of the radiolabeled WBC. (**b**) Planar spot views of the thorax (anterior, left panel; posterior, right panel) acquired at 4 h (top) and at 20 h (bottom), showing no abnormalities. (**c**) Transaxial SPECT/CT sections (SPECT, left; CT, middle; fused SPECT/CT, right) acquired at 4 h, showing increased WBC accumulation at the deep component of the ICD pocket and at the intravascular portion of the ICD lead

Conclusion/Teaching Point

^{99m}Tc-HMPAO-WBC scintigraphy identified the presence ICD infection.

References

1. Kollef MH, Sharpless L, Vlasnik J, Pasque C, Murphy D, Fraser VJ. The impact of nosocomial infections on patient outcomes following cardiac surgery. Chest. 1997;112(3):666–75.
2. Brown PP, Kugelmass AD, Cohen DJ, Reynolds MR, Culler SD, Dee AD, et al. The frequency and cost of complications associated with coronary artery bypass grafting surgery: results from the United States Medicare program. Ann Thorac Surg. 2008;85(6):1980–6.
3. Edwards JR, Peterson KD, Mu Y, Banerjee S, Allen-Bridson K, Morrell G, et al. National Healthcare Safety Network (NHSN) report: data summary for 2006 through 2008, issued December 2009. Am J Infect Control. 2009;37(10):783–805.
4. Dudeck MA, Weiner LM, Allen-Bridson K, Malpiedi PJ, Peterson KD, Pollock DA, et al. National Healthcare Safety Network (NHSN) report, data summary for 2012, Device-associated module. Am J Infect Control. 2013;41(12):1148–66.
5. Gelijns AC, Moskowitz AJ, Acker MA, Argenziano M, Geller NL, Puskas JD, et al. Management practices and major infections after cardiac surgery. J Am Coll Cardiol. 2014;64(4):372–81.
6. Donlan RM. Biofilms and device-associated infections. Emerg Infect Dis. 2001;7(2):277–81.
7. Zimmerli W, Sendi P. Pathogenesis of implant-associated infection: the role of the host. Semin Immunopathol. 2011;33(3):295–306.
8. Habib G, Hoen B, Tornos P, Thuny F, Prendergast B, Vilacosta I, et al. Guidelines on the prevention, diagnosis, and treatment of infective endocarditis (new version 2009): the Task Force on the Prevention, Diagnosis, and Treatment of Infective Endocarditis of the European Society of Cardiology (ESC). Endorsed by the European Society of Clinical Microbiology and Infectious Diseases (ESCMID) and the International Society of Chemotherapy (ISC) for Infection and Cancer. Eur Heart J. 2009;30(19):2369–413.
9. Hoen B, Alla F, Selton-Suty C, Béguinot I, Bouvet A, Briançon S, et al. Changing profile of infective endocarditis: results of a 1-year survey in France. JAMA. 2002;288(1):75–81.
10. Selton-Suty C, Célard M, Le Moing V, Doco-Lecompte T, Chirouze C, Iung B, et al. Preeminence of Staphylococcus aureus in infective endocarditis: a 1-year population-based survey. Clin Infect Dis. 2012;54(9):1230–9.
11. Habib G, Erba PA, Iung B, Donal E, Cosyns B, Laroche C, et al. Clinical presentation, aetiology and outcome of infective endocarditis. Results of the ESC-EORP EURO-ENDO (European infective endocarditis) registry: a prospective cohort study. Eur Heart J. 2019;40(39):3222–32.
12. Murdoch DR, Corey GR, Hoen B, Miró JM, Fowler VG, Bayer AS, et al. Clinical presentation, etiology, and outcome of infective endocarditis in the 21st century: the International Collaboration on Endocarditis-Prospective Cohort Study. Arch Intern Med. 2009;169(5):463–73.
13. Tornos P, Iung B, Permanyer-Miralda G, Baron G, Delahaye F, Gohlke-Bärwolf C, et al. Infective endocarditis in Europe: lessons from the Euro heart survey. Heart. 2005;91(5):571–5.

14. Tornos P, Gonzalez-Alujas T, Thuny F, Habib G. Infective endocarditis: the European viewpoint. Curr Probl Cardiol. 2011;36(5):175–222.
15. Nkomo VT. Epidemiology and prevention of valvular heart diseases and infective endocarditis in Africa. Heart. 2007;93(12):1510–9.
16. Letaief A, Boughzala E, Kaabia N, Ernez S, Abid F, Ben Chaabane T, et al. Epidemiology of infective endocarditis in Tunisia: a 10-year multicenter retrospective study. Int J Infect Dis. 2007;11(5):430–3.
17. Steckelberg JM, Wilson WR. Risk factors for infective endocarditis. Infect Dis Clin N Am. 1993;7(1):9–19.
18. Grover FL, Cohen DJ, Oprian C, Henderson WG, Sethi G, Hammermeister KE. Determinants of the occurrence of and survival from prosthetic valve endocarditis. Experience of the veterans affairs cooperative study on valvular heart disease. J Thorac Cardiovasc Surg. 1994;108(2):207–14.
19. Graves MK, Soto L. Left-sided endocarditis in parenteral drug abusers: recent experience at a large community hospital. South Med J. 1992;85(4):378–80.
20. Cabell CH, Jollis JG, Peterson GE, Corey GR, Anderson DJ, Sexton DJ, et al. Changing patient characteristics and the effect on mortality in endocarditis. Arch Intern Med. 2002;162(1):90–4.
21. Bayer AS, Bolger AF, Taubert KA, Wilson W, Steckelberg J, Karchmer AW, et al. Diagnosis and management of infective endocarditis and its complications. Circulation. 1998;98(25):2936–48.
22. Pérez de Isla L, Zamorano J, Lennie V, Vázquez J, Ribera JM, Macaya C. Negative blood culture infective endocarditis in the elderly: long-term follow-up. Gerontology. 2007;53(5):245–9.
23. Thuny F, Di Salvo G, Disalvo G, Belliard O, Avierinos JF, Pergola V, et al. Risk of embolism and death in infective endocarditis: prognostic value of echocardiography: a prospective multicenter study. Circulation. 2005;112(1):69–75.
24. Durack DT, Lukes AS, Bright DK. New criteria for diagnosis of infective endocarditis: utilization of specific echocardiographic findings. Duke Endocarditis Service. Am J Med. 1994;96(3):200–9.
25. Hubert S, Thuny F, Resseguier N, Giorgi R, Tribouilloy C, Le Dolley Y, et al. Prediction of symptomatic embolism in infective endocarditis: construction and validation of a risk calculator in a multicenter cohort. J Am Coll Cardiol. 2013;62(15):1384–92.
26. Li JS, Sexton DJ, Mick N, Nettles R, Fowler VG, Ryan T, et al. Proposed modifications to the Duke criteria for the diagnosis of infective endocarditis. Clin Infect Dis. 2000;30(4):633–8.
27. Habib G, Lancellotti P, Antunes MJ, Bongiorni MG, Casalta JP, Del Zotti F, et al. 2015 ESC Guidelines for the management of infective endocarditis: The Task Force for the Management of Infective Endocarditis of the European Society of Cardiology (ESC). Endorsed by: European Association for Cardio-Thoracic Surgery (EACTS), the European Association of Nuclear Medicine (EANM). Eur Heart J. 2015;36(44):3075–128.
28. Saby L, Laas O, Habib G, Cammilleri S, Mancini J, Tessonnier L, et al. Positron emission tomography/computed tomography for diagnosis of prosthetic valve endocarditis: increased valvular ^{18}F-fluorodeoxyglucose uptake as a novel major criterion. J Am Coll Cardiol. 2013;61(23):2374–82.
29. Bruun NE, Habib G, Thuny F, Sogaard P. Cardiac imaging in infectious endocarditis. Eur Heart J. 2014;35(10):624–32.
30. Erba PA, Conti U, Lazzeri E, Sollini M, Doria R, De Tommasi SM, et al. Added value of ^{99m}Tc-HMPAO-labeled leukocyte SPECT/CT in the characterization and management of patients with infectious endocarditis. J Nucl Med. 2012;53(8):1235–43.
31. Erba PA, Lancellotti P, Vilacosta I, Gaemperli O, Rouzet F, Hacker M, et al. Recommendations on nuclear and multimodality imaging in IE and CIED infections. Eur J Nucl Med Mol Imaging. 2018;45(10):1795–815.
32. Sollini M, Berchiolli R, Delgado Bolton RC, Rossi A, Kirienko M, Boni R, et al. The "3M" approach to cardiovascular infections: multimodality, multitracers, and multidisciplinary. Semin Nucl Med. 2018;48(3):199–224.
33. Fournier PE, Casalta JP, Habib G, Messana T, Raoult D. Modification of the diagnostic criteria proposed by the Duke Endocarditis Service to permit improved diagnosis of Q fever endocarditis. Am J Med. 1996;100(6):629–33.
34. Habib G, Derumeaux G, Avierinos JF, Casalta JP, Jamal F, Volot F, et al. Value and limitations of the Duke criteria for the diagnosis of infective endocarditis. J Am Coll Cardiol. 1999;33(7):2023–9.
35. Lamas CC, Eykyn SJ. Suggested modifications to the Duke criteria for the clinical diagnosis of native valve and prosthetic valve endocarditis: analysis of 118 pathologically proven cases. Clin Infect Dis. 1997;25(3):713–9.
36. Delahaye F, Rial MO, de Gevigney G, Ecochard R, Delaye J. A critical appraisal of the quality of the management of infective endocarditis. J Am Coll Cardiol. 1999;33(3):788–93.
37. Brouqui P, Raoult D. New insight into the diagnosis of fastidious bacterial endocarditis. FEMS Immunol Med Microbiol. 2006;47(1):1–13.
38. Winslow T, Foster E, Adams JR, Schiller NB. Pulmonary valve endocarditis: improved diagnosis with biplane transesophageal echocardiography. J Am Soc Echocardiogr. 1992;5(2):206–10.
39. Roe MT, Abramson MA, Li J, Heinle SK, Kisslo J, Corey GR, et al. Clinical information determines the impact of transesophageal echocardiography on the diagnosis of infective endocarditis by the duke criteria. Am Heart J. 2000;139(6):945–51.
40. Jacob S, Tong AT. Role of echocardiography in the diagnosis and management of infective endocarditis. Curr Opin Cardiol. 2002;17(5):478–85.
41. Hill EE, Herijgers P, Claus P, Vanderschueren S, Peetermans WE, Herregods MC. Abscess in infective endocarditis: the value of transesophageal echocardiography and outcome: a 5-year study. Am Heart J. 2007;154(5):923–8.
42. Habib G, Badano L, Tribouilloy C, Vilacosta I, Zamorano JL, Galderisi M, et al. Recommendations for the practice of echocardiography in infective endocarditis. Eur J Echocardiogr. 2010;11(2):202–19.
43. Baddour LM, Wilson WR, Bayer AS, Fowler VG, Tleyjeh IM, Rybak MJ, et al. Infective endocarditis in adults: diagnosis, antimicrobial therapy, and management of complications: a scientific statement for healthcare professionals from the American Heart Association. Circulation. 2015;132(15):1435–86.
44. Grob A, Thuny F, Villacampa C, Flavian A, Gaubert JY, Raoult D, et al. Cardiac multidetector computed tomography in infective endocarditis: a pictorial essay. Insights Imaging. 2014;5(5):559–70.
45. Feuchtner GM, Stolzmann P, Dichtl W, Schertler T, Bonatti J, Scheffel H, et al. Multislice computed tomography in infective endocarditis: comparison with transesophageal echocardiography and intraoperative findings. J Am Coll Cardiol. 2009;53(5):436–44.
46. Rouzet F, Chequer R, Benali K, Lepage L, Ghodbane W, Duval X, et al. Respective performance of ^{18}F-FDG PET and radiolabeled leukocyte scintigraphy for the diagnosis of prosthetic valve endocarditis. J Nucl Med. 2014;55(12):1980–5.
47. Hyafil F, Rouzet F, Lepage L, Benali K, Raffoul R, Duval X, et al. Role of radiolabelled leucocyte scintigraphy in patients with a suspicion of prosthetic valve endocarditis and inconclusive echocardiography. Eur Heart J Cardiovasc Imaging. 2013;14(6):586–94.
48. Kestler M, Muñoz P, Rodríguez-Créixems M, Rotger A, Jimenez-Requena F, Mari A, et al. Role of ^{18}F-FDG PET in patients with infectious endocarditis. J Nucl Med. 2014;55(7):1093–8.
49. Kouijzer IJ, Vos FJ, Janssen MJ, van Dijk AP, Oyen WJ, Bleeker-Rovers CP. The value of ^{18}F-FDG PET/CT in diagnosing infectious endocarditis. Eur J Nucl Med Mol Imaging. 2013;40(7):1102–7.

50. Granados U, Fuster D, Pericas JM, Llopis JL, Ninot S, Quintana E, et al. Diagnostic accuracy of ^{18}F-FDG PET/CT in infective endocarditis and implantable cardiac electronic device infection: a cross-sectional study. J Nucl Med. 2016;57(11):1726–32.
51. Pizzi MN, Roque A, Fernández-Hidalgo N, Cuéllar-Calabria H, Ferreira-González I, Gonzàlez-Alujas MT, et al. Improving the diagnosis of infective endocarditis in prosthetic valves and intracardiac devices with ^{18}F-fluordeoxyglucose positron emission tomography/computed tomography angiography: initial results at an infective endocarditis referral center. Circulation. 2015;132(12):1113–26.
52. Roque A, Pizzi MN, Cuéllar-Calàbria H, Aguadé-Bruix S. F-FDG-PET/CT angiography for the diagnosis of infective endocarditis. Curr Cardiol Rep. 2017;19(2):15.
53. Gomes A, Glaudemans AWJM, Touw DJ, van Melle JP, Willems TP, Maass AH, et al. Diagnostic value of imaging in infective endocarditis: a systematic review. Lancet Infect Dis. 2017;17(1):e1–e14.
54. Ricciardi A, Sordillo P, Ceccarelli L, Maffongelli G, Calisti G, Di Pietro B, et al. 18-Fluoro-2-deoxyglucose positron emission tomography-computed tomography: an additional tool in the diagnosis of prosthetic valve endocarditis. Int J Infect Dis. 2014;28:219–24.
55. Bartoletti M, Tumietto F, Fasulo G, Giannella M, Cristini F, Bonfiglioli R, et al. Combined computed tomography and fluorodeoxyglucose positron emission tomography in the diagnosis of prosthetic valve endocarditis: a case series. BMC Res Notes. 2014;7:32.
56. Fagman E, van Essen M, Fredén Lindqvist J, Snygg-Martin U, Bech-Hanssen O, Svensson G. ^{18}F-FDG PET/CT in the diagnosis of prosthetic valve endocarditis. Int J Cardiovasc Imaging. 2016;32(4):679–86.
57. Salomäki SP, Saraste A, Kemppainen J, Bax JJ, Knuuti J, Nuutila P, et al. ^{18}F-FDG positron emission tomography/computed tomography in infective endocarditis. J Nucl Cardiol. 2017;24(1):195–206.
58. Pizzi MN, Dos-Subirà L, Roque A, Fernández-Hidalgo N, Cuéllar-Calabria H, Pijuan Domènech A, et al. ^{18}F-FDG-PET/CT angiography in the diagnosis of infective endocarditis and cardiac device infection in adult patients with congenital heart disease and prosthetic material. Int J Cardiol. 2017;248:396–402.
59. San Román JA, Vilacosta I, López J, Revilla A, Arnold R, Sevilla T, et al. Role of transthoracic and transesophageal echocardiography in right-sided endocarditis: one echocardiographic modality does not fit all. J Am Soc Echocardiogr. 2012;25(8):807–14.
60. Morokuma H, Minato N, Kamohara K, Minematsu N. Three surgical cases of isolated tricuspid valve infective endocarditis. Ann Thorac Cardiovasc Surg. 2010;16(2):134–8.
61. Winslow TM, Redberg RF, Foster E, Schiller NB. Transesophageal echocardiographic detection of abnormalities of the tricuspid valve in adults associated with spontaneous closure of perimembranous ventricular septal defect. Am J Cardiol. 1992;70(9):967–9.
62. San Román JA, Vilacosta I. Role of transesophageal echocardiography in right-sided endocarditis. Echocardiography. 1995;12(6):669–72.
63. Vilacosta I, Sarriá C, San Román JA, Jiménez J, Castillo JA, Iturralde E, et al. Usefulness of transesophageal echocardiography for diagnosis of infected transvenous permanent pacemakers. Circulation. 1994;89(6):2684–7.
64. Sohail MR, Uslan DZ, Khan AH, Friedman PA, Hayes DL, Wilson WR, et al. Infective endocarditis complicating permanent pacemaker and implantable cardioverter-defibrillator infection. Mayo Clin Proc. 2008;83(1):46–53.
65. Duval X, Delahaye F, Alla F, Tattevin P, Obadia JF, Le Moing V, et al. Temporal trends in infective endocarditis in the context of prophylaxis guideline modifications: three successive population-based surveys. J Am Coll Cardiol. 2012;59(22):1968–76.
66. Vilacosta I, Graupner C, San Román JA, Sarriá C, Ronderos R, Fernández C, et al. Risk of embolization after institution of antibiotic therapy for infective endocarditis. J Am Coll Cardiol. 2002;39(9):1489–95.
67. Habib G. Embolic risk in subacute bacterial endocarditis: determinants and role of transesophageal echocardiography. Curr Cardiol Rep. 2003;5(2):129–36.
68. Di Salvo G, Habib G, Pergola V, Avierinos JF, Philip E, Casalta JP, et al. Echocardiography predicts embolic events in infective endocarditis. J Am Coll Cardiol. 2001;37(4):1069–76.
69. Steckelberg JM, Murphy JG, Ballard D, Bailey K, Tajik AJ, Taliercio CP, et al. Emboli in infective endocarditis: the prognostic value of echocardiography. Ann Intern Med. 1991;114(8):635–40.
70. García-Cabrera E, Fernández-Hidalgo N, Almirante B, Ivanova-Georgieva R, Noureddine M, Plata A, et al. Neurological complications of infective endocarditis: risk factors, outcome, and impact of cardiac surgery: a multicenter observational study. Circulation. 2013;127(23):2272–84.
71. Goldberger Z, Lampert R. Implantable cardioverter-defibrillators: expanding indications and technologies. JAMA. 2006;295(7):809–18.
72. Wilkoff BL, Auricchio A, Brugada J, Cowie M, Ellenbogen KA, Gillis AM, et al. HRS/EHRA expert consensus on the monitoring of cardiovascular implantable electronic devices (CIEDs): description of techniques, indications, personnel, frequency and ethical considerations: developed in partnership with the Heart Rhythm Society (HRS) and the European Heart Rhythm Association (EHRA); and in collaboration with the American College of Cardiology (ACC), the American Heart Association (AHA), the European Society of Cardiology (ESC), the Heart Failure Association of ESC (HFA), and the Heart Failure Society of America (HFSA). Endorsed by the Heart Rhythm Society, the European Heart Rhythm Association (a registered branch of the ESC), the American College of Cardiology, the American Heart Association. Europace. 2008;10(6):707–25.
73. Uslan DZ, Tleyjeh IM, Baddour LM, Friedman PA, Jenkins SM, St Sauver JL, et al. Temporal trends in permanent pacemaker implantation: a population-based study. Am Heart J. 2008;155(5):896–903.
74. Neelankavil JP, Thompson A, Mahajan A. Managing Cardiovascular Implantable Electronic Devices (CIEDs) during perioperative care. The Anesthesia Patient Safety Foundation. 2013. http://www.apsf.org/newsletters/html/2013/fall/01_cieds.htm.
75. Podoleanu C, Deharo JC. Management of cardiac implantable electronic device infection. Arrhythm Electrophysiol Rev. 2014;3(3):184–9.
76. Thuny F, Grisoli D, Collart F, Habib G, Raoult D. Management of infective endocarditis: challenges and perspectives. Lancet. 2012;379(9819):965–75.
77. DeSimone DC, Sohail MR. Management of bacteremia in patients living with cardiovascular implantable electronic devices. Heart Rhythm. 2016;13(11):2247–52.
78. Baddour LM, Epstein AE, Erickson CC, Knight BP, Levison ME, Lockhart PB, et al. Update on cardiovascular implantable electronic device infections and their management: a scientific statement from the American Heart Association. Circulation. 2010;121(3):458–77.
79. Voigt A, Shalaby A, Saba S. Rising rates of cardiac rhythm management device infections in the United States: 1996 through 2003. J Am Coll Cardiol. 2006;48(3):590–1.
80. Margey R, McCann H, Blake G, Keelan E, Galvin J, Lynch M, et al. Contemporary management of and outcomes from cardiac device related infections. Europace. 2010;12(1):64–70.
81. Baman TS, Gupta SK, Valle JA, Yamada E. Risk factors for mortality in patients with cardiac device-related infection. Circ Arrhythm Electrophysiol. 2009;2(2):129–34.

82. Da Costa A, Lelièvre H, Kirkorian G, Célard M, Chevalier P, Vandenesch F, et al. Role of the preaxillary flora in pacemaker infections: a prospective study. Circulation. 1998;97(18):1791–5.
83. Uslan DZ, Sohail MR, St Sauver JL, Friedman PA, Hayes DL, Stoner SM, et al. Permanent pacemaker and implantable cardioverter defibrillator infection: a population-based study. Arch Intern Med. 2007;167(7):669–75.
84. Darouiche RO. Device-associated infections: a macroproblem that starts with microadherence. Clin Infect Dis. 2001;33(9):1567–72.
85. Hussein AA, Baghdy Y, Wazni OM, Brunner MP, Kabbach G, Shao M, et al. Microbiology of cardiac implantable electronic device infections. JACC Clin Electrophysiol. 2016;2(4):498–505.
86. Mangram AJ, Horan TC, Pearson ML, Silver LC, Jarvis WR. Guideline for prevention of surgical site infection, 1999. Hospital Infection Control Practices Advisory Committee. Infect Control Hosp Epidemiol. 1999;20(4):250–78; quiz 79-80.
87. Mond HG, Irwin M, Ector H, Proclemer A. The world survey of cardiac pacing and cardioverter-defibrillators: calendar year 2005 an International Cardiac Pacing and Electrophysiology Society (ICPES) project. Pacing Clin Electrophysiol. 2008;31(9):1202–12.
88. Klug D, Wallet F, Lacroix D, Marquié C, Kouakam C, Kacet S, et al. Local symptoms at the site of pacemaker implantation indicate latent systemic infection. Heart. 2004;90(8):882–6.
89. Bongiorni MG, Burri H, Deharo JC, Starck C, Kennergren C, Saghy L, et al. 2018 EHRA expert consensus statement on lead extraction: recommendations on definitions, endpoints, research trial design, and data collection requirements for clinical scientific studies and registries: endorsed by APHRS/HRS/LAHRS. Europace. 2018;20(7):1217.
90. Cacoub P, Leprince P, Nataf P, Hausfater P, Dorent R, Wechsler B, et al. Pacemaker infective endocarditis. Am J Cardiol. 1998;82(4):480–4.
91. Klug D, Lacroix D, Savoye C, Goullard L, Grandmougin D, Hennequin JL, et al. Systemic infection related to endocarditis on pacemaker leads: clinical presentation and management. Circulation. 1997;95(8):2098–107.
92. Lennerz C, Vrazic H, Haller B, Braun S, Petzold T, Ott I, et al. Biomarker-based diagnosis of pacemaker and implantable cardioverter defibrillator pocket infections: a prospective, multicentre, case-control evaluation. PLoS One. 2017;12(3):e0172384.
93. Cornelissen CG, Frechen DA, Schreiner K, Marx N, Krüger S. Inflammatory parameters and prediction of prognosis in infective endocarditis. BMC Infect Dis. 2013;13:272.
94. Peacock JE, Stafford JM, Le K, Sohail MR, Baddour LM, Prutkin JM, et al. Attempted salvage of infected cardiovascular implantable electronic devices: are there clinical factors that predict success? Pacing Clin Electrophysiol. 2018;41(5):524–31.
95. Lebeaux D, Fernández-Hidalgo N, Chauhan A, Lee S, Ghigo JM, Almirante B, et al. Management of infections related to totally implantable venous-access ports: challenges and perspectives. Lancet Infect Dis. 2014;14(2):146–59.
96. Kusumoto FM, Schoenfeld MH, Wilkoff BL, Berul CI, Birgersdotter-Green UM, Carrillo R, et al. 2017 HRS expert consensus statement on cardiovascular implantable electronic device lead management and extraction. Heart Rhythm. 2017;14(12):e503–e51.
97. Blomström-Lundqvist C, Traykov V, Erba PA, Burri H, Nielsen JC, Bongiorni MG, et al. European Heart Rhythm Association (EHRA) international consensus document on how to prevent, diagnose, and treat cardiac implantable electronic device infections-endorsed by the Heart Rhythm Society (HRS), the Asia Pacific Heart Rhythm Society (APHRS), the Latin American Heart Rhythm Society (LAHRS), International Society for Cardiovascular Infectious Diseases (ISCVID) and the European Society of Clinical Microbiology and Infectious Diseases (ESCMID) in collaboration with the European Association for Cardio-Thoracic Surgery (EACTS). Europace. 2020;22(4):515–49.
98. Gould FK, Denning DW, Elliott TS, Foweraker J, Perry JD, Prendergast BD, et al. Guidelines for the diagnosis and antibiotic treatment of endocarditis in adults: a report of the Working Party of the British Society for Antimicrobial Chemotherapy. J Antimicrob Chemother. 2012;67(2):269–89.
99. Golzio PG, Errigo D, Peyracchia M, Gallo E, Frea S, Castagno D, et al. Prevalence and prognosis of lead masses in patients with cardiac implantable electronic devices without infection. J Cardiovasc Med (Hagerstown). 2019;20(6):372–8.
100. Downey BC, Juselius WE, Pandian NG, Estes NA, Link MS. Incidence and significance of pacemaker and implantable cardioverter-defibrillator lead masses discovered during transesophageal echocardiography. Pacing Clin Electrophysiol. 2011;34(6):679–83.
101. Bongiorni MG, Di Cori A, Soldati E, Zucchelli G, Arena G, Segreti L, et al. Intracardiac echocardiography in patients with pacing and defibrillating leads: a feasibility study. Echocardiography. 2008;25(6):632–8.
102. Narducci ML, Pelargonio G, Russo E, Marinaccio L, Di Monaco A, Perna F, et al. Usefulness of intracardiac echocardiography for the diagnosis of cardiovascular implantable electronic device-related endocarditis. J Am Coll Cardiol. 2013;61(13):1398–405.
103. Chang D, Gabriels J, Laighold S, Williamson AK, Ismail H, Epstein LM. A novel diagnostic approach to a mass on a device lead. Heart Rhythm Case Rep. 2019;5(6):306–9.
104. Diemberger I, Biffi M, Lorenzetti S, Martignani C, Raffaelli E, Ziacchi M, et al. Predictors of long-term survival free from relapses after extraction of infected CIED. Europace. 2018;20(6):1018–27.
105. Goodman LR, Almassi GH, Troup PJ, Gurney JW, Veseth-Rogers J, Chapman PD, et al. Complications of automatic implantable cardioverter defibrillators: radiographic, CT, and echocardiographic evaluation. Radiology. 1989;170(2):447–52.
106. Kelly PA, Wallace S, Tucker B, Hurvitz RJ, Ilvento J, Mirabel GS, et al. Postoperative infection with the automatic implantable cardioverter defibrillator: clinical presentation and use of the gallium scan in diagnosis. Pacing Clin Electrophysiol. 1988;11(8):1220–5.
107. Bhadelia RA, Oates E. Early cardioverter defibrillator infection: value of indium-111 leukocyte imaging. Ann Thorac Surg. 1997;63(1):236–8.
108. Almirante B, Miró JM. Infections associated with prosthetic heart valves, vascular prostheses, and cardiac pacemakers and defibrillators. Enferm Infecc Microbiol Clin. 2008;26(10):647–64.
109. Litzler PY, Manrique A, Etienne M, Salles A, Edet-Sanson A, Vera P, et al. Leukocyte SPECT/CT for detecting infection of left-ventricular-assist devices: preliminary results. J Nucl Med. 2010;51(7):1044–8.
110. Schiavo R, Ricci A, Pontillo D, Bernardini G, Melacrinis FF, Maccafeo S. Implantable cardioverter-defibrillator lead infection detected by ^{99m}Tc-sulesomab single-photon emission computed tomography/computed tomography 'fusion' imaging. J Cardiovasc Med (Hagerstown). 2009;10(11).
111. Ploux S, Riviere A, Amraoui S, Whinnett Z, Barandon L, Lafitte S, et al. Positron emission tomography in patients with suspected pacing system infections may play a critical role in difficult cases. Heart Rhythm. 2011;8(9):1478–81.
112. Vos FJ, Bleeker-Rovers CP, Sturm PD, Krabbe PF, van Dijk AP, Cuijpers ML, et al. ^{18}F-FDG PET/CT for detection of metastatic infection in gram-positive bacteremia. J Nucl Med. 2010;51(8):1234–40.
113. Abikhzer G, Turpin S, Bigras JL. Infected pacemaker causing septic lung emboli detected on FDG PET/CT. J Nucl Cardiol. 2010;17(3):514–5.

114. Costo S, Hourna E, Massetti M, Belin A, Bouvard G, Agostini D. Impact of F-18 FDG PET-CT for the diagnosis and management of infection in JARVIK 2000 device. Clin Nucl Med. 2011;36(12):e188–91.
115. Bensimhon L, Lavergne T, Hugonnet F, Mainardi JL, Latremouille C, Maunoury C, et al. Whole body [18F]fluorodeoxyglucose positron emission tomography imaging for the diagnosis of pacemaker or implantable cardioverter defibrillator infection: a preliminary prospective study. Clin Microbiol Infect. 2011;17(6):836–44.
116. Sarrazin JF, Philippon F, Tessier M, Guimond J, Molin F, Champagne J, et al. Usefulness of fluorine-18 positron emission tomography/computed tomography for identification of cardiovascular implantable electronic device infections. J Am Coll Cardiol. 2012;59(18):1616–25.
117. Juneau D, Golfam M, Hazra S, Zuckier LS, Garas S, Redpath C, et al. Positron emission tomography and single-photon emission computed tomography imaging in the diagnosis of cardiac implantable electronic device infection: a systematic review and meta-analysis. Circ Cardiovasc Imaging. 2017;10(4):pii: e005772.
118. Matsushita K, Tsuboi N, Nanasato M, Takefuji M, Inoue N, Okada T, et al. Intravenous vegetation of methicillin-resistant Staphylococcus aureus induced by central venous catheter in a patient with implantable cardioverter-defibrillator: a case report. J Cardiol. 2002;40(1):31–5.
119. Memmott MJ, James J, Armstrong IS, Tout D, Ahmed F. The performance of quantitation methods in the evaluation of cardiac implantable electronic device (CIED) infection: a technical review. J Nucl Cardiol. 2016;23(6):1457–66.
120. Erba PA, Sollini M, Conti U, Bandera F, Tascini C, De Tommasi SM, et al. Radiolabeled WBC scintigraphy in the diagnostic workup of patients with suspected device-related infections. JACC Cardiovasc Imaging. 2013;6(10):1075–86.
121. Ahmed FZ, James J, Cunnington C, Motwani M, Fullwood C, Hooper J, et al. Early diagnosis of cardiac implantable electronic device generator pocket infection using 18F-FDG-PET/CT. Eur Heart J Cardiovasc Imaging. 2015;16(5):521–30.
122. Amraoui S, Tlili G, Sohal M, Berte B, Hindié E, Ritter P, et al. Contribution of PET imaging to the diagnosis of septic embolism in patients with pacing lead endocarditis. JACC Cardiovasc Imaging. 2016;9(3):283–90.
123. Diemberger I, Bonfiglioli R, Martignani C, Graziosi M, Biffi M, Lorenzetti S, et al. Contribution of PET imaging to mortality risk stratification in candidates to lead extraction for pacemaker or defibrillator infection: a prospective single center study. Eur J Nucl Med Mol Imaging. 2019;46(1):194–205.
124. Paparoupa M, Spineli L, Framke T, Ho H, Schuppert F, Gillissen A. Pulmonary embolism in pneumonia: still a diagnostic challenge? Results of a case-control study in 100 patients. Dis Markers. 2016;2016:8682506.
125. Holman WL, Naftel DC, Eckert CE, Kormos RL, Goldstein DJ, Kirklin JK. Durability of left ventricular assist devices: Interagency Registry for Mechanically Assisted Circulatory Support (INTERMACS) 2006 to 2011. J Thorac Cardiovasc Surg. 2013;146(2):437–41.e1.
126. Xie A, Phan K, Yan TD. Durability of continuous-flow left ventricular assist devices: a systematic review. Ann Cardiothorac Surg. 2014;3(6):547–56.
127. Wickline SA, Fischer KC. Can infections be imaged in implanted devices? ASAIO J. 2000;46(6):S80–1.
128. Siméon S, Flécher E, Revest M, Niculescu M, Roussel JC, Michel M, et al. Left ventricular assist device-related infections: a multicentric study. Clin Microbiol Infect. 2017;23(10):748–51.
129. Koval CE, Rakita R, Practice AIDCo. Ventricular assist device related infections and solid organ transplantation. Am J Transplant. 2013;13(Suppl 4):348–54.
130. Dell'Aquila AM, Mastrobuoni S, Alles S, Wenning C, Henryk W, Schneider SR, et al. Contributory role of fluorine 18-fluorodeoxyglucose positron emission tomography/computed tomography in the diagnosis and clinical management of infections in patients supported with a continuous-flow left ventricular assist device. Ann Thorac Surg. 2016;101(1):87–94.
131. Avramovic N, Dell'Aquila AM, Weckesser M, Milankovic D, Vrachimis A, Sindermann JR, et al. Metabolic volume performs better than SUVmax in the detection of left ventricular assist device driveline infection. Eur J Nucl Med Mol Imaging. 2017;44(11):1870–7.
132. Erba PA, Leo G, Sollini M, Tascini C, Boni R, Berchiolli RN, et al. Radiolabelled leucocyte scintigraphy versus conventional radiological imaging for the management of late, low-grade vascular prosthesis infections. Eur J Nucl Med Mol Imaging. 2014;41(2):357–68.
133. Osborne MT, Hulten EA, Murthy VL, Skali H, Taqueti VR, Dorbala S, et al. Patient preparation for cardiac fluorine-18 fluorodeoxyglucose positron emission tomography imaging of inflammation. J Nucl Cardiol. 2017;24(1):86–99.
134. Jamar F, Buscombe J, Chiti A, Christian PE, Delbeke D, Donohoe KJ, et al. EANM/SNMMI guideline for 18F-FDG use in inflammation and infection. J Nucl Med. 2013;54(4):647–58.
135. Rabkin Z, Israel O, Keidar Z. Do hyperglycemia and diabetes affect the incidence of false-negative 18F-FDG PET/CT studies in patients evaluated for infection or inflammation and cancer? A Comparative analysis. J Nucl Med. 2010;51(7):1015–20.
136. Scholtens AM, van Aarnhem EE, Budde RP. Effect of antibiotics on FDG-PET/CT imaging of prosthetic heart valve endocarditis. Eur Heart J Cardiovasc Imaging. 2015;16(11):1223.
137. Raplinger K, Chandler K, Hunt C, Johnson G, Peller P. Effect of steroid use during chemotherapy on SUV levels in PET/CT. J Nucl Med. 2012;53(suppl 1):2718.
138. Mikail N, Benali K, Ou P, Slama J, Hyafil F, Le Guludec D, et al. Detection of mycotic aneurysms of lower limbs by whole-body 18F-FDG-PET. JACC Cardiovasc Imaging. 2015;8(7):859–62.
139. Caldarella C, Leccisotti L, Treglia G, Giordano A. Which is the optimal acquisition time for FDG PET/CT imaging in patients with infective endocarditis? J Nucl Cardiol. 2013;20(2):307–9.
140. Leccisotti L, Perna F, Lago M, Leo M, Stefanelli A, Calcagni ML, et al. Cardiovascular implantable electronic device infection: delayed vs standard FDG PET-CT imaging. J Nucl Cardiol. 2014;21(3):622–32.
141. Scholtens AM, Swart LE, Verberne HJ, Budde RPJ, Lam MGEH. Dual-time-point FDG PET/CT imaging in prosthetic heart valve endocarditis. J Nucl Cardiol. 2018;25(6):1960–7.
142. Bucerius J, Mani V, Moncrieff C, Machac J, Fuster V, Farkouh ME, et al. Optimizing 18F-FDG PET/CT imaging of vessel wall inflammation: the impact of 18F-FDG circulation time, injected dose, uptake parameters, and fasting blood glucose levels. Eur J Nucl Med Mol Imaging. 2014;41(2):369–83.
143. Swart LE, Gomes A, Scholtens AM, Sinha B, Tanis W, Lam MGEH, et al. Improving the diagnostic performance of 18F-fluorodeoxyglucose positron-emission tomography/computed tomography in prosthetic heart valve endocarditis. Circulation. 2018;138(14):1412–27.
144. Fan CM, Fischman AJ, Kwek BH, Abbara S, Aquino SL. Lipomatous hypertrophy of the interatrial septum: increased uptake on FDG PET. AJR Am J Roentgenol. 2005;184(1):339–42.
145. Keidar Z, Pirmisashvili N, Leiderman M, Nitecki S, Israel O. 18F-FDG uptake in noninfected prosthetic vascular grafts: incidence, patterns, and changes over time. J Nucl Med. 2014;55(3):392–5.
146. Pizzi MN, Roque A, Cuéllar-Calabria H, Fernández-Hidalgo N, Ferreira-González I, González-Alujas MT, et al. F-FDG-PET/CTA of prosthetic cardiac valves and valve-tube grafts: infec-

tive versus inflammatory patterns. JACC Cardiovasc Imaging. 2016;9(10):1224–7.
147. Schouten LR, Verberne HJ, Bouma BJ, van Eck-Smit BL, Mulder BJ. Surgical glue for repair of the aortic root as a possible explanation for increased F-18 FDG uptake. J Nucl Cardiol. 2008;15(1):146–7.
148. Mathieu C, Mikaïl N, Benali K, Iung B, Duval X, Nataf P, et al. Characterization of ^{18}F-fluorodeoxyglucose uptake pattern in noninfected prosthetic heart valves. Circ Cardiovasc Imaging. 2017;10(3):e005585.
149. Sochowski RA, Chan KL. Implication of negative results on a monoplane transesophageal echocardiographic study in patients with suspected infective endocarditis. J Am Coll Cardiol. 1993;21(1):216–21.
150. Salaun E, Aldebert P, Jaussaud N, Spychaj JC, Maysou LA, Collart F, et al. Early endocarditis and delayed left ventricular pseudoaneurysm complicating a transapical transcatheter mitral valve-in-valve implantation: percutaneous closure under local anesthesia and echocardiographic guidance. Circ Cardiovasc Interv. 2016;9(10):pii:e003886.
151. Nishimura RA, Otto CM, Bonow RO, Carabello BA, Erwin JP, Guyton RA, et al. 2014 AHA/ACC guideline for the management of patients with valvular heart disease: executive summary: a report of the American College of Cardiology/American Heart Association Task Force on Practice Guidelines. Circulation. 2014;129(23):2440–92.
152. Baddour LM, Wilson WR, Bayer AS, Fowler VG, Bolger AF, Levison ME, et al. Infective endocarditis: diagnosis, antimicrobial therapy, and management of complications: a statement for healthcare professionals from the Committee on Rheumatic Fever, Endocarditis, and Kawasaki Disease, Council on Cardiovascular Disease in the Young, and the Councils on Clinical Cardiology, Stroke, and Cardiovascular Surgery and Anesthesia, American Heart Association: endorsed by the Infectious Diseases Society of America. Circulation. 2005;111(23):e394–434.

Nuclear Medicine Imaging of Fever of Unknown Origin

10

Elena Lazzeri, Roberta Zanca, and Martina Sollini

Contents

Learning Objectives

- To understand the pathophysiologic mechanisms that determine different patterns of uptake/accumulation of the different radiopharmaceuticals used in the diagnostic approach to patients with FUO
- To learn the usefulness of radionuclide imaging to evaluate the whole body with a single scan, compared to radiological imaging that usually investigates some a priori defined target regions of the body
- To learn how [18F]FDG-PET/CT can be used to diagnose infection/inflammation as well as oncologic conditions—a property that potentially reduces its specificity in patients with FUO
- To learn how labeled leukocyte scintigraphy can identify infection and inflammation—without however clearly discriminating these two conditions
- To understand the rationale of preferring the use of [18F]FDG PET/CT in patients with low probability that FUO is caused by infection
- To understand the rationale of preferring the use of labeled leukocyte scintigraphy in patients with high probability that FUO is caused by infection

Originally described in 1961 as a separate disease condition, the classification of fever of unknown origin (FUO) has been revised in 1996, according to four categories [1]:

- Classic presentation with fever that is higher than 38.3 °C on several occasions of at least 3 weeks duration and an uncertain diagnosis after 3 days of hospitalization, three outpatient visits or 1 week of “intelligent and invasive” ambulatory investigation.
- The nosocomial form.
- The immune deficient (neutropenic) form.
- The HIV-related form.

E. Lazzeri (✉) · R. Zanca
Regional Center of Nuclear Medicine, University Hospital of Pisa, Pisa, Italy
e-mail: e.lazzeri@ao-pisa.toscana.it

M. Sollini
Department of Biomedical Sciences, Humanitas University, Milan, Italy

E. Lazzeri et al. (eds.), *Radionuclide Imaging of Infection and Inflammation*, https://doi.org/10.1007/978-3-030-62175-9_10

With the latest definition of FUO, the four categories have been more recently modified as follows [2]:

- Temperature ≥ 38.3 °C (101 °F) on at least two occasions.
- Duration of illness ≥3 weeks or multiple febrile episodes in ≥3 weeks.
- Without reduction of immune defence, defined as neutropenia for at least 1 week in the 3 months before, known HIV infection, known hypogammaglobulinemia, or use of 10-mg prednisone or equivalent for at least 2 weeks in the 3 months before.
- Uncertain diagnosis despite thorough history-taking, physical examination, and the following investigations: erythrocyte sedimentation rate (ESR) or C-reactive protein (CRP), hemoglobin, platelet count, leukocyte count and differentiation, electrolytes, creatinine, total serum protein, protein electrophoresis, alkaline phosphatase, aspartate aminotransferase, alanine aminotransferase, lactate dehydrogenase, creatine kinase, ferritin, antinuclear antibodies, rheumatoid factor, microscopic urinalysis, three blood cultures, urine culture, chest X-ray, abdominal ultrasonography, and tuberculin skin test or interferon gamma release assay.

The main causes of FUO can be infections (21–54%), malignancies (6–31%), and noninfectious inflammatory diseases (13–24%) [3–5]. Detailed history, physical examination, and the search for potentially diagnostic clues (PDCs) are the most important steps in the diagnostic workup of FUO [4]. FUO is diagnosed in about 69.2% of the cases by noninvasive methods, whereas invasive methods are required in 30.8% of the cases [6].

Radiological imaging modalities (US, CT, and MRI) often constitute the first diagnostic imaging in the workup of patients with FUO. However, these imaging modalities can evaluate localized regions of the body and may yield negative results in an early phase of infective disease, because of the lack of substantial anatomical changes at this time. The differential diagnosis between active infectious from inflammatory lesions following treated processes or surgery is sometimes difficult by radiological techniques. These considerations explain the limitations of radiological imaging that is not rarely less sensitive than functional imaging methods such as those based on radionuclide imaging [7].

In patients with FUO, the nuclear medicine imaging procedures currently available include scintigraphy with ^{67}Ga-citrate, labeled autologous leukocytes, or anti-granulocyte monoclonal antibodies, and PET/CT with [^{18}F]FDG. Although these imaging methods possess high diagnostic accuracy, they are usually utilized as a second-line investigation in the diagnostic workup of FUO [7–10], somewhat as a problem-solving diagnostic test.

^{67}Ga-citrate scintigraphy is one of the earliest nuclear medicine techniques employed to identify acute and chronic infections that shows however quite low sensitivity (67%) and specificity (78%) [10]; these suboptimal diagnostic parameters are due to its property to localize both in inflammatory sites and in tumor lesions [11, 12]. The low specificity of ^{67}Ga-citrate scintigraphy for infection may however represent an advantage, because it may allow the detection of a large spectrum of diseases possibly causing FUO. The disadvantages of ^{67}Ga-citrate include a high burden radiation to patients, relatively poor imaging quality (due to the gamma emissions of 67 Ga that are suboptimal for gamma camera imaging), and long acquisition time (up to 48–72 h post injection of the tracer) [11, 12].

Scintigraphy with labeled autologous leukocytes (WBC) shows higher sensitivity (60–85% and 96% for ^{111}In-oxine-WBC and for ^{99m}Tc-HMPAO-WBC, respectively) and specificity (78–94% for ^{111}In-oxine-WBC and for ^{99m}Tc-HMPAO-WBC, respectively) in the evaluation of patients with FUO [13–15]. This imaging technique represents the first-choice nuclear medicine imaging modality in patients with FUO with high probability of infectious origin.

In some patients with FUO, PET/CT with autologous leukocytes labeled in vitro with [^{18}F]FDG [16] showed higher spatial resolution imaging than single-photon imaging. However, the short physical half-life of ^{18}F represents an important drawback to this technique when evaluating leukocyte diapedesis over time in infection sites (at least 24 h); thus, the short time-window for acquisition of [^{18}F]FDG-leukocyte PET imaging does not permit to distinguish inflammatory from septic foci of accumulation.

The use of ^{111}In-labeled human immunoglobulin as an infection imaging agent has been investigated in patients with FUO, showing an overall 60% sensitivity and 83% specificity, yielding diagnostic information in a small percentage (about 18%) of the patients [17]; originally reported for this application in 1997, this tracer is no longer available for routine clinical use.

In the 1990s, it was reported that a murine anti-CEA monoclonal antibody that had originally been developed as a tumor-seeking agent (anti-NCA-95 IgG or compound BW 250/183), actually bound quite firmly to circulating granulocytes upon its i.v. administration; thus, administration of this agent resulted in an in vivo labeling of the patient's leukocytes. When evaluated in patients with FUO, ^{99m}Tc-anti-NCA-IgG (BW 250/183) identified infectious sites as the cause of FUO with 40–73% sensitivity and 92–97% specificity [18–20]. The main disadvantage for the clinical application of this monoclonal antibody is the possible generation of human anti-mouse antibodies (HAMA); for this reason, it can be safely used only once in the patient's lifetime.

Since both inflammatory cells and tumor cells have an increased glucometabolic demand, PET/CT with [^{18}F]FDG can usefully be performed in patients with FUO, especially in those with low probability of infection as the cause of FUO. The increased GLUT expression and upregulation of hexokinase enzymes in inflammatory and neoplastic cells allows the entry of [^{18}F]FDG that accumulates in all cells with a high glycolytic rate. All populations of activated leukocytes show increased [^{18}F]FDG uptake, thus preventing the possibility of [^{18}F]FDG imaging to discriminate between inflammation and infection, as well as between acute and chronic infection [2].

Additional limitations of [^{18}F]FDG PET/CT concern infection imaging in the brain or exploration of the urinary tract, because of the high physiologic [^{18}F]FDG uptake in the brain and urinary excretion of the tracer, respectively. When investigating the heart (searching for, e.g., infectious endocarditis), it is mandatory to suppress [^{18}F]FDG uptake in the myocardium by following a previous high-fat and low-carbohydrate diet for at least 24 h before the scan [2].

The main advantages of [^{18}F]FDG PET/CT are its high-quality imaging, short time required for imaging, and its high diagnostic accuracy for infections affecting the spine, as well as for chronic low-grade infections. The usefulness of [^{18}F]FDG PET/CT for investigating the source of fever has been demonstrated in many studies, where the site of infection causing FUO has been identified in 42–67% of patients [21–40]; such diagnostic performance is clinically nonnegligible, considering that in all such patients the traditional imaging modalities (US, CT, and MRI) had failed to identify the cause of FUO.

A comparative study between [^{18}F]FDG PET and ^{111}In-oxine-WBC scintigraphy in patients with FUO showed better diagnostic accuracy of WBC (71% sensitivity, 92% specificity, 85% positive and negative predictive values) compared to [^{18}F]FDG PET (50% sensitivity, 46% specificity, 30% positive and 67% negative predictive values) [41]. Whereas, in a more recent study in 58 patients with FUO, Hung et al. compared the diagnostic performance of [^{18}F]FDG PET/CT and of ^{67}Ga-citrate scintigraphy with SPECT/CT, the two radionuclide scans being performed within 7 days one from each other. This study showed that [^{18}F]FDG PET/CT provided clinically useful information in a significantly higher proportion of patients than ^{67}Ga-citrate SPECT/CT (57% versus 33%, $P < 0.05$) [42].

Based on extensive review of the literature, [^{18}F]FDG PET/CT is currently considered the radionuclide diagnostic procedure of choice for patients with FUO with low or intermediate probability of infection, because of its high negative-predictive value. Labeled leukocyte scintigraphy is instead the diagnostic procedure of choice in patients with FUO with high probability of infection as the cause of FUO; in this regard, the EANM acquisition modalities and interpretation criteria are highly recommended [43].

Key Learning Points

- Scintigraphy with ^{67}Ga-citrate is no longer recommended because of important drawbacks in terms of radiation burden to patients, generally poor image quality, and long-time interval between administration and acquisition of diagnostic quality images.
- PET/CT with [^{18}F]FDG is especially useful to identify the sites of infection/inflammation, without discriminating however between infection and inflammation.
- Especially if integrated with SPECT/CT acquisition, leukocyte scintigraphy can identify infection as the cause of FUO, also providing useful information for distinguishing infection from inflammation.
- Leukocyte scintigraphy is not recommended to evaluate patients with FUO with suspected spine infection.

Imaging in Patients with Fever of Unknown Origin

Clinical Cases

Case 10.1

Elena Lazzeri

Background

A 65-year-old man with fever, pain in the epigastric region, and jaundice. The CT scan of the abdomen showed a rather diffuse enlargement in size of the pancreas, without clear signs of focal lesion(s) (Fig. 10.15a). MRI confirmed the increase of pancreas size, but also visualized a focal lesion (about 3 cm in size) in the head of pancreas (Fig. 10.15b).

Based on these findings, the patient was referred for [^{18}F]FDG PET/CT for suspected pancreatic cancer. Contrary to expectation, the [^{18}F]FDG PET/CT scan only showed diffuse, mildly increased uptake of the pancreas parenchyma (Fig. 10.15c). Based on this pattern, the hypothesis of pancreatic cancer was ruled out, as the findings were consistent with pancreatitis. The final diagnosis was autoimmune pancreatitis.

Suspected Site of Disease

Pancreas.

Radiopharmaceutical Activity

[^{18}F]FDG, 270 MBq.

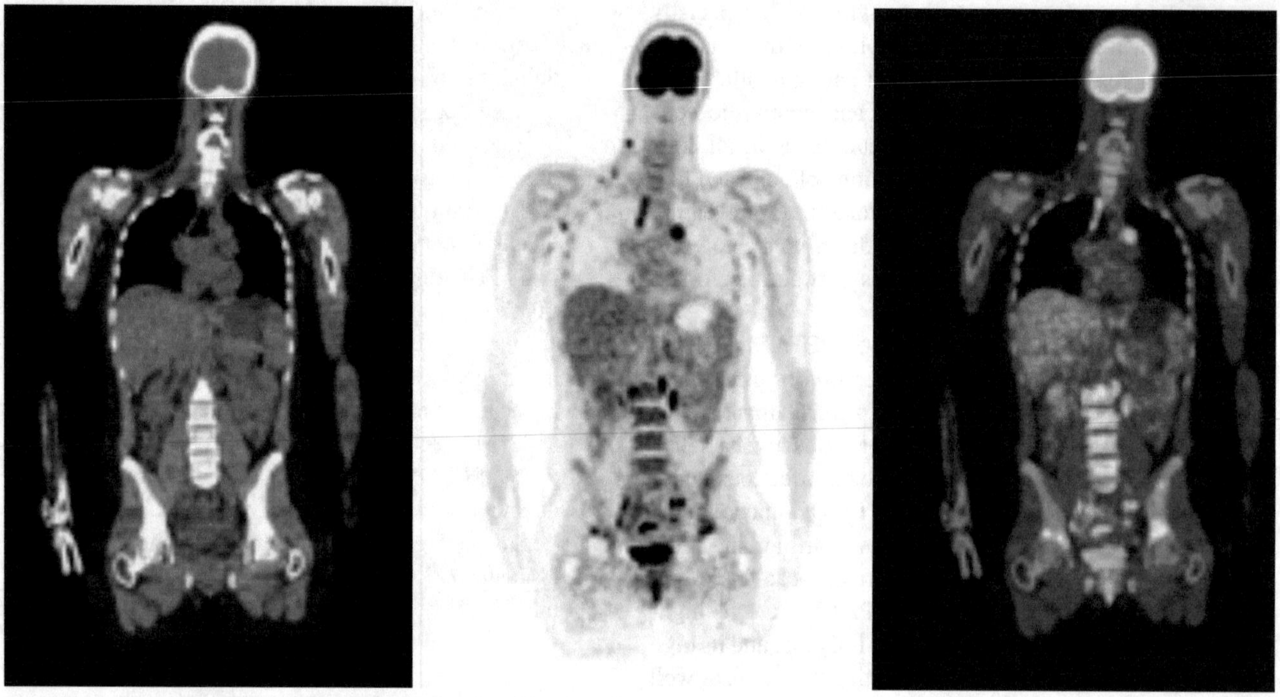

Fig. 10.1 [18F]FDG PET/CT in a patient with FUO: the coronal sections (CT, left; PET, middle; fused PET/CT, right) show increased [18F]FDG uptake in the right cervical, axillary, and mediastinal lymph nodes. The spleen is markedly increased in size. Lymph node biopsy demonstrated that a lymphoma was responsible for fever

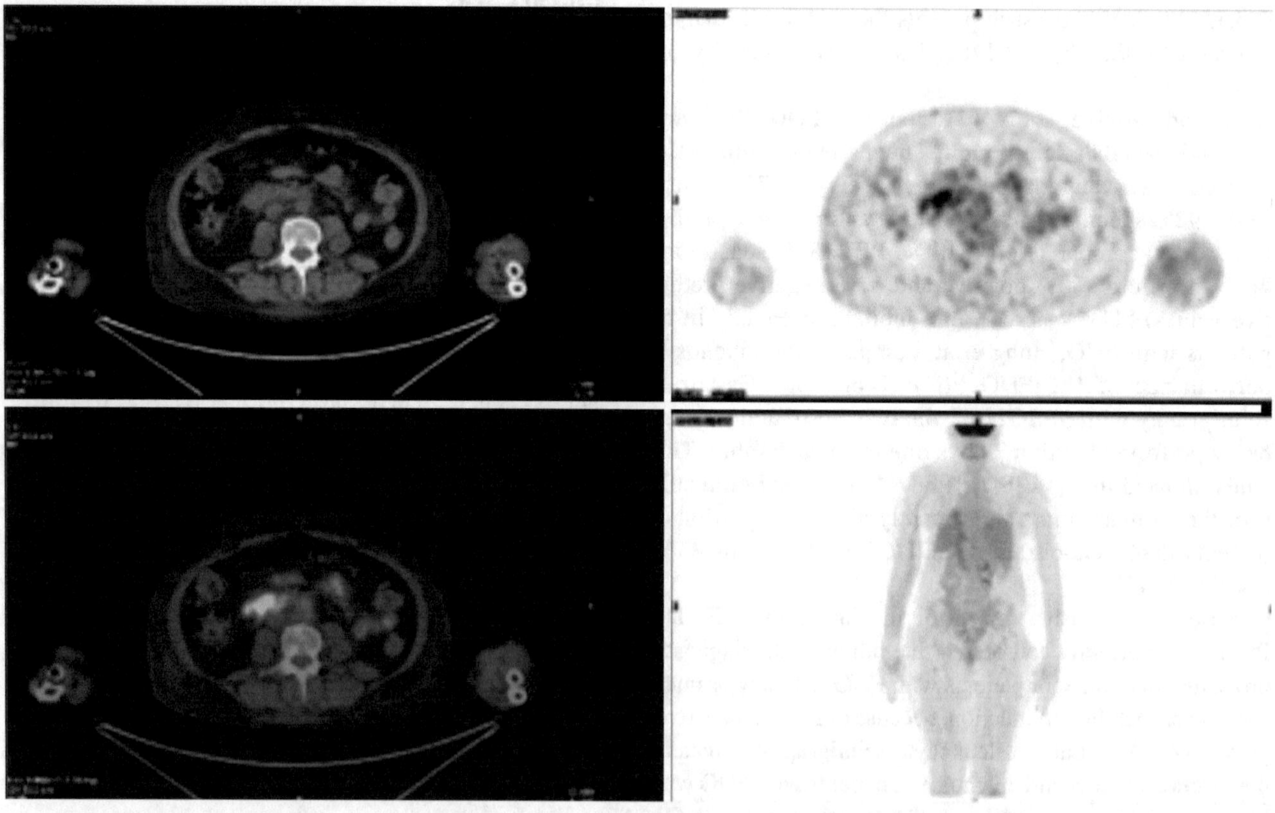

Fig. 10.2 [18F]FDG PET/CT in a patient with FUO: the transaxial sections (CT, upper left; PET, upper right; fused PET/CT, lower left; MIP, lower right) show increased [18F]FDG uptake in the head of pancreas head. Final diagnosis was acute pancreatitis

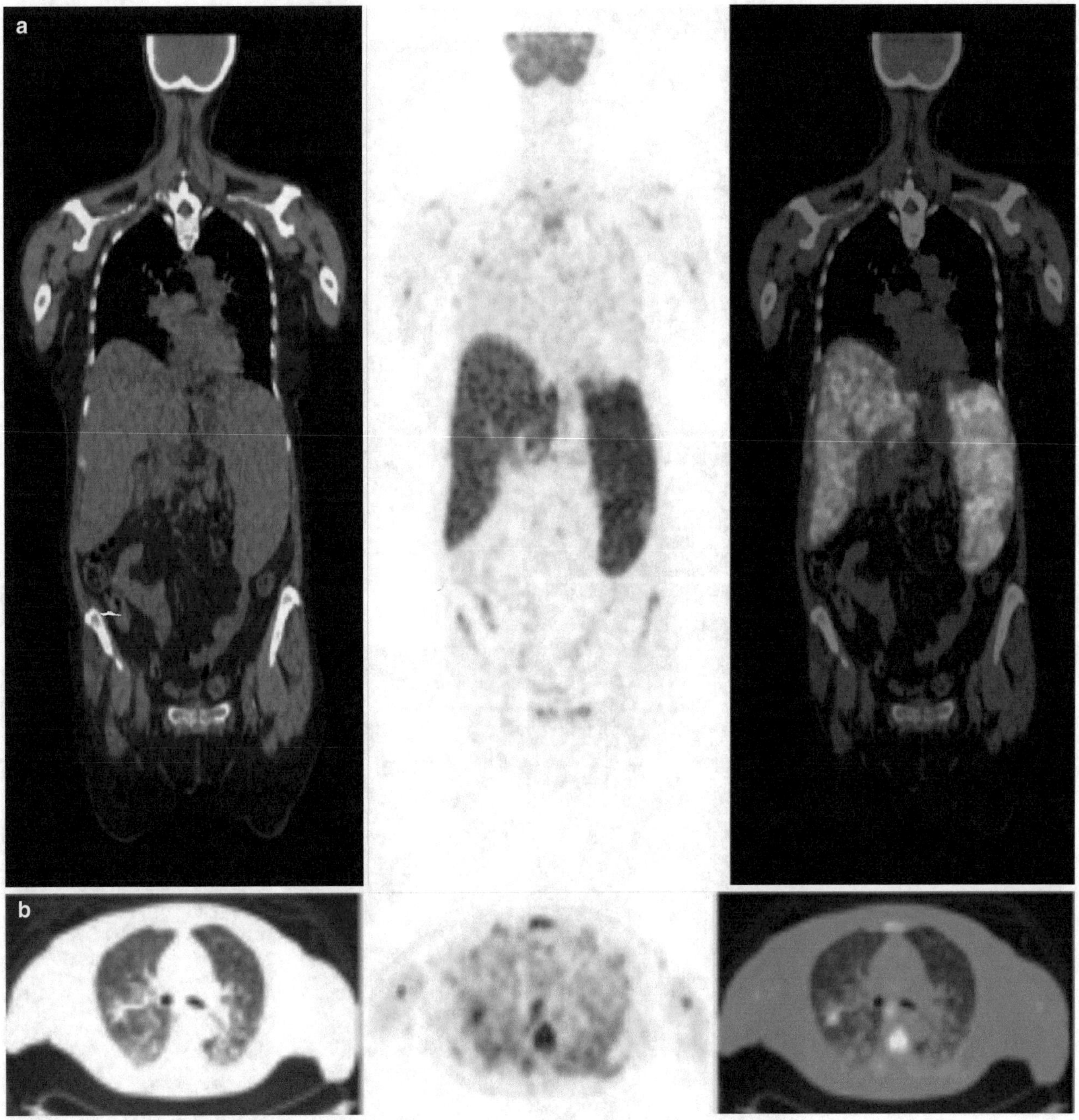

Fig. 10.3 [^{18}F]FDG PET/C in a patient with FUO: (**a**) the coronal sections (CT, left; PET, middle; fused PET/CT, right) show diffuse, markedly increased [^{18}F]FDG uptake in the spleen and liver that are also enlarged in size (especially the spleen). (**b**) The transaxial midthoracic sections (CT, left; PET, middle; fused PET/CT, right) show irregularly increased [^{18}F]FDG uptake in the right lung, where the low-dose CT image demonstrates the presence of cavitations, as well as bronchohilar and centrolobular opacities; enlarged lymph nodes are also present both above and below the diaphragm. Final diagnosis was diffuse tubercular infection

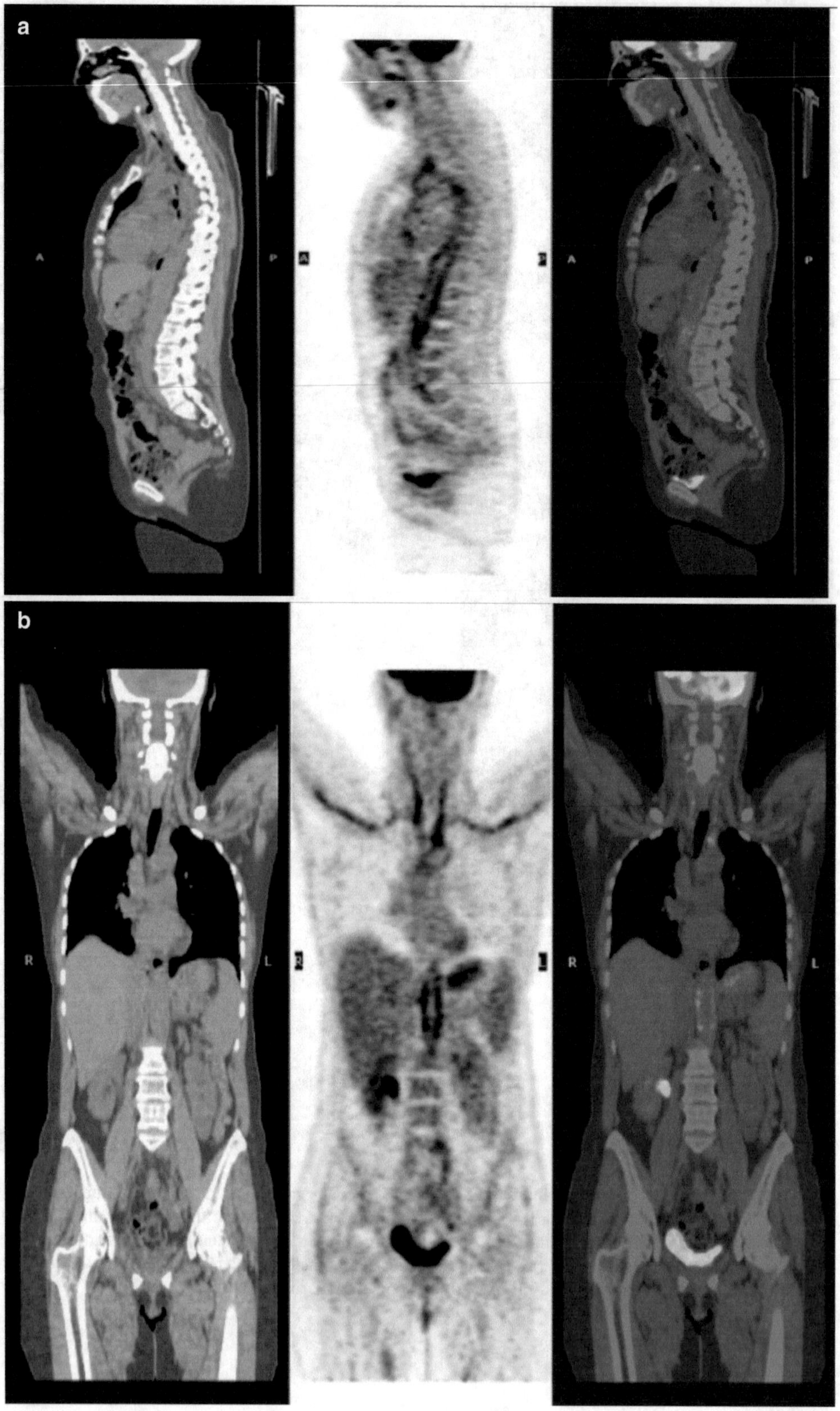

Fig. 10.4 [^{18}F]FDG PET/CT in a patient with FUO: (**a**) the sagittal sections (CT, left; PET, middle; fused PET/CT, right) show increased [^{18}F]FDG uptake in the wall of thoracic aorta. (**b**) The coronal sections (CT, left; PET, middle; fused PET/CT, right) show increased [^{18}F]FDG uptake, greater than liver uptake, in the epiaortic vessels and bilateral succlavia. Final diagnosis was acute Takayasu vasculitis

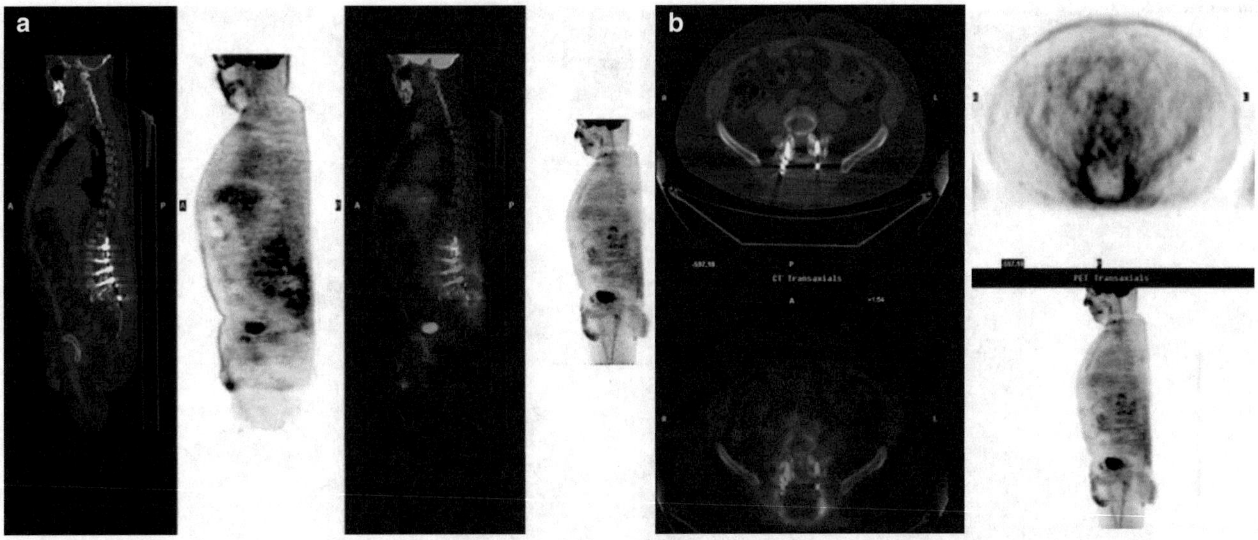

Fig. 10.5 [^{18}F]FDG PET/CT in a patient with FUO who had been submitted to surgery of the lumbar spine with implantation of metallic hardware: (**a**) the sagittal sections (from left to right: CT; PET; fused PET/CT; MIP) and the transaxial sections (**b**) (CT, upper left; PET, upper right; fused PET/CT, lower left; MIP image, lower right) show increased [^{18}F]FDG uptake in posterior tissues near to the vertebral implant. This post-surgical infection was responsible for fever

Imaging

[^{18}F]FDG PET/CT acquired 60 min post injection, including CT scout view (120 kV, 10 mA), whole-body CT scan (140 kV, 80 mA), and PET (3 min/FOV). Images were reconstructed with and without attenuation correction using the low-dose transmission CT scan.

Conclusion/Teaching Point

[^{18}F]FDG PET/CT ruled out the presence of neoplastic disease of pancreas and identified the origin of FUO and jaundice as autoimmune pancreatitis.

Case 10.2

Viviana Frantellizzi

(Nuclear Medicine Department, University "La Sapienza", Rome, Italy
viviana.frantellizzi@uniroma1.it).

Background

A 31-year-old woman with autosomic dominant hyper-IgE syndrome (a rare form of congenital, non-X-linked severe immune deficiency) was referred for remittent FUO. Medical history included right nephrectomy at the age of 8 years because of abscess, as well as abdominal abscesses at multiple sites and recurrent bronchopneumonia; the patient was kept on chronic antibiotic therapy.

MRI of the upper (coronal T2-STIR images in Fig. 10.16a) showed multiple focal roundish lesions in the liver parenchyma with regular wall and inhomogeneous fluid content; numerous foci of lung parenchymal consolidation and bronchiectasis on the basal region of the right lung were also detected. These findings were consistent with the clinical suspicion of multiple abscess localizations.

^{99m}Tc-HMPAO-WBC scintigraphy was performed to better characterize the focal lesions detected on MRI. The scan showed mild but increasing over time accumulation of labeled leukocytes in the antero-basal region of the right lung and in the upper region of the liver (Fig. 10.16b), matching the MRI findings and confirming the diagnosis of multiple abscess localizations in the liver and in the lower lobe of right lung.

Suspected Site of Infection

Lung and liver.

Radiopharmaceutical Activity

^{99m}Tc-HMPAO-WBC scintigraphy: acquisition of planar imaging at 1 h, 4 h, and 20 h.

Conclusion/Teaching Point

^{99m}Tc-HMPAO-WBC scintigraphy detected multiple sites of labeled leukocyte accumulation matching the MRI findings, therefore confirming the diagnosis of multiple abscess localizations in the liver and in the lower lobe of right lung.

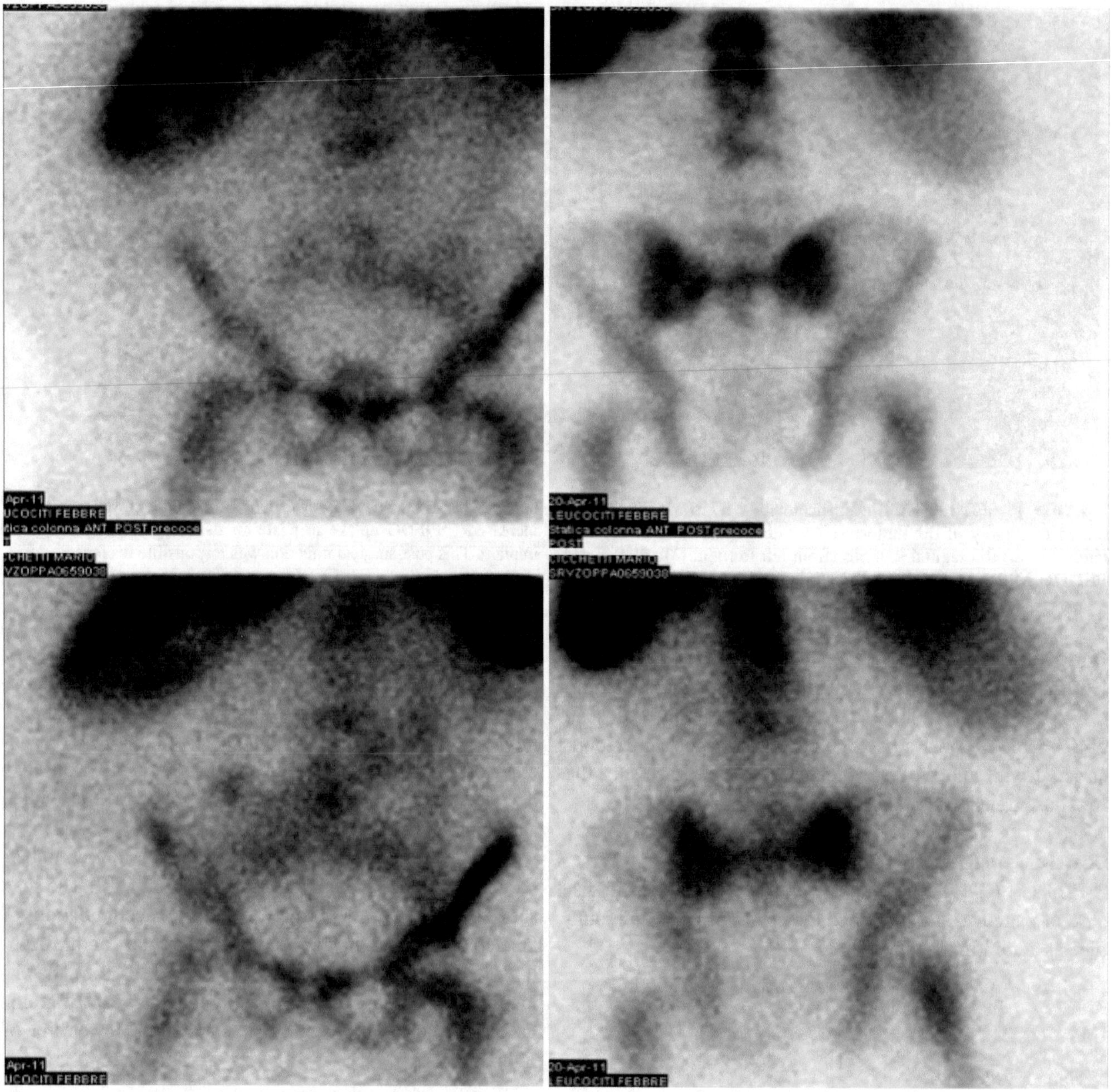

Fig. 10.6 ^{99m}Tc-HMPAO-WBC scintigraphy in a patient with FUO: the planar anterior and posterior views at 2 h (upper panel) and 24 (bottom panel) clearly show an area of reduced accumulation of labeled leukocytes in the lumbar vertebral region (L3–L5). MRI confirmed the presence of spine infection, as suspected on the basis of the scintigraphic pattern, as the cause of fever

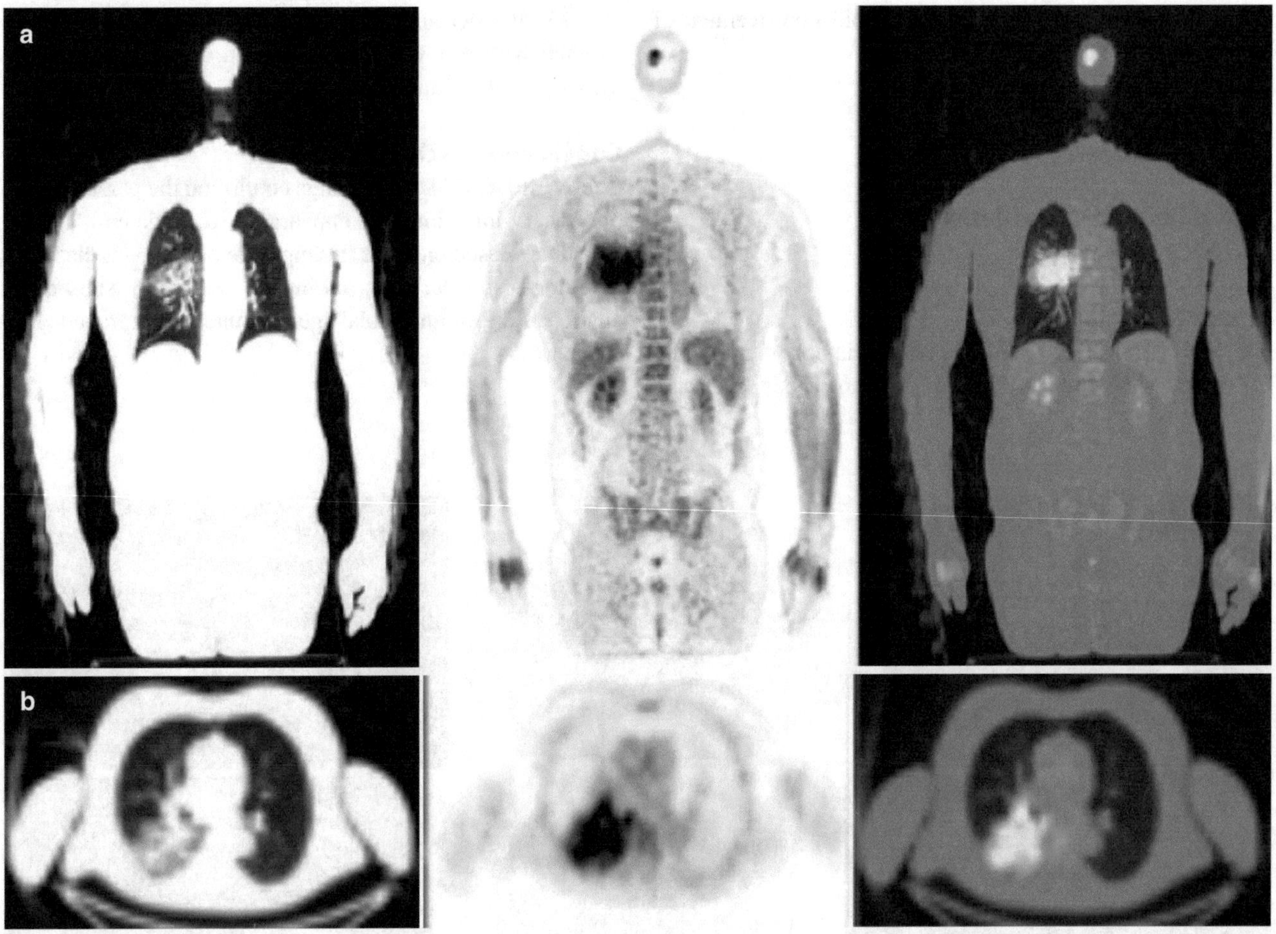

Fig. 10.7 [^{18}F]FDG PET/CT in a patient with FUO: (**a**) the coronal slices (CT, left; PET, middle; fused PET/CT, right) show markedly increased [^{18}F]FDG uptake in the mid-portion of right lung. (**b**) The transaxial sections (CT, left; PET, middle; fused PET/CT, right) localize such area of focally increased tracer uptake in the posterior region of right lung. The low-dose CT images show diffuse ground-glass opacities corresponding to the areas of increased [^{18}F]FDG uptake. Fever was due to bacterial pneumonia

Case 10.3

Elena Lazzeri

Background

A 56-year-old man with prior diagnosis of lung infection (but without certain etiology), undergoing long-lasting antibiotic treatment. Fever and coughing persisted despite antimicrobial therapy; moreover, lumbar back pain appeared.

The patient was referred for [^{18}F]FDG PET/CT to evaluate the presence and extension of lung infection. The PET/CT scan showed diffuse, increased [^{18}F]FDG uptake in pulmonary parenchyma, bilaterally (Fig. 10.17). PET images showed, furthermore, increased [^{18}F]FDG uptake in the lumbar spine, corresponding to L4–L5. The findings were consistent with the persistence of lung infection and appearance of infection in the lumbar spine. A subsequent MRI scan confirmed lumbar L4–L5 spondylodiscitis. Change in the antibiotic treatment plan resulted in rapid improvement of the patient's clinical conditions.

Suspected Site of Infection

Lungs.

Radiopharmaceutical Activity

[^{18}F]FDG, 184 MBq.

Imaging

[^{18}F]FDG PET/CT acquired 60 min post injection, including CT scout view (120 kV, 10 mA), whole-body CT scan (140 kV, 80 mA), and PET (3 min/FOV). Images were reconstructed with and without attenuation correction using the low-dose transmission CT scan.

Conclusion/Teaching Point

The [^{18}F]FDG PET/CT findings confirmed the persistence of pulmonary infection with appearance of septic embolism in the spine. Based on these findings, the patient was classified as "non-responder" to antibiotic treatment; subsequent change of the antimicrobial agent resulted in improved clinical status.

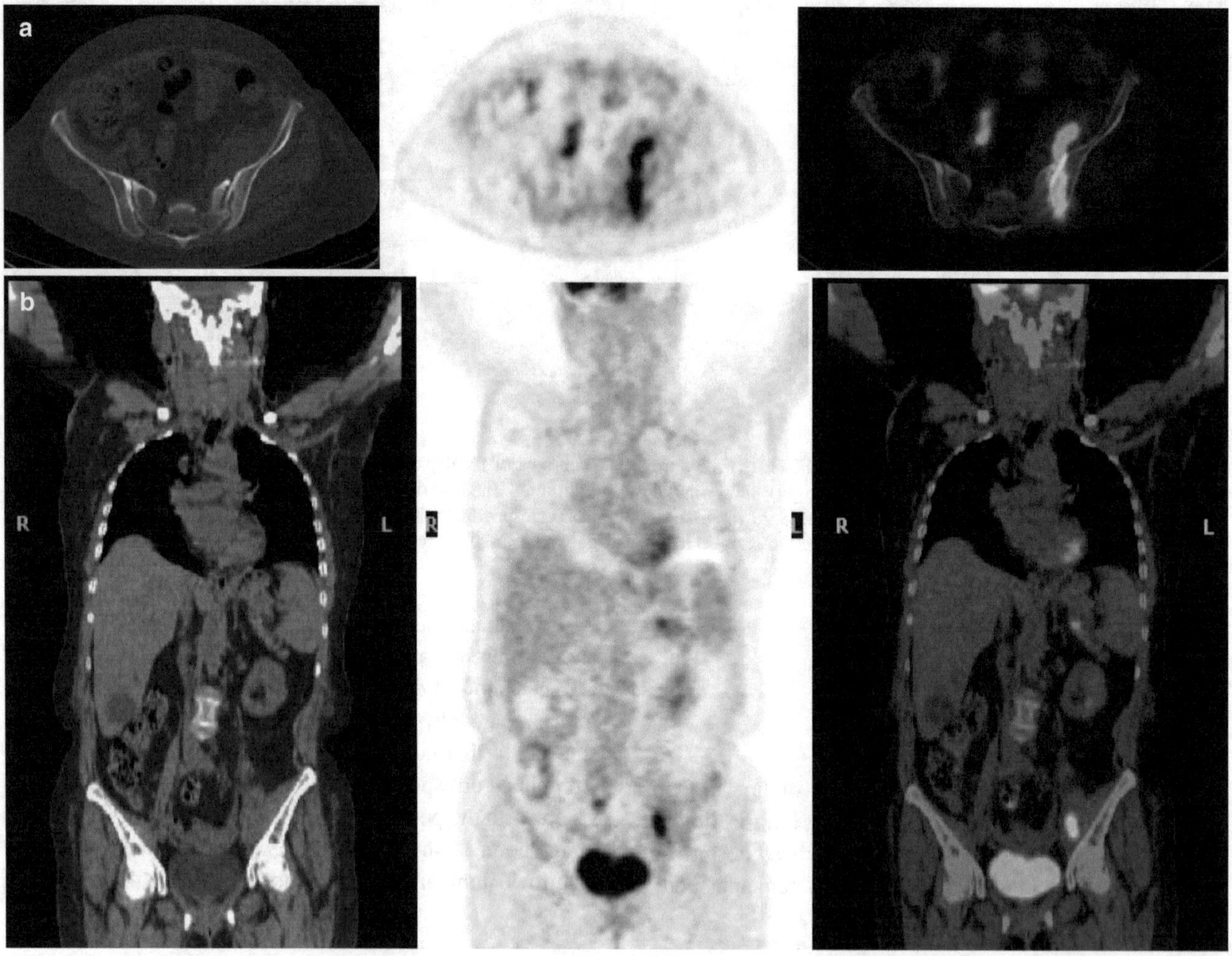

Fig. 10.8 [^{18}F]FDG PET/CT in a patient with FUO: (**a**) the transaxial sections (CT, left; PET, middle; fused PET/CT, right) show increased [^{18}F]FDG uptake at the left sacroiliac joint, with involvement also of the adjacent iliopsoas muscle. (**b**) and (**c**): Two coronal sections in different planes visualize extension of the infection along the whole anterior portion of the iliopsoas muscle. (**d**) Sagittal sections better visualize markedly increased [^{18}F]FDG uptake involving simultaneously the left sacroiliac joint and the left iliopsoas muscle. Final diagnosis was fever caused by infection of the left sacroiliac joint with soft tissue involvement

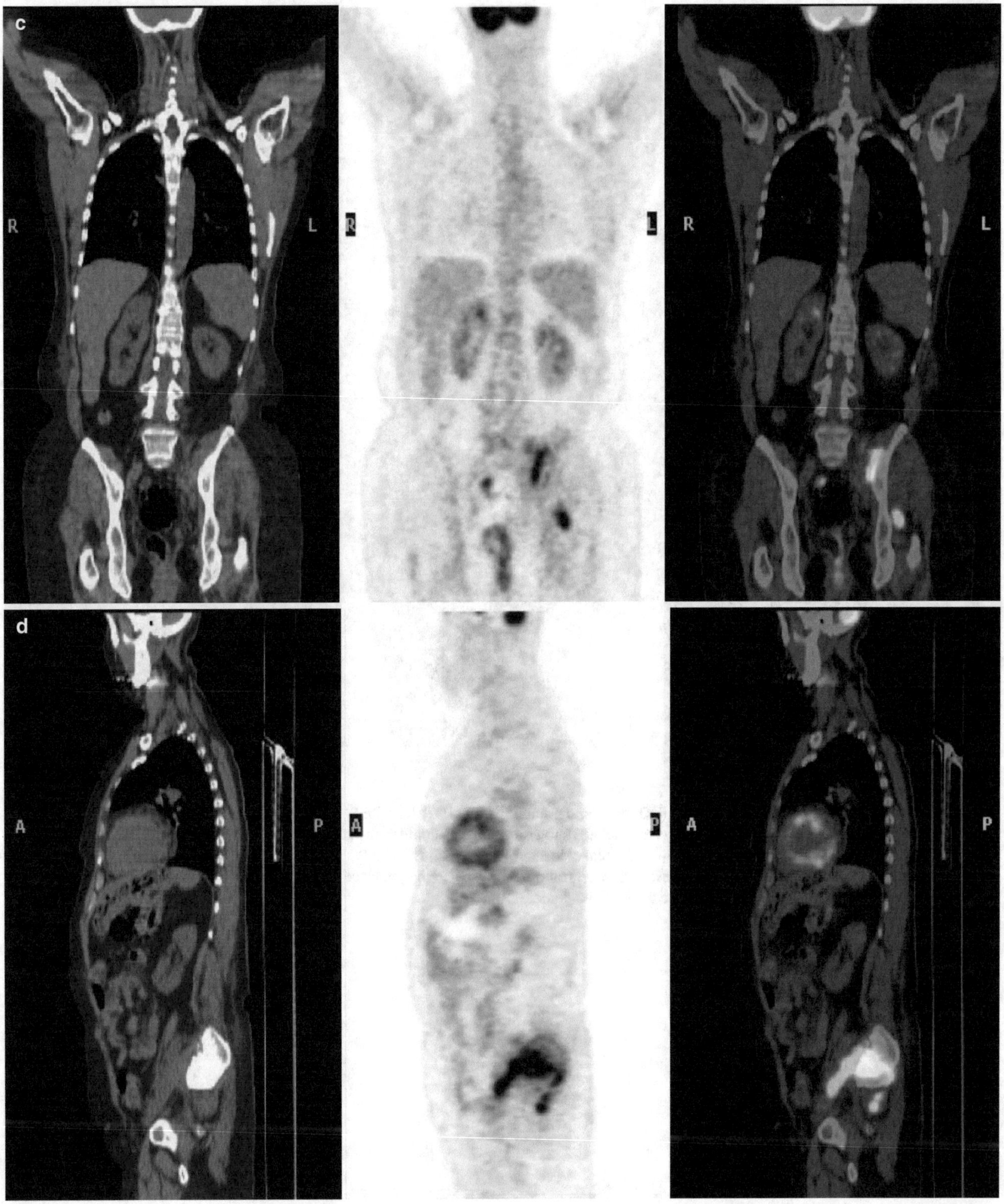

Fig. 10.8 (continued)

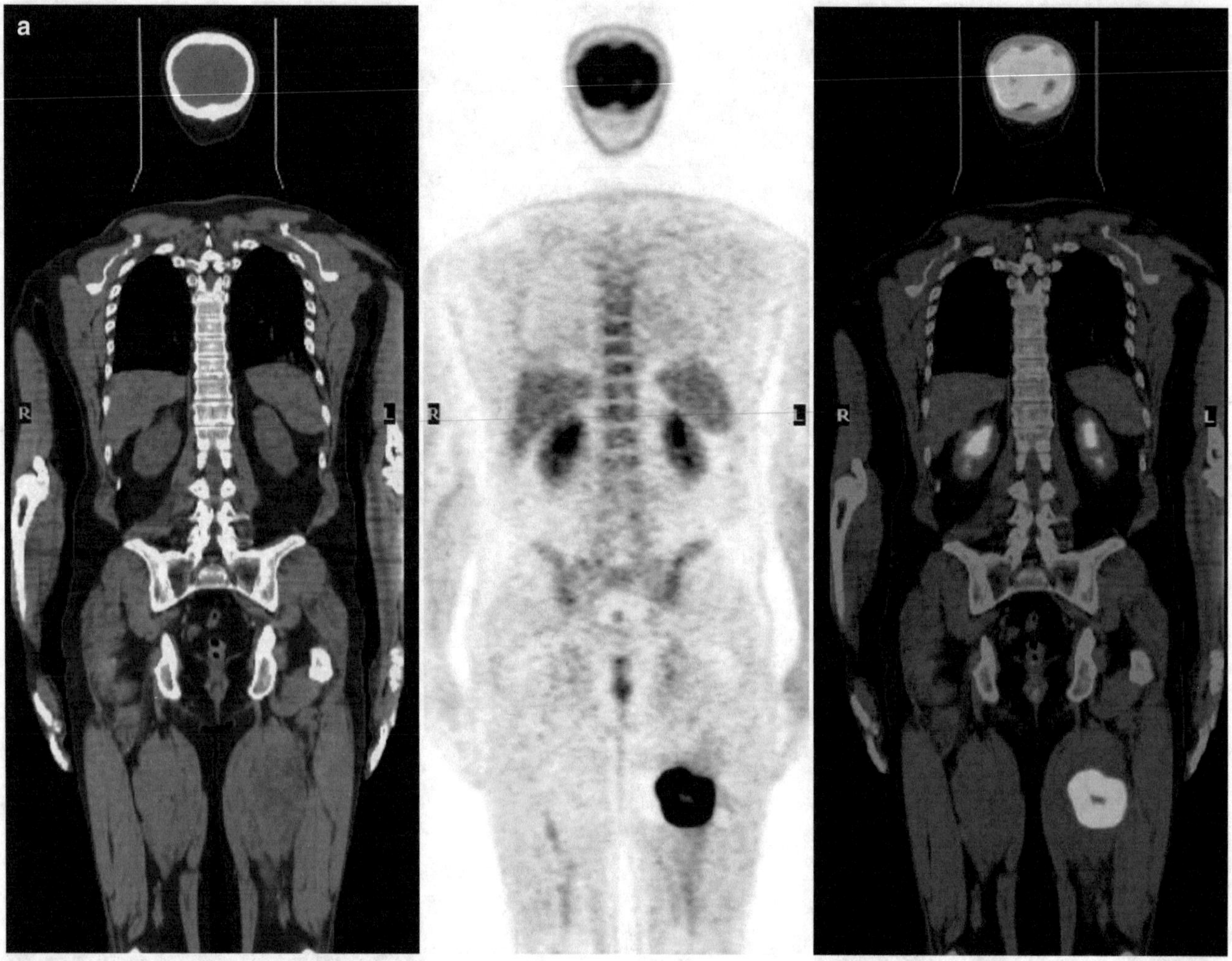

Fig. 10.9 [18F]FDG PET/CT in a patient with FUO: the tomographic images (shown in (**a**, coronal), (**b**, sagittal), and (**c**, transaxial)) shows a well-defined focus of markedly increased [18F]FDG uptake located between the quadriceps and the sartorius muscles, with a central area with reduced/absent uptake; there is no involvement of the femoral bone (CT, left; PET, middle; fused PET/CT, right). The low-dose CT images confirm the presence of a mass with mildly reduced and inhomogeneous density. Histology of a biopsy sample from the mass revealed the presence of sarcoma

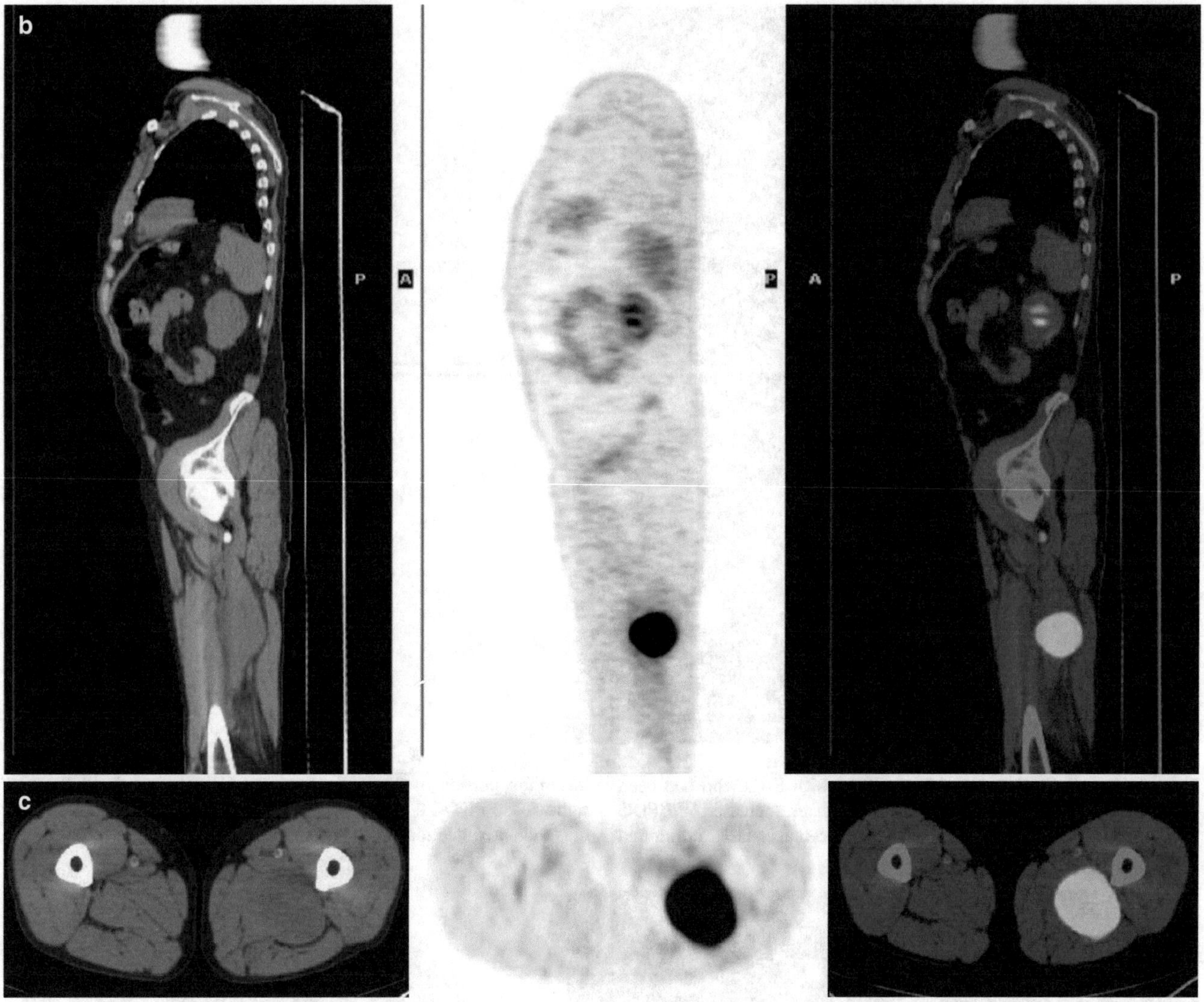

Fig. 10.9 (continued)

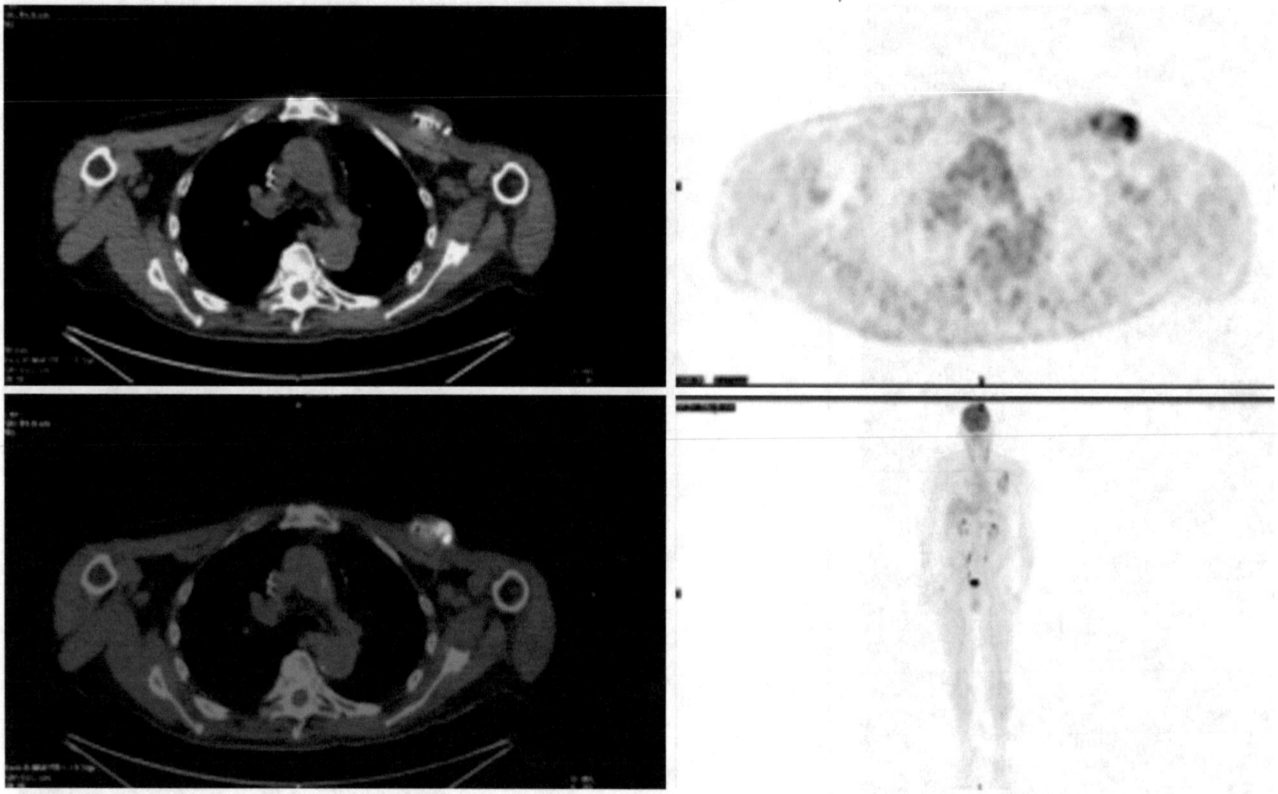

Fig. 10.10 [¹⁸F]FDG PET/CT in a patient with FUO who had been submitted to implantation of a cardiac pacemaker. Increased [¹⁸F]FDG uptake was observed in the subcutaneous pacemaker task and around the initial portion of the lead (transaxial CT, upper left; PET, upper right; fused PET/CT, lower left; MIP image, lower right). These findings indicate infection of the pacemaker task as the cause of fever

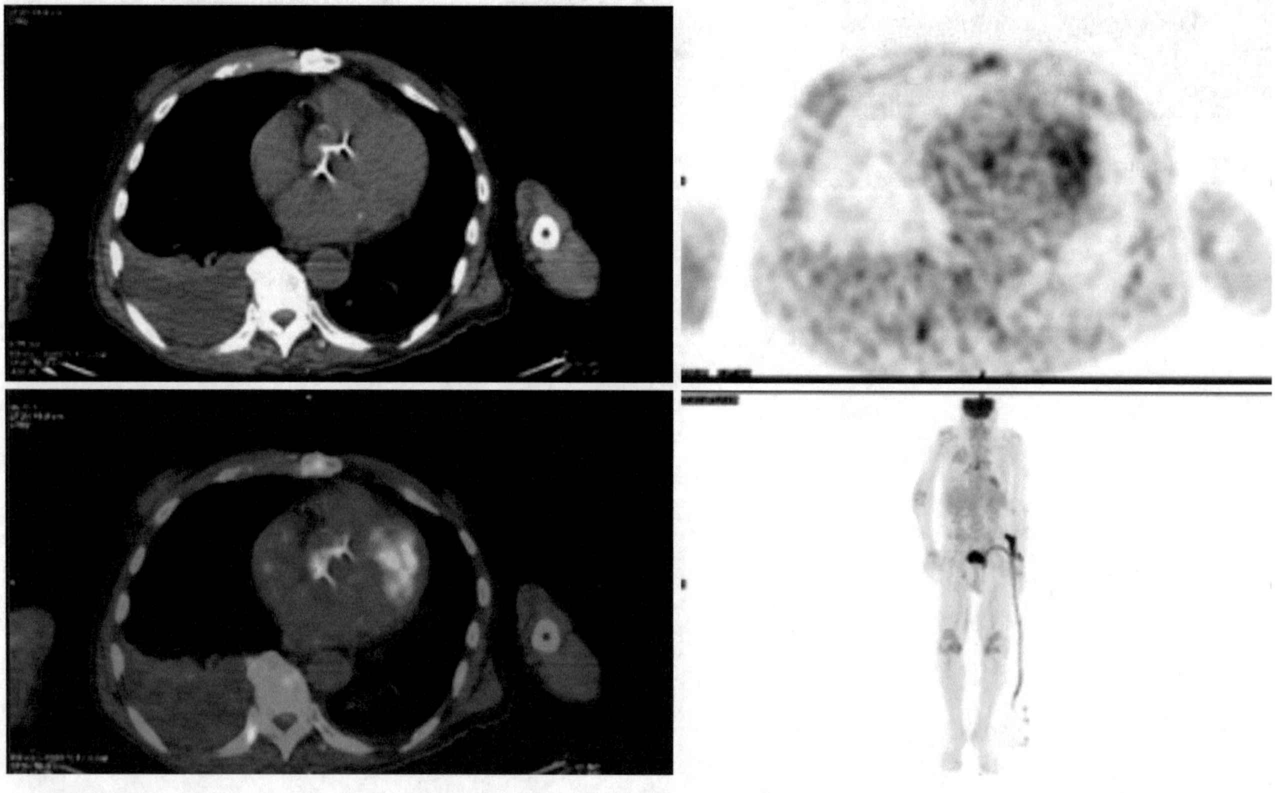

Fig. 10.11 [¹⁸F]FDG PET/CT in a patient with FUO who had been submitted to implantation of a prosthetic aortic valve. Increased [¹⁸F]FDG uptake was observed at the prosthetic aortic valve, well identified by the metallic artifact in the low-dose CT component of the scan (transaxial CT, upper left; PET, upper right; fused PET/CT, lower left; MIP image, lower right). These findings indicate infective endocarditis as the cause of fever

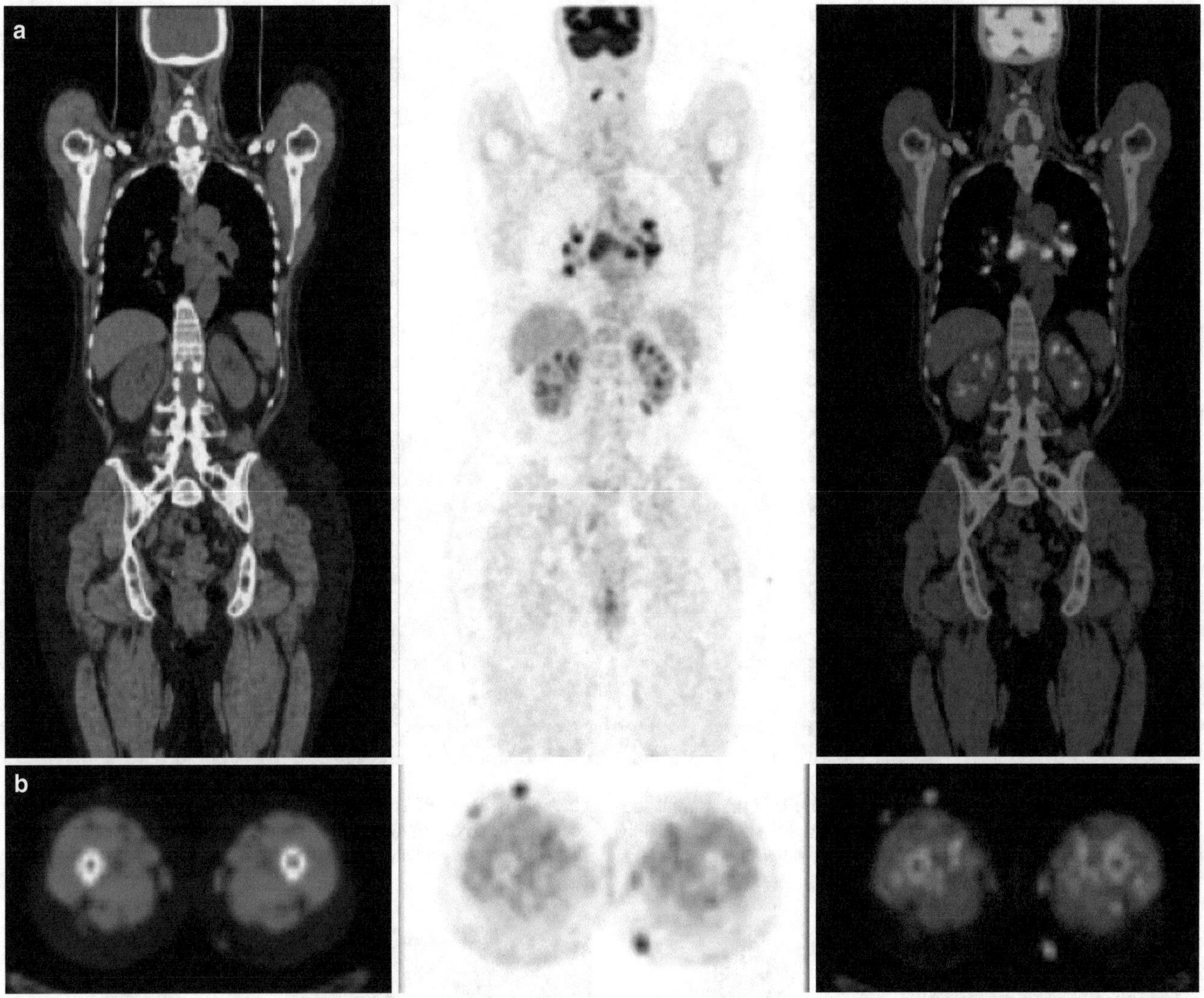

Fig. 10.12 [^{18}F]FDG PET/CT in a patient with FUO: (**a**) the coronal sections (CT, left; PET, middle; fused PET/CT, right) show markedly increased [^{18}F]FDG uptake involving at many mediastinal lymph nodes that appear as bilateral peri-hilar consolidations. In addition, transaxial sections of the lower limbs (**b**) show increased tracer uptake at multiple subcutaneous nodules. Flare of sarcoidosis was responsible for fever

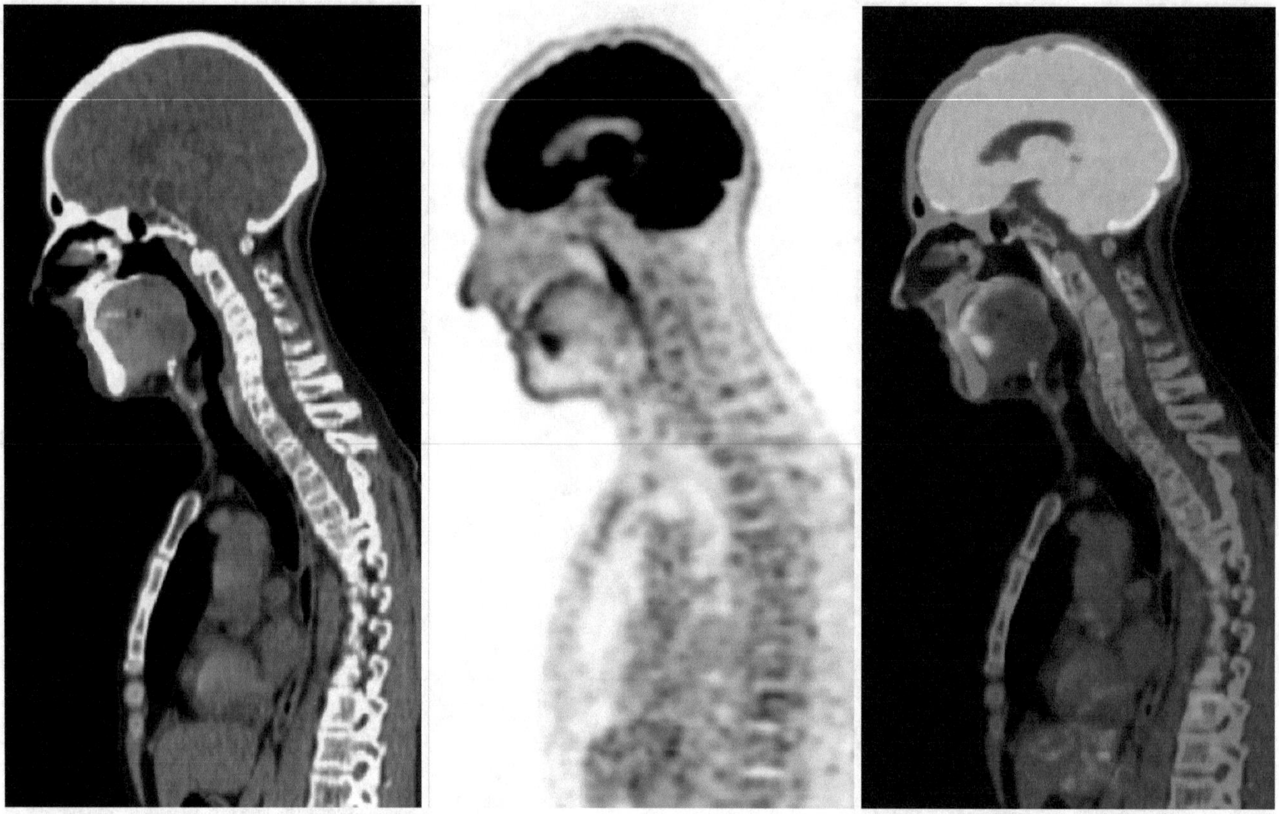

Fig. 10.13 [^{18}F]FDG PET/CT in a patient with FUO: the sagittal sections (CT, left; PET, middle; fused PET/CT, right) show moderately increased [^{18}F]FDG uptake at the nasopharynx, suggesting acute nasopharyngitis. These PET/CT findings turned out to be false positive, since acute nasopharyngitis was not present; the moderately increased [^{18}F]FDG uptake was probably due to a nonspecific inflammatory condition

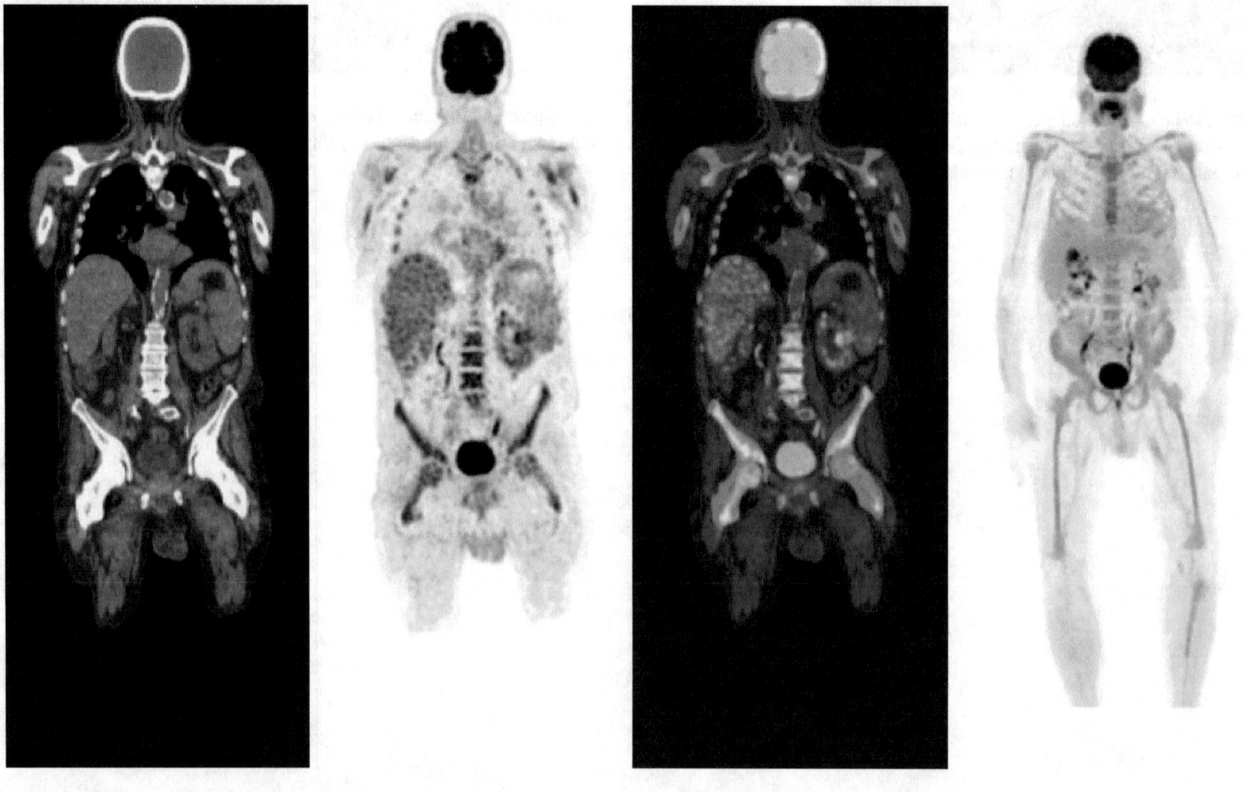

Fig. 10.14 [^{18}F]FDG PET/CT in a patient with FUO: coronal sections (from left to right: CT, PET, fused PET/CT, MIP image) showing markedly increased [^{18}F]FDG uptake in the bone marrow. Final diagnosis was myelodysplasia as the cause of fever

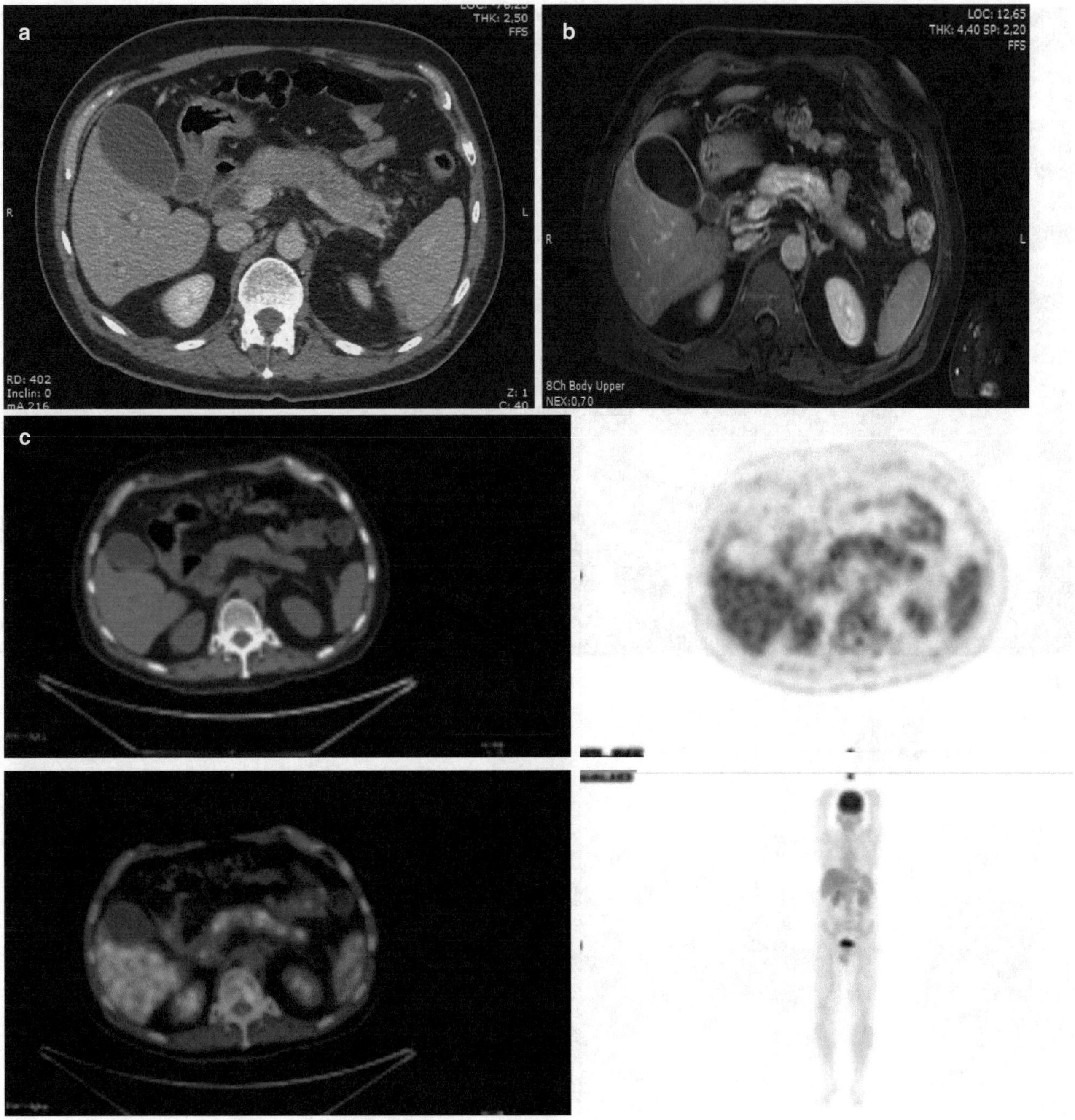

Fig. 10.15 (**a**) Abdominal CT showing diffuse enlargement of pancreas, with a somewhat inhomogeneous parenchyma. (**b**) Abdominal MRI showing the increase of contrast enhancement of the head and body of pancreas. (**c**) Transaxial sections of [^{18}F]FDG PET/CT (CT, upper left; PET, upper right; fused PET/CT, lower left; MIP image, lower right), showing diffuse, mildly increased tracer uptake in the whole pancreas. These findings are consistent with pancreatitis

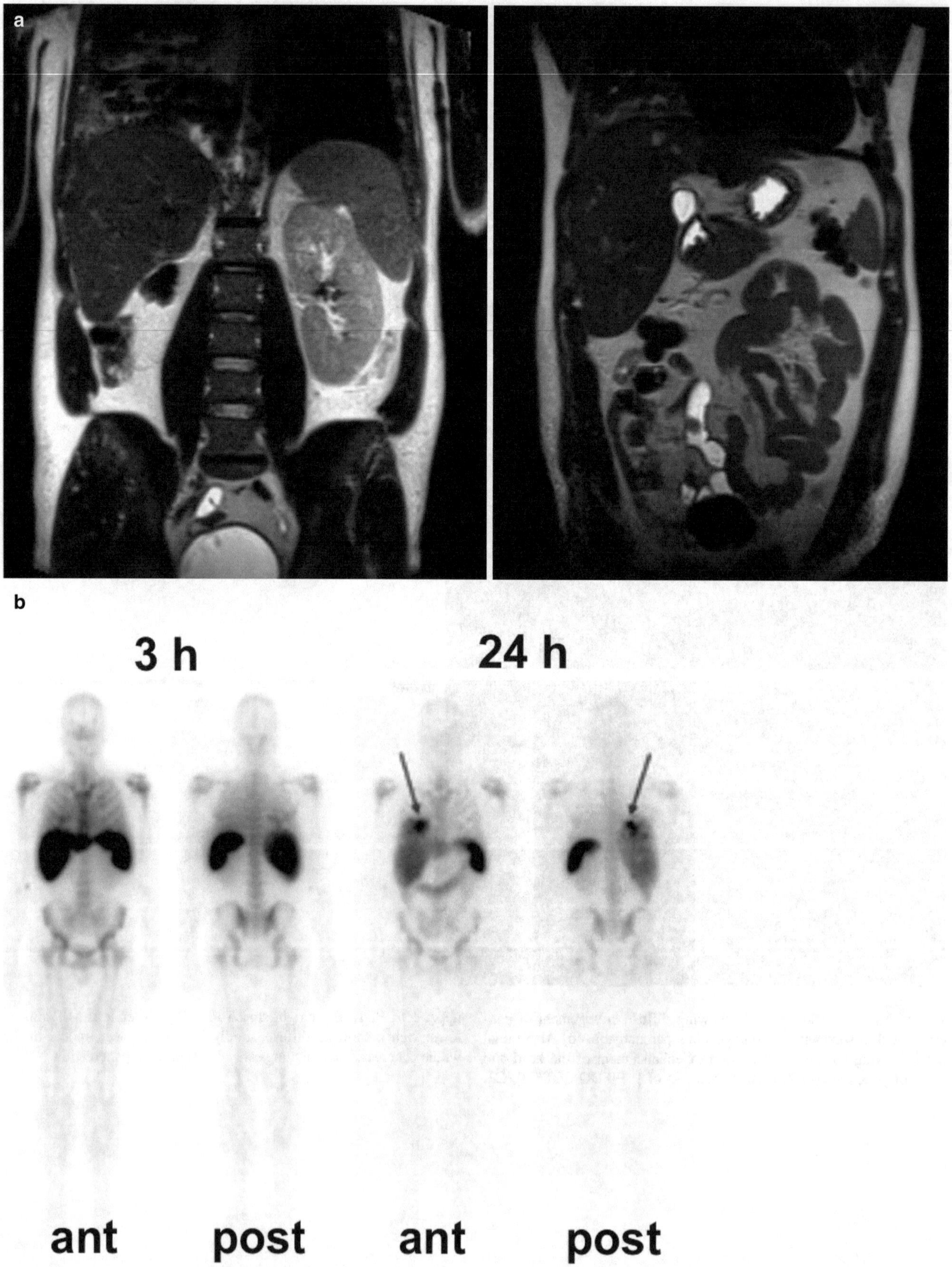

Fig. 10.16 (**a**) Coronal MR images in two different planes showing focal lesions in the upper portion of liver, associated with "honeycomb-type" changes in the anterior and basal regions of right lung; both changes are consistent with infection. (**b**) ^{99m}Tc-HMPAO-WBC scintigraphy (anterior and posterior planar whole-body views acquired at 3 h and 24 h) showing abnormal accumulation of labeled leukocytes at the base of right lung and upper liver, increasing over time and matching the MRI findings. The overall imaging results indicated the presence of multiple abscesses in right lung and liver

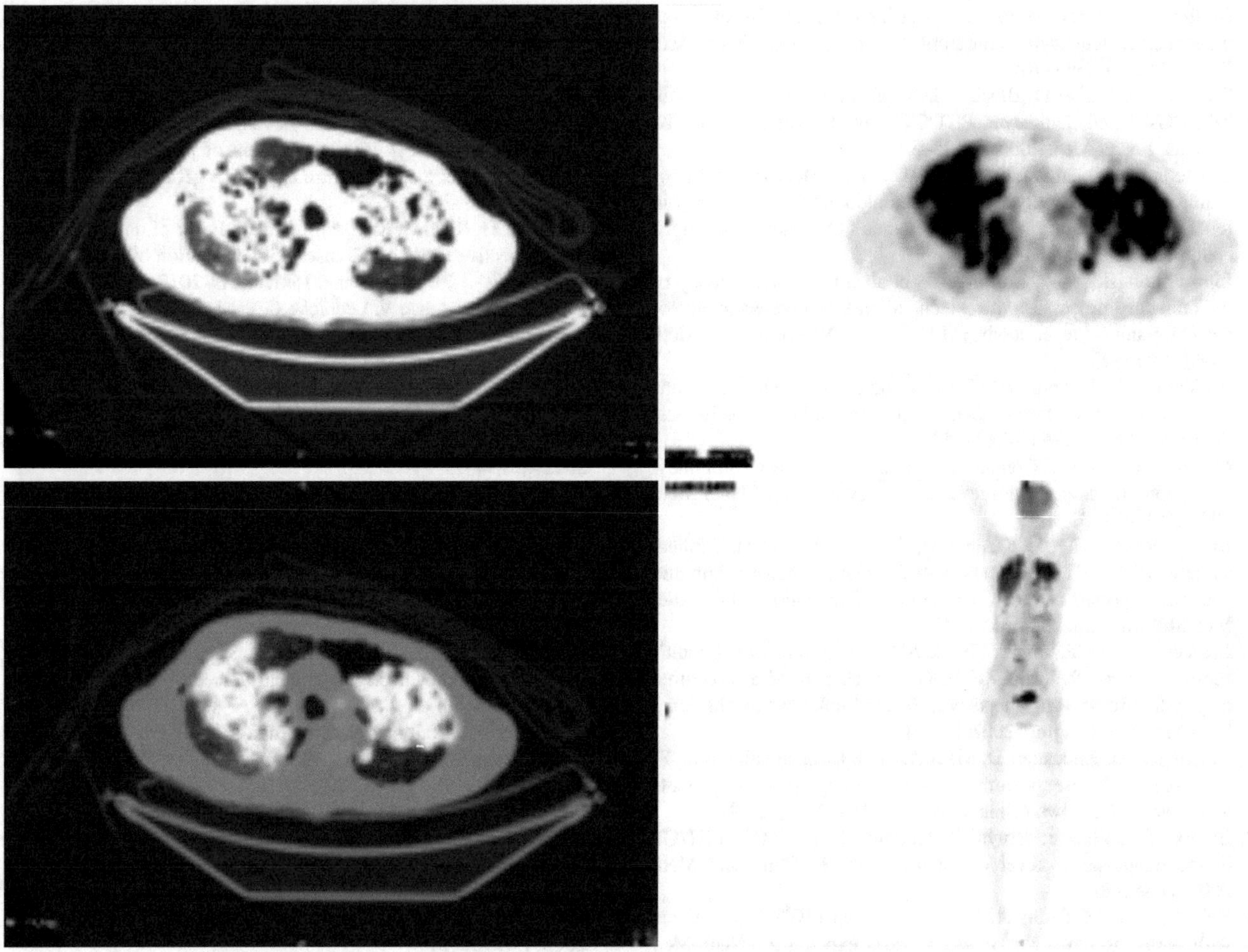

Fig. 10.17 [18F]FDG PET/CT: the transaxial sections (CT, upper left; PET, upper right; fused PET/CT, lower left; MIP image, lower right) show markedly increased [18F]FDG uptake in both lungs (upper and middle lobes of right lung, upper lobe of left lung) associated with irregularly shaped consolidation areas detected in the low dose CT scan. Increased [18F]FDG uptake was also noted in the lumbar spine (see MIP image; tomographic images not shown here). These findings, obtained after prolonged antibiotic therapy, classified the patient as "no responder" to the antibiotic regimen employed and led to change the antimicrobial agent

References

1. Konecny P, Davidson RN. Pyrexia of unknown origin in the 1990s: time to redefine. Br J Hosp Med. 1996;56:21–4.
2. Kouijzeri IJE, Mulders-Manders CM, Bleeker-Rovers CP, et al. Fever of unknown origin: the value of FDG-PET/CT. Semin Nucl Med. 2018;48:100–7.
3. Tabak F, Mert A, Celik AD, et al. Fever of unknown origin in Turkey. Infection. 2003;31:417–20.
4. Bleeker-Rovers CP, Vos FJ, de Kleijn EM, et al. A prospective multi-center study on fever of unknown origin: the yield of a structured diagnostic protocol. Medicine (Baltimore). 2007;86:26–38.
5. Mourad O, Palda V, Detsky AS. A comprehensive evidence-based approach to fever of unknown origin. Arch Intern Med. 2003;163:545–51.
6. Peters AM. Nuclear medicine imaging in fever of unknown origin. Q J Nucl Med. 1999;43:61–73.
7. Gaeta GB, Fusco FM, Nardiello S. Fever of unknown origin: a systematic review of the literature for 1995-2004. Nucl Med Commun. 2006;27:205–11.
8. Corstens FH, van der Meer JW. Nuclear medicine's role in infection and inflammation. Lancet. 1999;354:765–70.
9. Cascini GL, de Palma D, Matteucci F, et al. Fever of unknown origin, infection of subcutaneous devices, brain abscesses and endocarditis. Nucl Med Commun. 2006;27:213–22.
10. Palestro CJ. The current role of gallium imaging in infection. Semin Nucl Med. 1994;24:128–41.
11. Knockaert DC, Mortelmans LA, De Roo MC, Bobbaers HJ. Clinical value of gallium-67 scintigraphy in evaluation of fever of unknown origin. Clin Infect Dis. 1994;18:601–5.
12. Meller J, Altenvoerde G, Munzel U, et al. Fever of unknown origin: prospective comparison of [18F]FDG imaging with a double-head coincidence camera and gallium-67 citrate SPET. Eur J Nucl Med. 2000;27:1617–25.
13. Kjaer A, Lebech AM. Diagnostic value of 111In-granulocyte scintigraphy in patients with fever of unknown origin. J Nucl Med. 2002;43:140–4.
14. MacSweeney JE, Peters AM, Lavender JP. Indium labelled leucocyte scanning in pyrexia of unknown origin. Clin Radiol. 1990;42:414–7.

15. Gutfilen B, Lopes de Souza SA, Martins FP, et al. Use of ^{99m}Tc-mononuclear leukocyte scintigraphy in nosocomial fever. Acta Radiol. 2006;47:699–704.
16. Dumarey N, Egrise D, Blocklet D, et al. Imaging infection with ^{18}F-FDG-labeled leukocyte PET/CT: initial experience in 21 patients. J Nucl Med. 2006;47:625–32.
17. de Kleijn EM, Oyen WJ, Corstens FH, van der Meer JW. Utility of indium-111-labeled polyclonal immunoglobulin G scintigraphy in fever of unknown origin. The Netherlands FUO Imaging Group. J Nucl Med. 1997;38:484–9.
18. Lind P, Langsteger W, Koltringer P, et al. Immunoscintigraphy of inflammatory processes with a technetium-99m-labeled monoclonal antigranulocyte antibody (MAb BW 250/183). J Nucl Med. 1990;31:417–23.
19. Becker W, Goldenberg DM, Wolf F. The use of monoclonal antibodies and antibody fragments in the imaging of infectious lesions. Semin Nucl Med. 1994;24:42–153.
20. Meller J, Ivancevic V, Conrad M, et al. Clinical value of immunoscintigraphy in patients with fever of unknown origin. J Nucl Med. 1998;39:1248–53.
21. Bleeker-Rovers CP, de Kleijn EM, Corstens FH, et al. Clinical value of FDG PET in patients with fever of unknown origin and patients suspected of focal infection or inflammation. Eur J Nucl Med Mol Imaging. 2004;31:29–37.
22. Bleeker-Rovers CP, Vos FJ, Mudde AH, et al. A prospective multi-centre study of the value of FDG-PET as part of a structured diagnostic protocol in patients with fever of unknown origin. Eur J Nucl Med Mol Imaging. 2007;34:694–703.
23. Blockmans D, Knockaert D, Maes A, et al. Clinical value of [^{18}F] fluoro-deoxyglucose positron emission tomography for patients with fever of unknown origin. Clin Infect Dis. 2001;32:191–6.
24. Balink H, Collins J, Bruyn G, Gemmel F. [^{18}F]FDG PET/CT in the diagnosis of fever of unknown origin. Clin Nucl Med. 2009;34:862–8.
25. Kei PL, Kok TY, Padhy AK, et al. [^{18}F]FDG PET/CT in patients with fever of unknown origin: a local experience. Nucl Med Commun. 2010;31:788–92.
26. Jasper N, Däbritz J, Frosch M, et al. Diagnostic value of [^{18}F]-FDG PET/CT in children with fever of unknown origin or unexplained signs of inflammation. Eur J Nucl Med Mol Imaging. 2010;37:136–45.
27. Dong MJ, Zhao K, Liu ZF, et al. A meta-analysis of the value of fluorodeoxyglucose-PET/PET-CT in the evaluation of fever of unknown origin. Eur J Radiol. 2001;80:834–44.
28. Federici L, Blondet C, Imperiale A, et al. Value of ^{18}F-FDG-PET/CT in patients with fever of unknown origin and unexplained prolonged inflammatory syndrome: a single centre analysis experience. Int J Clin Pract. 2010;64:55–60.
29. Ferda J, Ferdova E, Zahlava J, et al. Fever of unknown origin: a value of ^{18}F-FDG-PET/CT with integrated full diagnostic isotropic CT imaging. Eur J Radiol. 2010;73:518–25.
30. Sheng JF, Sheng ZK, Shen XM, et al. Diagnostic value of fluorine-18 fluoro-deoxyglucose positron emission tomography/computed tomography in patients with fever of unknown origin. Eur J Intern Med. 2011;22:112–6.
31. Pelosi E, Skanjeti A, Penna D, et al. Role of integrated PET/CT with [^{18}F]-FDG in the management of patients with fever of unknown origin: a single-centre experience. Radiol Med (Torino). 2011;116:809–20.
32. Pedersen TI, Roed C, Knudsen LS, et al. Fever of unknown origin: a retrospective study of 52 cases with evaluation of the diagnostic utility of FDG-PET/CT. Scand J Infect Dis. 2012;44:18–23.
33. Crouzet J, Boudousq V, Lechiche C, et al. Place of ^{18}F-FDG-PET with computed tomography in the diagnostic algorithm of patients with fever of unknown origin. Eur J Clin Microbiol Infect Dis. 2012;31:1727–33.
34. Kim YJ, Kim SI, Hong KW, et al. Diagnostic value of ^{18}F-FDG PET/CT in patients with fever of unknown origin. Intern Med J. 2012;42:834–7.
35. Manohar K, Mittal BR, Jai S, et al. F-18 FDG-PET/CT in evaluation of patients with fever of unknown origin. Jpn J Radiol. 2013;31:320–7.
36. Tokmak H, Ergonul O, Demirkol O, et al. Diagnostic contribution of ^{18}F-FDG-PET/CT in fever of unknown origin. Int J Infect Dis. 2014;19:53–8.
37. Buch-Olsen KM, Andersen RV, Hess S, et al. ^{18}F-FDG-PET/CT in fever of unknown origin: clinical value. Nucl Med Commun. 2014;35:955–60.
38. Gafter-Gvili A, Raibman S, Grossman A, et al. [^{18}F]FDG-PET/CT for the diagnosis of patients with fever of unknown origin. QJM. 2015;108:289–98.
39. Pereira AM, Husmann L, Sah BR, et al. Determinants of diagnostic performance of ^{18}F-FDG PET/CT in patients with fever of unknown origin. Nucl Med Commun. 2016;37:57–65.
40. Keidar Z, Gurman-Balbir A, Gaitini D, et al. Fever of unknown origin: the role of ^{18}F-FDG PET/CT. J Nucl Med. 2008;49:1980–5.
41. Kjaer A, Lebech AM, Eigtved A, Højgaard L. Fever of unknown origin: prospective comparison of diagnostic value of ^{18}F-FDG PET and ^{111}In-granulocyte scintigraphy. Eur J Nucl Med Mol Imaging. 2004;31:622–6.
42. Hung BT, Wang PW, Su YJ, et al. The efficacy of ^{18}F-FDG PET/CT and ^{67}Ga SPECT/CT in diagnosing fever of unknown origin. Int J Infect Dis. 2017;62:10–7.
43. Signore A, Jamar F, Israel O, et al. Clinical indications, image acquisition and data interpretation for white blood cells and anti-granulocyte monoclonal antibody scintigraphy: an EANM procedural guideline. Eur J Nucl Med Mol Imaging. 2018;45:1816–31.

Nuclear Medicine Imaging of Abdominal Infections and Inflammations

11

Alberto Signore, Tiziana Lanzolla, and Chiara Lauri

Contents

Learning Objectives

- To learn the most frequent abdominal infections
- To understand the role of nuclear medicine procedures in these patients
- To show several clinical cases and pictures to help physicians to correctly acquire and interpret nuclear medicine images

A. Signore (✉)
Department of Medical-Surgical Sciences and of Translational Medicine, Sapienza University of Rome, Rome, Italy

Nuclear Medicine Unit, AOU Sant'Andrea, Rome, Italy
e-mail: alberto.signore@uniroma1.it

C. Lauri
Department of Medical-Surgical Sciences and of Translational Medicine, Sapienza University of Rome, Rome, Italy

Nuclear Medicine Unit, AOU Sant'Andrea, Rome, Italy

T. Lanzolla
Nuclear Medicine Unit, AOU Sant'Andrea, Rome, Italy

11.1 Introduction

Several different clinical conditions can cause abdominal infectious/inflammatory diseases, and they usually present with general symptoms such as abdominal pain, general discomfort, fever and diarrhoea. When investigating patients with acute abdominal pain, the main diagnostic tests remain radiological and endoscopic explorations; nonetheless, also nuclear medicine imaging has a role in the management of such patients, as some of the conditions causing abdominal inflammation and/or infection can be investigated with non-invasive nuclear medicine imaging techniques; in this regard, there are different radiopharmaceuticals that can be helpful to the physician for the management of patients with abdominal infectious or inflammatory diseases, from diagnosis to therapy follow-up. Nevertheless, it should be noted that most of the nuclear medicine examinations do not provide a quick diagnosis in acute abdominal pain with signs of perforation and, therefore, they are not applied as first-line examinations.

Positron emission tomography (PET) and single-photon emission computed tomography (SPECT), preferably acquired with hybrid positron emission tomography/computed tomography (PET/CT) or SPECT/CT cameras, are however increasingly used to diagnose, characterize and

E. Lazzeri et al. (eds.), *Radionuclide Imaging of Infection and Inflammation*, https://doi.org/10.1007/978-3-030-62175-9_11

monitor disease activity in the setting of inflammatory diseases of known and unknown aetiology.

This chapter focuses on the following conditions: intra-abdominal infections (IAI), inflammatory bowel disease (IBD), including ulcerative colitis and Crohn's disease, abdominal abscesses and acute cholecystitis and cholangitis.

11.2 Intra-abdominal Infections and Abscesses

Intra-abdominal infections (IAIs) constitute a major challenge in clinical practice. They are the main cause of postoperative morbidity after abdominal surgery and the most common cause of admission to a surgical intensive care unit, representing a frequent cause of severe sepsis [1, 2].

The clinical spectrum of IAIs is extremely wide, ranging from an uncomplicated appendicitis to a diffuse peritonitis due to perforation of the gastrointestinal (GI) tract, or to an ischemic bowel. A prompt and reliable clinical and microbiological diagnosis is crucial in these patients. On the other hand, the clinical symptoms and signs do not always match severity of the underlying conditions, sometimes delaying appropriate diagnosis and treatment. Risk stratification is therefore important as soon as we evaluate a patient with suspected IAI.

From the clinical point of view, the two major types of IAIs are: (1) 'uncomplicated IAIs', when the infectious process involves a single organ and no anatomical disruption is present, and (2) 'complicated IAIs', when the infectious process proceeds beyond the organ that is the source of infection and causes either localized or diffuse peritonitis, depending on the ability of the host to limit the process. In uncomplicated IAIs, treatment generally includes antimicrobial therapy (occasionally associated with limited surgical resection—when indicated), whereas in complicated IAIs, a more invasive surgical procedure is more often required in association with antimicrobial therapy [3–7].

As a first approach to a patient with a suspected IAI, an initial diagnostic evaluation should include a detailed clinical history, a physical examination and laboratory tests which will identify most patients with suspected IAI for whom further evaluation and management is warranted.

For selected patients with inconclusive/equivocal physical examination findings (such as impaired mental status or spinal cord injury or immunosuppression due to disease or therapy), intra-abdominal infection should be considered if the patient presents with evidence of infection from an undetermined source. Further diagnostic imaging is unnecessary in patients with obvious signs of diffuse peritonitis and in whom immediate surgical intervention must be performed. In adult patients not undergoing immediate laparotomy, computed tomography (CT) scan is the imaging modality of choice to determine the presence of an IAI and its source [8].

The underutilization of nuclear medicine imaging in this clinical scenario is probably due to the emergency of the examination, considering that in most cases nuclear medicine departments do not operate on a 24-h basis.

The most promising nuclear medicine technique for the diagnosis of IAIs is [^{18}F]-fluorodeoxyglucose positron emission tomography/computed tomography [^{18}F]FDG PET/CT, even if only a few case reports have been published—but consistently showing the ability of [^{18}F]FDG PET/CT to identify the location of the on-going infection [9–11]. Thus, [^{18}F]FDG PET/CT imaging is a promising technique for identifying foci of abdominal infections and for guiding biopsy (Fig. 11.1). Further studies and controlled clinical trials will allow for a better definition of the clinical impact of [^{18}F]FDG PET/CT imaging in the clinical setting of infection imaging of the abdomen.

Scintigraphy with autologous radiolabelled leukocytes (WBC), most often labelled with ^{99m}Tc-HMPAO, is still considered the gold standard nuclear medicine technique for imaging intra-abdominal abscesses. Early and late acquisitions are mandatory, preferably acquired with SPECT/CT imaging in order to better recognize physiologic gut transit of ^{99m}Tc-HMPAO, a problem that does not occur when using ^{111}In-oxine-WBC.

Key Learning Points

- Nuclear medicine procedures can be useful in patients with suspected abdominal infection, when conventional radiologic imaging cannot localize the site and extent of the infection.
- Different radiopharmaceutical preparations have been described to explore abdominal infection and/or inflammation including ^{99m}Tc-HMPAO- or ^{111}In-oxine-labelled WBC, ^{99m}Tc-anti-granulocute antibodies and [^{18}F]FDG.

11.3 Inflammatory Bowel Diseases (IBD)

Inflammatory bowel diseases (IBD), including Crohn's disease (CD) and ulcerative colitis (UC), are chronic relapsing inflammatory diseases predominantly affecting the GI tract whose pathogenesis is not completely known. The incidence of IBD is very high.

Although CD and UC are different clinical entities, they share many clinical aspects. The clinical course of CD and UC is chronically relapsing, alternating periods of remission and exacerbation, which profoundly impair the patient's

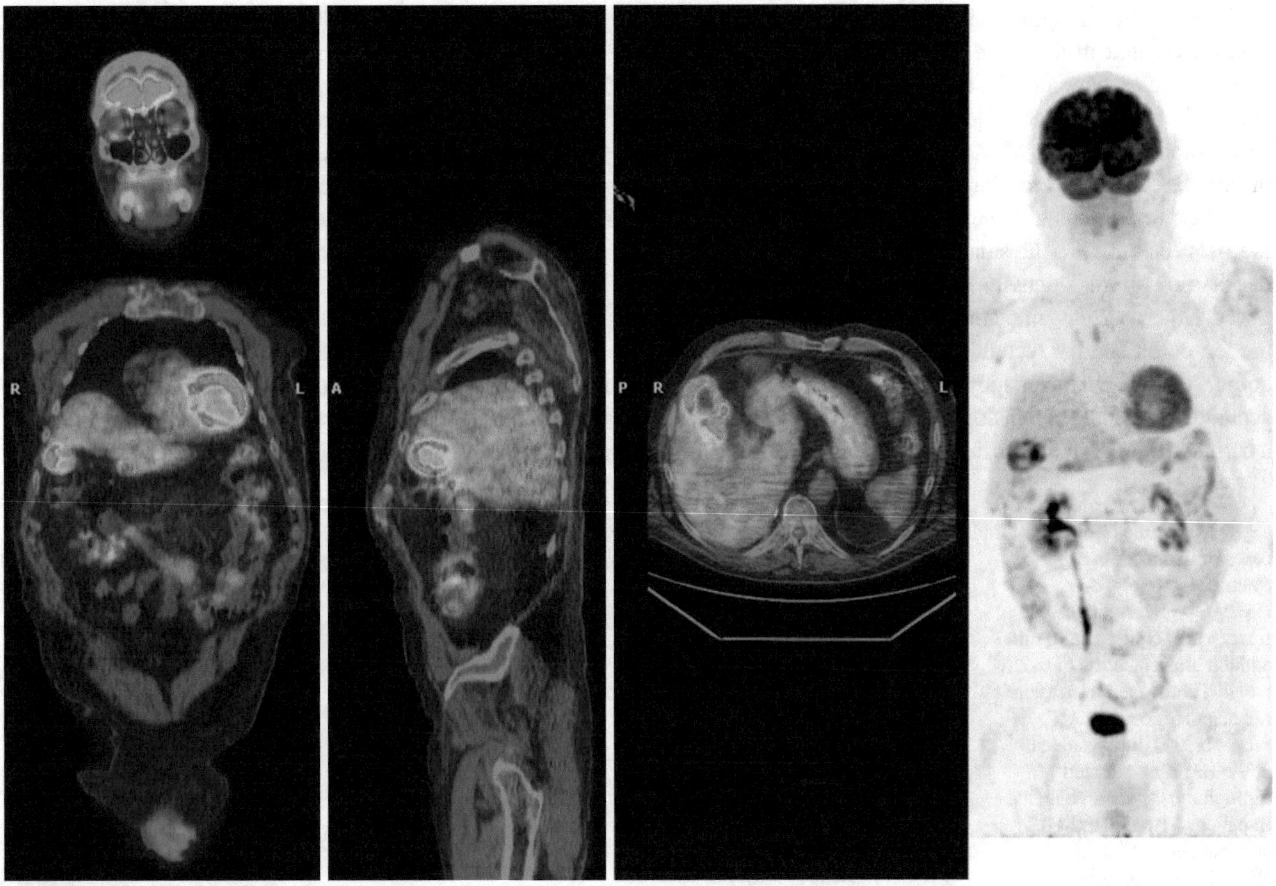

Fig. 11.1 Transaxial, coronal and sagittal views of [^{18}F]FDG PET/CT in a patient with acute cholecystitis. Images show avid [^{18}F]FDG uptake in the gallbladder wall. Differential diagnosis with a neoplasm of the gallbladder is based on the pattern of diffuse wall uptake rather than a focal uptake

quality of life. Cardinal symptom of UC is bloody diarrhoea. Associate symptoms can be abdominal pain, urgency or tenesmus. Symptoms of CD are more variable and heterogeneous, but commonly include diarrhoea for more than 6 weeks, abdominal pain and/or weight loss. Systemic symptoms, malaise, anorexia and fever, can be present but are more common in CD. The diagnosis of IBD should be based on clinical suspicion supported by appropriate colonoscopy findings, typical histological findings on biopsy, negative stool test for infectious agents and biochemical investigations. Medical management depends on disease activity and extent. It is critical to be able to evaluate disease activity when initiating as well as assessing the adequacy of therapy for both UC and CD; in this regard, unfortunately clinical and endoscopic scoring systems are either indirect or too invasive. Thus, an accurate non-invasive method of assessing disease activity would constitute a significant advance in the care of these patients.

Debate is still ongoing about the best diagnostic technique to be used in IBD, since different clinical presentations are possible and different stages of the diseases can be characterized by different findings. Overall, magnetic resonance imaging (MRI) is the most complete technique for staging a patient at the time of diagnosis, together with endoscopy. During follow-up and to address more specific questions, CT, ultrasound and nuclear medicine imaging have well-defined roles, as described in the recent ECCO-ESGAR-EANM guidelines [12–16].

Scintigraphy with radiolabelled autologous WBC (considered the nuclear medicine gold standard technique) constitutes a second-line imaging technique in the diagnostic assessment of IBD patients and it must be therefore applied when radiological and/or endoscopic examinations are inconclusive. This imaging method has a well-defined role in the characterization of strictures, in the evaluation of disease activity, in the follow-up of patients after therapy and for early identification of sub-clinical relapses.

Since scintigraphy with ^{99m}Tc-HMAPO-WBC or with ^{111}In-oxine-WBC is a highly sensitive technique for the diagnosis of IBD, the absence of abdominal accumulation of radiolabelled leukocytes excludes IBD. However, specificity of the scan is not equally high, since the presence of abnormal WBC accumulation in patients with symptoms suggesting IBD can be due to several other disorders.

Scintigraphic imaging using radiolabelled WBC is not contra-indicated in the acute phase and well tolerated, and several studies have demonstrated its reliability in patients with IBD [16]. This technique can be useful to distinguish IBD from UC and CD, where the pattern and localization of the uptake can address the diagnosis towards one condition or the other; in particular, if radiolabelled WBC accumulate in the ileocecal area, in the small bowel, and there is a patchy distribution of radioactivity, the diagnosis of CD is more likely. Otherwise, accumulation of the labelled leukocytes in the left colon and the rectum, or diffuse accumulation in the colon, is more characteristic for UC. When the scan shows accumulation in the colon alone, it is not possible to establish a certain differential diagnosis (Figures 11.2, 11.3, and 11.4).

Leukocytes have been labelled in vitro also with [^{18}F] FDG, which provides a good alternative to ^{111}In-oxine or ^{99m}Tc-HMPAO-WBC in patients with IBD, since in this condition there is no need of acquiring delayed images. In fact, [^{18}F]FDG PET/CT images can be acquired at 1–2 h or, based on a dual imaging point protocol, at 1 h and 3 h after administration. This protocol enables to identify early migration of the labelled cells in the affected tissues and co-localize the uptake with anatomical regions detected with CT (Fig. 11.5).

^{99m}Tc-Sn-fluoride-labelled leukocytes have also been used successfully to investigate patients with IBD [17] based on the fact that free ^{99m}Tc-Sn-fluoride (from labelling or released from labelled cells) is trapped in the endothelial reticular system (mainly in liver and bone morrow) without being

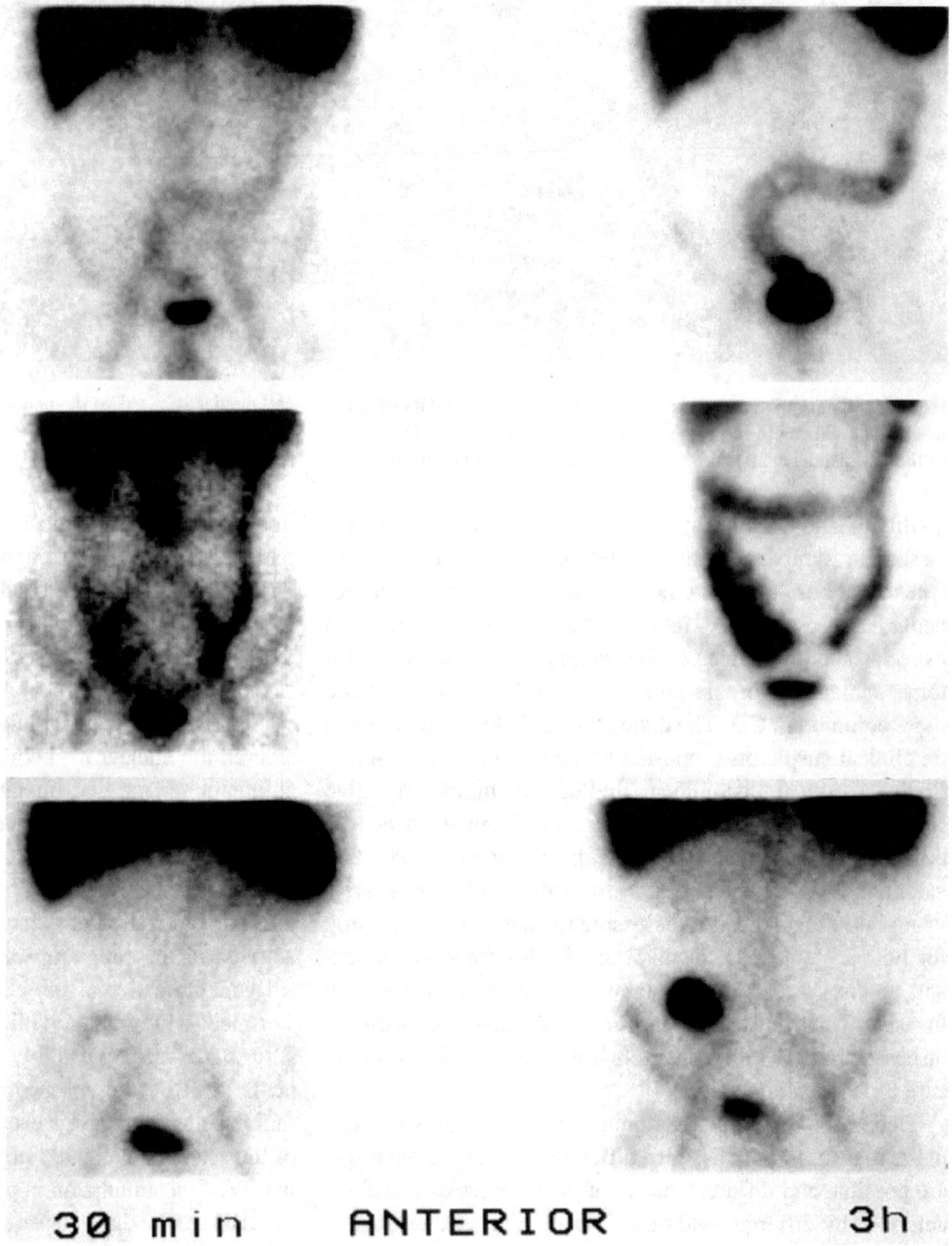

Fig. 11.2 Three different cases of Crohn's disease evaluated with ^{99m}Tc-HMPAO-WBC scintigraphy. Images are acquired at 30 min and 3 h after injection of the labelled cells; later images are not acquired to avoid false-positive findings due to ^{99m}Tc-HMPAO excreted through the GI tract. Note that in patient 1 (top images) the accumulation of labelled WBC is detected only in descending colon. This pattern could have been mistakenly interpreted as due ulcerative colitis and final diagnosis can only be based on biopsy. In patient 2 (middle images) the radiolabelled cells accumulate in the whole colon, cecum and terminal ileum that are more typical regions for colonic CD. In patient 3 (bottom images) the scan shows an abdominal abscess as consequence of the disease in the terminal ileum

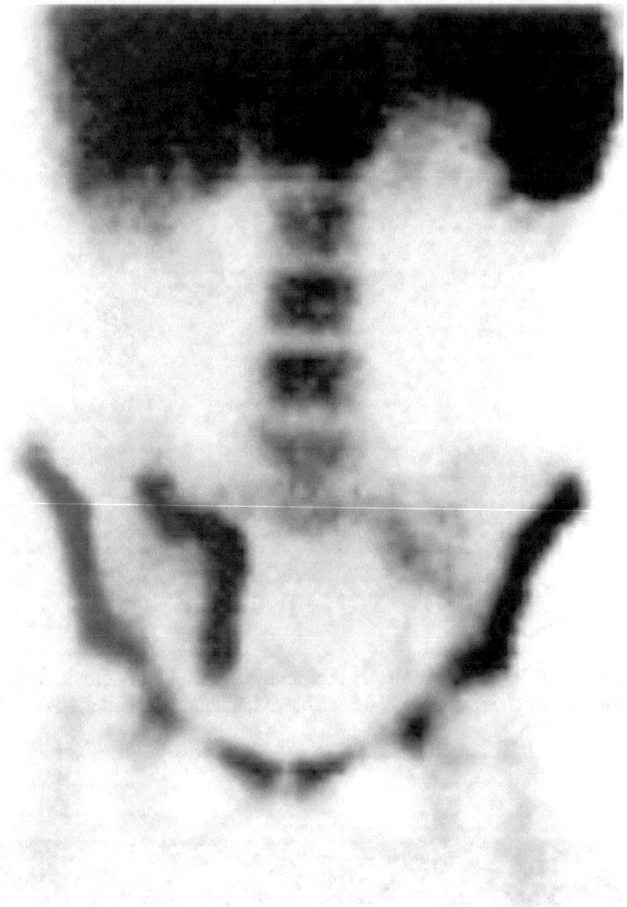

Fig. 11.3 A patient with active ileal Crohn's disease evaluated with ^{99m}Tc-HMPAO-WBC scintigraphy. Image is acquired at 3 h after injection of the radiolabelled cells. Higher accumulation in the left iliac crest (that would be reported as grade 1) than in the right iliac crest (that would be reported as grade 3) due to slight rotation of the patient. In this case, the average value between the two iliac bones should be considered with a final score of 2

excreted in the bowel through the gallbladder, differently from ^{99m}Tc-HMPAO. In practice, this feature allows to acquire images at later time points (20–24 h) without any interference from nonspecific bowel activity.

The clinical role of [^{18}F]FDG PET/CT in patients with IBD has not yet been defined. Since the physiological uptake of [^{18}F]FDG by the bowel can be extremely variable both in distribution and intensity due to several factors (e.g., fasting) [18, 19], the visual (qualitative) and semi-quantitative analysis does not always allow the characterization or lesions. The physiological [^{18}F]FDG uptake in the bowel is typically isolated, rather than diffuse with an SUV of less than 4, but intense uptake (SUV as high as 10) can occur, particularly in the right colon. The pathophysiology of [^{18}F]FDG uptake in the GI tract is not completely elucidated.

Several studies have evaluated the role of [^{18}F]FDG PET/CT in IBD, showing very high sensitivity and a high accuracy, diagnostic features combined with the important advantages of non-invasiveness, relatively low radiation exposure compared to other radiological studies (4–6 mSv) and possibility to study the small intestine.

Furthermore, the new hybrid PET/MRI systems, thanks to the superior soft tissue resolution and co-registration, can identify signs of disease activity such as vessel dilation, wall thickening, wall stratification with thickening of the submucosa, wall and mesenteric increased vascularity, lymph node enlargement and enhancement. Most relevant is the differential diagnosis between fibrotic strictures and inflammatory strictures that require different therapeutic approach (Figs. 11.6, 11.7, and 11.8) [20, 21].

For the evaluation of disease activity, several other radiopharmaceuticals have also been developed. Most of them are still in experimental phase, whereas two of these, ^{99m}Tc-interleukin-2 (^{99m}Tc-IL2) and ^{99m}Tc-anti-tumor necrosis

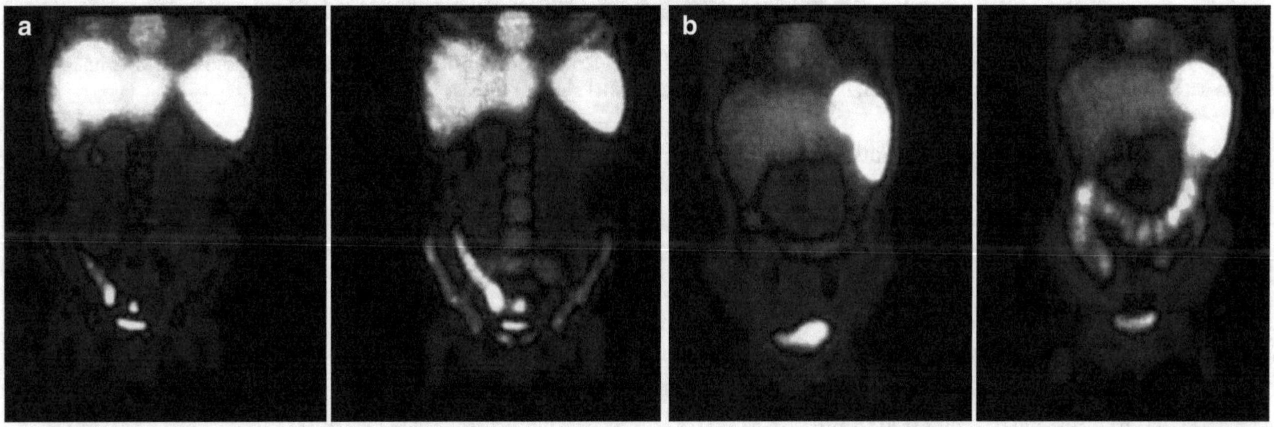

Fig. 11.4 Two cases of active Crohn's disease evaluated with ^{99m}Tc-HMPAO-WBC scintigraphy. Images are acquired at 30 min and 3 h after injection of the labelled cells. (**a**) Patient with involvement of the terminal ileum. (**b**) Patient with colitis. The accumulation of labelled leukocytes in the affected sites increases with time, and spleen activity is always higher than liver activity

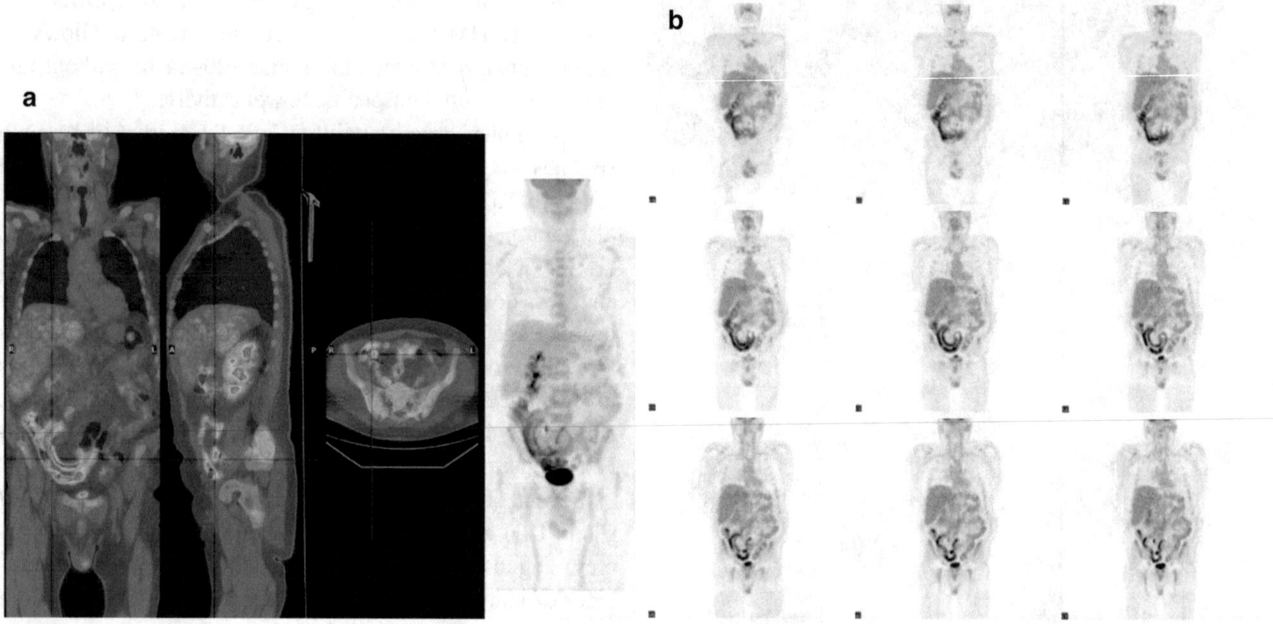

Fig. 11.5 [^{18}F]FDG PET/CT in a patient with active Chron's disease. (**a**) Fused transaxial, coronal and sagittal PET/CT sections. (**b**) Sequential coronal PET sections. Images show increased [^{18}F]FDG uptake in the terminal ileum, right colon flexure and ascending colon: the [^{18}F]FDG uptake is clearly seen in the gut wall and not within the lumen, which is not always detectable at the ileum and better observed at the colon

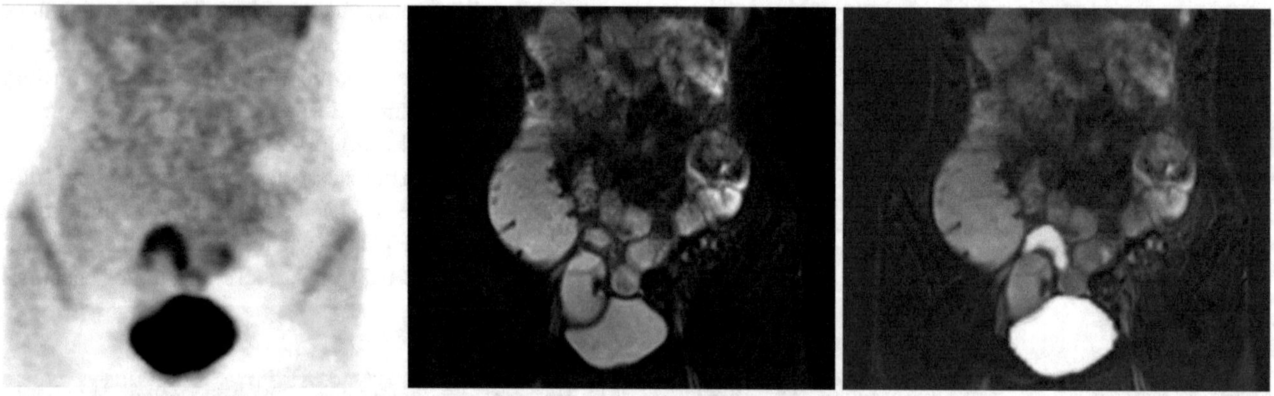

Fig. 11.6 PET scan with [^{18}F]FDG (left) in a patient with Crohn's disease. Co-registered MRI image (centre) and fused PET/MRI image (left) shows active high [^{18}F]FDG uptake in the distal ileum without significant MRI signs of disease

factor alpha (TNFα) monoclonal antibodies (^{99m}Tc-anti-TNF-mAb), have also been produced as GMP kits for commercial purposes [22]. These imaging agents appear to be highly specific for activated T cells and for TNFα, respectively, being, therefore, able to provide important in vivo histological information on the affected gut (Fig. 11.9). In particular, ^{99m}Tc-IL2 has shown to predict long-term disease relapse more accurately than radiolabelled WBC scintigraphy [23] and to allow early evaluation of the efficacy of steroid therapy [24]. ^{99m}Tc-anti-TNF-mAb has shown to predict the success of biological therapies based on anti-TNFα molecules (Fig. 11.10) [25].

Key Learning Points

- Nuclear medicine procedures are not usually the method of choice for the diagnosis of IBD, even if they play an important role (when other examinations remain inconclusive) and for therapy follow-up.
- Several radiopharmaceuticals have been developed to investigate patients with IBD, which emphasize the different aspects of the inflammation process.
- Radiolabelled WBC scintigraphy can differentiate between Crohn's disease (CD) and ulcerative colitis

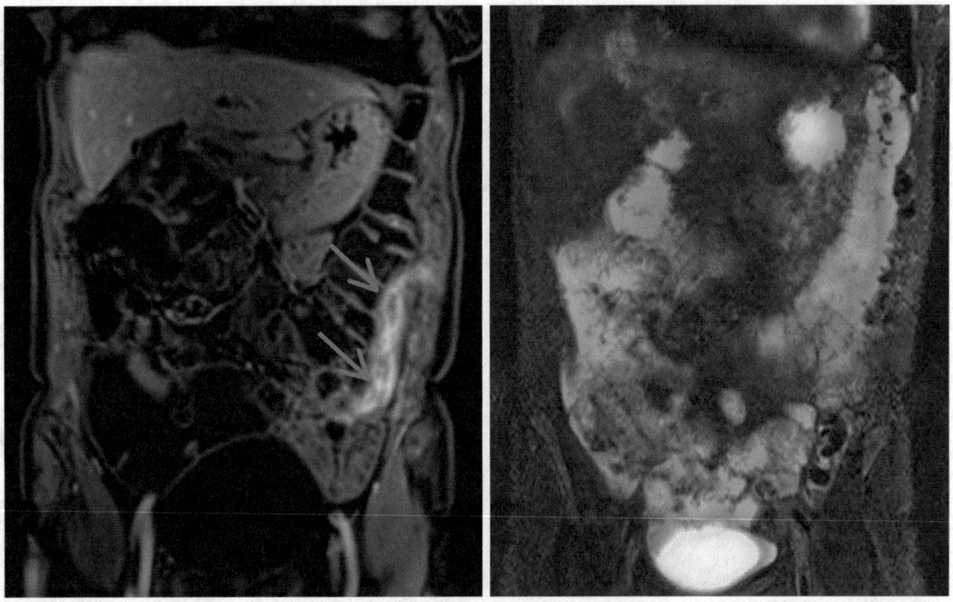

Fig. 11.7 [18F]FDG PET/MRI in a patient with Crohn's disease. The MR image (left) shows oedema with some strictures, suggesting the presence of inflammation. Whereas, the PET image (right) clearly shows the absence of [18F]FDG uptake, thus indicating a fibrotic stricture

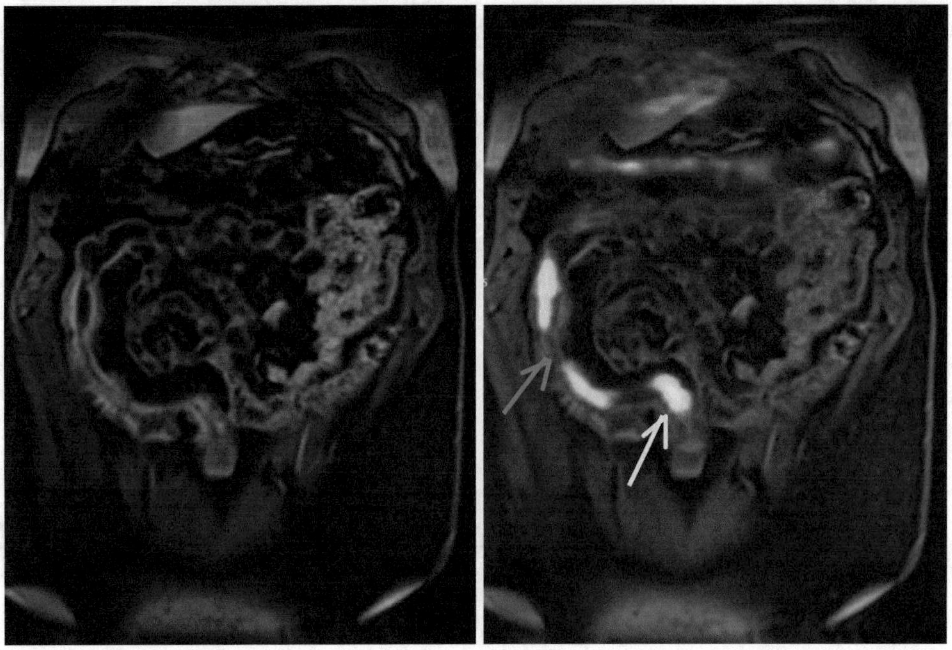

Fig. 11.8 [18F]FDG PET/MRI in a patient with Crohn's disease. The MR image (left) shows oedema, comb sign and some strictures, thus suggesting the presence of inflammation. The PET image (right) clearly shows the presence of [18F]FDG uptake in a stricture (yellow arrow), thus indicating the presence of an inflammatory stricture, but also the presence of a fibrotic stricture (blue arrow) where no [18F]FDG uptake is detectable. The other two sites of [18F]FDG uptake (before and after the fibrotic stricture) are due to inflammation of the gut wall

(UC) and can detect, in a non-invasive way, exacerbation of the disease. Images should be taken at 30 min and 2 h post-injection, although later time points may be useful to define infected fistulae.

- [18F]FDG PET/CT is not routinely used in IBD, but as a pan-inflammatory marker, it has been recently re-evaluated for the evaluation of early therapy efficacy and for the differential diagnosis between fibrotic and inflammatory strictures.
- The novel hybrid PET/MR imaging is a highly promising modality for the evaluation of activity and extent of disease.

11.4 Idiopathic Retroperitoneal Fibrosis

Retroperitoneal fibrosis (RPF) is a rare condition characterized by the presence of a retroperitoneal mass of fibro-inflammatory tissue, which can compress the ureters (thus creating obstructions) and other abdominal organs. The most frequent localization of the mass is around the abdominal aorta and the iliac arteries, extending to the retro-peritoneum. In most patients, the cause of RPF remains unknown and therefore idiopathic (idiopathic retroperitoneal fibrosis—IRF), but it can also be secondary to known factors such as the use of certain drugs, malignant diseases, infections and surgery. Symptoms and signs of RPF are unfortunately non-

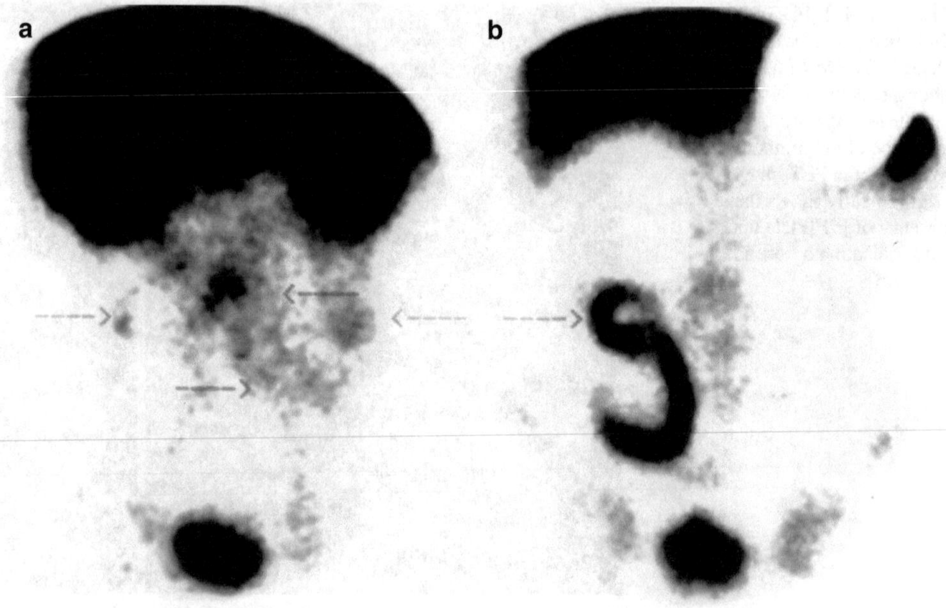

Fig. 11.9 Scintigraphy with ^{99m}Tc-IL2 (**a**) and with ^{99m}Tc-HMPAO-WBC (**b**) in a patient with active Chron's disease. It can be seen that the areas affected by autoimmune infiltration of activated T cells are not the same as those infiltrated by neutrophils

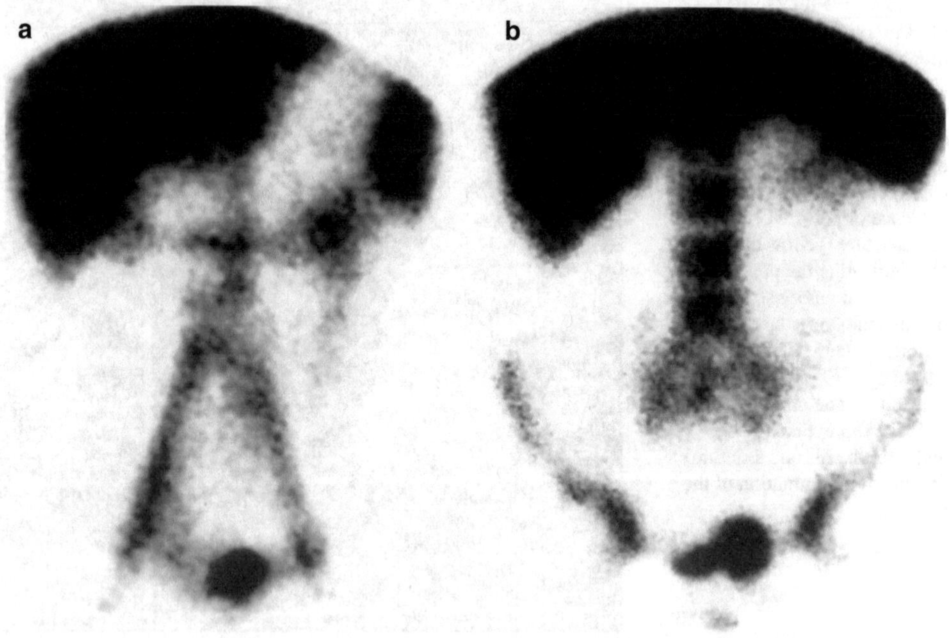

Fig. 11.10 Scintigraphy with ^{99m}Tc-anti-TNFα (**a**) and with ^{99m}Tc-HMPAO-WBC (**b**) in a patient with active Chron's disease. It can be seen that, despite a negative WBC scan, there is significant uptake of anti-TNF in the transverse colon, indicating the presence of an ongoing autoimmune process. Furthermore, a positive ^{99m}Tc-anti-TNFα scan suggests that the patient can most likely benefit from biological therapy

specific, making the diagnosis difficult and requiring a high clinical suspect. The definitive diagnosis is based on biopsy findings.

CT and MR imaging are the modalities of choice, because they allow a good anatomical identification of the extent of the retroperitoneal masses. [^{18}F]FDG PET/CT can be useful in the evaluation of patients with IRF, as it provides information about disease activity and the extent of the active mass; this imaging modality may also predict response to treatment in patients with IRF (Fig. 11.11) [26, 27].

Key Learning Points

- Radiolabelled WBC scintigraphy is not routinely used in the study of retroperitoneal fibrosis.
- [^{18}F]FDG PET/CT is the 'gold standard' in the evaluation of disease activity and the extent of the inflammation process and for assessing response to therapy.

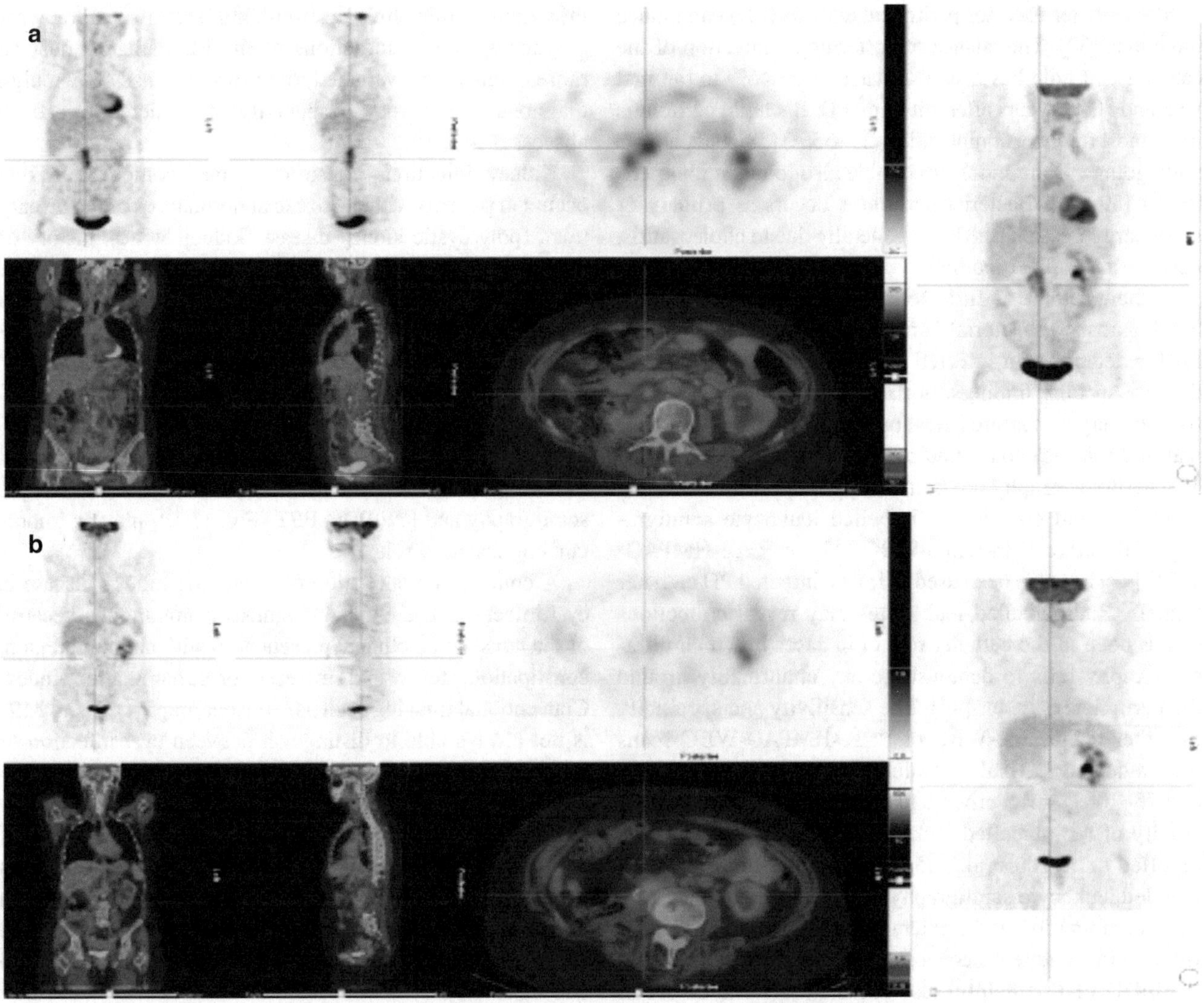

Fig. 11.11 Patient with histological diagnosis of fibro-inflammatory tissue surrounding the right kidney, ascertained after nephrectomy due to massive hydro-ureteronephrosis. Transaxial, coronal and sagittal slices and MIP images of [^{18}F]FDG PET/CT performed before (**a**) and after (**b**) corticosteroids therapy. The baseline scan clearly shows an abnormal hypodense tissue that surrounds the inferior vena cava, associated with intense [^{18}F]FDG uptake (**a**), that disappears on the PET scan performed 8 months later after steroid therapy (**b**)

11.5 Miscellaneous Abdominal Infections

Mesh infection can follow either open or laparoscopic ventral incisional hernia repair. The reported incidence after open repair ranges from 6 to 10%, whereas it is lower after laparoscopic repairs (0–3.6%) [28, 29]. Infections that occur early in the post-operative period are more likely to be associated with an entero-cutaneous fistula or a superficial incisional surgical site infection [30]. CT imaging is the prevailing standard of reference for the diagnosis of intra-abdominal abscess (with 76–94% sensitivity) [31]; however, although radiologic imaging (ultrasound, CT, or MRI) is useful in some cases for diagnosing mesh infection, fluid surrounding the mesh can be a normal benign finding [32].

The main advantage of radionuclide imaging techniques over radiological imaging is their ability to distinguish, non-invasively, infection from benign fluid collections and to evaluate the whole body in a single examination [33]. Radiopharmaceuticals available for imaging abdominal infection include ^{67}Ga-citrate, radiolabelled leukocytes or radiolabelled anti-granulocyte antibodies [34–36]. Although radiolabelled leukocyte imaging is generally the preferred radionuclide method to evaluate postoperative patients, ^{67}Ga-citrate imaging should not be totally discarded. When tested to diagnose late mesh infection, ^{99m}Tc-antigranulocyte antibody scintigraphy showed higher sensitivity than both ultrasound and CT imaging (100% versus 71% and 76%, respectively) for the detection of clinically 'silent' abdominal wall infections after surgery.

The catheter used for peritoneal dialysis (PD) can induce infections [37]. The chance of suffering an infection of the catheter exit hole has been estimated to be 46% in the first year and 70% 3 years after initiating PD. Bacterial peritonitis is the most frequent complication (15–35%) [38], but patients undergoing PD are more susceptible also to tubercular peritonitis [39, 40]. Bacterial peritonitis occurs as primary or secondary infection (the latter generally due to cholecystitis, pancreatitis or diverticulitis).

Although there is little role for imaging modalities in the diagnosis of bacterial peritonitis, imaging may be useful for detecting an infected fluid collection [41]. Due to the non-specific findings, in case of tuberculous peritonitis, the imaging features must be correlated with both clinical and microbiologic findings. Ultrasound, CT and CT/MR peritoneography are particularly helpful for detecting loculated fluid collections. Labelled leukocyte scintigraphy with either ^{111}In-oxine-WBC [42] or ^{99m}Tc-HMPAO-WBC [43] has also been used to image infected PD catheter tunnels. Radiolabelled leukocytes may reveal collections of pus deep in the catheter tunnel in cases in which ultrasonography fails to demonstrate any abnormality around the peritoneal catheter [44]. The sensitivity and specificity of either ^{111}In-oxine-WBC or ^{99m}Tc-HMPAO-WBC scans for diagnosing PD catheter infection range around 70–83% and 75–100%, respectively. In case of peritonitis, the sensitivity of radiolabelled leukocytes scintigraphy has been reported to be 100% [43, 45]. An advantage of the use of labelled leukocyte scintigraphy is represented by the accurate determination of the extent of infection, which is helpful also in treatment decision-making [46]. Imaging with [^{18}F]FDG PET is helpful also for the diagnosis of occult infections in this clinical setting; although its accuracy for diagnosing tunnel infections of the PD catheter must be more extensively evaluated, the procedure has shown high diagnostic, accuracy especially for detecting deep abscesses [47, 48].

Kidney infections constitute a rare complication that occurs in patients with anatomic abnormalities of the urinary tract, (poly)cystic kidney disease, kidney stones, history of urological surgery, trauma and diabetes mellitus. Pyelonephritis can often result in a kidney abscess, due to vasospasm and inflammatory response that leads to tissue necrosis and abscess formation. The diagnostic workup of kidney infection is mainly based on laboratory tests, including blood inflammation index and urinalysis and culture. CT is the most accurate radiologic modality for diagnosis and follow-up of the abscess. However, radiolabelled leukocyte scintigraphy and [^{18}F]FDG PET (Fig. 11.12) play an important confirmatory role.

A common complication of polycystic kidney disease is cyst infection. The clinical diagnosis is not simple, because of the nonspecific clinical presentation with abdominal pain, constipation, fever and increase of inflammation index. Conventional imaging such us ultrasonography, CT and MRI is not always able to distinguish between cyst infection or haemorrhage or pyelonephritis and nephrolithiasis complication; furthermore, in patients with polycystic kidney disease, renal function is usually reduced and the use of radiological contrast agents is prohibited. For the diagnosis of cyst infection, several studies have demonstrated a high diagnostic accuracy of [^{18}F]FDG PET/CT (Fig. 11.13), with sensitivity ranging from 77% to 95% and specificity close to 100% [49–52].

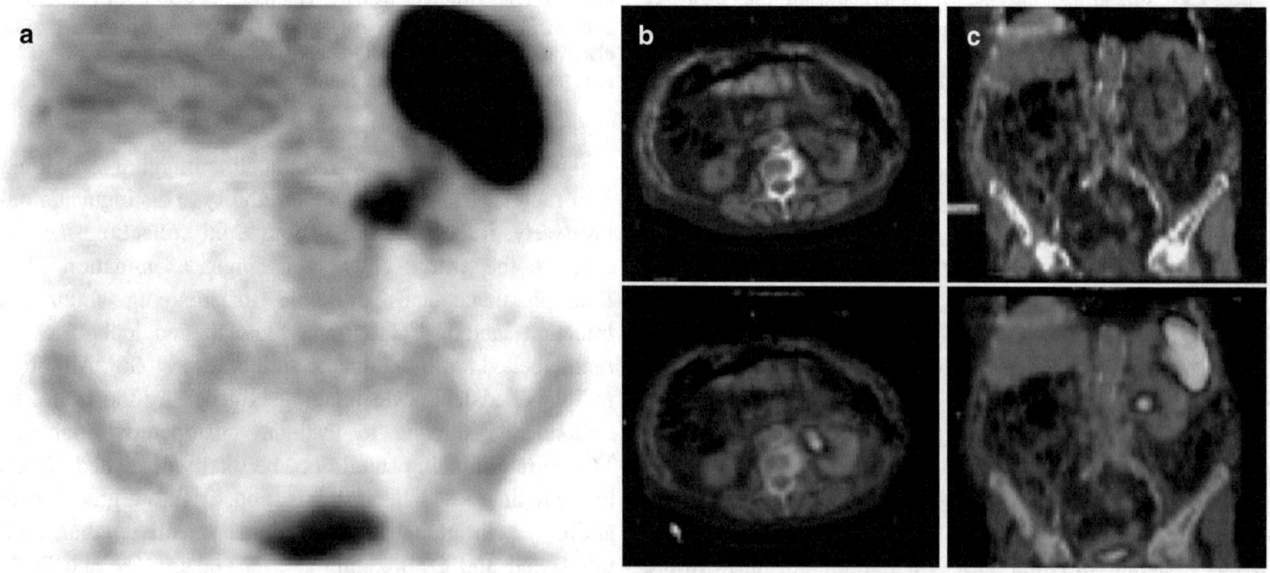

Fig. 11.12 Patient with renal abscess. (**a**) Planar ^{99m}Tc-HMPAO-WBC scintigraphy acquired 3 h p.i.; (**b**) and (**c**) fused SPECT/CT transaxial and coronal sections showing a pathological persistent accumulation of the radiolabelled cells in the left kidney

Key Learning Points

- Radiolabelled WBC scintigraphy and [^{18}F]FDG PET/CT play an important role in the diagnosis of peritoneal and/or kidney infections.
- ^{111}In-oxine-WBC should be preferred to ^{99m}Tc-HMPAO-WBC because of lower urinary excretion of the radionuclide moiety.
- [^{18}F]FDG PET/CT has higher sensitivity, but lower specificity than radiolabelled WBC scintigraphy.

Clinical Cases

Case 11.1

Paola A. Erba

Female, age 45 years. 25 November 2010: Bilateral hystero-annessiectomy because of endometrial adenocarcinoma (G1, PT1a, Stage IA). 29 November 2011: Spleno-pancreatectomy, partial gastrectomy, partial hepatic resection: nonmucinous adenocarcinoma (G2 pT3pN1 (1/5)).

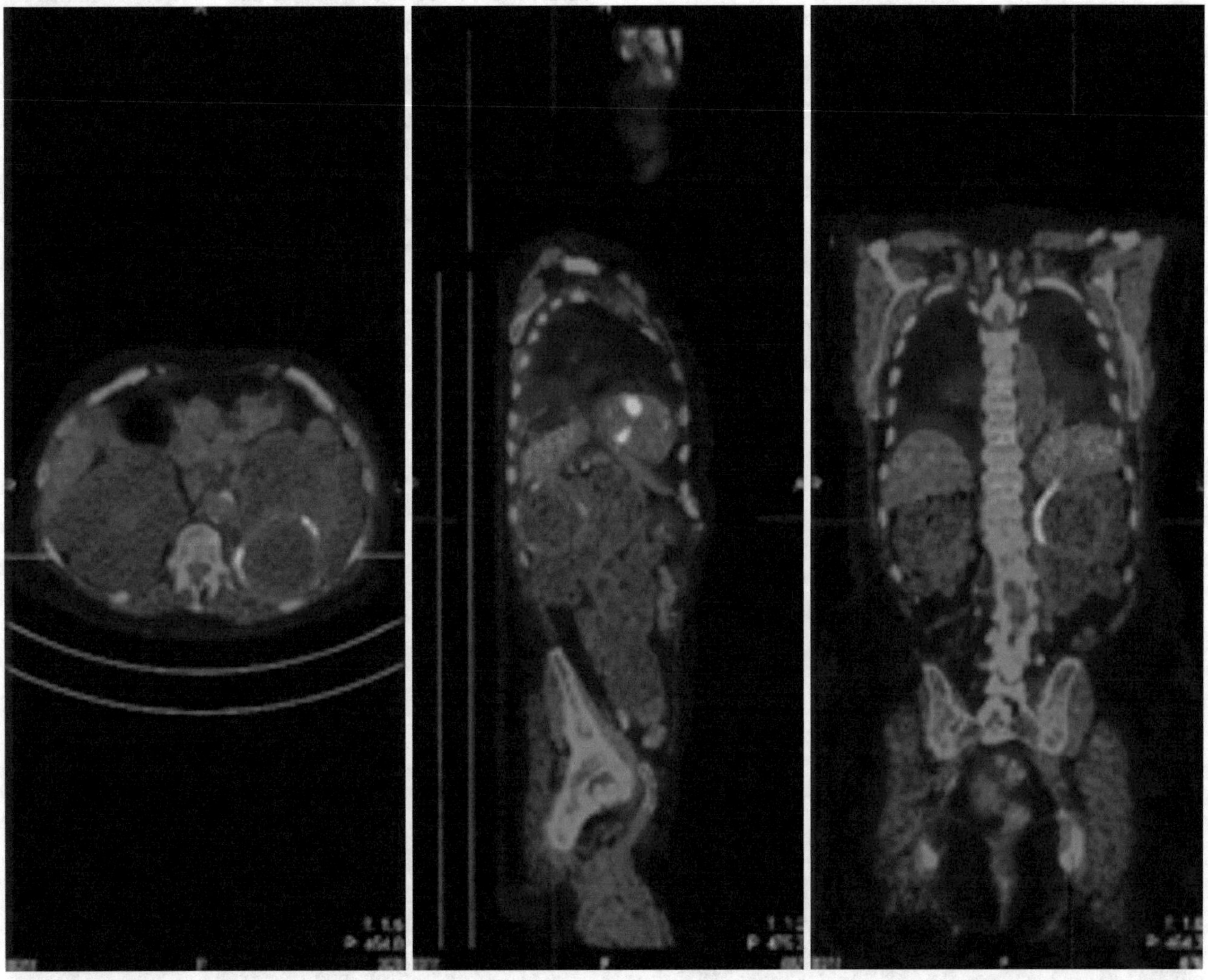

Fig. 11.13 Fused transaxial, coronal and sagittal [^{18}F]FDG PET/CT images in a patient with infected renal cyst. Markedly [^{18}F]FDG uptake with a ring-type pattern, indicating infection around the cyst

Since February 2012: Asthenia, anorexia, septic fever.

CT, 16 February 2012: Hypodense fluid-colliquative lesions in the liver with hyperdense peripheral ring.

PET, 21 February 2012: Focal hepatic lesions in segments VI and VIII with peripheral ring uptake associated with multiple lesions outside the liver.

Whole-body radiolabelled autologous WBC scintigraphy with SPECT/CT: Heterogeneous uptake in the liver due to the presence of cold areas (liver metastases); no uptake outside the liver.

Suspected Site of Infection

Differential diagnosis between liver metastases and liver abscesses.

Radiopharmaceutical Activity

^{111}In-oxine WBC, injected activity 19 MBq.

Imaging

Static planar spot images (4 min/image; 128 × 128 matrix). SPECT/CT images of the abdomen: dual head SPECT, matrix size 64 × 64, 35 s/step, 360° rotation, 5 mm/slice, low-dose CT slice thickness: 5 mm (Fig. 11.14). Planar imaging acquisition after 6 h and after 24 h. SPECT/CT images of the abdomen after 24 h.

Conclusion/Teaching Point

In the presence of suspected residual disease, on anatomic imaging or PET/CT and clinical signs of sepsis, relapse of disease should be considered after a negative labelled-WBC scan. Before starting chemotherapy, it is important to exclude septic focal lesions.

Case 11.2

Alberto Biggi✠

Male, age 64 years. 13 October 2011: Nephrectomized for clear cell renal carcinoma. Residual mild renal failure. During the follow-up, because of persistent abdominal pain and asthenia, an MRI (9 February 2012) was performed that showed a solid mass (4 × 4 cm) T1-hypo, T2-hyper in the surrenalic left area. For differential diagnosis between an abscess and a tumour relapse, an [^{18}F]FDG PET/CT was also performed (16 February 2012) that showed a clear focal uptake in the solid mass, suggesting tumour metastases.

Nevertheless, the patient was hospitalized due to septic fever associated with abnormal laboratory findings and a

✠ Dr. Alberto Biggi died prematurely on October 29, 2019.

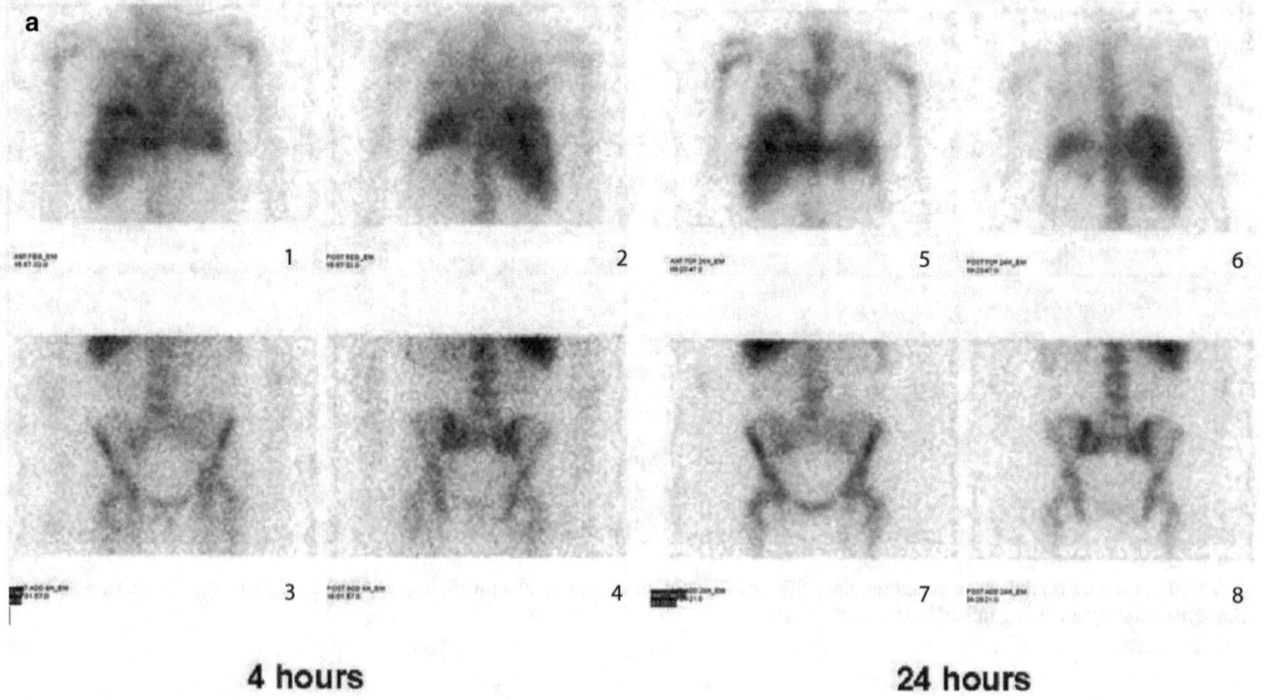

Fig. 11.14 (**a**) ^{111}In-oxine-WBC scintigraphy: planar imaging show normal biodistribution of the labelled WBCs in the thorax and abdomen (*1* and *5* anterior chest, *2* and *6* posterior chest, *3* and *7* anterior abdomen, *4* and *8* posterior abdomen); the uptake in the liver is heterogeneous with areas of focal uptake, suspicious for infection, identified in VI and VIII segments. (**b**) SPECT/CT images (CT, *upper*; fused images, *lower*): cold areas in correspondence of the focal lesions with a peripheral ring of increased activity identified by PET/CT. (**c**) [^{18}F]FDG PET/CT was performed 1 h after 402 MBq of [^{18}F]FDG administration. Transaxial images (CT, *upper*; fused images, *lower*) showed focal lesions with peripheral ring uptake were observed in the liver (SVI and SVIII)

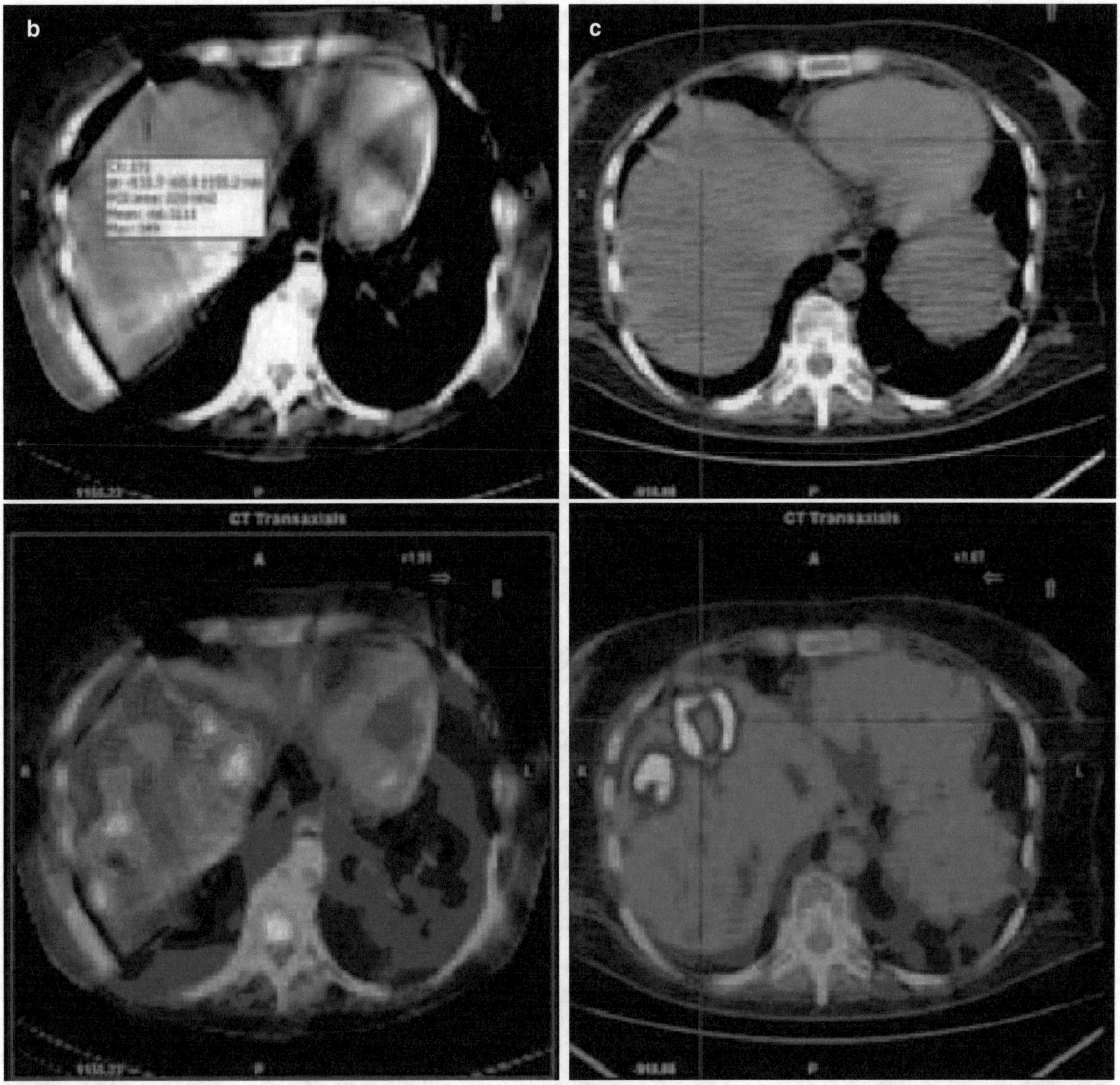

Fig. 11.14 (continued)

radiolabelled WBC whole body scan was performed (29 February 2012) that showed no uptake in the mass, which confirmed its neoplastic nature.

Suspected Site of Infection

Surrenalic left area.

Radiopharmaceutical Activity

^{111}In-oxine-WBC, injected activity 13 MBq, planar imaging acquisition after 6 h and after 24 h.

Imaging

Static planar spot images (4 min/image; 128 × 128 matrix). SPECT/CT images of the abdomen: dual head SPECT, matrix size 64 × 64, 35 s/step, 360° rotation, 5 mm/slice, low-dose CT slice thickness: 5 mm (Fig. 11.15).

Conclusion/Teaching Point

After surgery, in the presence of suspected residual disease, on anatomic imaging and clinical signs of sepsis, relapse of disease should be considered after a negative labelled WBC

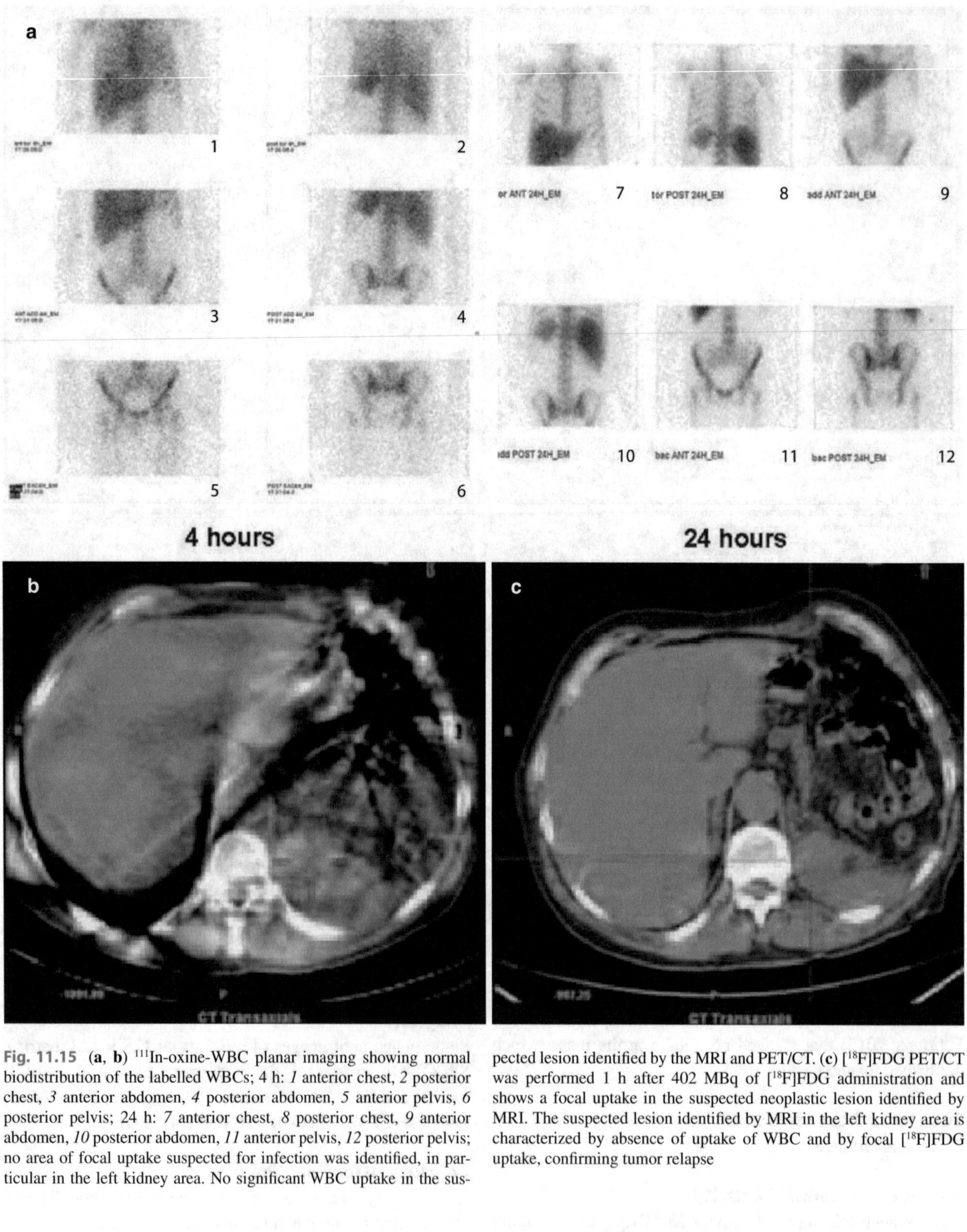

Fig. 11.15 (**a**, **b**) ^{111}In-oxine-WBC planar imaging showing normal biodistribution of the labelled WBCs; 4 h: *1* anterior chest, *2* posterior chest, *3* anterior abdomen, *4* posterior abdomen, *5* anterior pelvis, *6* posterior pelvis; 24 h: *7* anterior chest, *8* posterior chest, *9* anterior abdomen, *10* posterior abdomen, *11* anterior pelvis, *12* posterior pelvis; no area of focal uptake suspected for infection was identified, in particular in the left kidney area. No significant WBC uptake in the suspected lesion identified by the MRI and PET/CT. (**c**) [^{18}F]FDG PET/CT was performed 1 h after 402 MBq of [^{18}F]FDG administration and shows a focal uptake in the suspected neoplastic lesion identified by MRI. The suspected lesion identified by MRI in the left kidney area is characterized by absence of uptake of WBC and by focal [^{18}F]FDG uptake, confirming tumor relapse

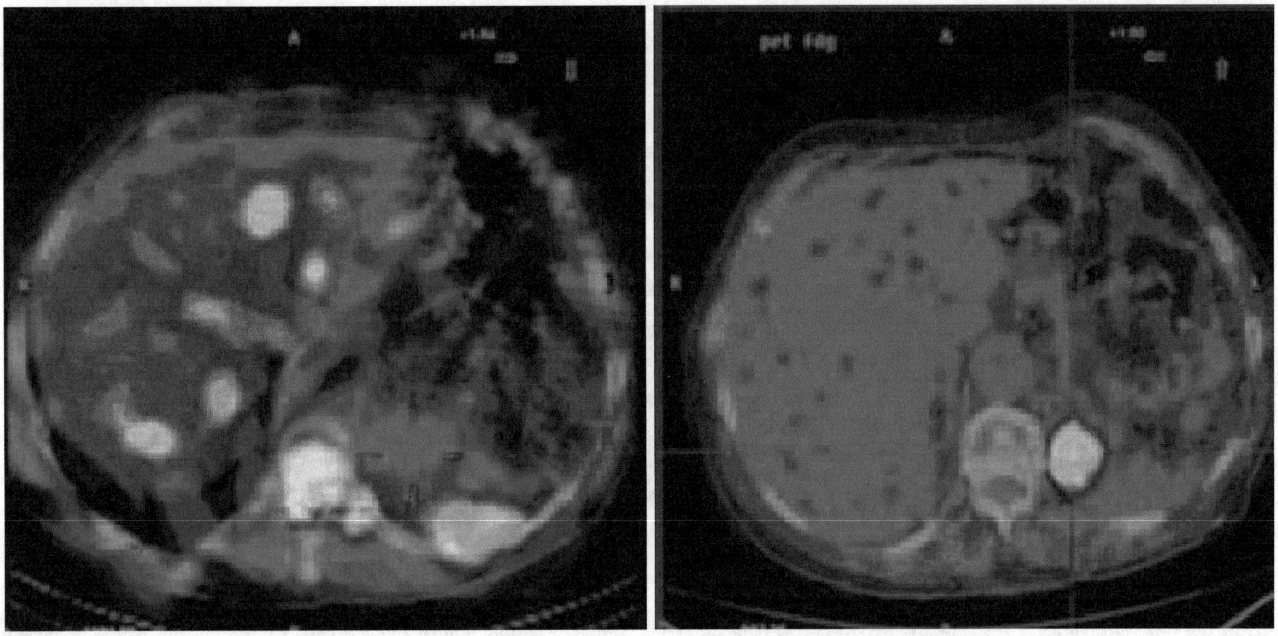

Fig. 11.15 (continued)

scan. The patient was finally operated on for relapse of clear cell renal carcinoma.

Case 11.3

Jose Martin-Comin

Male, age 48 years, presenting with bloody diarrhoea, abdominal pain, showed general laboratory data for inflammatory disease, and was referred to colonoscopy that showed a normal colonic mucosa and multiple biopsies compatible with Crohn's disease. He was then referred to nuclear medicine for a radiolabelled WBC scan in order to confirm disease and evaluate its activity and extent.

Scintigraphy confirmed the colonic location of the disease with severe activity and no complications, and steroid treatment was started. After 1 year, the colonoscopy was repeated and was normal again, but due to an increase of pain and subobstruction, stronger immunosuppression was added to the therapy. After 3 months, symptoms and subobstruction disappeared, but the Crohn's disease activity index (CDAI) was still 300. Therefore, a new radiolabelled WBC scan was requested.

Scintigraphy showed very mild colonic uptake, in contrast with elevated CDAI. Therapy was discontinued and CDAI decreased with time to normal values.

The patient had no clinical relapse for 7 years, and no other colonoscopies were performed. After 7 years, abdominal pain started again. CDAI increased to 250 and a new colonoscopy was again normal with normal biopsies. For the correct evaluation of the disease activity and the extent, a third radiolabelled WBC scan was requested. Scintigraphy identified a diffused ileal accumulation of WBC without colonic involvement. In these 7 years, the disease evolved from colon to ileum. The radiolabelled scan always correctly identified disease activity, differently from colonoscopy and CDAI measurement.

Suspected Site of Disease

Colonic Crohn's disease.

Radiopharmaceutical Activity

^{99m}Tc-HMPAO-WBC (550–625 MBq) was administered on each occasion.

Imaging

Planar anteroposterior images were acquired for 300–500 s, 2 h after cell administration (Fig. 11.16).

Conclusion/Teaching Point

Radiolabelled WBC scintigraphy can help in the evaluation of Crohn's disease extent and evaluate its activity. It is a useful method in addition to colonoscopy and allows the examination of all bowel segments.

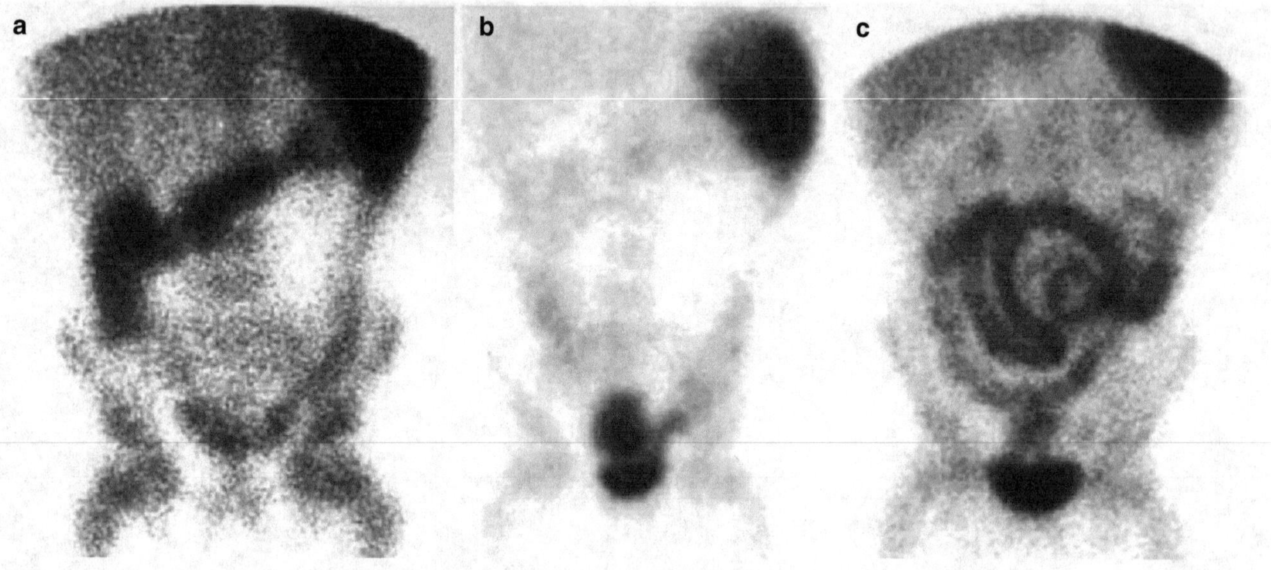

Fig. 11.16 ^{99m}Tc-HMPAO-leukocyte scintigraphy in Crohn's disease. (**a**) At the time of diagnosis, a severe colonic disease is detected. (**b**) One year later, patient was in remission with very mild and diffused colonic activity. (**c**) After 7 years, the patient had a clinical disease relapse and images showed moderate to severe pan-ileitis. Note physiologic accumulation of labeled cells by the spleen, which is always higher than liver accumulation; this is a sign of undamaged labeled cells

References

1. Krukowski ZH, Matheson NA. Ten-year computerized audit of infection after abdominal surgery. Br J Surg. 1988;75:857–61.
2. Weiss G, Meyer F, Lipper H. Infectivological diagnostic problems in tertiary peritonitis. Langenbeck's Arch Surg. 2006;391:437–82.
3. Solomkin JS, Mazuski JE, Baron EJ, et al. Guidelines for the selection of anti-infective agents for complicated intra-abdominal infections. Clin Infect Dis. 2003;37:997–1005.
4. Cheadle WG, Spain DA. The continuing challenge of intra-abdominal infection. Am J Surg. 2003;186:15S–22S.
5. Christou NV, Barie PS, Dellinger EP, et al. Surgical Infection Society intra-abdominal infection study. Prospective evaluation and management techniques and outcome. Arch Surg. 1993;128:193–8.
6. Bohnen J, Boulanger M, Meakins JL, et al. Prognosis in generalized peritonitis. Relation to cause and risk factors. Arch Surg. 1983;118:285–90.
7. Mazuski JE, Sawyer RG, Nathens AB, et al. The Surgical Infection Society guidelines on antimicrobial therapy for intra-abdominal infections: evidence for the recommendations. Surg Infect. 2002;3:175–233.
8. Solomkin JS, Mazuski JE, Bradley JS, et al. Diagnosis and management of complicated intra-abdominal infection in adults and children: guidelines by the Surgical Infection Society and the Infectious Diseases Society of America. Surg Infect (Larchmt). 2010;11:79–109.
9. Ogawa S, Itabashi M, Kameoka S. Significance of FDG-PET in identification of diseases of the appendix—based on experience of two cases falsely positive for FDG accumulation. Case Rep Gastroenterol. 2009;3:125–30.
10. Koff SG, Sterbis JR, Davison JM, Montilla-Soler JL. A unique presentation of appendicitis: F-18 FDG PET/CT. Clin Nucl Med. 2006;31:704–6.
11. Tahara T, Ichiya Y, Kuwabara Y, et al. High [^{18}F]-fluorodeoxyglucose uptake in abdominal abscesses: a PET study. J Comput Assist Tomogr. 1989;13:829–31.
12. Signore A, Jamar F, Israel O, et al. Clinical indications, image acquisition and data interpretation for white blood cells and anti-granulocyte monoclonal antibody scintigraphy: an EANM procedural guideline. Eur J Nucl Med Mol Imaging. 2018;45:1816–31.
13. Jamar F, Buscombe J, Chiti A, et al. EANM/SNMMI guideline for ^{18}F-FDG use in inflammation and infection. J Nucl Med. 2013;54:647–58.
14. Panes J, Bouhnik Y, Reinisch W, et al. Imaging techniques for assessment of inflammatory bowel disease: joint ECCO and ESGAR evidence-based consensus guidelines. J Crohns Colitis. 2013;7:556–85.
15. Viscido A, Aratari A, Maccioni F, et al. Inflammatory bowel diseases: clinical update of practical guidelines. Nucl Med Commun. 2005;26:649–55.
16. Annovazzi A, Bagni B, Burroni L, et al. Nuclear medicine imaging of inflammatory/infective disorders of the abdomen. Nucl Med Commun. 2005;26:657–64.
17. Peacock K, Porn U, Howman-Giles R, et al. ^{99m}Tc-Stannous colloid white cell scintigraphy in childhood inflammatory bowel disease. J Nucl Med. 2004;45:261–5.
18. de Groot M, Meeuwis AP, Kok PJ, et al. Influence of blood glucose level, age and fasting period on non-pathological FDG uptake in heart and gut. Eur J Nucl Med Mol Imaging. 2005;32:98–101.
19. Toriihara A, Yoshida K, Umehara I, Shibuya H. Normal variants of bowel FDG uptake in dual-time-point PET/CT imaging. Ann Nucl Med. 2011;25:173–8.
20. Glaudemans AWJM, Quintero AM, Signore A. PET/MRI in infectious and inflammatory diseases: will it be a useful improvement? Eur J Nucl Med Mol Imaging. 2012;39:745–9.
21. Sollini M, Berchiolli R, Kirienko M, et al. PET/MRI in infection and inflammation. Semin Nucl Med. 2018;48:225–41.
22. Karczmarczyk U, Garnuszek P, Maurin M, et al. Investigation of ^{99m}Tc-labelling of recombinant human interleukin-2 via hydrazinenicotinamide. Nucl Med Biol. 2010;37:795–803.
23. Signore A, Chianelli M, Annovazzi A, et al. ^{123}I-Interleukin-2 scintigraphy for the in vivo assessment of intestinal mononuclear cell infiltration in Crohn's disease. J Nucl Med. 2000;4:242–9.

24. Annovazzi A, Biancone L, Caviglia R, et al. ^{99m}Tc-interleukin-2 and ^{99m}Tc-HMPAO granulocyte scintigraphy in patients with inactive Crohn's disease. Eur J Nucl Med Mol Imaging. 2003;30:374–82.
25. D'Alessandria C, Malviya G, Viscido A, et al. Use of a ^{99m}Tc labeled anti-TNF-alpha monoclonal antibody in Crohn's disease: in vitro and in vivo studies. Q J Nucl Med Mol Imaging. 2007;51:334–42.
26. Versari A, et al. FDG-PET in idiopathic retroperitoneal fibrosis [abstract]. J Nucl Med. 2007;48(Suppl 2):288P.
27. Morin G, Mageau A, Benali K, et al. Persistent FDG/PET CT uptake in idiopathic retroperitoneal fibrosis helps identifying patients at a higher risk for relapse. Eur J Intern Med. 2019;62:67–71.
28. Cobb WS, Carbonell AM, Kalbaugh CL, et al. Infection risk of open placement of intraperitoneal composite mesh. Am Surg. 2009;75:762–8.
29. Vix J, Meyer C, Rohr S, et al. The treatment of incisional and abdominal hernia with a prosthesis in potentially infected tissues: a series of 47 cases. Hernia. 1997;1:157–61.
30. Petersen S, Henke G, Freitag M, et al. Deep prosthesis infection in incisional hernia repair: predictive factors and clinical outcome. Eur J Surg. 2001;167:453–7.
31. Eriksen JR, Gogenur T, Rosenberg J. Choice of mesh for laparoscopic ventral hernia repair. Hernia. 2007;11:481–92.
32. Sanchez VM, Abi-Haidar YE, Itani KM. Mesh infection in ventral incisional hernia repair: incidence, contributing factors, and treatment. Surg Infect. 2011;12:205–10.
33. Zuvela M, Antic A, Bajec D, et al. Diagnosis of mesh infection after abdominal wall hernia surgery—role of radionuclide methods. Hepato-Gastroenterology. 2011;58(110–111):1455–60.
34. Lin WY, Chao TH, Wang SJ. Clinical features and gallium scan in the detection of post-surgical infection in the elderly. Eur J Nucl Med Mol Imaging. 2002;29:371–5.
35. Datz FL. Abdominal abscess detection: gallium, ^{111}In-, and ^{99m}Tc-labeled leukocytes, and polyclonal and monoclonal antibodies. Semin Nucl Med. 1996;26:51–64.
36. Palestro CJ, Love C, Tronco GG, Tomas MB. Role of radionuclide imaging in the diagnosis of postoperative infection. Radiographics. 2000;20:1649–60.
37. Thodis E, Passadakis P, Lyrantzopooulos N, et al. Peritoneal catheters and related infections. Int Urol Nephrol. 2005;37:379–93.
38. Vargemezis V. Prevention and management of peritonitis and exit-site infection in patients on continuous ambulatory peritoneal dialysis. Nephrol Dial Transplant. 2001;16(Suppl 6):106–8.
39. Quantrill SJ, Woodhead MA, Bell CE, et al. Peritoneal tuberculosis in patients receiving continuous ambulatory peritoneal dialysis. Nephrol Dial Transplant. 2001;16:1024–7.
40. Stuart S, Booth TC, Cash CJ, et al. Complications of continuous ambulatory peritoneal dialysis. Radiographics. 2009;29:441–60.
41. Sheikh M, Abu-Zidan F, al-Hilaly M, Behbehani A. Abdominal tuberculosis: comparison of sonography and computed tomography. J Clin Ultrasound. 1995;23:413–7.
42. Kipper SL, Steiner RW, Wilztum KF, et al. In-111-leukocyte scintigraphy for detection of infection associated with peritoneal dialysis catheters. Radiology. 1984;151:491–4.
43. Ruiz Solis S, Garcia Vicente A, et al. Diagnosis of the infectious complications of continuous ambulatory peritoneal dialysis by ^{99m}Tc-HMPAO labeled leucocytes [Spanish]. Rev Esp Med Nucl. 2004;23:403–13.
44. Gibel LJ, Hartshorne MF, Tzamaloukas AH. Indium-111 oxine leukocyte scan in the diagnosis of peritoneal catheter tunnel infections. Perit Dial Int. 1998;18:234–5.
45. Gibel LJ, Quintana BJ, Tzamaloukas AH, Garcia DL. Soft tissue complications of Tenckhoff catheters. Adv Perit Dial. 1989;5:229–33.
46. Carlos MG, Juliana R, Matilde N, et al. Hidden clotted vascular access infection diagnosed by fluorodeoxyglucose positron emission tomography. Nephrology (Carlton). 2008;13:264–5.
47. Singh P, Wiggins B, Sun Y, et al. Imaging of peritoneal catheter tunnel infection using positron-emission tomography. Adv Perit Dial. 2010;26:96–100.
48. Mahfouz T, Miceli MH, Saghafifar F, et al. ^{18}F-Fluorodeoxyglucose positron emission tomography contributes to the diagnosis and management of infections in patients with multiple myeloma: a study of 165 infectious episodes. J Clin Oncol. 2005;23:7857–63.
49. Sallée M, Rafat C, Zahar JR, et al. Cyst infections in patients with autosomal dominant polycystic kidney disease. Clin J Am Soc Nephrol. 2009;4:1183–9.
50. Balbo BE, Sapienza MT, Ono CR, et al. Cyst infection in hospital-admitted autosomal dominant polycystic kidney disease patients is predominantly multifocal and associated with kidney and liver volume. Braz J Med Biol Res. 2014;47:584–93.
51. Bobot M, Ghez C, Gondouin B, et al. Diagnostic performance of [^{18}F]fluorodeoxyglucose positron emission tomography-computed tomography in cyst infection in patients with autosomal dominant polycystic kidney disease. Clin Microbiol Infect. 2016;22:71–7.
52. Pijl JP, Kwee TC, Slart RHJA, Glaudemans AWJM. FDG-PET/CT for diagnosis of cyst infection in autosomal dominant polycystic kidney disease. Clin Transl Imaging. 2018;6:61–7.

Nuclear Medicine Imaging of Diabetic Foot

12

Napoleone Prandini and Andrea Bedini

Contents

Learning Objectives

- To acquire basic knowledge of the clinical problems of diabetic foot complications and their management
- To understand the pathophysiologic bases of the development of the infection in diabetic foot and of the Charcot neuroarthropathy
- To become familiar with the diagnosis of diabetic foot infection using radionuclide imaging techniques
- To become familiar with the most common imaging presentations of diabetic foot infection

Diabetes is an increasing public health concern with an estimated 422 million adults living with diabetes in 2014; its increase in prevalence occurs at a faster rate in low- and middle-income countries [1]. Approximately 25% of the patients with diabetes will develop diabetic foot ulcers (DFUs) in their lifetime [2], with an incidence of 2–7% per year; 60% of DFUs become infected during the course of treatment, with 20% of infected patients developing osteomyelitis. Infected diabetic foot ulcerations are one of the most common reasons for hospitalization and are associated with an increased risk of multiple hospitalizations and of limb amputation [3–5] (Fig. 12.1). The impact of individual factors on the outcome of DFUs varies across communities and across countries. Of note, 80% of people with diabetes live in low- and middle-income countries [1], where many diagnostic techniques are not easily available—and are not expected to become so in the near future.

Diabetic foot is a condition where predisposing factors such as peripheral vascular disease and/or diabetic neuropathy affect function and/or structure of the lower limbs in a diabetic patient [6]. There are generally two or more risk factors that concur to the development of a foot ulcer in diabetic patients:

- Neuropathic foot: It is caused by diabetic neuropathy with involvement of sensory and/or motor nerve fibers.
- Vascular or ischemic foot: It is caused by peripheral artery disease, which represents a major factor in the evolution of the ulcer.

N. Prandini (✉)
Nuclear Medicine Department, Azienda Ospedaliero-Universitaria di Modena, Modena, Italy

A. Bedini
Infectious Diseases Unit, Department of Medical and Surgical Sciences for Children and Adults, University Hospital "Policlinico di Modena", Modena, Italy

E. Lazzeri et al. (eds.), *Radionuclide Imaging of Infection and Inflammation*, https://doi.org/10.1007/978-3-030-62175-9_12

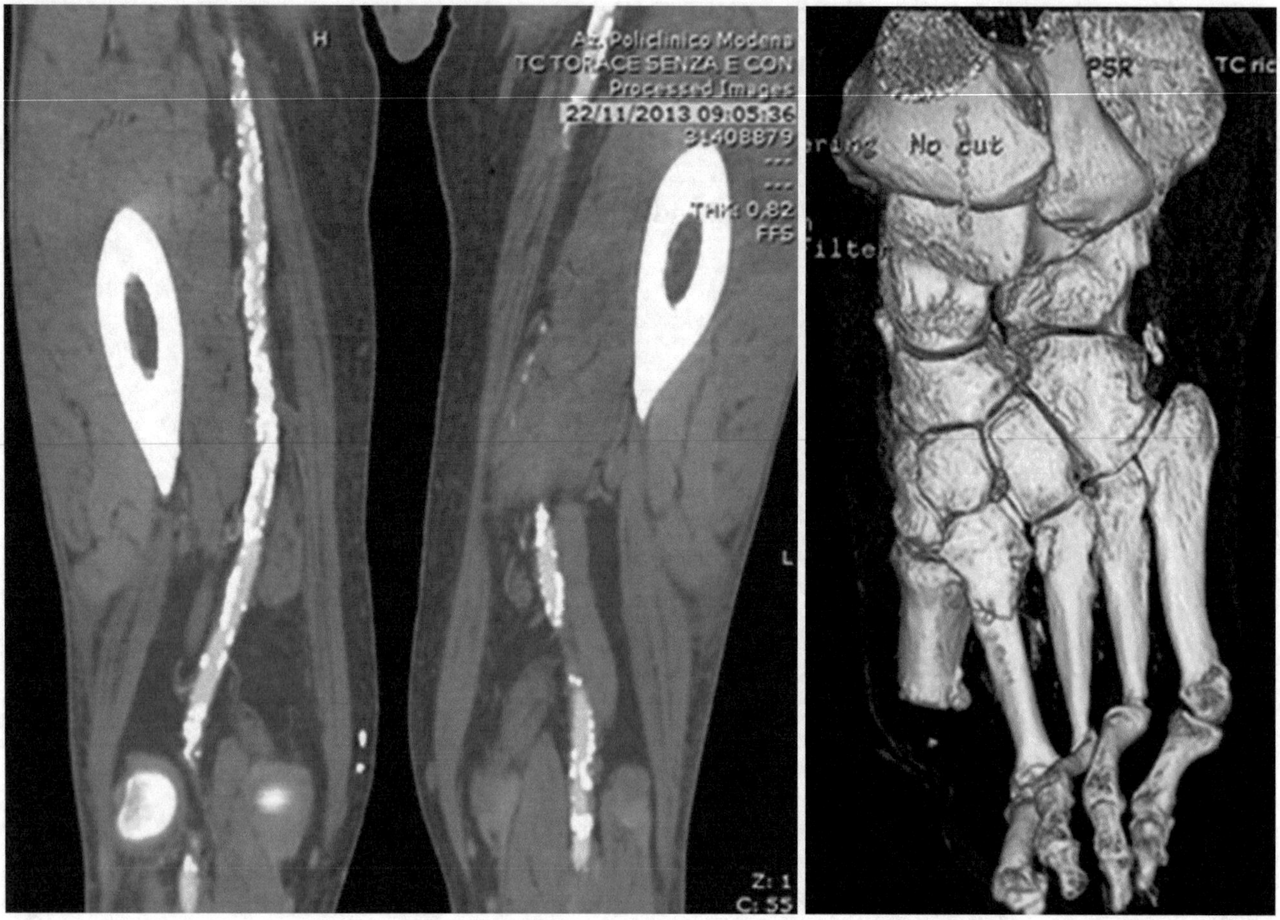

Fig. 12.1 CT images of the lower limbs of a patient with long-standing diabetes. Coronal section of the thighs displayed in left panel shows diffuse and intense calcification of the femoral arteries on both sides. The right panel displays the 3D surface volume rendering of left foot (with bone window), showing amputation of first toe

- Other conditions causing atherosclerotic lesions, such as hyperlipidemia, arterial hypertension, obesity, smoking, and hereditary factors associated with diabetes.

Although numerous classifications have been developed for DFUs, the International Working Group on Diabetic Foot recommends using the SINBAD system (Ischemia, Neuropathy, Bacterial Infection, Area, and Depth) [7] for better communication among health professionals about the characteristics of the ulcer in people with diabetes [8]. The SINBAD system is simple and quick to use, requiring no sophisticated equipment beyond clinical examination alone, and contains the necessary information to allow for triage by a specialists' team. The SINBAD system grades area, depth, sepsis, arteriopathy, and denervation plus site as either 0 or 1 point (Table 12.1); such easy-to-use scoring system generates a score that can achieve a maximum of 6 points. This classification has successfully been validated for prognostic purposes to predict both ulcer healing and amputation [9, 10].

Table 12.1 Clinical parameters included in the SINBAD scoring system (Ischemia, Neuropathy, Bacterial Infection, Area, and Depth)

Category	Definition	Score
Site	Forefoot	0
	Midfoot and hindfoot	1
Ischemia	Pedal blood flow intact: at least one palpable pulse	0
	Clinical evidence of reduced pedal flow	1
Neuropathy	Protective sensation intact	0
	Protective sensation lost	1
Bacterial infection	None	0
	Present	1
Area	Ulcer <1 cm^2	0
	Ulcer ≥1 cm^2	1
Depth	Ulcer confined to skin and subcutaneous tissue	0
	Ulcer reaching muscle, tendon, or deeper	1
Total possible score		6

12.1 Diabetic Foot Infection

It is a most serious condition, in which an infection develops in a foot with both sensitive and vascular impairment [11]. In acute diabetic foot infection, cellulitis and abscess, wet gangrene or gas-forming microorganisms, and necrotizing fasciitis may not only be a risk for the limb but also as a life-threatening condition. In the case of a chronic diabetic foot infection, the infection may involve only soft tissues (cellulitis and phlegmon) or the deeper tissues and bone (osteomyelitis).

In 2019, the Infectious Diseases Society of America (IDSA) proposed a further update of the classification of diabetic foot infection (DFI) [12], previously published in 2004 and already updated in 2012 [13, 14]. The new classification is based on a four-tier system that is subdivided into "No infection," "Mild infection," "Moderate infection," and "Severe infection" based on the extent and severity of local clinical signs (mild and moderate) and on the presence of systemic signs of infection (moderate or severe) (Table 12.2). In the moderate and severe infection tiers, superficial infection, deep infection or abscess, and bone infection can be grouped together.

Table 12.2 Most recent classification system proposed by the Infectious Diseases Society of America (IDSA)

Diabetic foot ulceration without any sign of infection	No infection
The infection is limited to skin or superficial subcutaneous tissues without local complication or systemic illness ≥2 Manifestations of: • Local swelling or induration • Erythema (any extending ≤2 cm around the ulceration) • Local tenderness or pain • Local warmth • Purulent discharge	Mild soft tissue infection
Either systemically stable or unstable patient with ≥1 of the following: erythema extending >2 cm from the ulceration, lymphangitis, spread beneath the fascia, deep tissue abscess, gangrene. Can involve muscle, tendon, and joint, but does not involve bone. This includes patients who meet criteria for moderate or severe infections: • Temperature >38 °C or <36 °C • Heart rate >90 beats/min • Respiratory rate >20 breaths/min, or $PaCO_2$ < 32 mmHg • White blood cell count >12,000 or <4000 cells/µL, or ≥10% immature (band) forms	Moderate/severe soft tissue infection
Any bone infection of the foot. This includes patients who meet criteria for moderate or severe infections as noted above including systemic signs: • Temperature >38 °C or <36 °C • Hart rate >90 beats/min • Respiratory rate >20 breaths/min or $PaCO_2$ < 32 mmHg • White blood cell count >12,000 or <4000 cells/µL, or ≥10% immature (band) forms	Moderate/severe foot osteomyelitis

Osteomyelitis is defined as the infection of bone and bone marrow, and it develops as a result of an ulcer with bone exposure [15]. It most frequently affects prominent bone sites (metatarsal heads and joint capsules). Acute osteomyelitis is characterized by an inflammatory infiltrate with neutrophils, edema, and vascular congestion with thrombosis of small vessels; within a few days bone necrosis occurs, caused by ischemia due to infection of peripheral tissues. Whereas, chronic osteomyelitis is an infection that has been present for some time and is therefore characterized by cells in the chronic phase of the inflammatory process, followed by a reactive healing phase with osteoclast activation, fibroblast proliferation, formation of new bone, demarcation of the necrotic bone, fragmentation of reactive bone, and formation of fistulas through which pus and necrotic material reach the skin surface.

The techniques for diagnosing osteomyelitis include "probe to bone" probing (i.e., probing with a speculum from the superficial lesion or the fistula to bone), standard X-ray, magnetic resonance imaging (MRI), bone scintigraphy, scintigraphy with radiolabeled leukocytes (especially if including SPECT/CT imaging, as shown in Fig. 12.1), and bone biopsy with microbiologic culture [16–19].

Plain radiographs and "probe to bone" may misclassify early cases of osteomyelitis. Instead, when MRI and leukocyte scintigraphy with SPECT/CT imaging are negative, false-negative cases are rather uncommon [20].

The IDSA recommendations for moderate soft tissue infection (STI) are for initial parenteral therapy followed by oral antibiotics for a total of 1–2 weeks. For severe STI, the recommended treatment duration is 2–4 weeks, for bone infection with no residual osteomyelitis, after surgery it is of 2–5 days of oral antibiotics, and for patients with residual infection with viable bone, it is of 4–6 weeks of antibiotic treatment [14].

12.2 Charcot Neuroarthropathy

The development of Charcot foot is a dreadful complication that can be associated with peripheral neuropathy [21]. It commonly affects the middle of the foot, hind–foot joints, the ankle, and forefoot joints, and it is believed to result from inflammation in the foot that becomes abnormally protracted due to the underlying neuropathy. Charcot foot should be suspected if a patient presents with a hot, red, swollen foot, and presence of neuropathy. These serious deformities significantly alter the biomechanical forces and cause overloads and areas of localized high pressure where ulcers develop and frequently recur despite treatment.

The gold standard of conservative management strategy for Charcot neuroarthropathy has been immobilization and non-weight bearing [22]. Patient education is an essential component of the long-term management, focusing on the importance of appropriate footwear, offloading, regular follow-up reviews, and the risk of further complications [23, 24]. Patients should be educated on regular self-examinations of their feet for skin breakdown, swelling, erythema, and ulcers.

In patients with a Charcot foot, the differential diagnosis between neuroarthropathy and acute osteomyelitis is extremely important, since treatment of these two different conditions requires different therapeutic strategies. Diagnostic techniques for identifying and characterizing a Charcot foot include standard X-ray, MRI (repeated every 2–3 weeks to monitor evolution of the disease), bone scintigraphy, scintigraphy with radiolabeled leukocytes (to exclude osteomyelitis), and bone biopsy [25]. Radiolabeled leukocytes do not accumulate in the uninfected neuropathic joint, but hematopoietically active bone marrow can be present; in these cases, dual-tracer scintigraphy (labeled leukocytes followed by a radiocolloid scan) or three-phase leukocyte scintigraphy is necessary to distinguish active bone marrow from infection [17, 26, 27]. Investigations in this field are very active and so are the proposals of new modalities [28–30].

12.3 Imaging of the Diabetic Foot

MRI identifies bone oedema with accurate anatomical localization as early as 3–5 days from the onset of infection and is considered the primary imaging modality in DFIs, also because of its high spatial resolution and soft tissue contrast (Fig. 12.2) [31].

Key Learning Points

- Unlike scintigraphy or PET, MRI does not expose the patient to ionizing radiation.
- MRI has a very high resolution, associated with sensitivity comparable to that of [^{18}F]FDG PET/CT or of scintigraphy with labeled leukocytes.
- MRI is a suitable technique to distinguish bone infection from soft tissues infection.

The earliest nuclear medicine imaging technique employed to diagnose infections and Charcot neuroarthropathy in diabetic foot is three-phase bone scintigraphy: a positive scan indicates involvement of bone, but it cannot distinguish osteomyelitis from neuroarthropathy.

The 2012 American College of Radiology guidelines suggest the use of scintigraphy with labeled autologous leukocytes (^{111}In-oxine-WBC, or more recently ^{99m}Tc-HMPAO-WBC) as the first-line nuclear medicine scan to evaluate patients with DFI (Figs. 12.3 and 12.4) [32]. In this regard, SPECT/CT imaging provides definite advantages over planar scintigraphy, such as improved spatial resolution, better soft tissue contrast, and anatomical localization of the infection (Figs. 12.5 and 12.6).

Key Learning Points

- A three-phase acquisition protocol is recommended also for investigating osteomyelitis in diabetic foot.
- A 20–24 h acquisition is required for identifying low-grade infections.
- A three-phase acquisition protocol is recommended also when investigating osteomyelitis in diabetic foot with ^{99m}Tc-HMPAO-WBC scintigraphy, with acquisitions at 1 h, 4 h, and 20–24 h.
- The scan can be considered complete when the infection site is clearly demonstrated in the 4 h acquisition, as in this case (the delayed 20–24 h acquisition is therefore not invariably necessary).
- The added value of SPECT/CT imaging over planar imaging is to correctly localize the infection site in bone or in soft tissue (or both); this information considerably changes the treatment plan.
- Infection does not respect the tissue boundaries and can spread from bone to soft tissues.

The most recent radionuclide imaging procedure, PET/CT with the glycometabolic tracer [^{18}F]FDG has been proposed to investigate both infection and osteomyelitis of diabetic foot, although its role is still undergoing clinical validation [33]. When reviewing the diagnostic performance of [^{18}F]FDG PET for detecting osteomyelitis related to DFI (Fig. 12.7), Treglia et al. estimated an average sen-

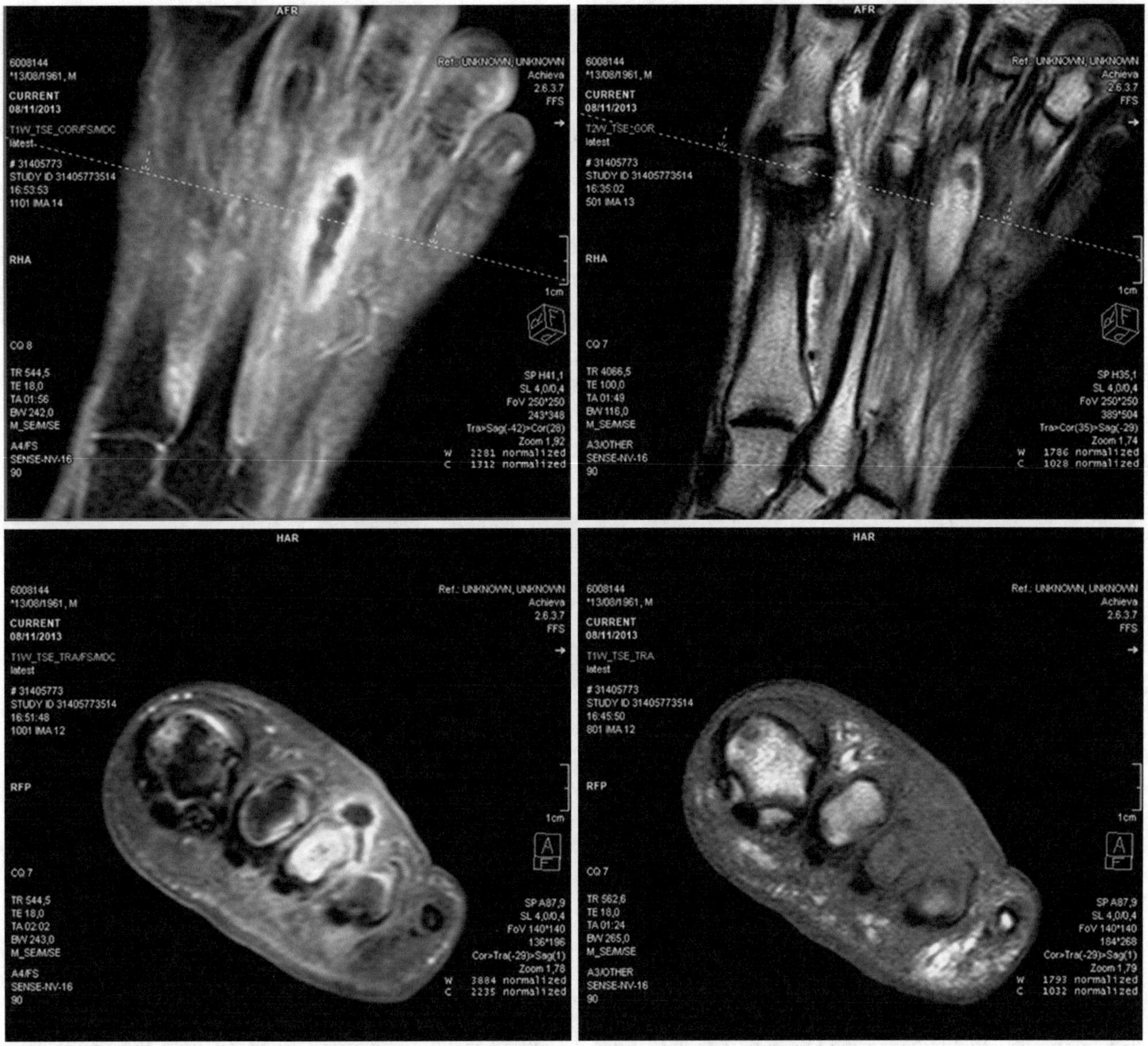

Fig. 12.2 MRI T1-weighted (left) and T2-weighted (right) images with axial reconstruction (upper row) and coronal reconstruction (lower row) of a patient with diabetic foot on the left side. Signal abnormality, characterized by hypointensity in T1 sequences, hyperintensity in T2 sequences, intense contrasting impregnation, is appreciable in the distal epiphysis and in the middle distal diaphysis of the III metatarsal. Fistula that reaches the ulnar side of the III metatarsal head from the cutaneous surface. These findings are consistent with osteomyelitis

sitivity ranging from 29 to 100%, with specificity ranged from 67 to 93% [34]. Other authors report lower values of specificity of [^{18}F]FDG PET, which is cannot distinguish between an infection (e.g., osteomyelitis), neoplasia, and sterile inflammation because of its accumulation in immune, bacterial, and tumoral cells. Furthermore, the uptake of glucose can remain abnormally high for 3–4 months after surgery or trauma. Nonetheless, [^{18}F]FDG PET is useful for the diagnosis of osteomyelitis in patients with DFI, because of its high spatial resolution and its ability to explore the whole body with fast results [35, 36].

Key Learning Point

- Imaging with [^{18}F]FDG PET/CT is very sensitive for assessing and localizing infection in diabetic foot.

In a more recent review and meta-analysis on the diagnostic approach to DFI, Lauri et al. reported that [^{18}F]FDG PET/CT and ^{99m}Tc-HMPAO-WBC scintigraphy each had the highest specificity (92%), followed by MRI and by ^{111}In-oxine–WBC scintigraphy (both 75%). Sensitivities were similar for all imaging modalities, that is, 93% for

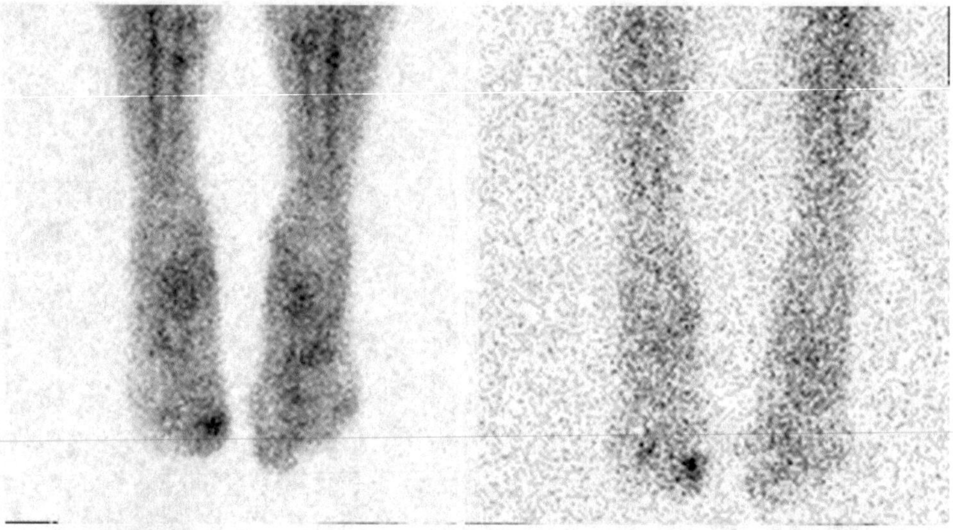

Fig. 12.3 Anterior views of ^{99m}Tc-HMPAO-WBC scintigraphy acquired at 4 h (left) and 20 h (right). The faint radioactivity accumulation in the first toe of right foot detectable in the 4 h image becomes a clear focal accumulation in the 20 h image

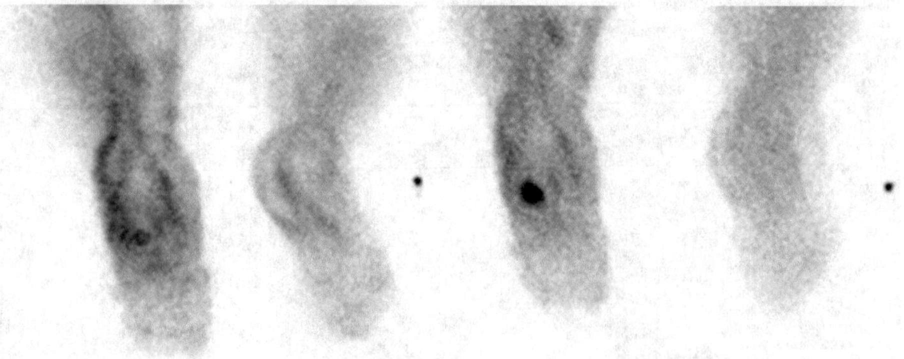

Fig. 12.4 ^{99m}Tc-HMPAO-WBC scintigraphy: planar posterior views acquired at 1 h (left) and 4 h (right) after administration. Faint radioactive accumulation in the middle of tarsum of left foot, barely detectable in the 1 h image, becomes a clear focus of accumulation in the 4 h image, with high target-to-background ratio

MRI, 92% for ^{111}In-oxine–WBC scintigraphy, 91% for ^{99m}Tc-HMPAO–WBC scintigraphy, and 89% for [^{18}F]FDG PET/CT [37].

All the imaging techniques mentioned above have proven to be quite accurate for diagnosing DFI and Charcot neuroarthropathy (Fig. 12.8). The clinician must approach the problem of the diabetic foot in several steps, starting from the simplest methods such as laboratory tests (ESR and PCR in the first place), moving on to the speculum and radiography for the simpler cases. The use of complex and expensive methods such as molecular analysis of samples, MRI, SPET/CT with labeled leukocytes, or PET/CT with [^{18}F]FDG must be considered within a multidisciplinary discussion of the most complex and controversial cases.

Clinical management of diabetic foot pathology involves many departments specialized in diabetes, infectious disease, radiology, clinical pathology, nuclear medicine, orthopedics, vascular surgery, and plastic surgery. A multidisciplinary discussion is therefore required to define a diagnostic and therapeutic path for the patients, selecting the most appropriate imaging test in each clinical situation. This will ensure the most cost-effective imaging method to allow accurate diagnosis with the lowest cost for the healthcare system (Fig. 12.9).

Key Learning Point

- [^{18}F]FDG PET/CT is a sensitive imaging method for assessing the Charcot neuroarthropathy involvement of the diabetic foot.
- Whole-body imaging acquired during [^{18}F]FDG PET/CT demonstrates the metastatic infectious foci that are often present in patients with diabetic foot infection.

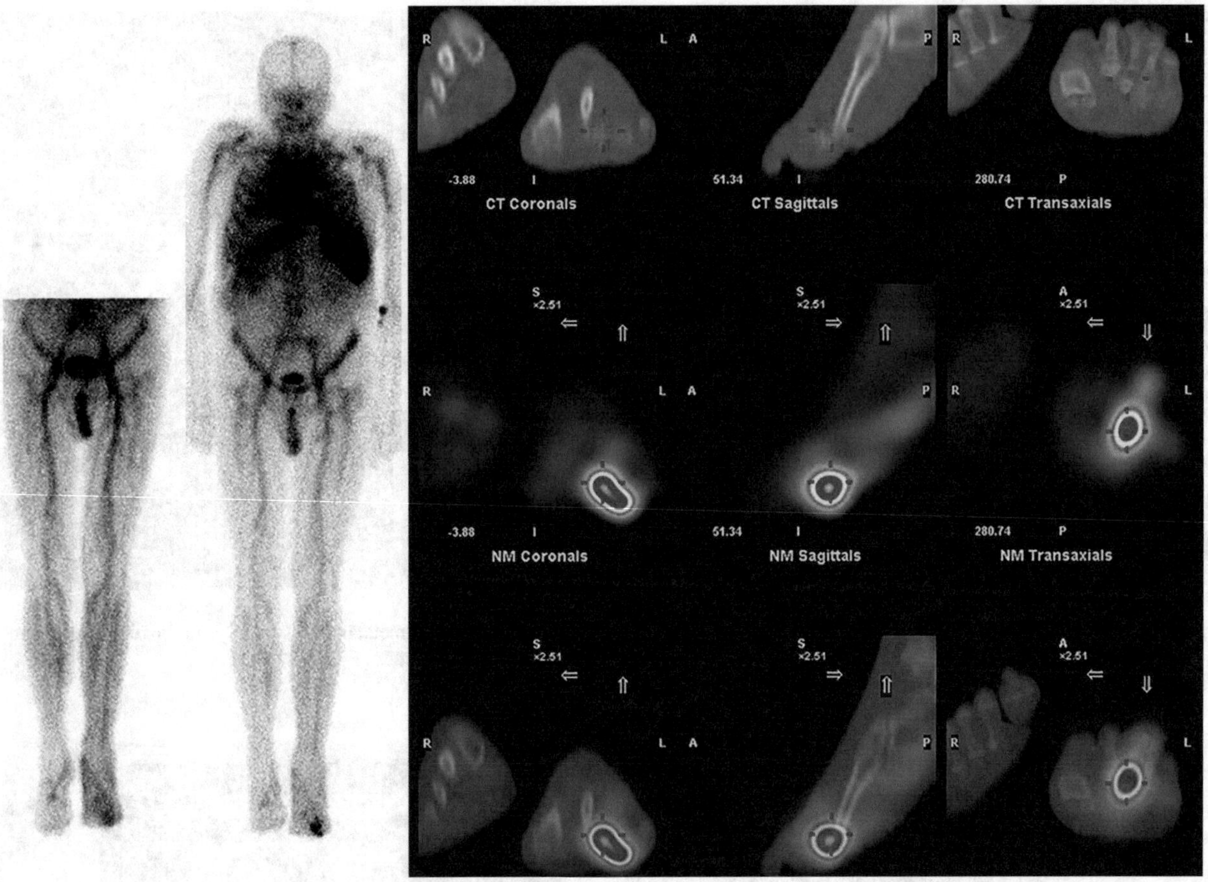

Fig. 12.5 ^{99m}Tc-HMPAO-WBC scintigraphy. Left panel displays the anterior planar views acquired at 1 and 4 h. Right panel shows the SPECT/CT sections of the feet in the three planes acquired at 4 h (low-dose CT in the upper row, SPECT in the middle row, fused SPECT/CT images in the lower row). The planar 1 h image shows increased perfusion in the left foot, with focal accumulation in the forefoot that becomes more evident in the 4 h image. SPECT/CT more precisely localizes osteomyelitis of the third and fourth toes of the left foot

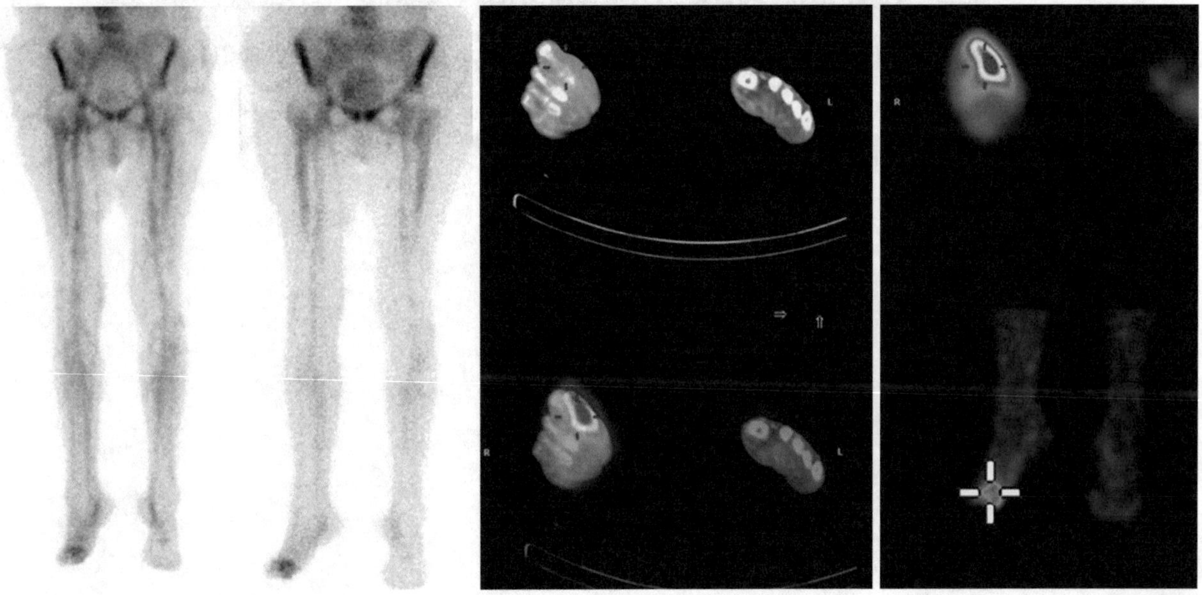

Fig. 12.6 ^{99m}Tc-HMPAO-WBC scintigraphy. Left panel displays the anterior planar views acquired at 1 and 4 h. Right panel shows coronal SPECT/CT sections of the feet (low-dose CT, upper left; SPECT, upper right; fused SPECT/CT image, lower left; MIP image, lower right). The planar 1 h image shows increased perfusion in right foot, with focal accumulation in the forefoot that becomes more evident in the 4 h image. SPECT/CT more precisely localizes infection mostly in the soft tissue of the first toe of the right foot

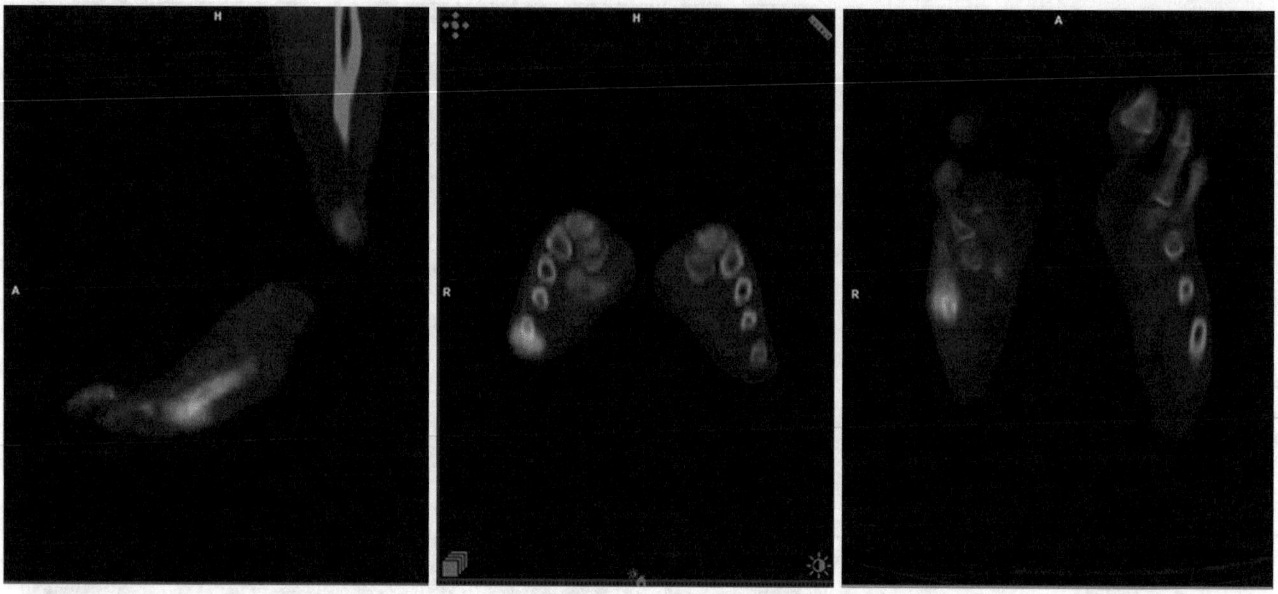

Fig. 12.7 [^{18}F]FDG PET/CT: fused sagittal section in the left panel, coronal section in the center panel, transaxial section in the right panel. A clear focus of increased [^{18}F]FDG uptake localizes correctly the infection in the fifth metatarsal-falangeal joint, involving both bone and surrounding soft tissues

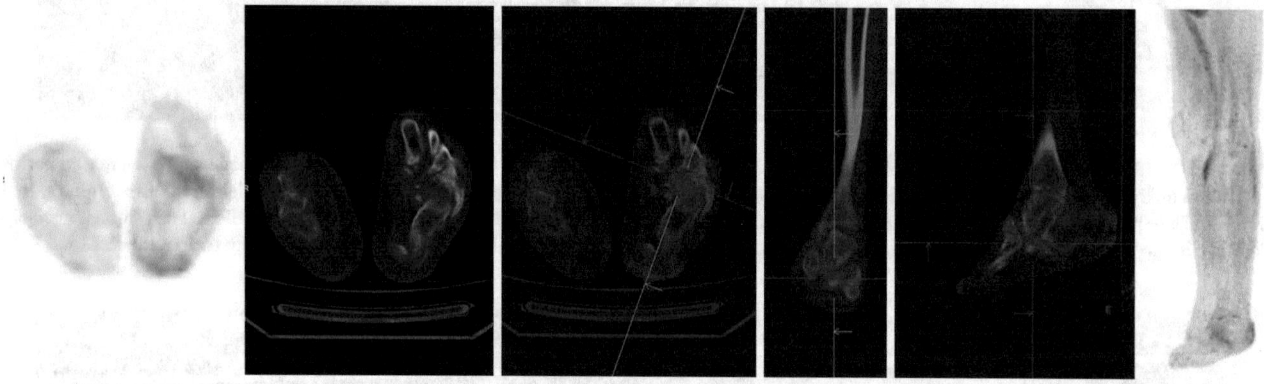

Fig. 12.8 [^{18}F]FDG PET/CT images from left to right: PET, low-dose CT, fused PET/CT coronal section, fused PET/CT sagittal section, MIP image. Diffuse moderately increased [^{18}F]FDG uptake in the mid foot and calcaneus, mostly in soft tissues, as typically observed in Charcot neuroarthropathy

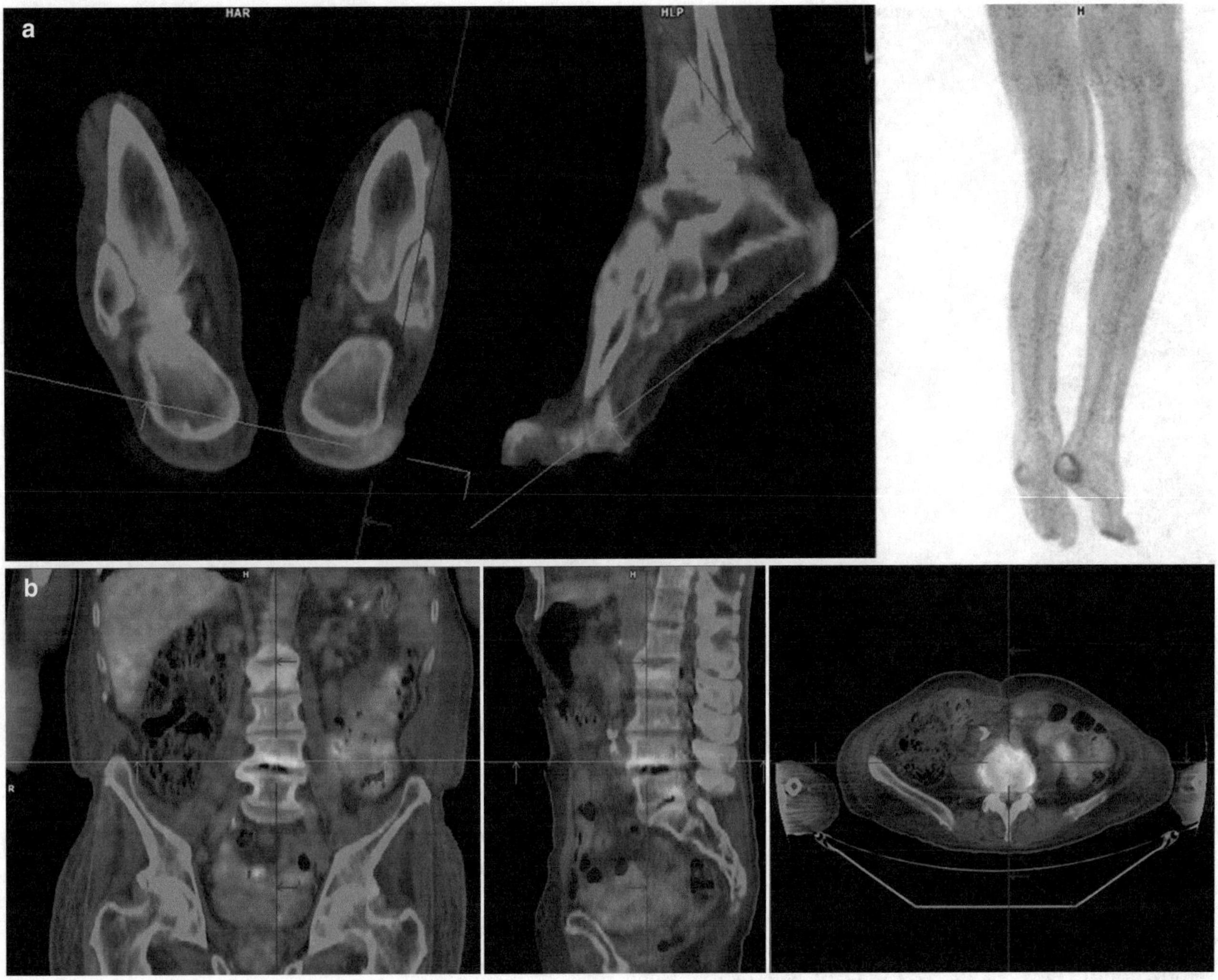

Fig. 12.9 [^{18}F]FDG PET/CT: (**a**) fused transaxial section (left), fused sagittal section of the right foot (center), MIP image (right), showing diffuse [^{18}F]FDG uptake in the calcaneal region corresponding to the skin ulcers that are better observed in the MIP image. (**b**) Fused coronal (left), sagittal (center), and transaxial sections (right), showing increased [^{18}F]FDG uptake at the lower portion of L5, with partial involvement of the perivertebral tissues. Final diagnosis was spondylodiscitis secondary to foot infection

Clinical Cases

Case 12.1

Chiara Peterle and Lorenzo Fantini

A 58-year-old female with history of type 1 diabetes (chronic therapy with insulin). Various amputations in the left foot (third and fourth metatarsal bones); weeping wound in the left foot treated by hyperbaric oxygen therapy and antibiotics (amoxicillin clavulanate + levofloxacin) until 10 days before bone scintigraphy (June 2011).

Clinical Presentation

Pain and loss of function of left foot; scar of previous weeping wound; red and swollen skin in left foot.

Previous Diagnostic Work-Up

X-rays of left foot; angio-CT and morphologic CT of the left foot; the patient needs a differential diagnosis between Charcot's foot and osteomyelitis (Figs. 12.10 and 12.11). MRI cannot be performed because of spinal cord implantable stimulator.

Suspected Site of Infection

Anterior part of left foot, near previous amputations.

Radiopharmaceutical Activity

Bone scan (740 MBq); ^{99m}Tc-HMPAO-leukocyte scan (814 MBq).

Imaging

Gamma camera type: Gamma camera that combines variable angle dual-detector with a dual slice CT scanner (Symbia-T2);

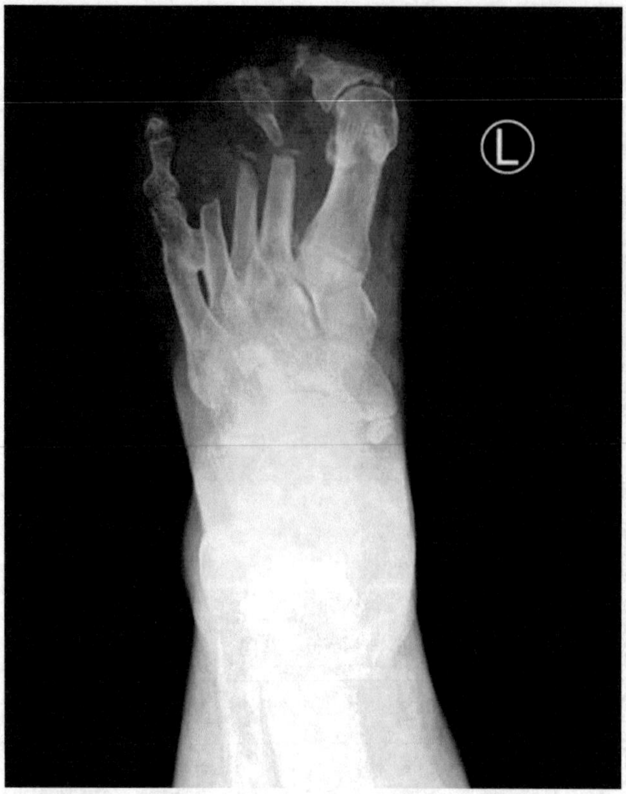

Fig. 12.10 X-ray of left foot: Previous bone amputations can be observed

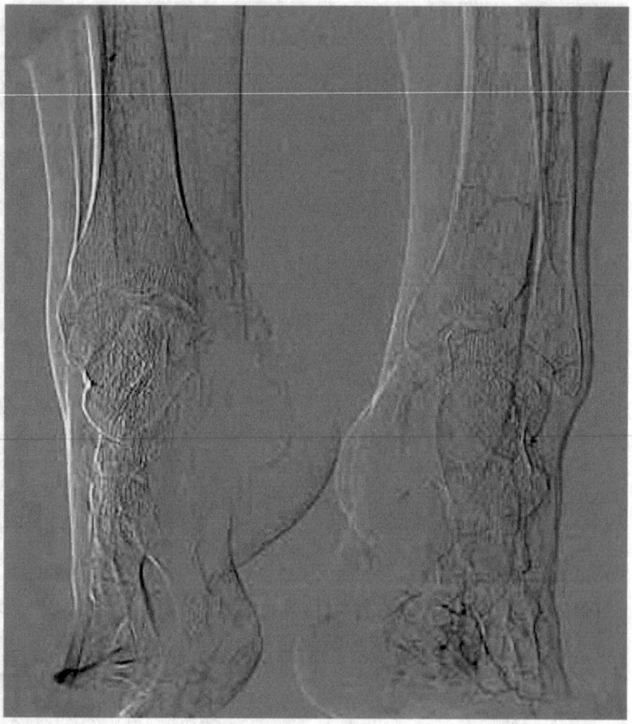

Fig. 12.11 Angio-CT: Increased vascularity near second metatarsal bone (sign of inflammation) can be observed

parallel holes collimator (low energy); Zoom: 1; SPECT matrix: 256 × 256. CT slice thickness: 1 mm. Display used for SPECT/CT fusion: 2D orthogonal MPR (multiplanar reformatting) (Figs. 12.12, 12.13, 12.14 and 12.15). Bone scan: (a) early scan (5 min after injection, 300 s) feet laid upon collimator; (b) late scan (3 h after injection, 498 s); leukocyte scan: (a) early scan, pool scan (1 h after injection, scan from pelvis to feet, 617 s); second scan (3 h after injection, scan from pelvis to feet, 928 s); late scan (20 h after injection, scan from pelvis to feet, 1856 s); SPECT/CT (20 h after injection).

Conclusion/Teaching Point

Since the patient only had inflammation of the left foot (Charcot's foot) with no infection, she did not go back to her hyperbaric and antibiotic therapy. She is still well now.

Case 12.2

Chiara Peterle and Ilaria Rambaldi

A 55-year-old male with the history of type 1 diabetes. Several amputations in both the feet; weeping wound in the left foot. Patient underwent no treatment until the examination was performed.

Clinical Presentation

Pain and loss of function of the left foot; red and swollen skin in the left foot.

Previous Diagnostic Work-Up

A tampon culture was performed; *Pseudomonas aeruginosa* was found. Patient needs a differential diagnosis, between infection of soft tissues only and osteomyelitis, to develop an appropriate treatment plan.

Suspected Site of Infection

Anterior part of the back of left foot, near previous amputations.

Radiopharmaceutical Activity

^{99m}Tc-HMPAO-leukocyte scintigraphy. Activity injected, 740 MBq.

Imaging

Gamma camera type: Gamma camera that combines variable angle dual-detector with a dual slice CT scanner (Symbia-T2); parallel holes collimator (low energy); Zoom, 1; SPECT matrix, 256 × 256; CT slice thickness,

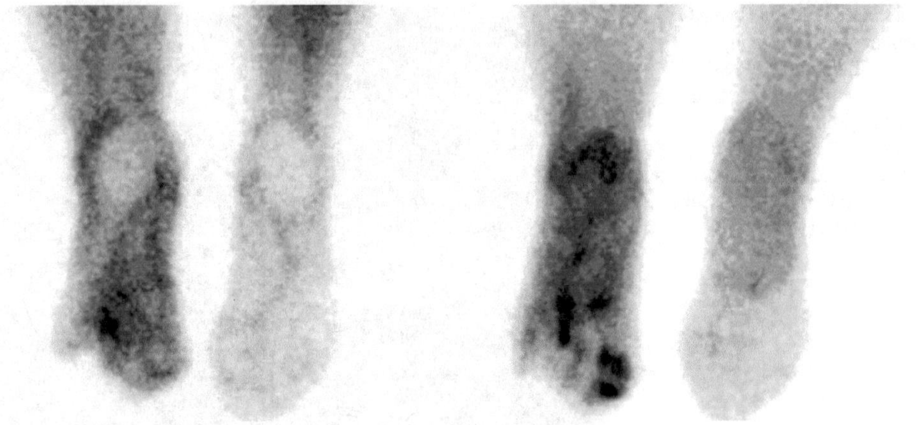

Fig. 12.12 ^{99m}Tc-MDP scintigraphy, planar posterior images of the feet. Two-phase bone scan: Increased vascularity in pool scan (*left*) and increased bone turnover in late scan (*right*); signs of inflammation (septic or aseptic?)

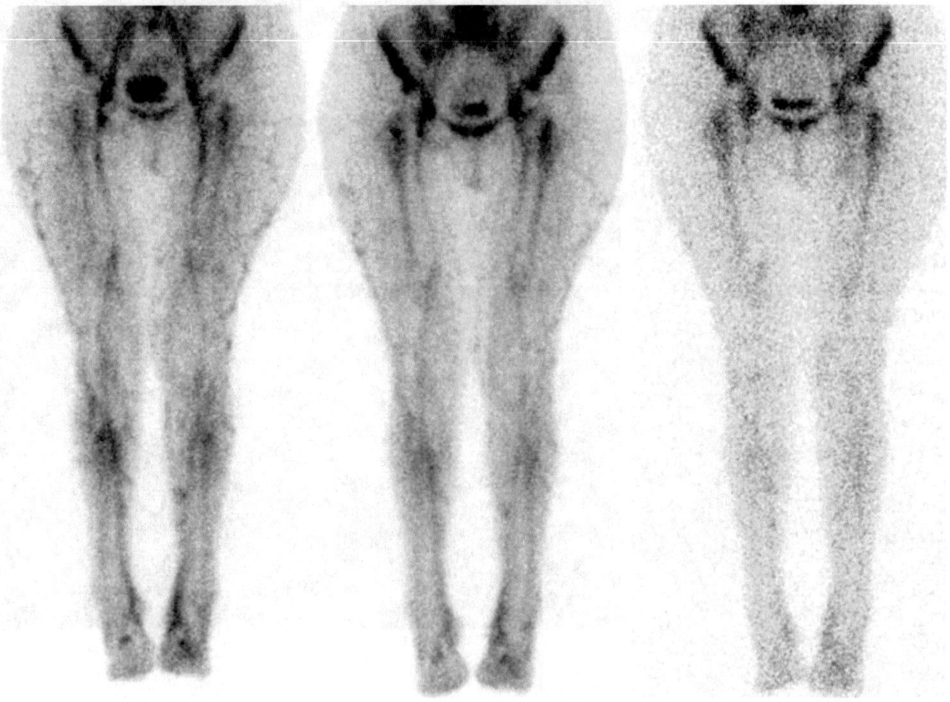

Fig. 12.13 ^{99m}Tc-HMPAO-leukocyte scintigraphy. Anterior scan images: In the first view on the left, we can see an increased uptake of leukocytes (inflammation) in the left foot that decreases in the 3 and 20 h scans (signs of aseptic inflammation, like in Charcot's foot disease)

1 mm; display used for SPECT/CT fusion, 2D orthogonal MPR (Figs. 12.16, 12.17, 12.18, and 12.19). Leukocyte scan: (a) early scan, pool scan (1 h after injection, scan from pelvis to feet, 636 s); second scan (3 h after injection, scan from pelvis to feet, 958 s); late scan (20 h after injection, scan from pelvis to feet, 1917 s); SPECT/CT (20 h after injection).

Conclusion/Teaching Point

Scintigraphy with radiolabeled leukocytes demonstrated osteomyelitis of the second metatarsal bone, in addition to the infection of soft tissues by *Pseudomonas aeruginosa*. The patient underwent an antibiotic specific therapy (imipenem + cilastatin). Finally, hyperbaric oxygen therapy was performed.

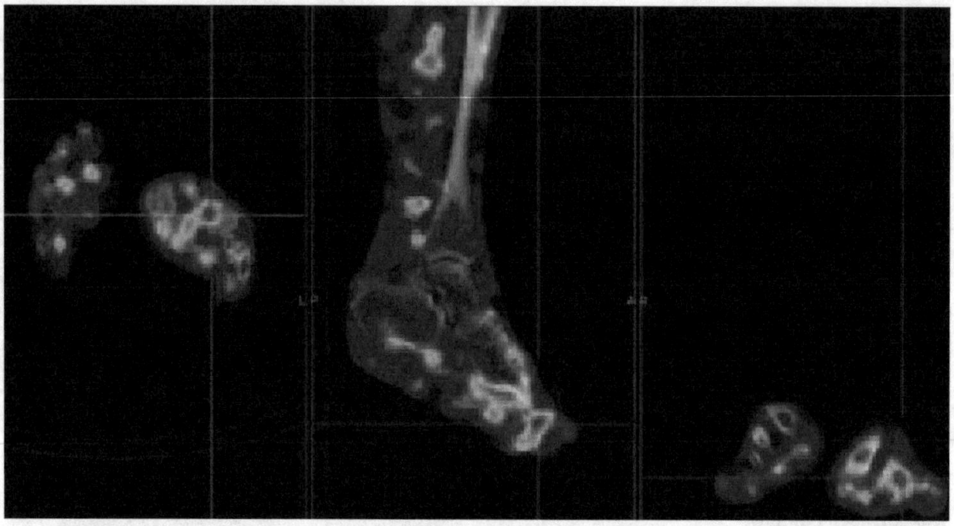

Fig. 12.14 ^{99m}Tc-HMPAO-leukocyte scintigraphy. 2D-orthogonal MPR SPECT/CT fused images (coronal, *left*; sagittal, *middle*; transaxial, *right*): A little uptake in soft tissues only, common in inflamed tissues can be observed

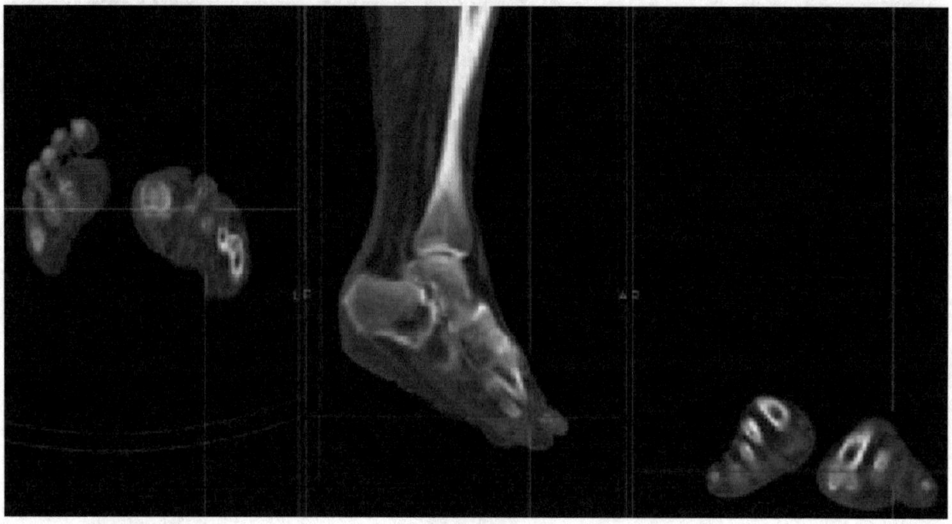

Fig. 12.15 ^{99m}Tc-HMPAO-leukocyte scintigraphy. 2D-orthogonal MPR SPECT/CT fusion: CT images (coronal, *left*; sagittal, *middle*; transaxial, *right*) only demonstrates the signs of amputation

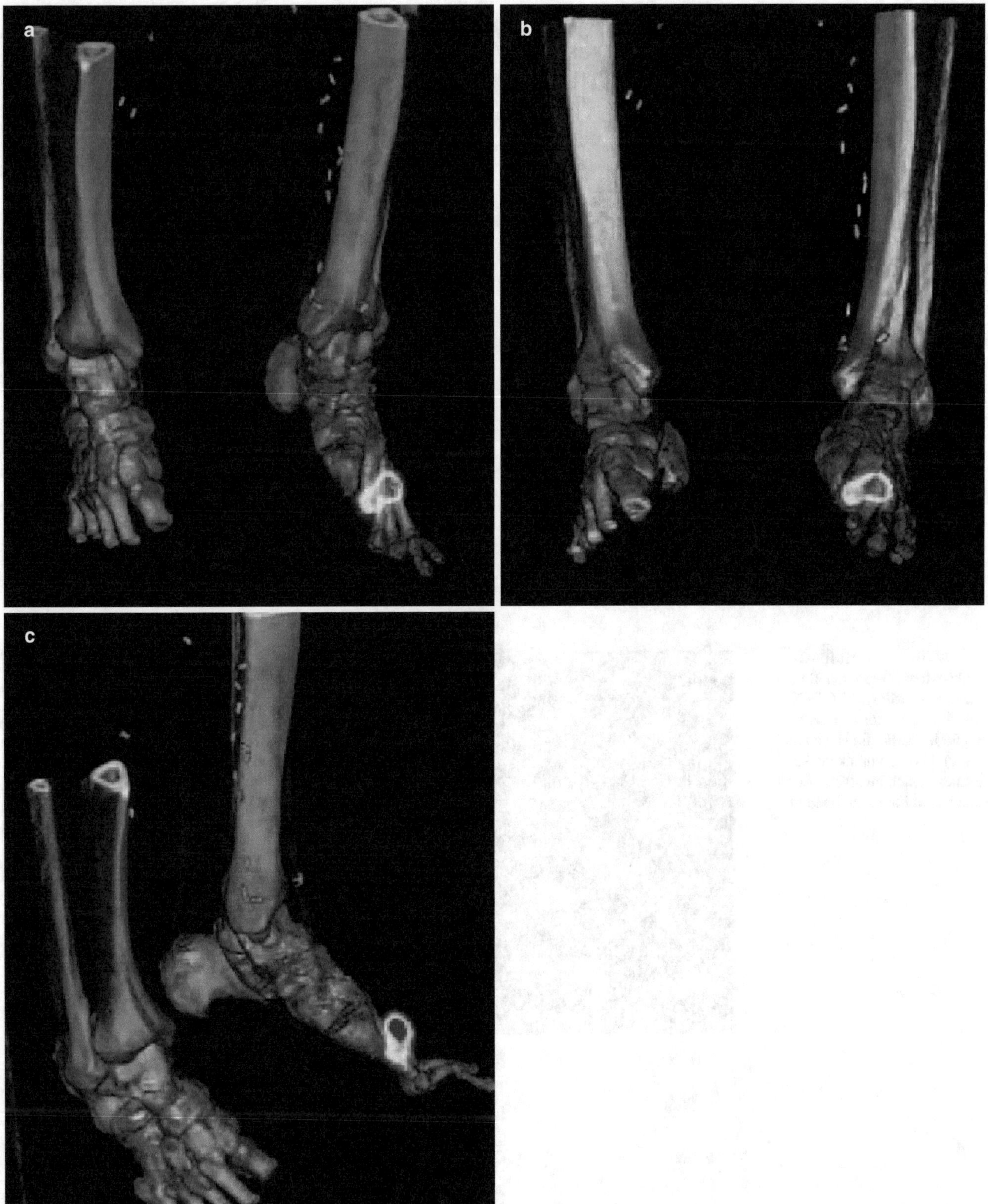

Fig. 12.16 ^{99m}Tc-HMPAO-leukocyte scintigraphy. 3D fusion volume rendering: (**a**) right anterior oblique view of the feet; (**b**) anterior view and (**c**) right lateral view of the feet. The spot in rainbow color shows site of infection. Bilateral amputations of bones in feet can be seen

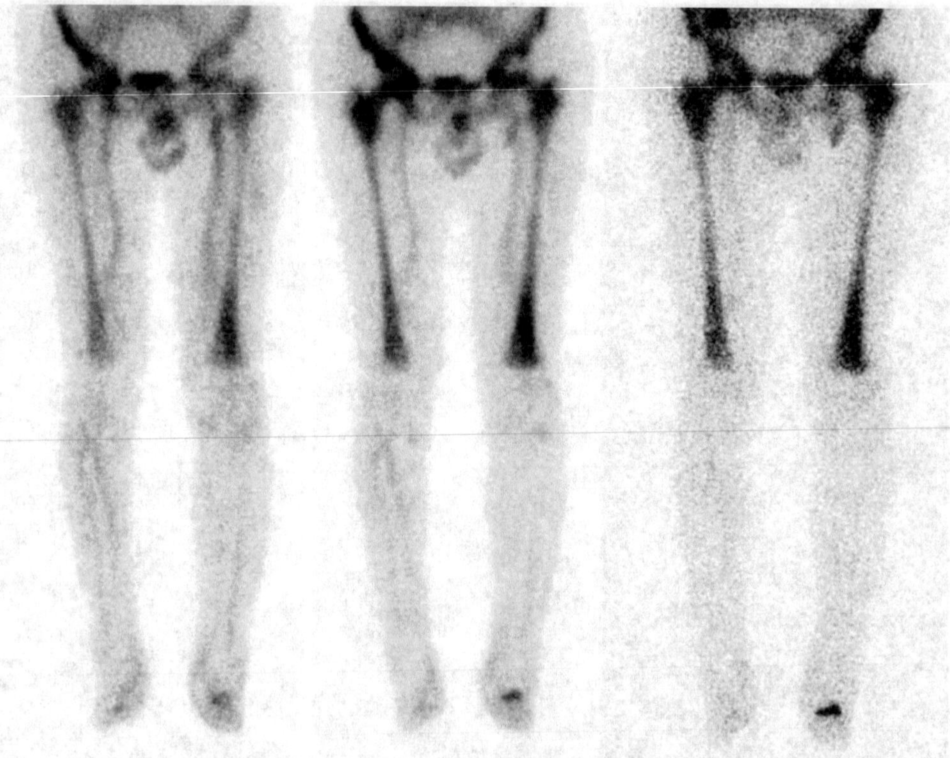

Fig. 12.17 ^{99m}Tc-HMPAO-leukocyte scintigraphy scan. An increased uptake of leukocytes (inflammation) can be seen (left) that rises and focuses in the 3 h (*middle*) and 20 h (*right*) scans in the left foot (signs of septic inflammation, as in osteomyelitis). In the left groin, we can see another spot of leukocytes in the 20 h scan, which may be reactive lymph nodes

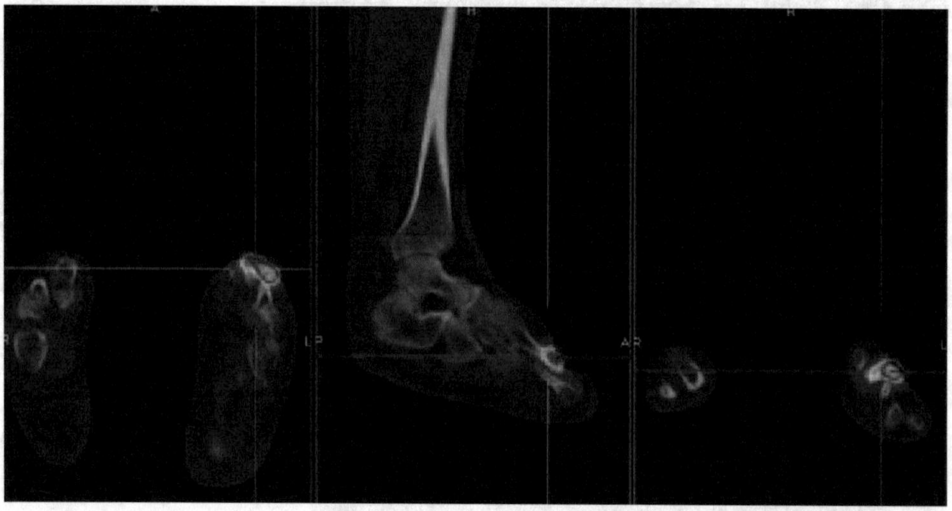

Fig. 12.18 ^{99m}Tc-HMPAO-leukocyte scintigraphy. 2D orthogonal MPR SPECT/CT fused images (coronal, *left*; sagittal, *middle*; transaxial, *right*): Focused uptake in soft tissues, which involves second metatarsal bone, can be seen

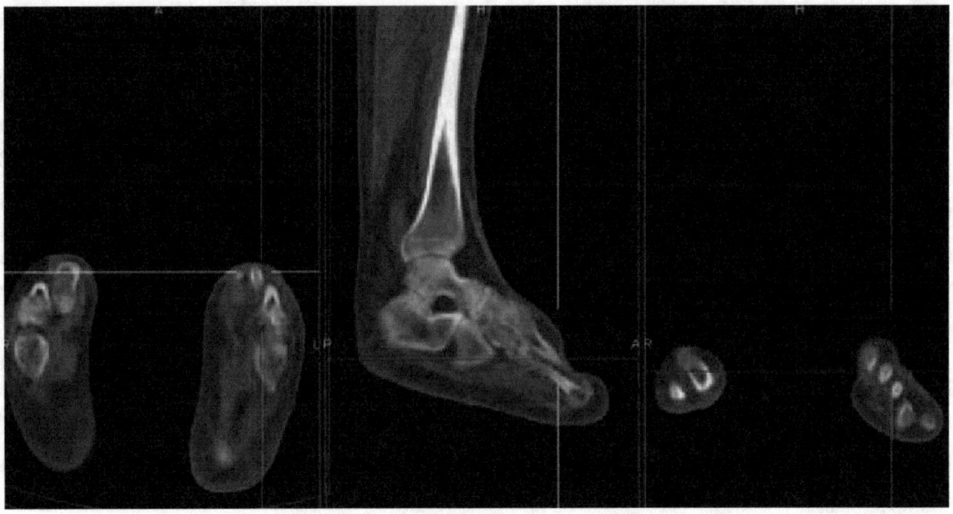

Fig. 12.19 2D orthogonal MPR SPECT/CT. CT images (coronal, *left*; sagittal, *middle*; transaxial, *right*) demonstrate the normal structure of bones in the foot

References

1. World Health Organization. Global report on diabetes. Geneva, Switzerland: World Health Organization; 2016. https://www.who.int/diabetes/global-report/en/
2. Armstrong DG, Boulton AJ, Bus SA. Diabetic foot ulcers and their recurrence. N Engl J Med. 2017;376:2367–75.
3. Lavery LA, Lavery DC, Hunt NA, La Fontaine J, Ndip A, Boulton AJ. Amputations and foot-related hospitalisations disproportionately affect dialysis patients. Int Wound J. 2015;12:523–6.
4. Lavery LA, Armstrong DG, Wunderlich RP, Mohler MJ, Wendel CS, Lipsky BA. Risk factors for foot infections in individuals with diabetes. Diabetes Care. 2006;29:1288–93.
5. Lavery LA, Armstrong DG, Wunderlich RP, Tredwell J, Boulton AJ. Diabetic foot syndrome: evaluating the prevalence and incidence of foot pathology in Mexican Americans and non-Hispanic whites from a diabetes disease management cohort. Diabetes Care. 2003;26:1435–8.
6. Boulton AJ, Vileikyte L, Ragnarson Tennvall G, Apelqvist J. The global burden of diabetic foot disease. Lancet. 2005;366:1719–24.
7. Ince P, Abbas ZG, Lutale JK, Basit A, Ali SM, Chohan F, et al. Use of the SINBAD classification system and score in comparing outcome of foot ulcer management on three continents. Diabetes Care. 2008;31:964–7.
8. https://iwgdfguidelines.org/wp-content/uploads/2019/05/IWGDF-Guidelines-2019.pdf
9. NHS. National Diabetes Foot Care Audit third annual report. In: Partnership HQI, editor. https://www.hqip.org.uk/resource/national-diabetes-footcare-audit-third-annual-report-2014-2017.
10. Bravo-Molina A, Linares-Palomino JP, Vera-Arroyo B, Salmerón-Febres LM, Ros-Díe E. Inter-observer agreement of the Wagner, University of Texas and PEDIS classification systems for the diabetic foot syndrome. Foot Ankle Surg. 2016;24:60–4.
11. Giurato L, Uccioli L. The diabetic foot: Charcot joint and osteomyelitis. Nucl Med Commun. 2006;27:745–9.
12. Lavery LA, Ryan EC, Ahn J, Crisologo PA, Oz OK, La Fontaine J, Wukich DK. The infected diabetic foot: re-evaluating the IDSA diabetic foot infection classification. Clin Infect Dis. 2020;70(8):1573–9.
13. Lipsky BA, Berendt AR, Embil J, De Lalla F. Diagnosing and treating diabetic foot infections. Diabetes Metab Res Rev. 2004;20(Suppl 1):S56–64.
14. Lipsky BA, Berendt AR, Cornia PB, Pile JC, Peters EJ, Armstrong DG, et al. Infectious Diseases Society of America. Infectious Diseases Society of America clinical practice guideline for the diagnosis and treatment of diabetic foot infections. Clin Infect Dis. 2012;54:e132–73.
15. Filippi L, Uccioli L, Giurato L, Schillaci O. Diabetic foot infection: usefulness of SPECT/CT for ^{99m}Tc-HMPAO-labeled leukocyte imaging. J Nucl Med. 2009;50:1042–6.
16. Tan PL, Teh J. MRI of the diabetic foot: differentiation of infection from neuropathic change. Br J Radiol. 2007;80:939–48.
17. Palestro CJ, Love C. Nuclear medicine and diabetic foot infections. Semin Nucl Med. 2009;39:52–65.
18. Capriotti G, Chianelli M, Signore A. Nuclear medicine imaging of diabetic foot infection: results of meta-analysis. Nucl Med Commun. 2009;27:757–64.
19. Sanders LJ, Frykberg RG. Charcot neuroarthropathy of the foot. In: Levin ME, O'Neal LW, Bowker JH, Pfeifer MA, editors. The diabetic foot. 6th ed. St Louis: Mosby; 2001. p. 439–65.
20. Butalia S, Palda VA, Sargeant RJ, Detsky AS, Mourad O. Does this patient with diabetes have osteomyelitis of the lower extremity? JAMA. 2008;299:806–13.
21. Apelqvist J, Bakker K, van Houtum WH, Nabuurs-Franssen MH, Schaper NC. International consensus on the diabetic foot & practical guidelines on the management and prevention of the diabetic foot, by the International Working Group on the Diabetic Foot. Diabetes Metab Res Rev. 2000;16(Suppl 1):s 84–92.
22. Clohisy DR, Thompson RC Jr. Fractures associated with neuropathic arthropathy in adults who have juvenile-onset diabetes. J Bone Joint Surg Am. 1988;70:1192–200.
23. Wraight PR, Lawrence SM, Campbell DA, Colman PG. Creation of a multidisciplinary, evidence based, clinical guideline for the assessment, investigation and management of acute diabetes related foot complications. Diabet Med. 2005;22:127–36.
24. Baglioni P, Malik M, Okosieme OE. Acute Charcot foot. BMJ. 2012;344:e1397.
25. Tan PL, Teh J. MRI of the diabetic foot: differentiation of infection from neuropathic change. Br J Radiol. 2001;80:939–48.
26. Palestro CJ, Mehta HH, Patel M, Freeman SJ, Harrington WN, Tomas MB, Marwin SE. Marrow versus infection in the Charcot joint: indium-111 leukocyte and technetium-99m sulfur colloid scintigraphy. J Nucl Med. 1998;39:346–50.
27. Prandini N, Lazzeri E, Rossi B, Erba P, Parisella MG, Signore A. Nuclear medicine imaging of bone infections. Nucl Med Commun. 2006;27:633–44.
28. Nawaz A, Torigian DA, Siegelman ES, Basu S, Chryssikos T, Alavi A. Diagnostic performance of FDG-PET, MRI, and plain film radi-

ography (PFR) for the diagnosis of osteomyelitis in the diabetic foot. Mol Imaging Biol. 2010;12:335–42.
29. Heiba SI, Kolker D, Mocherla B, Kapoor K, Jiang M, Son H, et al. The optimized evaluation of diabetic foot infection by dual isotope SPECT/CT. Imaging protocol. J Foot Ankle Surg. 2010;49:529–36.
30. Ruiz-Bedoya CA, Gordon O, Mota F, Abhishek S, Tucker EW, Ordonez AA, Jain SK. Molecular imaging of diabetic foot infections: new tools for old questions. Int J Mol Sci. 2019;20(23):5984. https://doi.org/10.3390/ijms20235984.
31. Eser Sanverdi S, Ergen B, Oznur A. Current challenges in imaging of the diabetic foot. Diabet Foot Ankle. 2012;3 https://doi.org/10.3402/dfa.v3i0.18754.
32. Beaman FD, von Herrmann PF, Kransdorf MJ, Adler RS, Amini B, Appel M, et al. ACR Appropriateness Criteria® suspected osteomyelitis, septic arthritis, or soft tissue infection (excluding spine and diabetic foot). J Am Coll Radiol. 2017;14:S326–37.
33. Basu S, Chryssikos T, Houseni M, Scot MD, Shah J, Zhuang H, et al. Potential role of FDG PET in the setting of diabetic neuro-osteoarthropathy: can it differentiate uncomplicated Charcot's neuroarthropathy from osteomyelitis and soft-tissue infection? Nucl Med Commun. 2007;28:465–72.
34. Treglia G, Sadeghi R, Annunziata S, Zakavi SR, Caldarella C, Muoio B, et al. Diagnostic performance of fluorine-18-fluorodeoxyglucose positron emission tomography for the diagnosis of osteomyelitis related to diabetic foot: a systematic review and a meta-analysis. Foot (Edinb). 2013;23:140–8.
35. Lipsky B, Senneville E, Abbas Z, Aragón-Sánchez J, Diggle M, Embil J. Guideline on the diagnosis and treatment of foot infection in persons with diabetes (WGDF 2019 update). Diabetes Metab Res Rev. 2020;36(Suppl 1):e3280. https://doi.org/10.1002/dmrr.3280.
36. Familiari D, Glaudemans AW, Vitale V, Prosperi D, Bagni O, Lenza A, et al. Can sequential ^{18}F-FDG PET/CT replace WBC imaging in the diabetic foot? J Nucl Med. 2011;52:1012–9.
37. Lauri C, Tamminga M, Glaudemans AW, Orozco LEJ, Erba PA, Jutte PC, et al. Detection of osteomyelitis in the diabetic foot by imaging techniques: a systematic review and meta-analysis comparing MRI, white blood cell scintigraphy, and FDG-PET. Diabetes Care. 2017;40:1111–20.

Nuclear Medicine Imaging of Lung Infection

13

Martina Sollini and Giuliano Mariani

Contents

Learning Objectives

- To become familiar with the pathophysiology and clinical presentation of the most frequent and potentially severe forms of lung infection
- To understand the principles of X-ray-based and radionuclide-based imaging for diagnosing/identifying sites of lung infection
- To learn the role of single-photon emitting agents for imaging lung infection: ^{67}Ga-citrate, ^{111}In-oxine-leukocytes, ^{99m}Tc-HMPAO-leukocytes
- To learn the role of the positron emitting agent, [^{18}F]FDG for imaging lung infection
- To learn the most common patterns of radionuclide imaging in patients with different forms of lung infection

M. Sollini
Department of Biomedical Sciences, Humanitas University, Milan, Italy

G. Mariani (✉)
Department of Translational Research and Advanced Technologies in Medicine and Surgery, Regional Center of Nuclear Medicine, University of Pisa, Pisa, Italy
e-mail: giuliano.mariani@med.unipi.it

13.1 Introductory Background

The definition of lung infection includes acute or chronic infection of the upper or lower respiratory tract caused by microorganisms such as bacteria, viruses, fungi, or parasites. This condition that causes discomfort and affects the day-to-day life of patients can become severely complicated if not properly treated [1]. Bronchitis is most commonly due to viruses rather than bacteria, while pneumonia (either it be community-acquired or a nosocomial infection) is most frequently

E. Lazzeri et al. (eds.), *Radionuclide Imaging of Infection and Inflammation*, https://doi.org/10.1007/978-3-030-62175-9_13

caused by *Streptococcus pneumoniae* [2, 3]. Symptoms, treatment, prevention, and prognosis differ depending on the cause of infection (bacterial, viral, fungal, or parasitic), the type of infection (acquired in a community environment, hospital, or nursing home), and the patient's status (immunocompetent or immunocompromised) [4]. The main signs and symptoms of lung infections are fever, shortness of breath, dry or productive coughing, fatigue (particularly in case of infection caused by Candida), production of mucus, tightness, pressure, and pain in the chest that worsens when breathing in deeply or coughing. In case of infection with methicillin-resistant *Staphylococcus aureus* (MRSA), concomitant skin or urinary infection may also be present [1].

The diagnosis of lung infection is generally based on clinical findings associated with the detection of parenchymal infiltrate at chest X-ray or CT scan [5]. High-resolution CT is the imaging method of choice to evaluate diffuse lung and small airway diseases [6], and it reliably detects infection also in the presence of an underlying chronic lung disease (such as bronchiectasis) [7, 8]. However, in some instances, radiological imaging alone cannot distinguish an acute exacerbation from sequela of a prior infection.

Cultures of both blood and sputum often identify the microorganism responsible for the infection, so that the most adequate antibiotic therapy can be planned, although false-positive as well as false-negative findings have been reported [9–11]. When infection from *Mycobacterium tuberculosis* (TB) or HIV-associated infection is suspected, specific recommendations and guidelines should be followed for a correct diagnosis [12].

Key Learning Points

- Acute or chronic infection of the upper or lower respiratory tract due to microorganisms causes discomfort, affects the day-to-day life of patients, and can become severely complicated.
- The diagnosis of lung infection is generally based on clinical findings associated with detection of parenchymal infiltrate at chest X-ray or CT scan.
- However, in some instances, radiological imaging alone cannot distinguish an acute exacerbation from sequela of a prior infection.

13.2 Imaging Lung Infection with Single-Photon Emitting Agents

Nuclear medicine imaging techniques have been extensively used in patients with lung infection, mostly for TB-associated or HIV-associated infections [13–16]. Following seminal work by Levenson et al. in patients with *Pneumocystis carinii* pneumonia [17], increased uptake of ^{67}Ga-citrate has been described in many conditions (besides *Pneumocystis carinii* pneumonia), such as abscess, TB or mycotic lesions, pneumoconiosis, and infection from cytomegalovirus, although false-negative results have been reported [16, 18–21]. One of the most important non-oncologic clinical applications of ^{67}Ga-citrate scintigraphy of the lungs is early detection of opportunistic infection; this imaging technique enables to detect diffusely increased uptake of the radiopharmaceutical in the lung even when the chest X-ray is normal [17, 22]. In this regard, although ^{67}Ga-citrate scintigraphy for pulmonary diseases is hampered by several drawbacks (such as its relative lack of specificity, delay between tracer injection and imaging time, and suboptimal imaging characteristics) [23], its sensitivity is higher than that of a chest X-ray in the detection of pulmonary TB [24] and of lung involvement from paracoccidioidomycosis [25]. In patients with TB, the intensity of pulmonary uptake of ^{67}Ga-citrate is directly related to the inflammation level and to the burden of *Mycobacterium tuberculosis* (assessed by semi-quantitation of sputum acid-fast bacillus) [26]. ^{67}Ga-citrate scintigraphy and high-resolution CT in sputum smear-negative patients with active TB perform equally well in the noninvasive diagnosis of TB, with high sensitivity (100% versus 93%) and specificity (83% versus 100%) [27].

Sequential ^{67}Ga-citrate scans are also helpful to monitor the response to treatment in patients with TB, chronic lung disease, or AIDS, in whom radiological findings can be equivocal because of the confounding effects of either chronic pulmonary fibrotic changes or poor inflammatory reaction due to immunodeficiency [28]. ^{67}Ga-citrate scintigraphy has also been employed to determine the most appropriate duration of treatment with different anti-TB regimens [26]. Pulmonary lesions in active TB compared to nontuberculous mycobacterial infection in acid-fast bacilli smear-positive non-HIV-infected patients have also been successfully evaluated with ^{67}Ga-citrate scintigraphy, demonstrating the usefulness of this technique in predicting active pulmonary TB in acid-fast bacilli smear-positive patients [29].

Scintigraphy with autologous leukocytes labeled with either ^{111}In-oxine (most recently reviewed in [30]) or ^{99m}Tc-HMPAO [31] detects infection with high diagnostic accuracy (sensitivity up to 95% for soft tissue infections). However, there have been only a limited number of investigations on the usefulness of this imaging method for diagnosing lung infections [32]. In patients with focal pulmonary bacterial infections, scintigraphy with labeled leukocytes is more sensitive than ^{67}Ga-citrate scintigraphy [33], and it is often positive before changes can even be seen on a plain chest X-ray [34]. Equivocal results have instead been reported for radiolabeled leukocyte scintigraphy in patients with bronchiectasis [32, 35].

It should be noted that interpretation of the images obtained with labeled leukocyte scintigraphy of the lungs can be problematic, because of interference from blood pool activity in the heart and great vessels and pulmonary blood background and because of the physiologic leukocyte margination along the walls of small pulmonary vessels early after reinfusion of labeled leukocytes. Furthermore, nonspecific inflammatory changes associated with congestive heart failure or with acute respiratory distress syndrome may mimic diffuse or focal pulmonary uptake in a similar manner as observed in patients with lung infection, making the distinction between infection and inflammation difficult [23, 36]. Nonetheless, if pulmonary accumulation of radiolabeled leukocytes is graded according to soft tissue, rib, and liver activities, specificity increases up to 100% for pulmonary and pleural infections, and a negative scan rules out pulmonary infection with high confidence [37]. Furthermore, in the current clinical practice, these methodological limitations can be largely overcome by SPECT/CT imaging.

A pathophysiologic limitation of radiolabeled leukocyte scintigraphy can be seen in lung infections where leukocyte infiltrations are less significant, as it occurs in granulomatous or nonpyogenic infections [23, 34, 38]. For similar reasons, labeled leukocyte scintigraphy is not routinely used for the characterization of TB patients since variable results (especially in the evaluation of small infectious foci) have been reported, probably due to the predominant type of cells involved (lymphocytes and macrophages, rather than granulocytes) [38]. Finally, in patients with AIDS radiolabeling of autologous leukocytes for scintigraphy can be technically unfeasible because of low white blood cell counts.

Scintigraphy with ^{67}Ga-citrate or with ^{99m}Tc-HMPAO-labeled leukocytes has been used in patients with occult sepsis in intensive care units. Although ^{67}Ga-citrate scintigraphy reliably identified extra-site(s) of infection, it did not accurately identify ventilator-associated pneumonia [39]. Instead, ^{99m}Tc-HMPAO-leukocyte scintigraphy demonstrated good sensitivity (95–96%) and specificity (84–91%) in detecting the occult source of sepsis [40, 41]. It should be noted, however, that in this critical clinical scenario, scintigraphy with ^{67}Ga-citrate or with labeled leukocytes has definite disadvantages (i.e., either amount of blood needed to harvest leukocytes for labeling or long time span between administration and scintigraphy) with respect to [^{18}F]FDG PET/CT (see further below).

Although both ^{201}Tl-chloride and ^{111}In-DTPA-octreotide have been employed to distinguish benign lung lesions (i.e., infection) from cancer, their clinical application in infection per se has been very limited [23], except for scanty reports concerning patients with fungal infection [42] or with TB infection [43]. In TB infection, ^{201}Tl-chloride scintigraphy seems to perform better than ^{67}Ga-citrate scintigraphy (sensitivity 88% versus 83%, specificity 82% versus 60%, accuracy 85% versus 75%) [44]. Similar results have been reported for ^{99m}Tc(V)-DMSA, suggesting that scintigraphy with this imaging agent might perform better than ^{67}Ga-citrate scintigraphy for assessing the overall burden and activity of TB [45]. Good diagnostic performance in patients with pulmonary TB has been reported also for ^{99m}Tc-sestamibi and ^{99m}Tc-tetrofosmin, with high sensitivity (96% and 94%, respectively) and specificity (86% and 88%, respectively) [46].

Key Learning Points

- Single-photon emitting agents employed for imaging lung infection include ^{67}Ga-citrate, ^{111}In-oxine-leukocytes, ^{99m}Tc-HMPAO-leukocytes.
- The preferred imaging modality is currently scintigraphy with ^{99m}Tc-HMPAO-leukocytes, preferably with SPECT/CT imaging.
- However, in some conditions, the diagnostic performance of ^{99m}Tc-HMPAO-leukocyte scintigraphy is suboptimal because of the predominant type of cells involved (lymphocytes and macrophages, rather than granulocytes, as in TB infection) or is technically unfeasible because of low white blood cell count, as in HIV-associated infections.
- In such conditions, conventional scintigraphy with ^{67}Ga-citrate can be usefully employed.
- Less validated agents include ^{201}Tl-chloride, ^{111}In-DTPA-octreotide, ^{99m}Tc(V)-DMSA, ^{99m}Tc-sestamibi, and ^{99m}Tc-tetrofosmin.

13.3 Imaging Lung Infection with Positron Emitting Agents

Although not specific for infection, PET imaging with [^{18}F]FDG can be particularly useful to identify site(s) and extent of infectious disease or to guide biopsy in doubtful cases [22, 47–50], even before the appearance of radiological abnormalities [51].

Different patterns of [^{18}F]FDG uptake have been reported in patients with lung infections. Bacterial, viral, fungal, or parasitic pneumonia may present with either a nodular or diffuse pattern of uptake [51–57], while TB may appear as lung or lymphatic patterns [14, 58], and cryptococcosis may present with a solitary pulmonary/scattered nodular or bronchopneumonic/single mass pattern [59].

A positive [^{18}F]FDG PET scan should be interpreted with caution when evaluating pulmonary nodules, especially in patients with predisposing factors for nontuberculous mycobacterial infections [60, 61]. In non-HIV-infected patients suffering from TB, [^{18}F]FDG PET and [^{18}F]FDG PET/CT performed better than contrast-enhanced CT, revealing more extensive involvement than CT [14, 62]. In HIV-positive patients, [^{18}F]FDG PET and PET/CT consistently demonstrate increased tracer uptake in active pulmonary and extrapulmonary TB; nevertheless, it is difficult to distinguish a malignancy from HIV infection and TB based only on the degree of [^{18}F]FDG uptake [63, 64], which is also related to viral load [65]. In this regard, it has been reported that dual-phase [^{18}F]FDG PET can distinguish inflammation from malignancy [64].

[^{18}F]FDG PET/CT has a promising role also in the diagnosis and identification of other HIV-associated infections (i.e., Pneumocystis pneumonia) [66, 67], as well as in fever of unknown origin (FUO) [68–70]. However, quite often increased [^{18}F]FDG uptake due to infection cannot be distinguished from increased uptake due to malignancy [71].

Similarly, when evaluating bronchiectasis in HIV-positive patients, [^{18}F]FDG PET/CT did not reliably predict disease exacerbation [72]. Nonetheless, although [^{18}F]FDG PET (currently PET/CT) alone does not have a definite role in identifying the cause of abnormalities, in patients with HIV it can be useful to detect or exclude the presence of abnormal [^{18}F]FDG uptake; furthermore, combining the CT anatomic landmarks with the PET findings allows the guidance of biopsy when histopathologic diagnosis is needed and therefore impacts on patient's management and clinical decision-making [73].

The use of [^{18}F]FDG PET can be helpful for assessing response to therapy in a variety of nonmalignant disorders and has therefore been proposed for evaluating the efficacy of therapy also in infectious diseases [74], especially anti-TB therapy [15]. The role of [^{18}F]FDG PET in monitoring the efficacy of therapy has been described also for patients with invasive candidiasis [54], cryptococcosis [59], aspergillosis [75], and *Pneumocystis carinii* pneumonia [66].

In over 85% of the cases, nosocomial pneumonia is associated with the use of respiratory assistance procedures, such as endotracheal tubes, tracheostomy/tracheotomy, nasal masks, and nebulization treatment. Ventilator-associated pneumonia (VAP), the most common nosocomial infection in the intensive care unit [76–78], occurs in 8–28% of patients receiving prolonged mechanical ventilation (>48 h) [79]. Also tracheostomy is associated with VAP [80], whereas nasotracheal intubation is more frequently associated with sinusitis [81] and otitis. Infection is caused by continuous tidal movements of air during artificial respiration, which determines some sort of "milking" into the adjacent structures along the nasopharyngeal path of microorganisms that cover the endotracheal tube. When suspecting VAP, endotracheal aspirates or samples collected bronchoscopically should be obtained for microbiological culture [82]. Although sensitive, chest X-ray is typically nonspecific [83], since lobar or subsegmental atelectasis, acute respiratory distress syndrome, alveolar hemorrhage, and/or infarction may be mistaken for pneumonia. Chest CT frequently shows pulmonary abnormalities consistent with atelectasis, pleural effusion, and infiltrates in mechanically ventilated patients. The metabolic information provided by [^{18}F]FDG PET has a definite added value in these patients; in fact, detecting increased metabolism in these lesions can be crucial in deciding whether or not the abnormalities found on the CT scan are actually sites of infection causing the symptoms and signs in patients [84]. An overall good diagnostic performance of [^{18}F]FDG PET/CT in mechanically ventilated patients with suspected lung infection has been reported, with 100% sensitivity, 79% specificity, and 91% overall accuracy; because of such extremely high sensitivity, a normal [^{18}F]FDG PET/CT scan could reliably rule out the presence of a focal active infectious process, thus excluding the need for prolonged antibiotic therapy or drainage [84].

The recent worldwide medical emergency associated with the pandemic caused by the Covid-19 (or SARS-CoV-2) virus has opened new opportunities for the use of [^{18}F]FDG PET/CT in patients with either asymptomatic or symptomatic infection with the virus [85–92]. Although in many of the cases reported so far, detection of increased [^{18}F]FDG uptake in areas exhibiting the CT pattern of interstitial pneumonia has been purely incidental, and it can reasonably be assumed that the use of [^{18}F]FDG PET/CT will provide helpful information to monitor the course of disease—and possibly to assess the efficacy of therapy.

Finally, PET imaging with other agents other than [^{18}F]FDG, such as [^{11}C]choline and ^{18}F-fluoroethyltyrosine, has also been explored in patients with lung infections [93]; in this regard, in patients with pulmonary TB and atypical lung mycobacterial infection, the uptake of [^{18}F]FDG at the infections sites has been reported to be higher than uptake of [^{11}C]choline [94].

Key Learning Points

- Although not specific for infection, PET imaging with [^{18}F]FDG can be particularly useful to identify site(s) and extent of infectious disease or to guide biopsy in doubtful cases.
- A positive [^{18}F]FDG PET scan should be interpreted with caution when evaluating pulmonary nodules, especially in patients with predisposing factors for nontuberculous mycobacterial infections.
- In HIV-positive patients, [^{18}F]FDG PET and PET/CT consistently demonstrate increased tracer uptake in active pulmonary and extrapulmonary TB.
- Increased [^{18}F]FDG uptake due to infection cannot be distinguished from increased uptake due to malignancy.
- By combining the CT anatomic landmarks with the PET findings, PET/CT imaging allows the guidance of biopsy when histopathologic diagnosis is needed and therefore impacts on patient's management and clinical decision making.
- [^{18}F]FDG PET/CT is especially useful for assessing patients with ventilator-associated pneumonia.
- The metabolic information provided by [^{18}F]FDG PET has a definite added value in deciding whether or not the abnormalities found on the CT scan are actually sites of infection.
- The most recent application of [^{18}F]FDG PET/CT is to be seen in patients with interstitial pneumonia, as observed during infection with the Covid-19 virus (SARS-CoV-2).

Acknowledgments Special thanks are due to Drs. Elena Lazzeri and Annibale Versari for providing images that have been included in this chapter.

Examples of Lung Infection Imaging

Chest X-ray and ^{99m}Tc-HMPAO-Leukocyte Scintigraphy in Patient with Lung Infection (Figs. 13.1, 13.2, and 13.3)

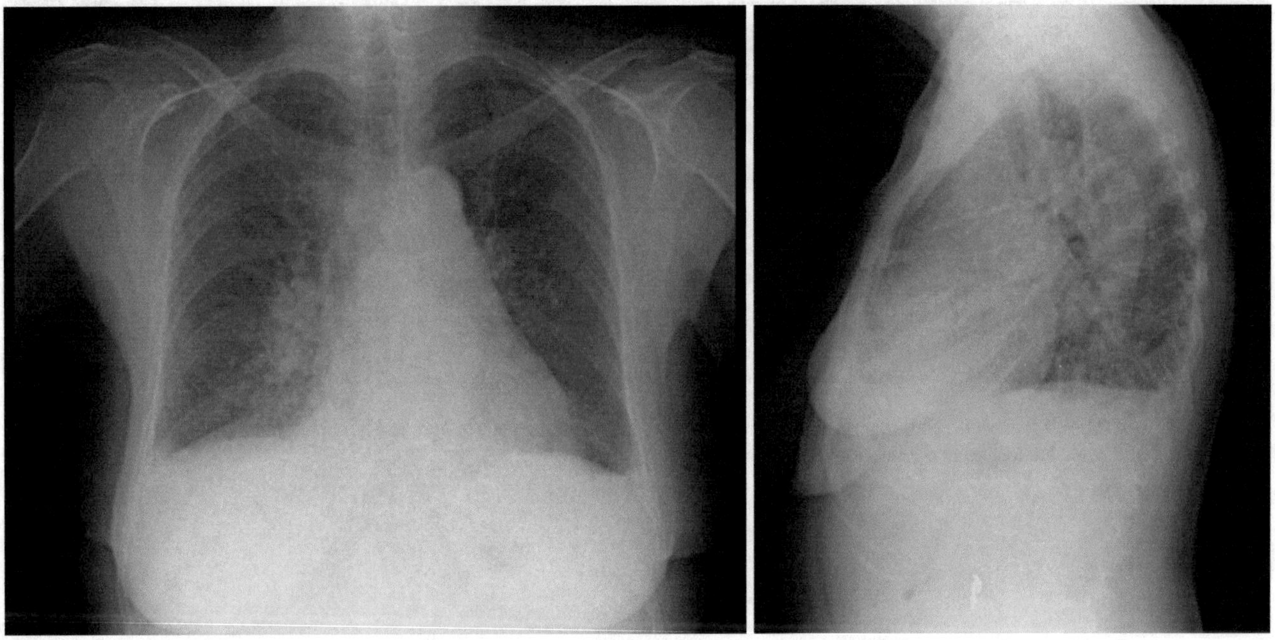

Fig. 13.1 Chest X-ray: posteroanterior (left) and lateral (right) projections

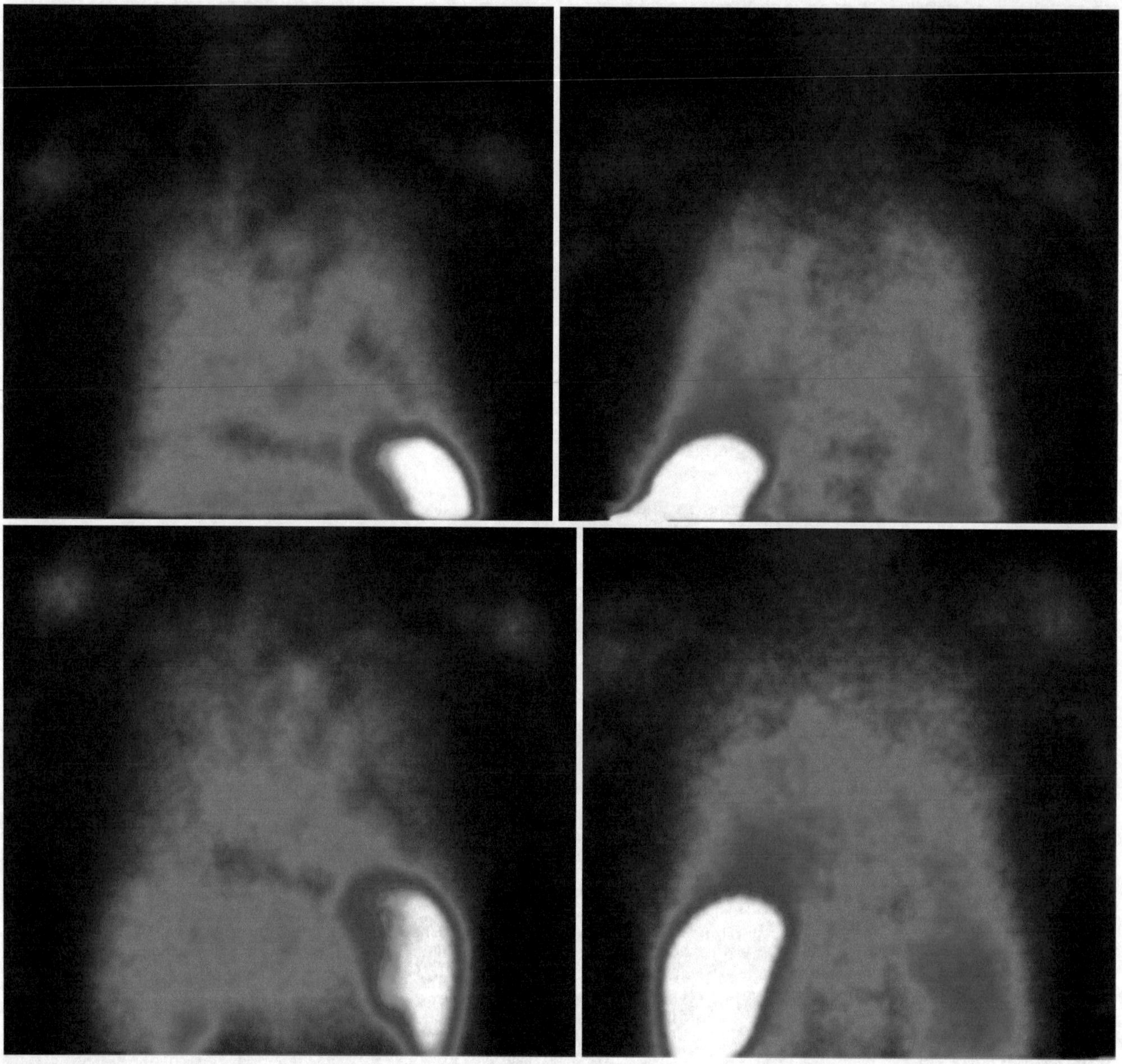

Fig. 13.2 ^{99m}Tc-HMPAO-leukocyte scintigraphy: planar anterior (right) and posterior (left) images at 4 h (upper) and 24 h (lower), showing a mild accumulation of labeled leukocytes in the inferior lobe of right lung

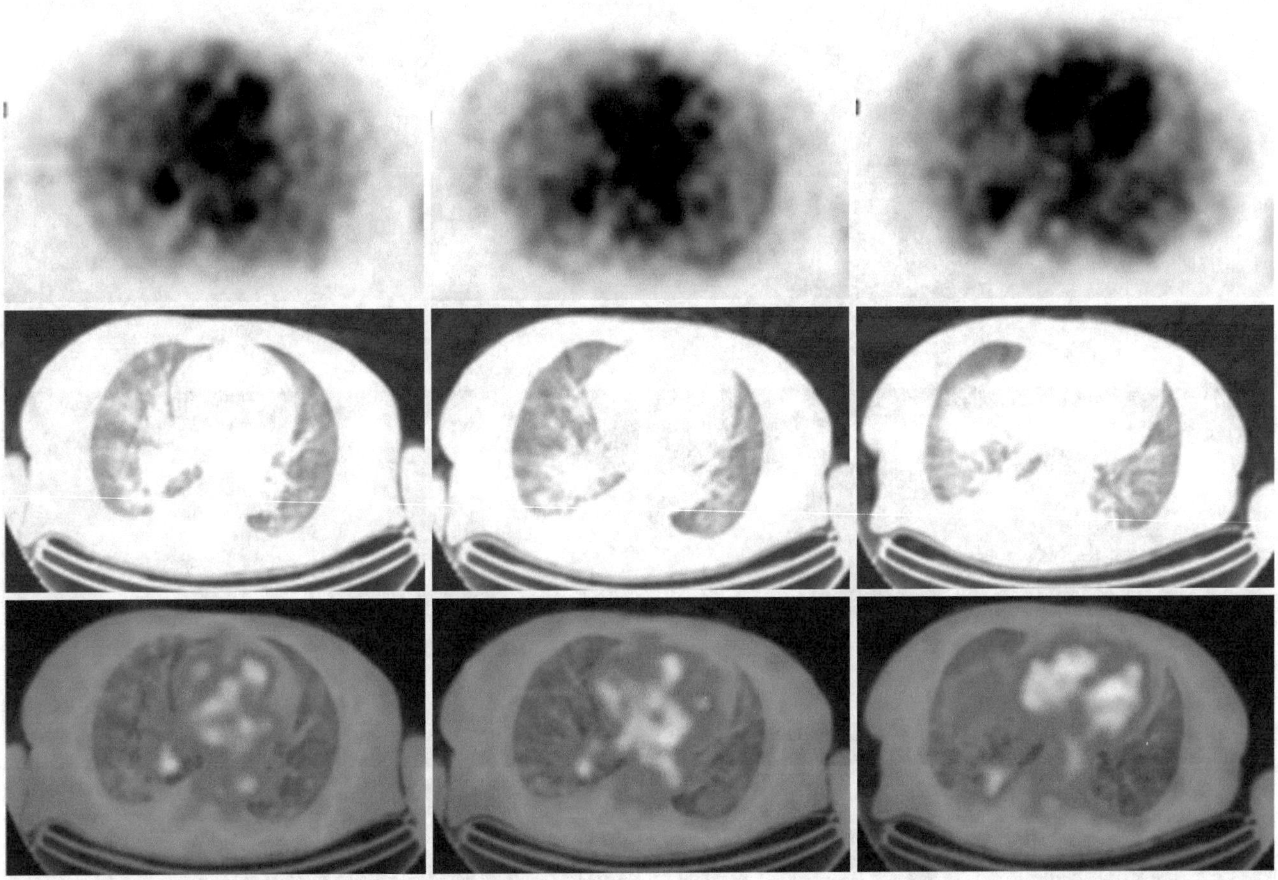

Fig. 13.3 ^{99m}Tc-HMPAO-leukocyte scintigraphy: transaxial SPECT (upper), CT (middle), and fused SPECT/CT sections (lower) allow the identification of the exact site of leukocyte accumulation

[^{18}F]FDG PET/CT in Patient with Tuberculosis Infection of Left Pleura (Figs. 13.4, 13.5, 13.6, and 13.7)

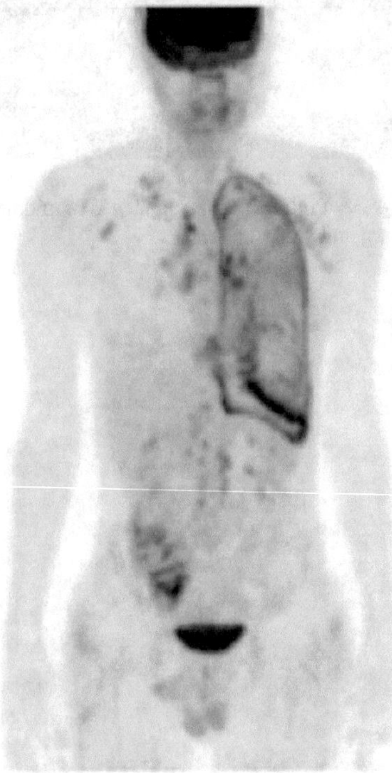

Fig. 13.4 [^{18}F]FDG PET/CT: maximum intensity projection (MIP), showing diffusely increased [^{18}F]FDG uptake in left chest and in mediastinum

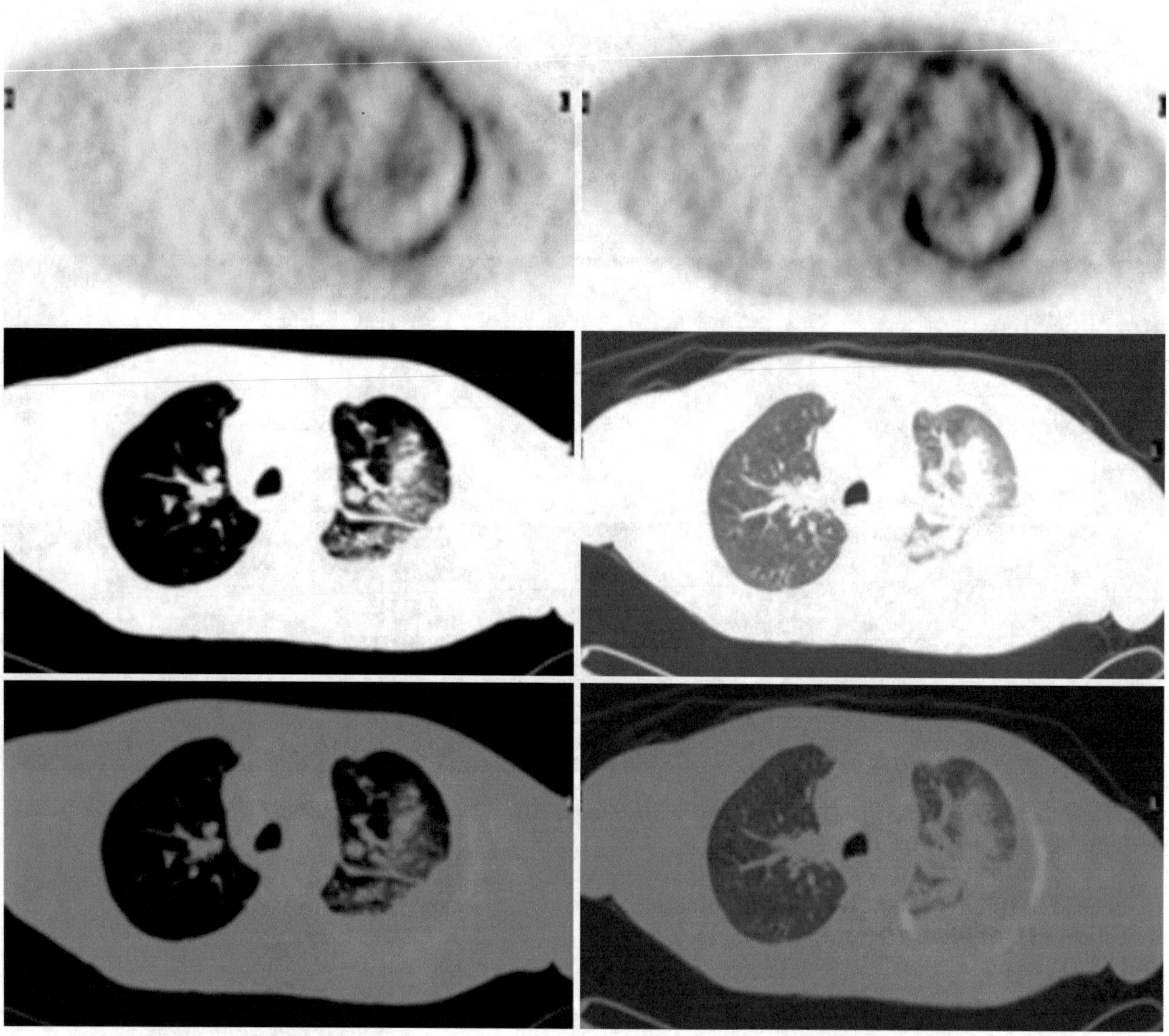

Fig. 13.5 [^{18}F]FDG PET/CT: PET (upper), CT (middle), and fused PET/CT (lower) transaxial sections of chest, showing increased [^{18}F]FDG uptake in left lung and pleural tissues

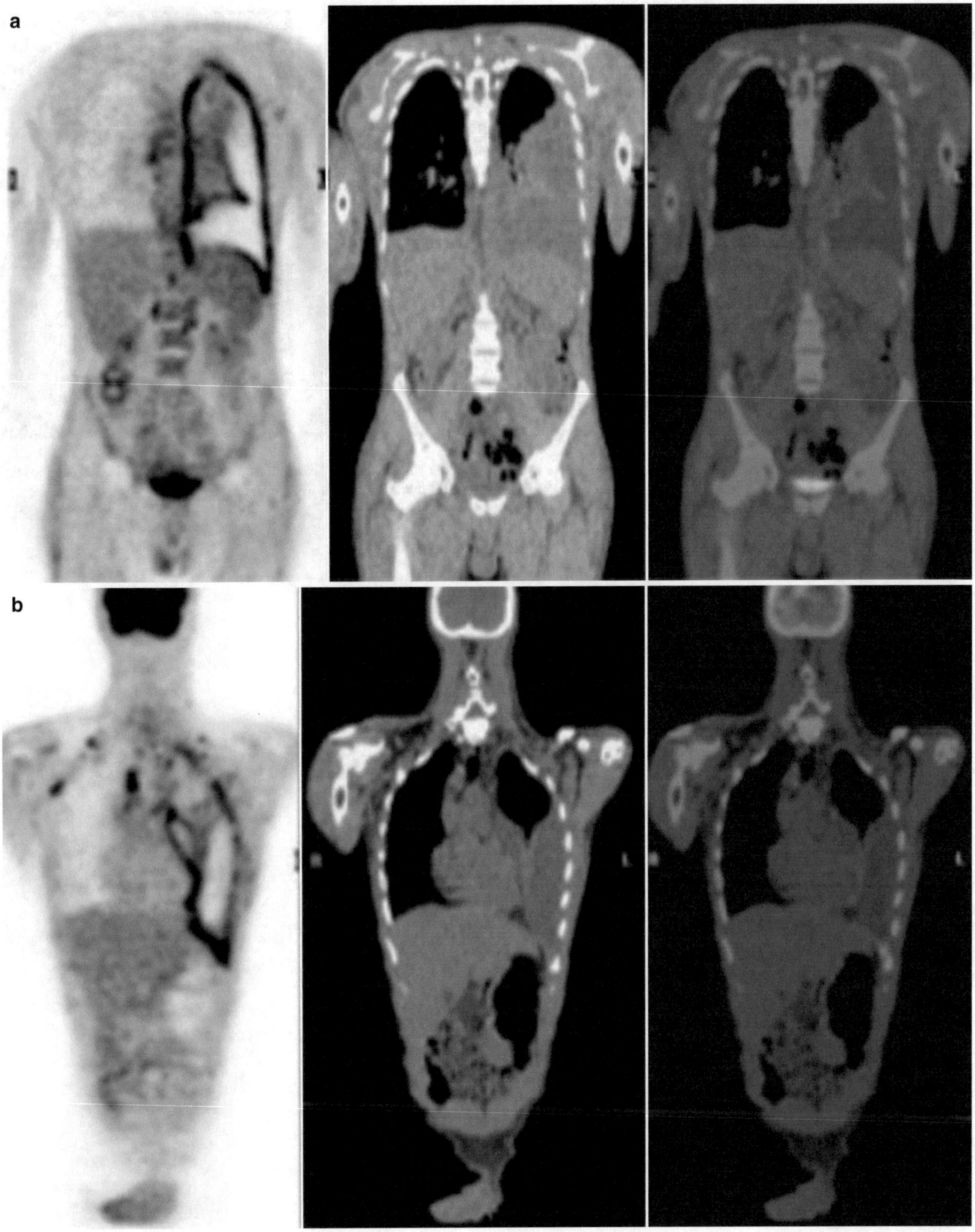

Fig. 13.6 [18F]FDG PET/CT: PET (left), CT (middle), and fused PET/CT (right) coronal sections of chest, showing increased [18F]FDG uptake in left lung and pleural tissues; [18F]FDG uptake is localized at left lung and at all left pleural tissues (**a**) while pleural effusion does not exhibit increased tracer uptake (**b**)

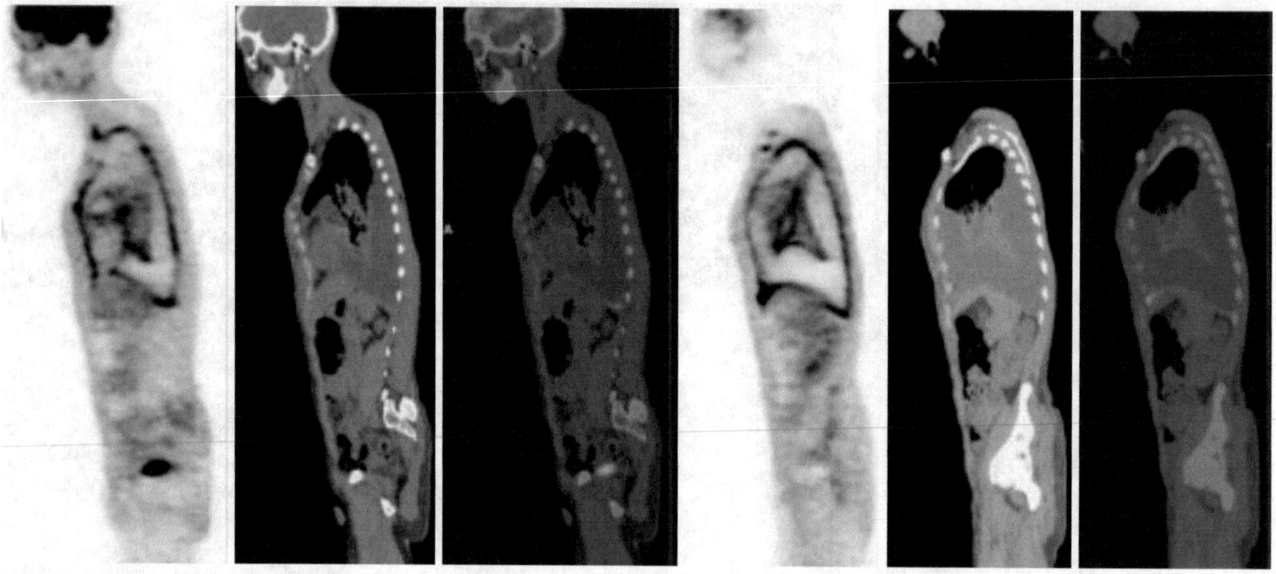

Fig. 13.7 [18F]FDG PET/CT: PET (left), CT (middle), and fused PET/CT (right) sagittal sections of chest, showing increased [18F]FDG uptake in left lung and pleural tissues; [18F]FDG uptake is localized at left lung and at all left pleural tissues (**a**) while pleural effusion does not exhibit increased tracer uptake (**b**)

[^{18}F]FDG PET/CT in Patient with "Ab Ingestis" Pneumonia (Fig. 13.8)

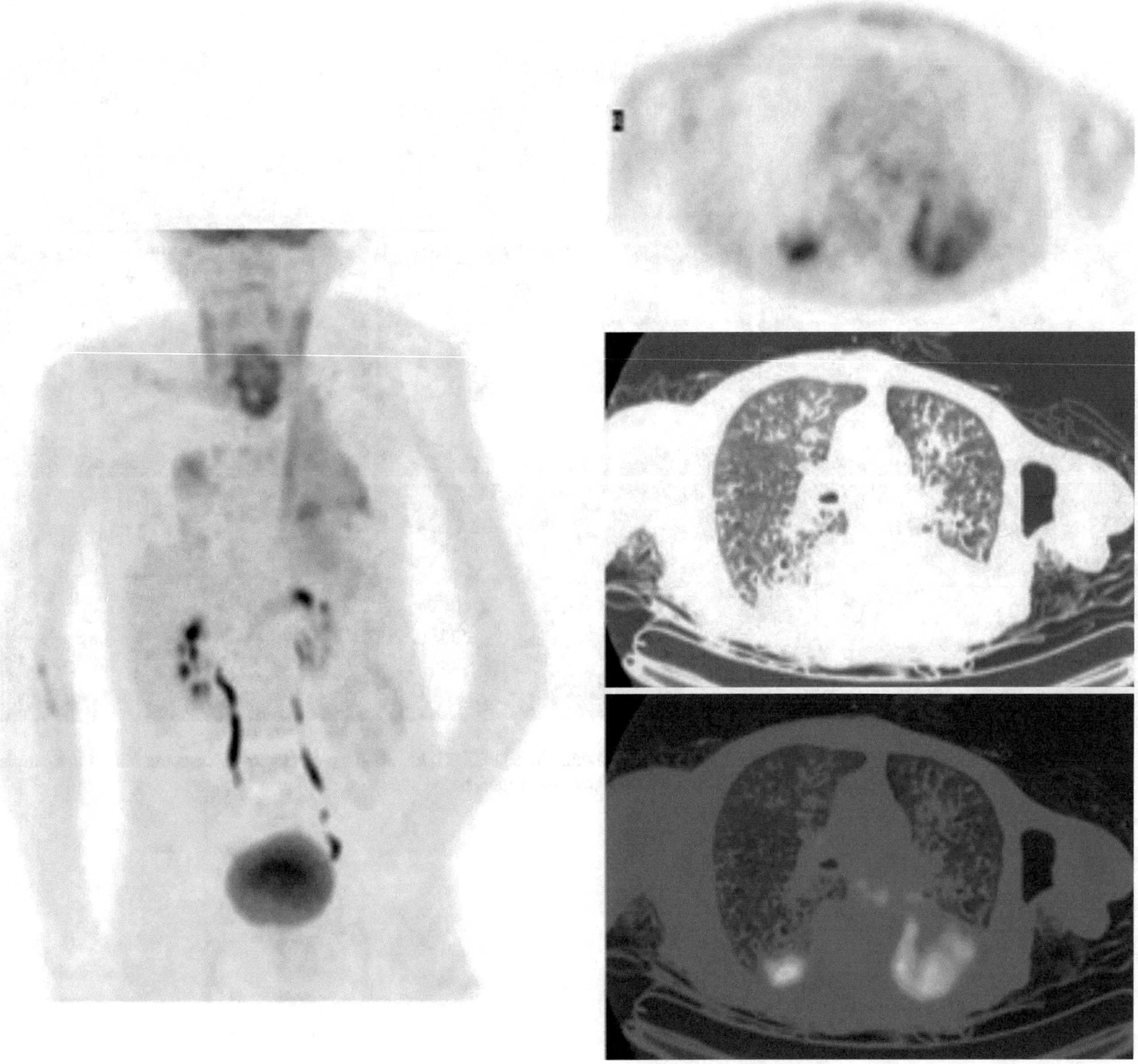

Fig. 13.8 [^{18}F]FDG PET/CT: (**left**) Maximum intensity projection (MIP) image and (**right**) transaxial section of PET (upper), CT (middle), and fused PET/CT (lower), showing increased tracer uptake in posterior fields of both lungs

[18F]FDG PET/CT in Patient with Hypereosinophilic Syndrome (Fig. 13.9)

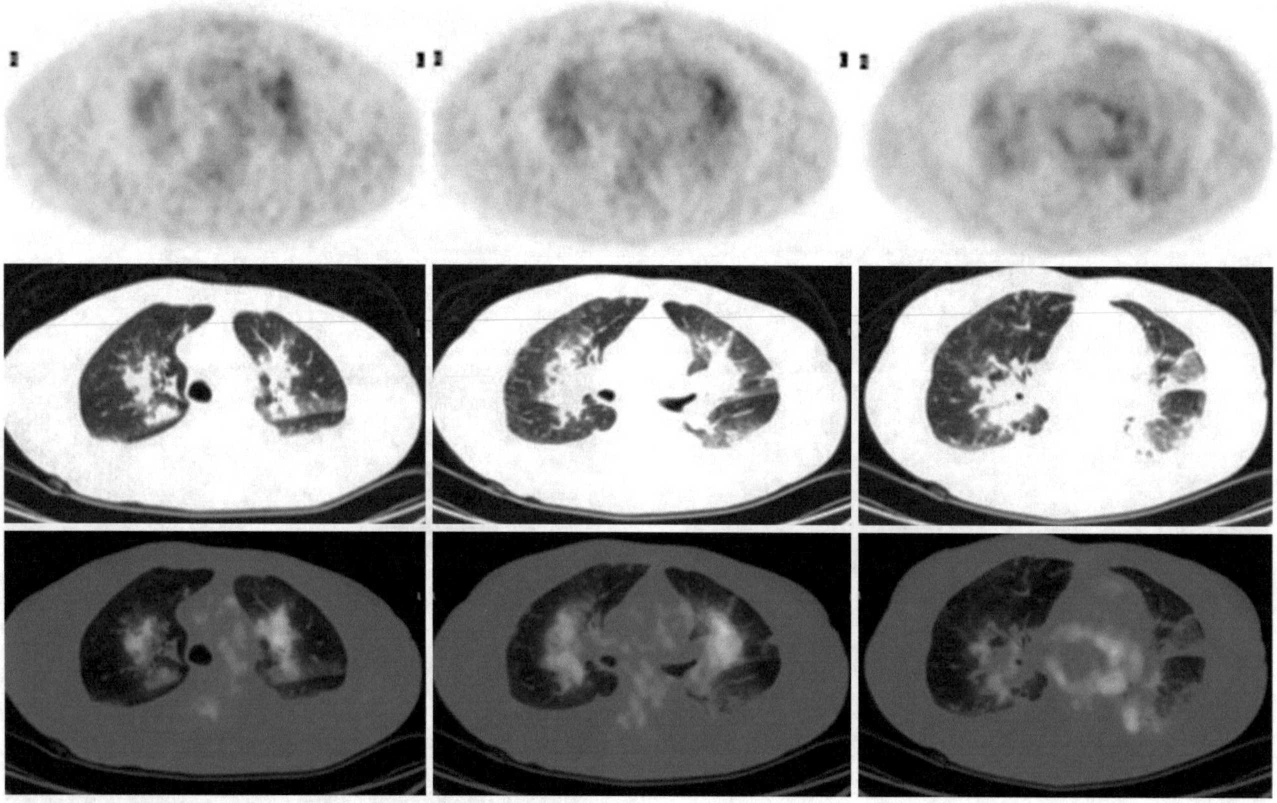

Fig. 13.9 Transaxial [18F]FDG PET/CT sections (PET, upper; CT, middle; fused PET/CT, lower) in a patient with pleuropericarditis and multiple pulmonary opacities, showing intense [18F]FDG uptake at both lungs; biopsy demonstrated hypereosinophilic syndrome

[^{18}F]FDG PET/CT in Patient with Atypical Mycobacteria Pneumonia (Fig. 13.10)

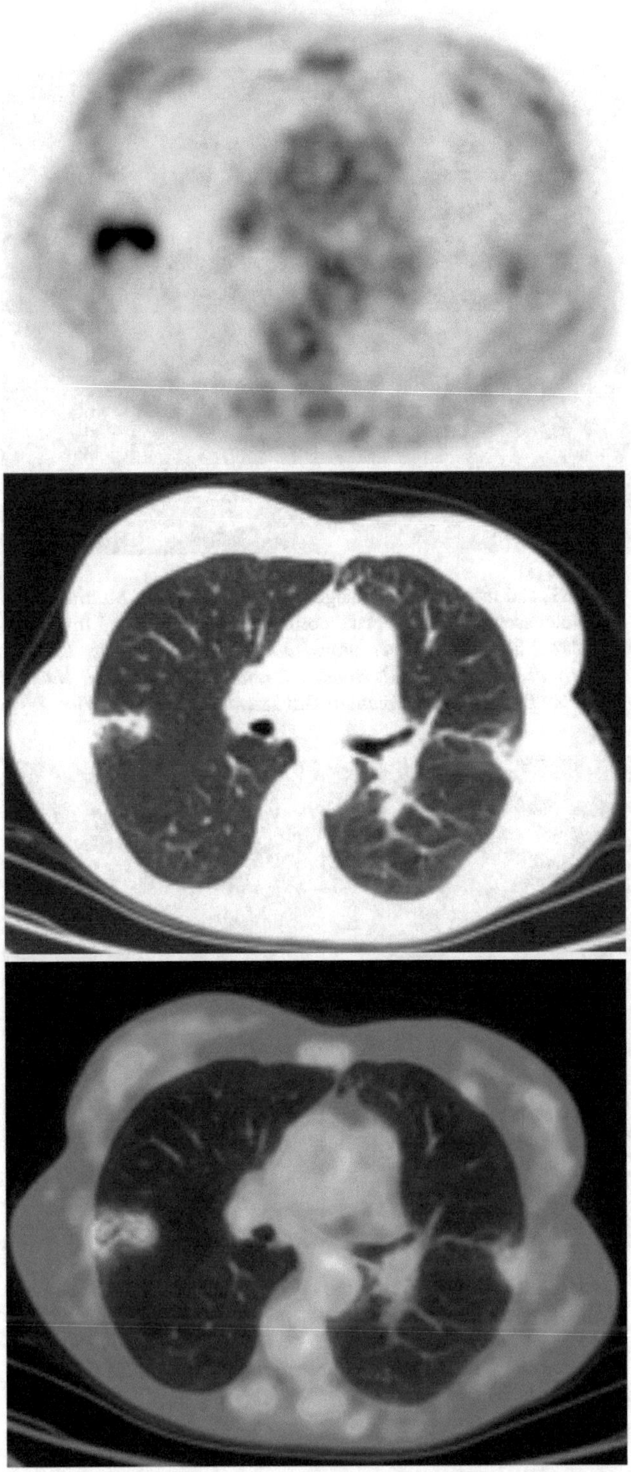

Fig. 13.10 Transaxial [^{18}F]FDG PET/CT sections (PET, top; CT, middle; fused PET/CT, bottom) in a woman with several episodes of pneumonia; biopsy performed after [^{18}F]FDG PET/CT revealed pneumonia sustained by atypical mycobacteria

[18F]FDG PET/CT in Patients with Incidentally Detected Interstitial Pneumonia Associated with the Covid-19 Virus (SARS-CoV-2)
(Figs. 13.11 and 13.12)

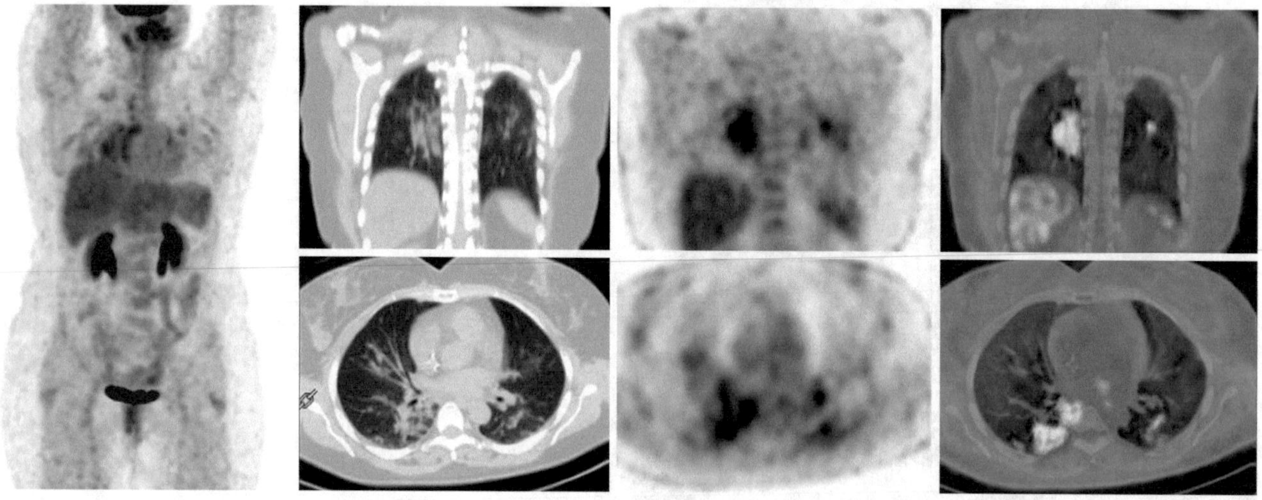

Fig. 13.11 [^{18}F]FDG PET/CT performed in a 45-year-old woman for restaging after chemotherapy for recurring colorectal cancer. The patient did not complain of fever, cough, or dyspnea, but lived in an area with very high incidence of Covid-19 infection. MIP image on the left. On the right: selected coronal (above) and transaxial slices (below) for CT, PET, and fused PET/CT images (from left to right). Multiple areas with increased [^{18}F]FDG uptake corresponding to bilateral interstitial alveolar infiltrates. (*Images provided by courtesy of Drs. L. Setti, M. Kirienko, SC Dalto, M. Bonacina, and E. Bombardieri, Nuclear Medicine Department, Humanitas Gavazzeni, Bergamo, Italy*)

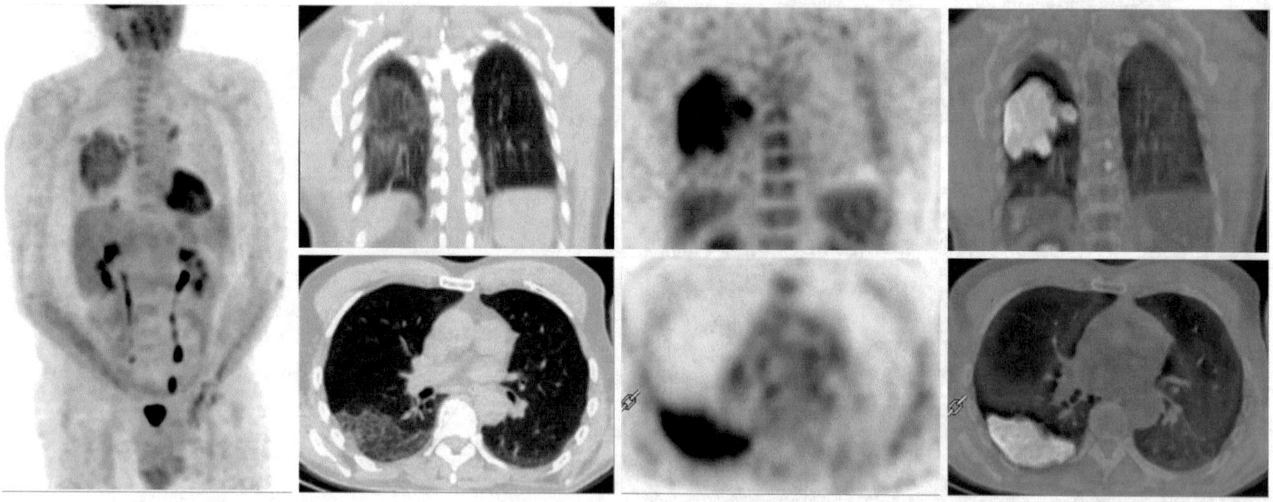

Fig. 13.12 [^{18}F]FDG PET/CT performed in a 70-year-old man for staging after the discovery of metastasis in cervical lymph nodes from a squamocellular cancer with unknown primary. The patient did not complain of fever cough or dyspnea but lived in an area with very high incidence of Covid-19 infection. MIP image on the left. On the right: selected coronal (above) and transaxial slices (below) for CT PET and fused PET/CT images (from left to right). Multiple areas with increased [^{18}F]FDG uptake consistent with viral pneumonia. (*Images provided by courtesy of Drs. L. Setti, M. Kirienko, SC Dalto, M. Bonacina, and E. Bombardieri, Nuclear Medicine Department, Humanitas Gavazzeni, Bergamo, Italy*)

Clinical Cases

Case 13.1

Josep Martin-Comin

Background

A 20-year-old man without previous history of illness or allergies was stabbed in the back. No signs or symptoms of TB were present. Chest X-ray and CT findings were: lung wound due to stab on the back and areas with opacification of air spaces within the lung parenchyma (in the left inferior lobe) associated with pleural effusion (bleeding) and left hilar and mediastinal lymphadenopathy. Passive atelectasis.

Differential Diagnosis

Lung neoplasm and granulomatous/infectious process.

Radiopharmaceutical Activity

[^{18}F]FDG 3.7 MBq/kg.

Imaging

PET/CT protocol acquisition: scan was performed for 60–120 min p.i. Acquisition of the scan included: (1) scout view (120 kV, 10 mA) in order to define the limits of body to explore, (2) whole-body CT scan (from skull base to proximal femur: 140 kV, 80 mA), and (3) craniocaudal whole-body PET (2D, 3–5 min/field of view, FOV). Images were reconstructed with soft tissue and lung filters using iterative OSEM, with and without attenuation correction using the low-dose transmission CT scan (Figs. 13.13, 13.14, and 13.15).

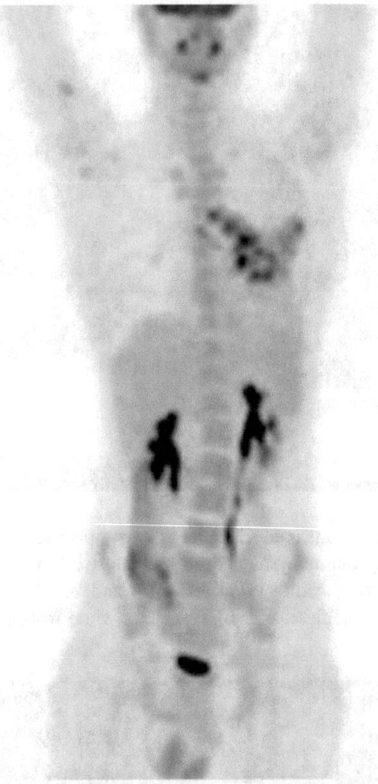

Fig. 13.13 Maximum intensity projection (MIP) image shows increased and heterogeneous [^{18}F]FDG uptake in the left inferior lung

Conclusion/Teaching Point

The conclusion of these findings is based on analyzing the characteristics of the morphometabolic changes, considering the young age of the patient. PET without CT cannot distinguish between tuberculosis and lung neoplasm, but CT findings of the hybrid PET/CT acquisition support the diagnosis of tuberculosis. The cutaneous purified protein derivative (PPD) test was positive (18 mm), and sputum smears were positive for *Mycobacterium tuberculosis*. The patient was treated with tuberculostatics.

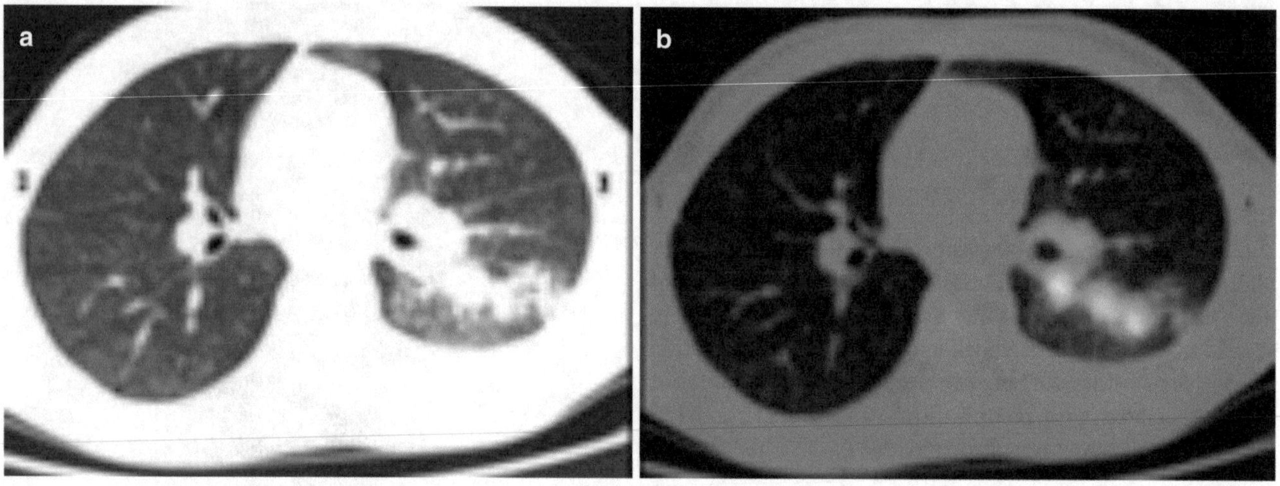

Fig. 13.14 (**a**) Transaxial CT slice shows opacification of airspaces within the lung parenchyma (in the left inferior lobe) associated with pleural effusion (bleeding) and left hilar and mediastinal lymphadenopathy. Passive atelectasis. (**b**) Transaxial slice from [^{18}F]FDG PET/CT fusion in lung window shows increased and heterogeneous [^{18}F]FDG uptake in the left inferior lung corresponding to multiple consolidation areas with cavity lesion, and subpleural nodules with poorly defined margins, associated with pleural effusion and stab wound

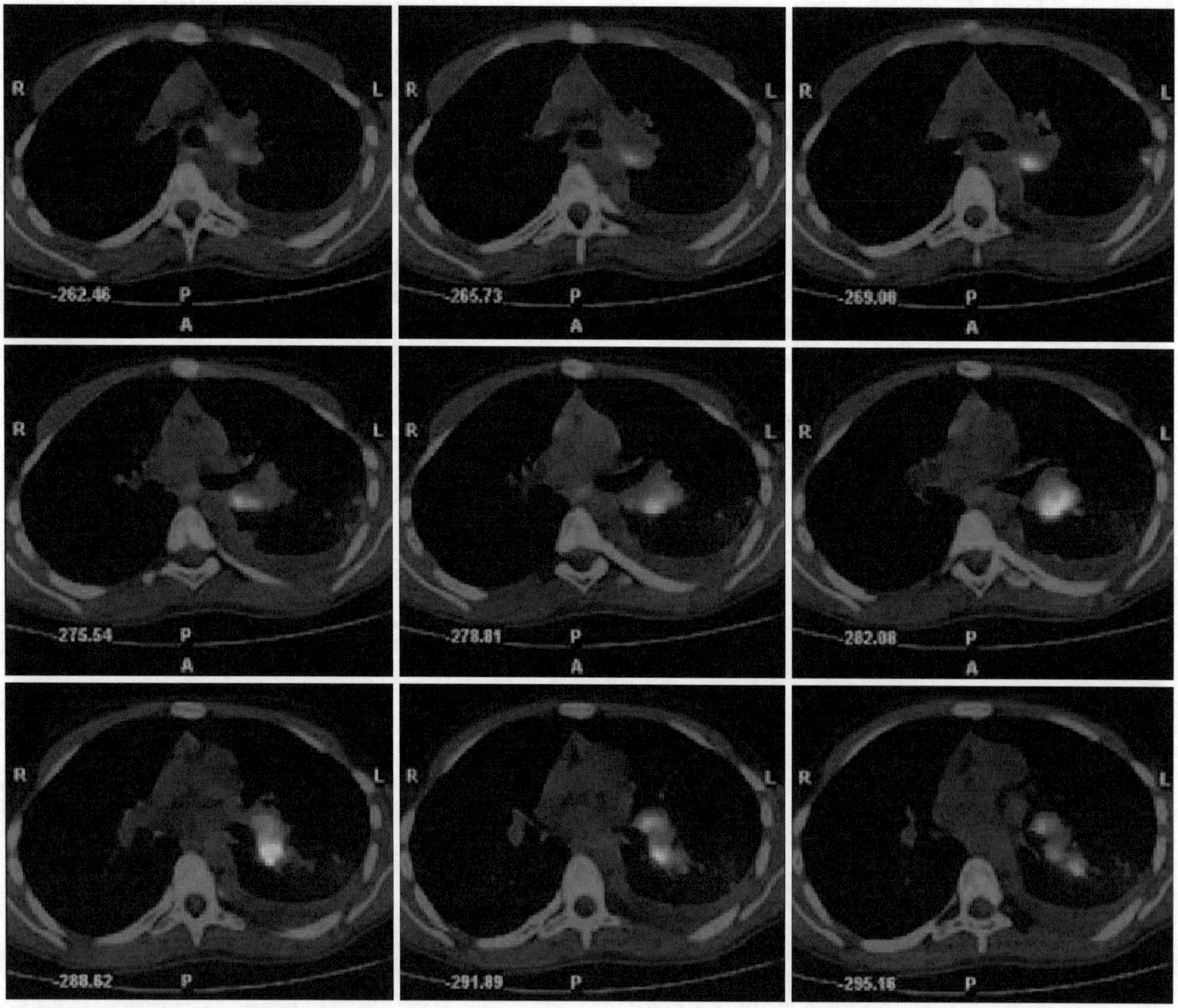

Fig. 13.15 Sequential transaxial slices from [^{18}F]FDG PET/CT fusion in mediastinum window demonstrate increased uptake of [^{18}F]FDG in the bilateral hilar and mediastinal nodes

Case 13.2

Paola A. Erba

Background

An 80-year-old man previously submitted to axillo-bifemoral vascular prosthesis presented with fever and cough. Abnormalities in the chest X-ray and CT: opacity in the superior lobe of the right lung of equivocal interpretation. Bronchoscopy with bronchoalveolar washing was inconclusive.

Due to persistence of fever associated with suspected vascular periprosthetic infection, [^{18}F]FDG PET/CT was performed (Fig. 13.16). Since the PET/CT findings were inconclusive, ^{99m}Tc-HMPAO-leukocyte scintigraphy was performed (Figs. 13.17, 13.18 and 13.19). ^{99m}Tc-HMPAO-leukocyte scintigraphy ruled out ongoing active infection.

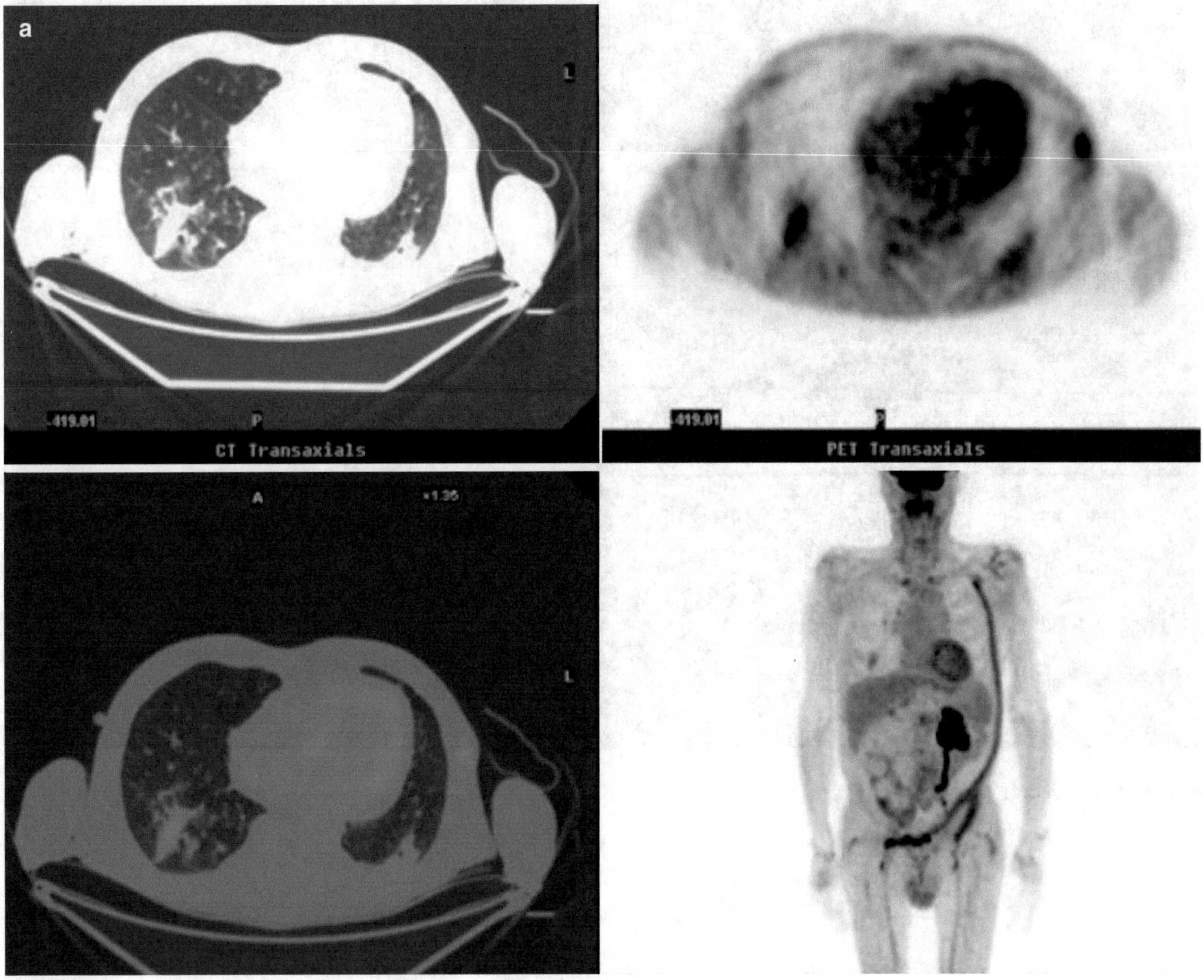

Fig. 13.16 [^{18}F]FDG PET/CT. Transaxial CT, PET, and fused PET/CT sections of chest (**a**) show increased [^{18}F]FDG uptake in the right lung. Transaxial CT, PET, and fused PET/CT sections of abdomen (**b**) show a mildly increased [^{18}F]FDG uptake in aortic region, site of previous surgery

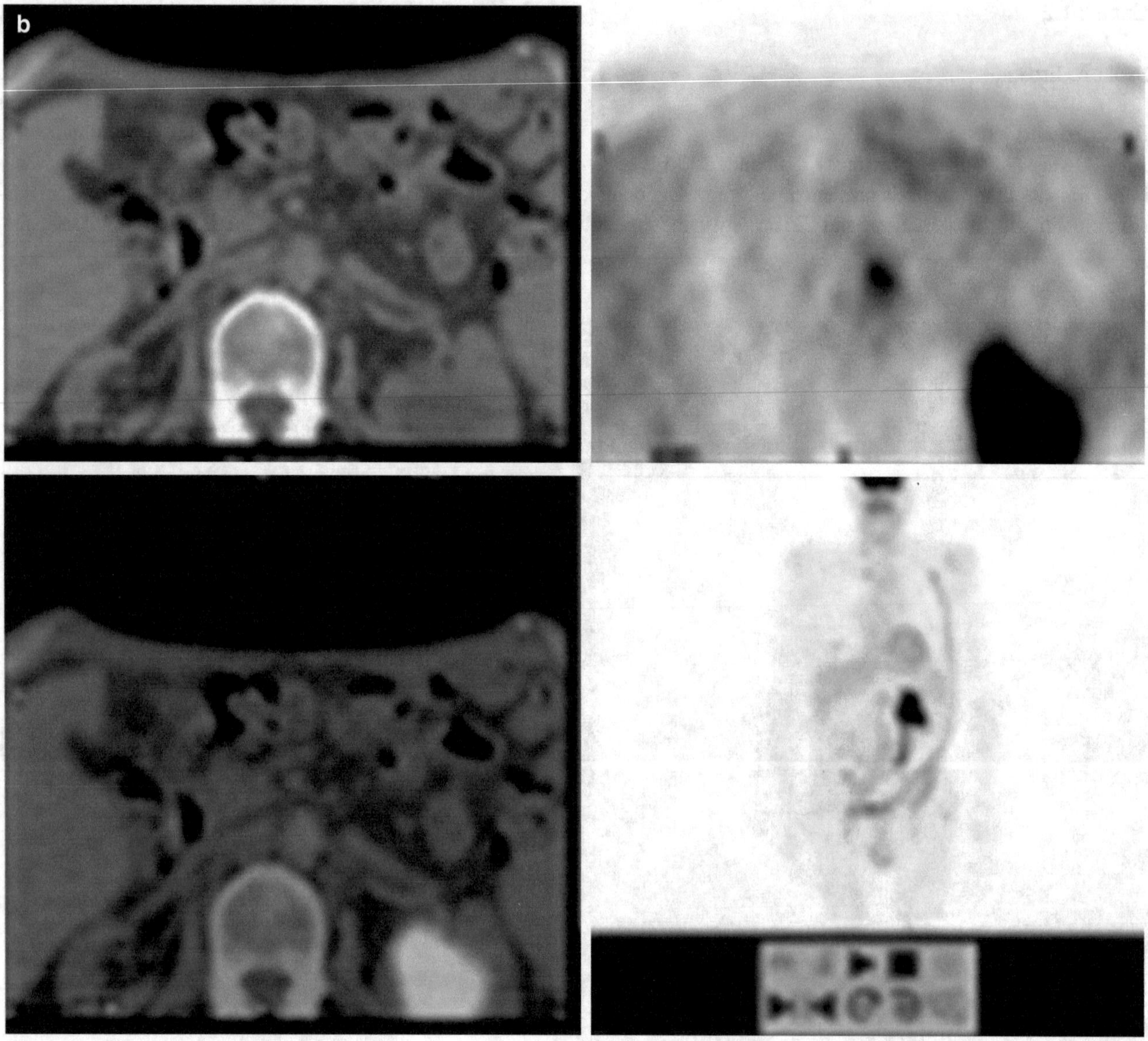

Fig. 13.16 (continued)

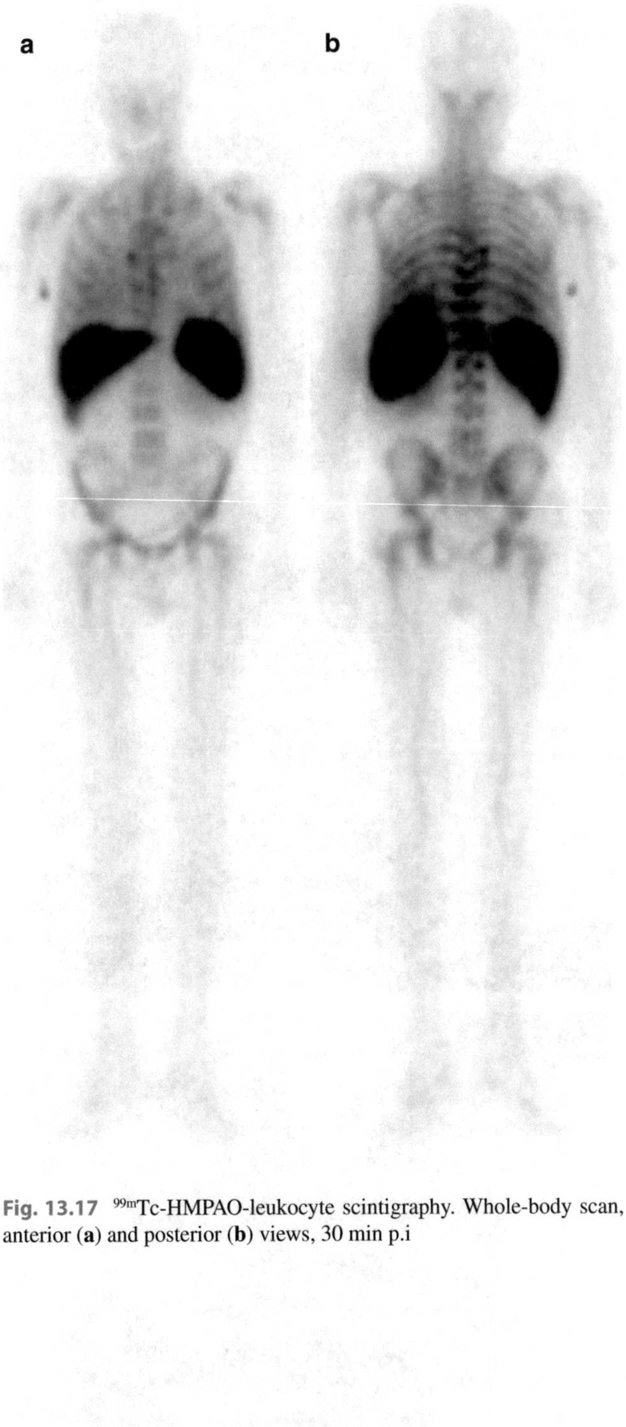

Fig. 13.17 ^{99m}Tc-HMPAO-leukocyte scintigraphy. Whole-body scan, anterior (**a**) and posterior (**b**) views, 30 min p.i

Differential Diagnosis

Lung neoplasm and infectious process.

Radiopharmaceutical Activity

[^{18}F]FDG, 3.7 MBq/kg; ^{99m}Tc-HMPAO-leukocytes, 640 MBq.

Imaging

PET/CT acquisition protocol: the scan was performed at 60–120 min p.i. Acquisition of the scan included: (1) scout view (120 kV, 10 mA) in order to define the limits of the body to explore, (2) whole-body CT scan (from skull base to proximal femur: 140 kV, 80 mA), and (3) whole-body PET (3D, 3 min/FOV).

^{99m}Tc-HMPAO-leukocyte scintigraphy: whole-body scan was performed 30 min p.i. Planar anterior and posterior acquisitions of the chest were acquired at 30 min, 4 h, and 24 h p.i. and SPECT/CT imaging of the abdomen was acquired 3 h, whereas SPECT/CT imaging of the chest was acquired at 24 h.

Conclusion/Teaching Point

This clinical case highlights the different specificity of [^{18}F] FDG PET/CT and of scintigraphy with radiolabeled leukocytes. [^{18}F]FDG allows the identification of inflammatory processes as well as infection; radiolabeled leukocytes allow the identification of only neutrophil-mediated processes, which are present in the majority of infections.

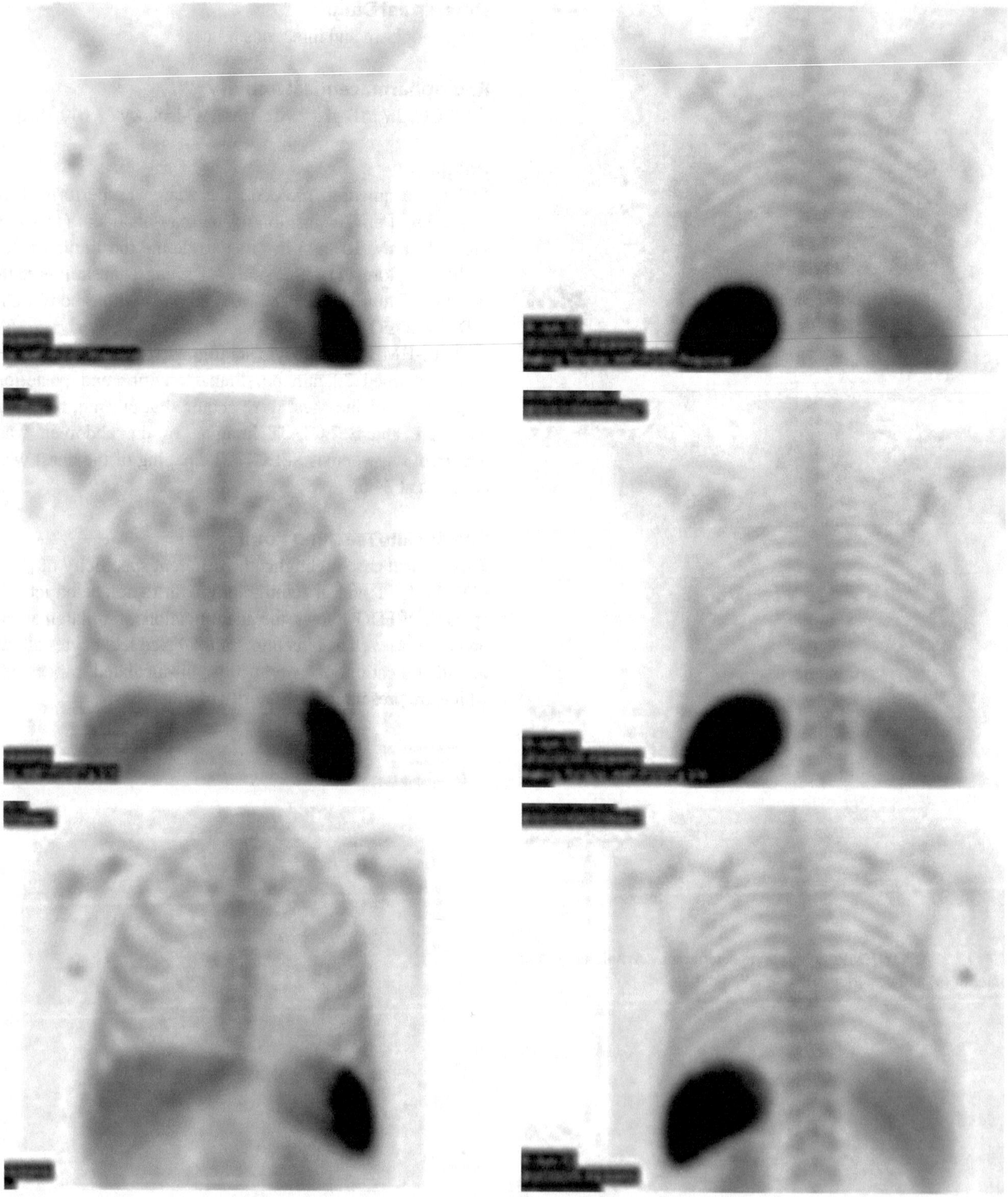

Fig. 13.18 ^{99m}Tc-HMPAO-leukocyte scintigraphy. Planar anterior (left) and posterior (right) images of chest, 30 min (upper), 4 h (middle), and 24 h (lower) p.i. The images show no pathologic accumulation in the lung region. The focal uptake of radiopharmaceutical in the axillary right region corresponds to the external portion of the central venous catheter

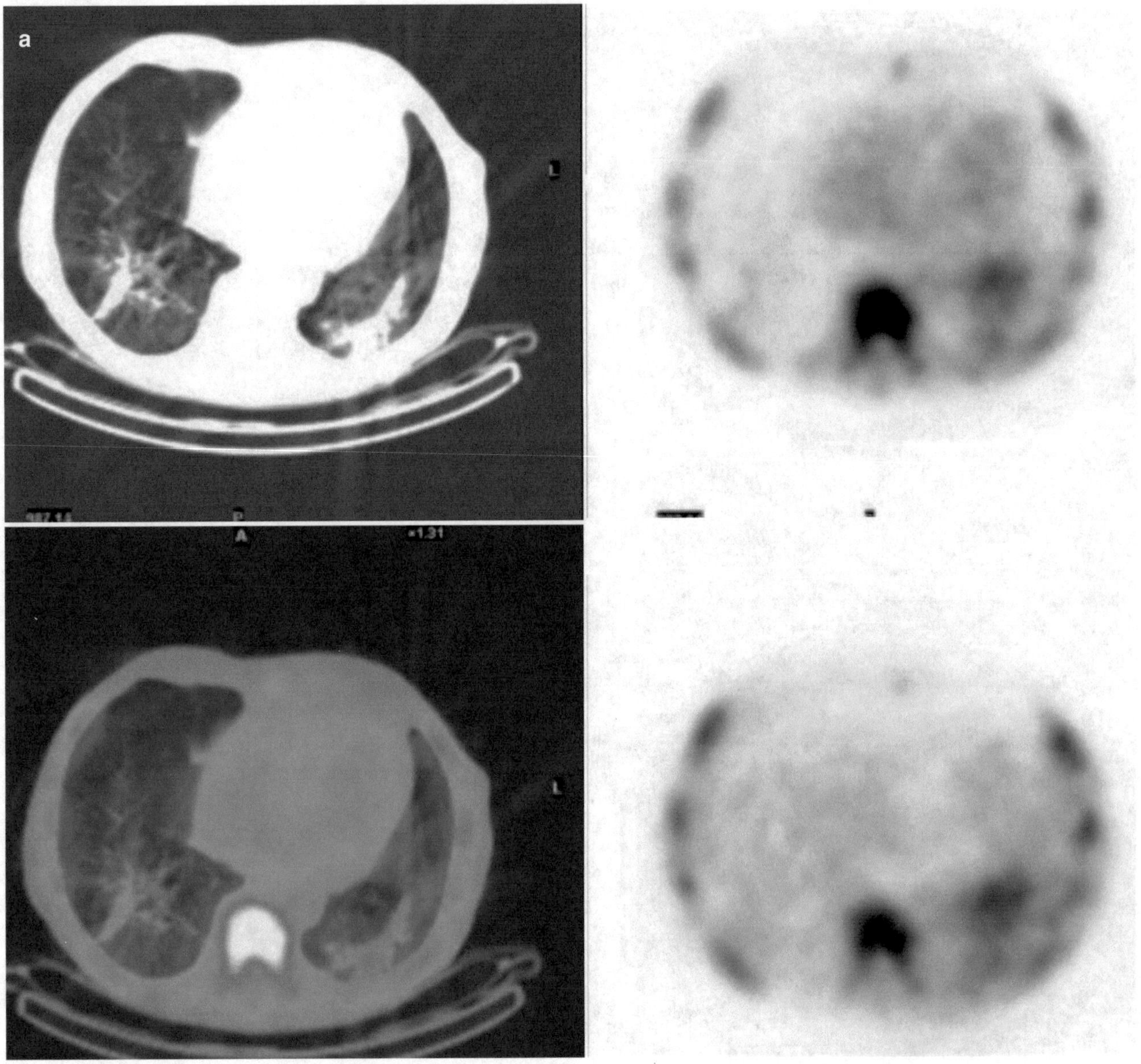

Fig. 13.19 ^{99m}Tc-HMPAO-leukocyte scintigraphy. SPECT/CT acquisitions of chest (**a**) and abdomen (**b**) do not show pathologic accumulation of labeled leukocytes (CT, upper left; SPECT, upper right; fused, bottom left)

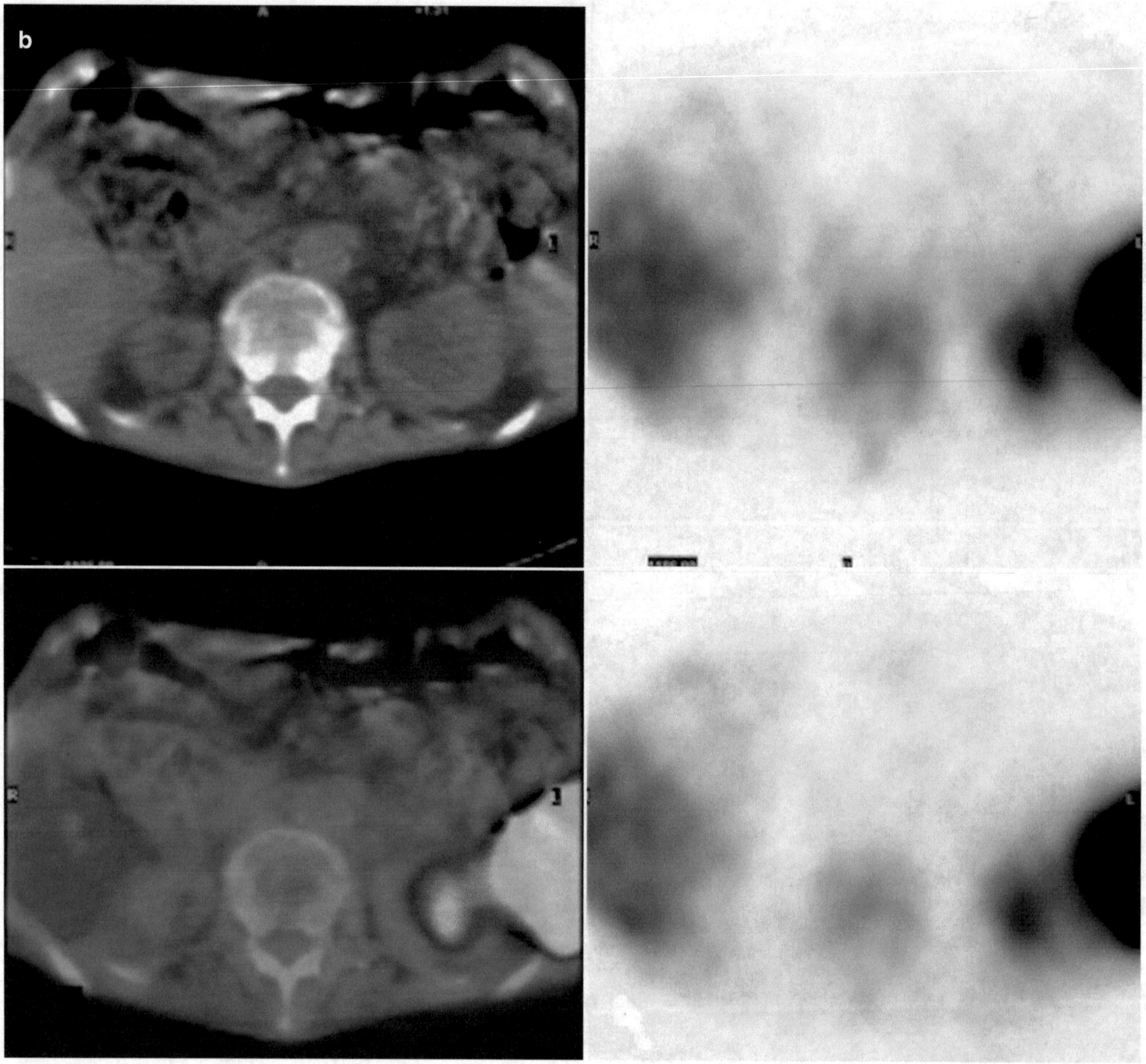

Fig. 13.19 (continued)

References

1. Driver C. Pneumonia part 1: pathology, presentation and prevention. Br J Nurs. 2012;21:103–6.
2. Anevlavis S, Bouros D. Community acquired bacterial pneumonia. Expert Opin Pharmacother. 2010;11:361–74.
3. Winther B. Rhinovirus infections in the upper airway. Proc Am Thorac Soc. 2011;8:79–89.
4. Rosen MJ. Epidemiology and risk of pulmonary disease. Semin Respir Infect. 1999;14:301–8.
5. Lynch T, Bialy L, Kellner JD, et al. A systematic review on the diagnosis of pediatric bacterial pneumonia: when gold is bronze. PLoS One. 2010;5(8):e11989. https://doi.org/10.1371/journal.pone.0011989.
6. Franquent T. Imaging techniques in the examination of the distal airways: asthma and COPD. Arch Bronconeumol. 2011;47:20–6.
7. Roberts HR, Wells AU, Milne DG, et al. Airflow obstruction in bronchiectasis: correlations between computed tomography features and pulmonary function test. Thorax. 2000;55:198–204.
8. Franquet T, Chung JH. Imaging of pulmonary infection. In: Hodler J, Kubik-Huch RA, von Schulthess GK, editors. Diseases of the chest, breast, heart and vessels 2019–2022: diagnostic and interventional imaging. Cham: Springer; 2019. p. 65–77.
9. Lim WS, Baudouin SV, George RC, et al. BTS guidelines for the management of community acquired pneumonia in adults: update 2009. Thorax. 2009;64(Suppl 3):iii1–55.
10. Haworth CS, Floto RA. Introducing the new BTS guideline: management of non-tuberculous mycobacterial pulmonary disease (NTM-PD). Thorax. 2017;72:969–70.
11. Haworth CS, Banks J, Capstick T, et al. British Thoracic Society guidelines for the management of non-tuberculous mycobacterial pulmonary disease (NTM-PD). Thorax. 2017;72(Suppl 2):ii1–ii64.

12. TB/HIV—a clinical manual. Geneva: World Health Organization; 2004. http://www.who.int/tb/publications/who_htm_tb_2004_329/en/index.html. Last Accessed 8 Apr 2020.
13. Prvulovich EM, Buscombe JR, Miller RF. The role of nuclear medicine in the investigation of patients with AIDS. Br J Hosp Med. 1996;55:549–53.
14. Ankrah AO, Glaudemans AWJM, Maes A, et al. Tuberculosis. Semin Nucl Med. 2018;48:108–30.
15. Sathekge MM, Ankrah AO, Lawal I, Vorster M. Monitoring response to therapy. Semin Nucl Med. 2018;48:166–81.
16. Vorster M, Buscombe J, Saad Z, Sathekge M. Past and future of Ga-citrate for infection and inflammation imaging. Curr Pharm Des. 2018;24:787–94.
17. Levenson SM, Warren RD, Richman SD, et al. Abnormal pulmonary gallium accumulation in P. carinii pneumonia. Radiology. 1976;19:395–8.
18. Niden AH, Mishkin FS, Khurana MML, et al. ^{67}Ga lung scan: an aid in the differential diagnosis of pulmonary embolism and pneumonitis. JAMA. 1977;237:1206–11.
19. Siemsen JK, Grebe SF, Waxman AD. The use of gallium-67 in pulmonary disorders. Semin Nucl Med. 1978;8:235–49.
20. Bekerman C, Hoffer PB, Bittran JD, et al. Gallium-67 citrate imaging studies of the lung. Semin Nucl Med. 1980;10:286–301.
21. Hoffer P. Gallium and infection. J Nucl Med. 1980;21:484–8.
22. Giraudo C, Evangelista L, Fraia AS, et al. Molecular imaging of pulmonary inflammation and infection. Int J Mol Sci. 2020;21(3):E894. https://doi.org/10.3390/ijms21030894.
23. Schuster DM, Alazraki N. Gallium and other agents in diseases of the lung. Semin Nucl Med. 2002;32:193–211.
24. Goldfarb CR, Colp C, Ongseng F, et al. Gallium scanning in the 'new' tuberculosis. Clin Nucl Med. 1997;22:470–4.
25. Yamaga LY, Benard G, Hironaka FH, et al. The role of gallium-67 scan in defining the extent of disease in an endemic deep mycosis, paracoccidioidomycosis: a predominantly multifocal disease. Eur J Nucl Med Mol Imaging. 2003;30:888–94.
26. Liu SF, Liu JW, Lin MC, et al. Monitoring treatment responses in patients with pulmonary TB using serial lung gallium-67 scintigraphy. AJR Am J Roentgenol. 2007;188:W403–8.
27. Lal FM, Liam CK, Paramsothy M, et al. The role of ^{67}gallium scintigraphy and high resolution computed tomography as predictors of disease activity in sputum smear-negative tuberculosis. Int J Tuberc Lung Dis. 1997;1:563–9.
28. Walsh TJ, Beckerman C, Chausow A, et al. The value of gallium-67 scanning in pulmonary tuberculosis. Am Rev Respir Dis. 1985;132:746747.
29. Yeh JJ, Huang YC, Teng WB, et al. The role of gallium-67 scintigraphy in comparing inflammatory activity between tuberculous and nontuberculous mycobacterial pulmonary diseases. Nucl Med Commun. 2011;32:392–401.
30. Herron T, Gossman W. 111 Indium white blood cell scan (indium leukocyte imaging, indium-111 scan). Treasure Island, FL: StatPearls Publishing; 2020.
31. Peters AM. The utility of [^{99m}Tc]HMPAO-leukocytes for imaging infection. Semin Nucl Med. 1994;24:110–27.
32. Altiay G, Cermik TF. ^{99m}Tc-HMPAO labeled white blood cell scintigraphy in the diagnosis and monitoring of response of the therapy in patients with active bronchiectasis. Rev Esp Med Nucl. 2012;31:9–14.
33. Kramer EL, Divgi CR. Pulmonary applications of nuclear medicine. Clin Chest Med. 1991;12:55–75.
34. Oates E, Ramberg K. Imaging of intrathoracic disease with indium-111-labeled leukocytes. J Thorac Imaging. 1990;5:78–88.
35. Currie DC, Saverymuttu SH, Peters AM, et al. Indium-111-labeled granulocyte accumulation in respiratory tract of patients with bronchiectasis. Lancet. 1987;1(8546):1335–9.
36. Fineman DS, Palestro CJ, Kim CK, et al. Detection of abnormalities in febrile AIDS patients with In-111-labeled leukocyte and Ga-67 scintigraphy. Radiology. 1989;170:677–80.
37. Segall GM, McDougall IR. Diagnostic value of lung uptake of indium-111 oxine-labeled white blood cells. AJR Am J Roentgenol. 1986;147:601–6.
38. Oyen WJ, Claessens RA, van der Meer JW, et al. Detection of subacute infectious foci with indium-111-labeled autologous leukocytes and indium-111-labeled human nonspecific immunoglobulin G: a prospective comparative study. J Nucl Med. 1991;32:1854–60.
39. Meduri GU, Belenchia JM, Massie JD, et al. The role of gallium-67 scintigraphy in diagnosing sources of fever in ventilated patients. Intensive Care Med. 1996;22:395–403.
40. Kao CH, Wang YL, Liao SQ, Wang SJ. Tc-99m HMPAO labelled WBCs in the detection of occult sepsis in the intensive care unit. Intensive Care Med. 1992;1:15–9.
41. Minoja G, Chiaranda M, Fachinetti A, et al. The clinical use of 99m-Tc-labeled WBC scintigraphy in critically ill surgical and trauma patients with occult sepsis. Intensive Care Med. 1996;9:867–71.
42. Slavin JD Jr, Sherigar RM, Spencer RP, et al. In-111 octreotide lung uptake in hypersensitive pneumonitis caused by fungal infection. Clin Nucl Med. 1998;23:847–8.
43. Vanhagen PM, Krenning EP, Reubi JC, et al. Somatostatin analogue scintigraphy in granulomatous diseases. Eur J Nucl Med. 1994;21:497–502.
44. Utsunomiya K, Narabayashi I, Nishigaki H, et al. Clinical significance of thallium-201 and gallium-67 scintigraphy in pulmonary tuberculosis. Eur J Nucl Med. 1997;24:252–7.
45. Gulaldi NC, Bayhan H, Ercan MT, et al. The visualization of pulmonary tuberculosis with Tc-99m(V)DMSA and Tc-99m citrate in comparison to Ga-67 citrate. Clin Nucl Med. 1995;20:1012–4.
46. Stefanescu C, Rusu V, Boişteanu D, et al. ^{99m}Tc isonitrils biophysical aspects in pulmonary tuberculosis. Part I. In vivo evaluation of ^{99m}T MIBI and ^{99m}T Tetrofosmin biophysical localization mechanisms. Rev Med Chir Soc Med Nat Iasi. 2006;110:944–9.
47. Vaidyanathan S, Patel CN, Scarsbrook AF, Chowdhury FU. FDG PET/CT in infection and inflammation—current and emerging clinical applications. Clin Radiol. 2015;70:787–800.
48. Dibble EH, Yoo DC, Baird GL, Noto RB. FDG PET/CT of infection: should it replace labeled leukocyte scintigraphy of inpatients? AJR Am J Roentgenol. 2019;213:1358–65.
49. Kung BT, Seraj SM, Zadeh MZ, et al. An update on the role of ^{18}F-FDG-PET/CT in major infectious and inflammatory diseases. Am J Nucl Med Mol Imaging. 2019;9:255–73.
50. Arnon-Sheleg E, Israel O, Keidar Z. PET/CT imaging in soft tissue infection and inflammation—an update. Semin Nucl Med. 2020;50:35–49.
51. Lorenzen J, Buchert M, Bleckmann C, et al. A search for the focus in patients with fever of unknown origin: is positron-emission tomography with F-18-fluorodeoxyglucose helpful? RöFo Fortschr Geb Rontgenstr Nuklearmed. 1999;171:49–53.
52. Watanabe S, Nakamura Y, Kariatsumari K, et al. Pulmonary paragonimiasis mimicking lung cancer on FDG–PET imaging. Anticancer Res. 2003;23:3437–40.
53. Wilkinson MD, Fulham MJ, McCaughan BC, et al. Invasive aspergillosis mimicking stage IIIA non-small-cell lung cancer on FDG positron emission tomography. Clin Nucl Med. 2003;28:234–5.
54. Bleeker-Rovers CP, Warris A, Drenth JP, et al. Diagnosis of Candida lung abscesses by ^{18}F-fluorodeoxyglucose positron emission tomography. Clin Microbiol Infect. 2005;11:493–5.
55. Chang JM, Lee HJ, Goo JM, et al. False positive and false negative FDG-PET scans in various thoracic diseases. Korean J Radiol. 2006;7:57–69.

56. Mascarenhas NB, Lam D, Lynch GR, et al. PET imaging of cerebral and pulmonary Nocardia infection. Clin Nucl Med. 2006;31:131–3.
57. Intriago B, Danùs M, Calvo N, et al. Influenza-like infection can result in diffuse fluorodeoxyglucose uptake in the lungs. Clin Nucl Med. 2009;34:737–8.
58. Soussan M, Brillet PY, Mekinian A, et al. Patterns of pulmonary tuberculosis on FDG-PET/CT. Eur J Radiol. 2012;81:2872–6.
59. Song KD, Lee KS, Chung MP, et al. Pulmonary cryptococcosis: imaging findings in 23 non-AIDS patients. Korean J Radiol. 2010;11:407–16.
60. Franzen D, Latshang T, Frauenfelder T, et al. [Be cautious with a prognosis!]. Ther Umsch. 2010;67:605–7.
61. Kawate E, Yamazaki M, Kohno T, et al. Two cases with solitary pulmonary nodule due to nontuberculous mycobacterial infection showing intense ^{18}F-fluorodeoxyglucose uptake on positron emission tomography scan. Geriatr Gerontol Int. 2010;10:251–4.
62. Sathekge M, Maes A, Kgomo M, et al. Impact of FDG PET on the management of TBC treatment: a pilot study. Nuklearmedizin. 2010;49:35–40.
63. Hadley GP, Naude F. Malignant solid tumor, HIV infection and tuberculosis in children: an unholy triad. Pediatr Surg Int. 2009;25:697–701.
64. Liu Y. Demonstrations of AIDS-associated malignancies and infections at FDG PET-CT. Ann Nucl Med. 2011;25:536–46.
65. Sathekge M, Goethals I, Maes A, et al. Positron emission tomography in patients suffering from HIV-1 infection. Eur J Nucl Med Mol Imaging. 2009;36:1176–84.
66. Win Z, Todd J, Al-Nahhas A. FDG-PET imaging in pneumocystis carinii pneumonia. Clin Nucl Med. 2005;30:690–1.
67. Sojan SM, Chew G. Pneumocystis carinii pneumonia on F-18 FDG PET. Clin Nucl Med. 2005;30:763–4.
68. Bharucha T, Rutherford A, Skeoch S, et al. Diagnostic yield of FDG-PET/CT in fever of unknown origin: a systematic review, meta-analysis, and Delphi exercise. Clin Radiol. 2017;72:764–71.
69. Kouijzer IJE, Mulders-Manders CM, Bleeker-Rovers CP, Oyen WJG. Fever of unknown origin: the value of FDG-PET/CT. Semin Nucl Med. 2018;48:100–7.
70. Schönau V, Vogel K, Englbrecht M, et al. The value of ^{18}F-FDG-PET/CT in identifying the cause of fever of unknown origin (FUO) and inflammation of unknown origin (IUO): data from a prospective study. Ann Rheum Dis. 2018;77:70–7.
71. Warwick JM, Sathekge MM. PET/CT scanning with a high HIV/AIDS prevalence. Transfus Apher Sci. 2011;44:167–72.
72. Masekela R, Gongxeka H, Green RJ. Positron emission tomography in the prediction of inflammation in children with human immunodeficiency virus related bronchiectasis. Hell J Nucl Med. 2012;15:23–7.
73. Davison JM, Subramaniam RM, Surasi DS, et al. FDG PET/CT in patients with HIV. AJR Am J Roentgenol. 2011;197:284–94.
74. Basu S, Saboury B, Werner T, et al. Clinical utility of FDG PET and PET/CT in non-malignant thoracic disorders. Mol Imaging Biol. 2011;13:1051–60.
75. Ozsahin H, von Planta M, Müller I, et al. Successful treatment of invasive aspergillosis in chronic granulomatous disease by bone marrow transplantation, granulocyte colony-stimulating factor-mobilized granulocytes, and liposomal amphotericin-B. Blood. 1998;92:2719–24.
76. Kalanuria AA, Ziai W, Mirski M. Ventilator-associated pneumonia in the ICU. Crit Care. 2014;18:208.
77. Chang I, Schibler A. Ventilator associated pneumonia in children. Paediatr Respir Rev. 2016;20:10–6.
78. Spalding MC, Cripps MW, Minshall CT. Ventilator-associated pneumonia: new definitions. Crit Care Clin. 2017;33:277–92.
79. Cook DJ, Kollef MH. Risk factors for ICU-acquired pneumonia. JAMA. 1998;279:1605–6.
80. Georges H, Leroy O, Guery B, et al. Predisposing factors for nosocomial pneumonia in patients receiving mechanical ventilation and requiring tracheotomy. Chest. 2000;118:767–74.
81. Holzapfel L, Chastang C, Demingeon G, et al. A randomized study assessing the systematic search for maxillary sinusitis in nasotracheally mechanically ventilated patients. Influence of nosocomial maxillary sinusitis on the occurrence of ventilator-associated pneumonia. Am J Respir Crit Care Med. 1999;159:695–701.
82. Fàbregas N, Ewig S, Torres A, et al. Clinical diagnosis of ventilator associated pneumonia revisited: comparative validation using immediate post-mortem lung biopsies. Thorax. 1999;54:867–73.
83. Wunderink RG, Woldenberg LS, Zeiss J, et al. The radiologic diagnosis of autopsy-proven ventilator-associated pneumonia. Chest. 1992;101:458–63.
84. Simons KS, Pickkers P, Bleeker-Rovers CP, et al. F-18-fluorodeoxyglucose positron emission tomography combined with CT in critically ill patients with suspected infection. Intensive Care Med. 2010;36:504–11.
85. Qin C, Liu F, Yen TC, Lan X. ^{18}F-FDG PET/CT findings of COVID-19: a series of four highly suspected cases. Eur J Nucl Med Mol Imaging. 2020;47:1281–6.
86. Zou S, Zhu X. FDG PET/CT of COVID-19. Radiology. 2020;296(2):E118. https://doi.org/10.1148/radiol.2020200770.
87. Joob B, Wiwanitkit V. ^{18}F-FDG PET/CT and COVID-19. Eur J Nucl Med Mol Imaging. 2020;47:1348.
88. Deng Y, Lei L, Chen Y, Zhang W. The potential added value of FDG PET/CT for COVID-19 pneumonia. Eur J Nucl Med Mol Imaging. 2020;47:1634–5.
89. Polverari G, Arena V, Ceci F, et al. ^{18}F-FDG uptake in asymptomatic SARS-CoV-2 (COVID-19) patient, referred to PET/CT for non-small cells lung cancer restaging. J Thorac Oncol. 2020;15:1078–80.
90. Albano D, Bertagna F, Bertolia M, et al. Incidental findings suggestive of Covid-19 in asymptomatic patients undergoing nuclear medicine procedures in a high prevalence region. J Nucl Med. 2020;61:632–6.
91. Lütje S, Marinova M, Kütting D, et al. Nuclear medicine in SARS-CoV-2 pandemia: ^{18}F-FDG-PET/CT to visualize COVID-19. Nuklearmedizin. 2020;59:276–80.
92. Setti L, Kirienko M, Dalto SC, et al. FDG-PET/CT findings highly suspicious for COVID-19 in an Italian case series of asymptomatic patients. Eur J Nucl Med Mol Imaging. 2020;47:1649–56.
93. Tian J, Yang X, Yu L, et al. A multicenter clinical trial on the diagnostic value of dual-tracer PET/CT in pulmonary lesions using 3′-deoxy-3′-^{18}F-fluorothymidine and ^{18}F-FDG. J Nucl Med. 2008;49:186–94.
94. Hara T, Kosaka N, Suzuki T, et al. Uptake rates of ^{18}F-fluorodeoxyglucose and ^{11}C-choline in lung cancer and pulmonary tuberculosis: a positron emission tomography study. Chest. 2003;124:893–901.

Nuclear Medicine Imaging in Chronic Inflammatory Diseases

14

Annibale Versari and Massimiliano Casali

Contents

Learning Objectives

- To acquire knowledge of the clinical applications of radiological and nuclear medicine techniques in patients with rheumatoid arthritis
- To define the role of [^{18}F]FDG PET/CT for the diagnosis, management, response to therapy, and follow-up of patients with large vessel vasculitis
- To become familiar with the applications of [^{18}F]FDG PET/CT for diagnosis and for monitoring response to therapy in patients with idiopathic retroperitoneal fibrosis
- To understand the comparative role of [^{18}F]FDG PET/CT versus ^{67}Ga-citrate scintigraphy for the diagnosis and monitoring response to therapy in patients with sarcoidosis
- To summarize the radiological and nuclear medicine applications, mainly sialoscintigraphy, in patients with the Sjögren syndrome
- To understand the pathophysiologic bases for the use of PET/CT with [^{18}F]FDG or ^{18}F-NaF for the evaluation of the atherosclerotic plaque

A. Versari (✉)
Nuclear Medicine, Azienda Unità Sanitaria Locale-IRCCS di Reggio Emilia, Reggio Emilia, Italy
e-mail: annibale.versari@ausl.re.it

M. Casali
Nuclear Medicine, Azienda Unità Sanitaria Locale-IRCCS of Reggio Emilia, Reggio Emilia, Italy

E. Lazzeri et al. (eds.), *Radionuclide Imaging of Infection and Inflammation*, https://doi.org/10.1007/978-3-030-62175-9_14

14.1 Introductory Background

Chronic inflammatory diseases include numerous, clinically heterogeneous immune-mediated disorders such as arthritis, large-vessel vasculitis, and sarcoidosis. Imaging has a key role in the workup of inflammatory disorders, being an excellent tool both for diagnosis and for monitoring disease activity. Standard conventional X-ray is inexpensive and widely available, but its sensitivity in this scenario is limited. Computerized tomography (CT) and magnetic resonance imaging (MRI) are more sensitive and more specific than plain radiography. However, they are more expensive, less available, and sometimes unable to define the full extent of the disease process; moreover, CT and MRI may not always reliably gauge disease activity.

Metabolic imaging with radiopharmaceuticals has the distinctive advantage of visualizing virtually the entire body, thus providing key information on the organs involved and even detecting occult sites of inflammation. In addition, metabolic imaging techniques lend themselves better to measure disease activity [1, 2]. In particular, positron emission tomography (PET) with [^{18}F]fluorodeoxyglucose ([^{18}F]FDG) has emerged over the last years as an increasingly useful technique both for diagnostic and for monitoring purposes in a host of inflammatory conditions. A major progress has been the combination of [^{18}F]FDG-PET with CT (or MRI), thus combining the high CT (or MR) anatomical spatial resolution for localizing sites of active inflammation with the PET characteristics of high sensitivity and marker of metabolic activity.

14.2 Rheumatoid Arthritis

Rheumatoid arthritis (RA) is a systemic progressive chronic autoimmune disease affecting principally the joints, which occur in 5–1.0% of the global population [3]. RA is characterized by a typical chronic mononuclear cell infiltration of the synovial membrane causing cartilage and bone erosion, leading eventually to joint ankylosis. Subcutaneous tissues are frequently involved and diffuse inflammation may also occur in the lungs and pleura, in the pericardium and in the sclera [4]. Pain, loss of function, and loss of mobility are the main clinical features. Laboratory tests including rheumatoid factor, anti-citrullinated protein antibodies, and antinuclear antibody determination are generally performed in conjunction with more common hematological and biochemical tests [5]. Early diagnosis and prompt treatment usually translate into better outcome [6].

Conventional plain X-ray has been the imaging modality most frequently used for several decades, despite its lack of sensitivity in detecting RA joint structural changes, especially in early stages of the disease [7].

MRI is superior to plain radiography (45% sensitivity for bone erosions versus 15% of X-ray), allowing a three-dimensional view and precise assessment of the bone and surrounding soft tissue involvement within a certain affected joint [8].

Musculoskeletal ultrasonography allows an in-depth analysis of soft tissue structures, but it cannot provide information on osteitis [9]. Being more sensitive than clinical examination in detecting joint inflammation, ultrasonography can be useful when the clinical features of synovitis and/or tenosynovitis are equivocal, or when subclinical disease is suspected, especially in early stage disease [10].

Traditionally, the contribution of imaging to RA prognosis has been based on the identification of radiographic erosions, while data on MRI and ultrasonography are not univocal [10–12].

Nuclear medicine imaging techniques have been extensively employed in the evaluation of RA [11]. Despite the high sensitivity (98–100%) reported for three-phase bone scintigraphy (Figs. 14.1 and 14.2) and its contribution to predict/assess the success of knee joint radiosynoviorthesis [12–14], at present the usefulness of this technique in the assessment of RA is limited, because of some discordance with clinical diagnosis (based on the American College of Rheumatology criteria) [15] and of its relative low-specificity and low-spatial resolution (especially when evaluating small joints). High-resolution multi-pinhole SPECT (MPH-SPECT) can be employed to increase the diagnostic accuracy of bone scintigraphy, to identify the uptake pattern more typical of early RA (central uptake) than of early osteoarthritis (eccentric uptake), and to recognize patterns of uptake that enable to distinguish RA from osteoarthritis [16]. However, in early RA MPH-SPECT, evaluation of the metacarpophalangeal joints performs worse than MRI [17, 18].

^{99m}Tc-nanocolloid scintigraphy has been compared to clinical data in the evaluation of RA patients considered to be in remission (according to the American College of Rheumatology and the European League Against Rheumatism criteria), resulting negative for active joint disease in 35% of the cases and positive in 65% of patients; 92% of the scintigraphy-positive patients were also sero-

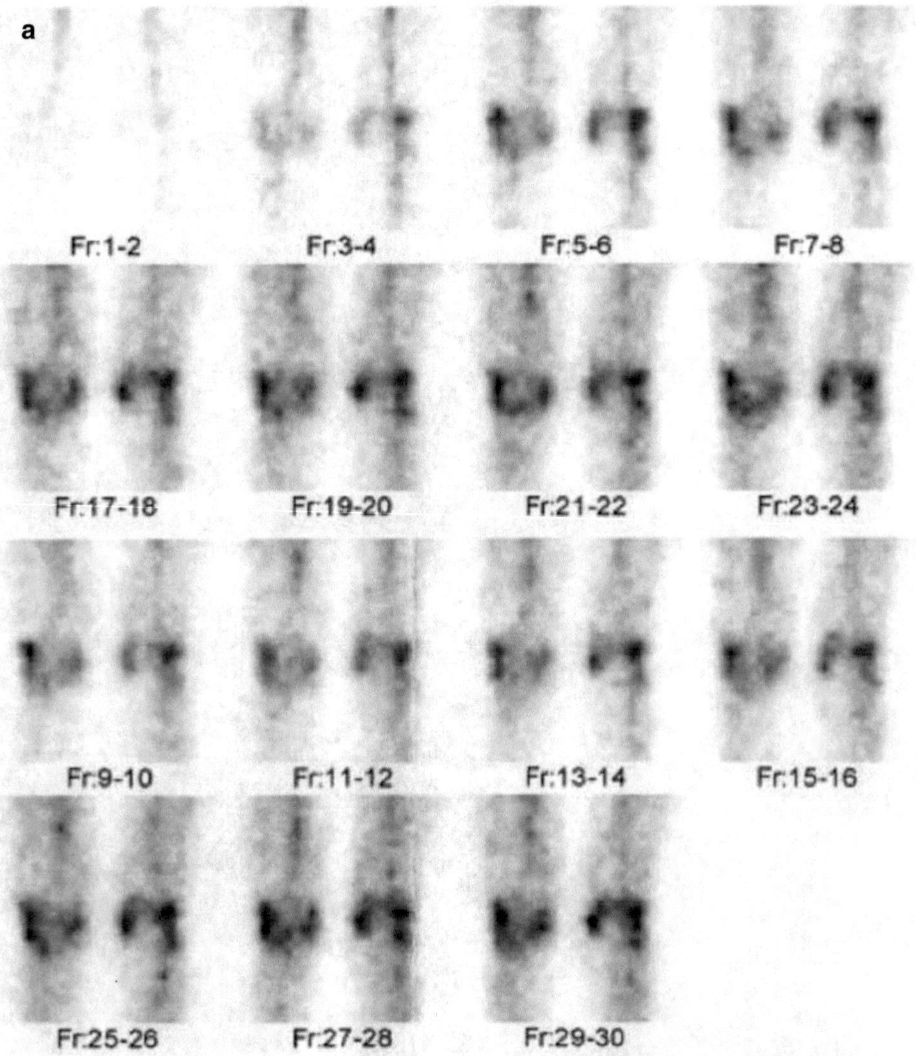

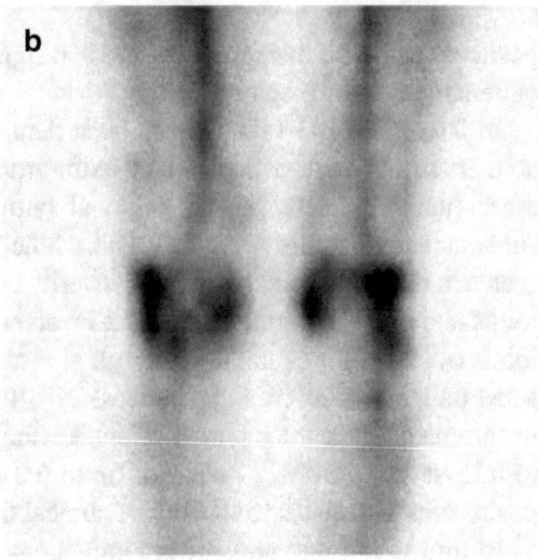

Fig. 14.1 ^{99m}Tc-MDP three-phase bone scintigraphy in a patient with RA. Images of the knees obtained in anterior view during the dynamic vascular phase (**a** and **b**) show an increased blood flow in both knees, as confirmed by images obtained in anterior and posterior views during the blood pool phase (**c**). Planar spot images (anterior, left; posterior, right) of knees obtained 3 h after radiopharmaceutical injection demonstrate intense ^{99m}Tc-MDP uptake (**d**) particularly in lateral region or joints

Fig. 14.1 (continued)

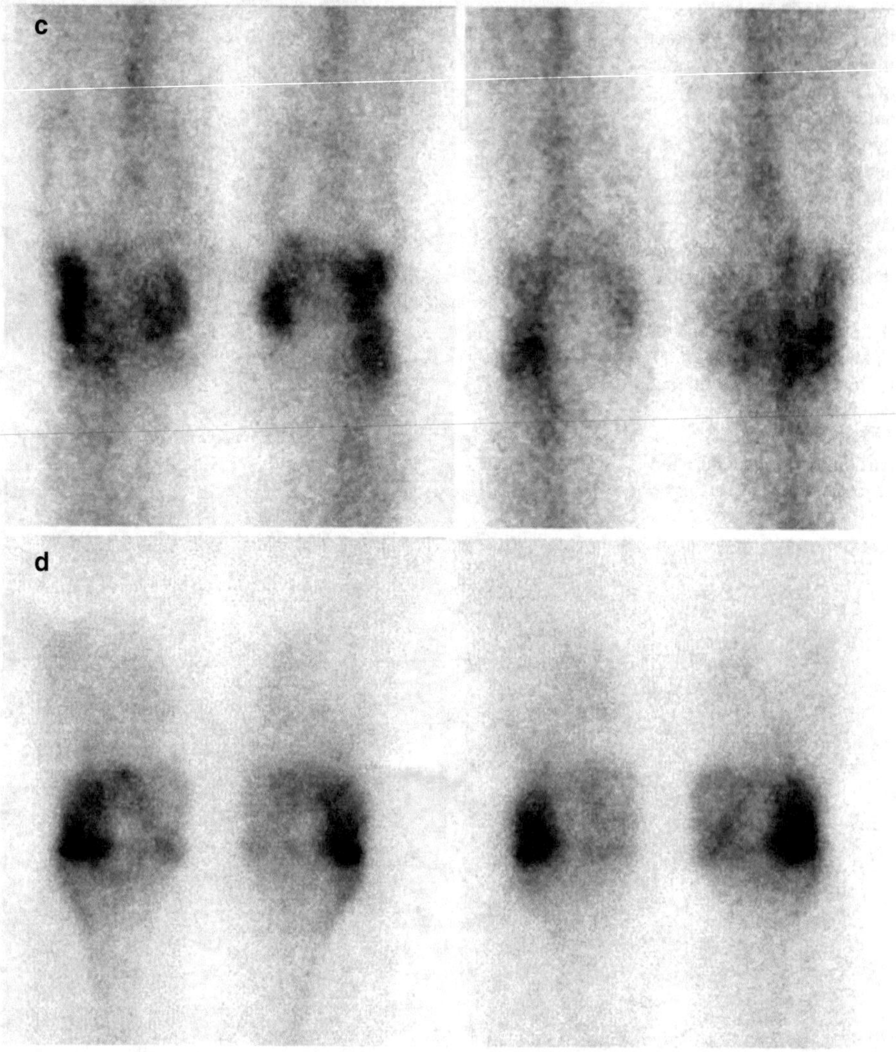

positive, while all except one of the scintigraphy-negative patients were sero-negative [19].

In RA, [^{18}F]FDG PET/CT has been demonstrated to be able to reveal both articular and extra-articular inflamed areas (tendon sheets, bursae, regional lymph nodes, and subcutaneous nodules) [20–22]. The whole-body PET/CT scan can delineate disease grade of severity among different joints and provide information about involvement of deeper joints (midfoot for example), difficult to evaluate clinically. Most patients with RA show increased [^{18}F]FDG uptake in the affected joints, the intensity of uptake ranging from mild to intense, with SUV_{max} values of up to 6.0 [23], and PET positivities, correlates to severity of clinical findings as well as to ultrasound measures of inflammations [24]. In addition, changes in the PET scan pattern shortly after commencing therapy have been shown to correlate with the clinical assessment [25] and to predict outcomes at later stages [26]. In this regard, [^{18}F]FDG-PET has proved more accurate than either conventional inflammatory markers or clinical examination [26]. The capacity of PET to identify active joint disease in RA has also been assessed in comparison to ultrasonography and MRI. In a study on 16 patients with an inflamed knee, [^{18}F]FDG PET was positive in 69% of the knees, while MRI and ultrasonography were positive in 69% and 75%, respectively [26]. PET-positive knees exhibited significantly higher SUVs, higher MRI activity scores, and greater synovial thickness compared with PET-negative knees. Posttreatment changes in SUV correlated with changes of MRI activity parameters and of serum C-reactive protein levels. These data suggest that PET can reliably gauge disease activity, including response to therapy in RA [26]. It remains to be established how cost-effective PET is compared to ultrasonography and MRI in assessing activity of arthritis.

Novel PET tracers such as [^{11}C]choline (for semi-quantitative imaging of inflammatory arthropathy), ^{68}Ga-DOTA-Siglec-9 (for synovitis evaluation), and ^{89}Zr-rituximab (for predicting responder to anti-B-cell therapy) have recently shown promising results that must however be further validated [27–30].

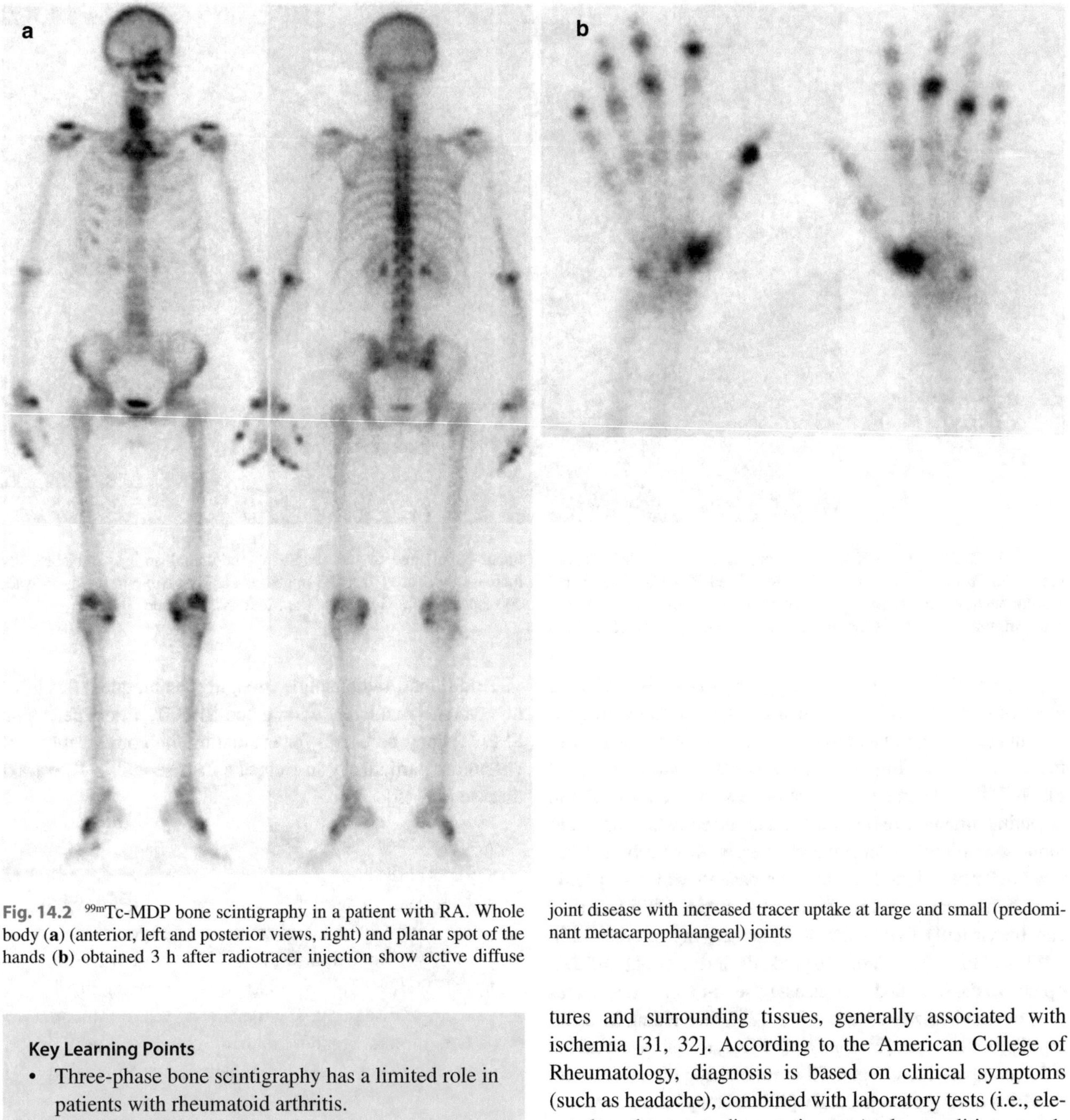

Fig. 14.2 ^{99m}Tc-MDP bone scintigraphy in a patient with RA. Whole body (**a**) (anterior, left and posterior views, right) and planar spot of the hands (**b**) obtained 3 h after radiotracer injection show active diffuse joint disease with increased tracer uptake at large and small (predominant metacarpophalangeal) joints

Key Learning Points

- Three-phase bone scintigraphy has a limited role in patients with rheumatoid arthritis.
- [^{18}F]FDG-PET/CT is able to reveal both articular and extra-articular inflamed areas, to define the grade of disease severity, to provide information about involvement of deeper joints, to monitor response to therapy, and to predict outcomes at later stages.

14.3 Vasculitis

Vasculitis is characterized by inflammation and necrosis with macrophages (M1 and M2) and with leukocyte infiltration of the vessel wall and reactive damage to mural structures and surrounding tissues, generally associated with ischemia [31, 32]. According to the American College of Rheumatology, diagnosis is based on clinical symptoms (such as headache), combined with laboratory tests (i.e., elevated erythrocyte sedimentation rate), abnormalities on palpation of temporal artery, and histologic changes of the temporal artery in case of giant cell vasculitis [33].

Doppler ultrasonography is highly sensitive (about 85%) for the detection of proximal arm and axillary vessels and carotid, finger, and temporal arteries (over 90% specificity when either edema, stenosis or occlusion are present) [34].

The typical MRI findings for diagnosing giant cell vasculitis are arterial wall thickening and increased gadolinium contrast enhancement (81% sensitivity, 97% specificity). However, high field strengths are required for imaging vasculitis with MRI [35].

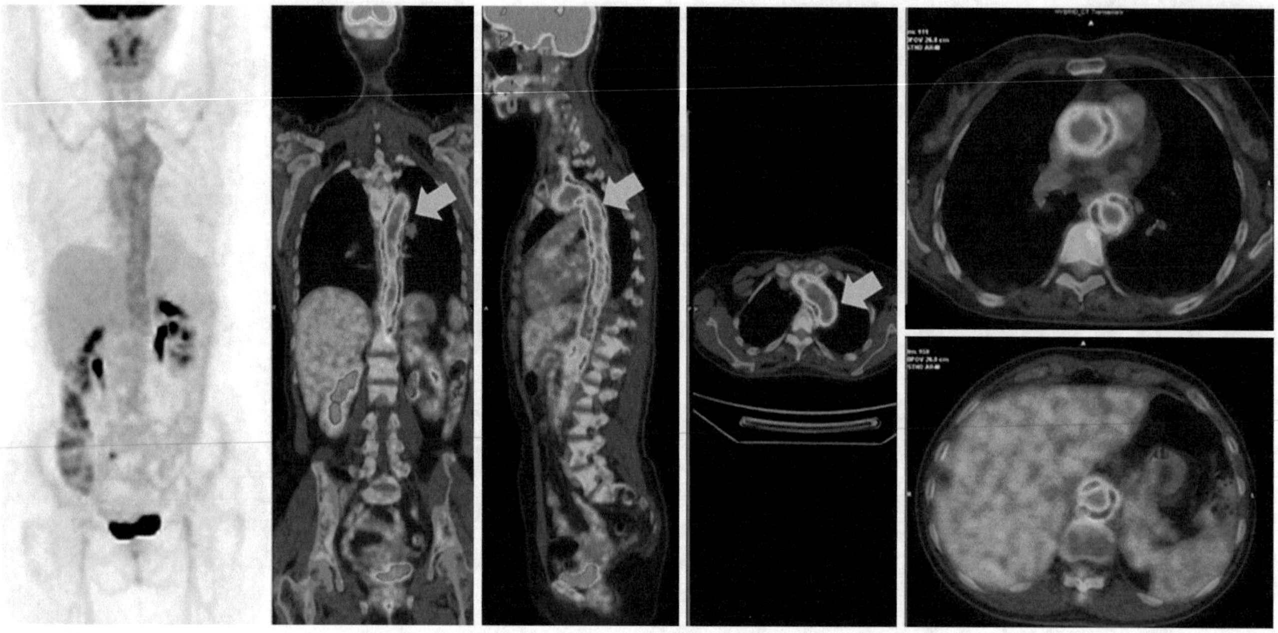

Fig. 14.3 PET/CT with [^{18}F]FDG in a patient with active large vessel vasculitis. From left to right: MIP image, fused PET/CT coronal and sagittal sections, transaxial section of upper chest (ascending aorta), and transaxial sections of the mid-chest (descending thoracic aorta in upper panel) and of the abdomen (abdominal aorta). The markedly increased, diffuse [^{18}F]FDG uptake is clearly visible in the aorta wall, corresponding to Grade 3 of the Meller visual scale

Radionuclide imaging of large vessel vasculitis, including giant cell arteritis and Takayasu arteritis, has resulted in great advantages for the management of patients with this inflammatory condition (Fig. 14.3). In large-vessel vasculitis, [^{18}F]FDG PET has been shown to be more sensitive than MRI in detecting inflamed vessels [36] and is currently the only technique that allows visualization of nearly all vessels that can potentially be affected [2]. In some patients with nonspecific complains, such as fever of unknown origin, [^{18}F]FDG PET can be virtually diagnostic of an underlying arteritis [37]. [^{18}F]FDG PET also enables to grade the intensity of [^{18}F]FDG uptake in the inflamed vessels using semi-quantitative scores [38] or standardized uptake values [39], thus aiding in defining disease severity [2]. Finally, [^{18}F]FDG PET has an added value compared to CT or MRI in monitoring disease activity by virtue of its greater accuracy [40] and may have a prognostic role in identifying patients at greater risk of developing vascular complications such as aneurysm or rupture [41]. Vasculitis can usually be differentiated from atherosclerosis on the basis of the vessel segments involved, of the intensity of [^{18}F]FDG uptake, and of the pattern of vascular uptake ("hot spots" in atherosclerosis versus smooth, linear uptake in vasculitis) [2]. PET also allows the evaluation of the response to pharmacological treatment (cortisone, immunosuppressants, biological drugs). In the first 3 months after the initiation of cortisone therapy, PET imaging demonstrates a drop of vascular uptake of [^{18}F]FDG that does not seem to undergo significant changes in the following months [42].

Additional radionuclide imaging techniques (such as myocardial perfusion with gated-SPECT, brain perfusion SPECT) may be useful for evaluating the complications of vasculitis, particularly in Behçet's disease and in Kawasaki disease [43–45].

Key Learning Points

- Metabolic imaging has an important role in the clinical management of patients with large vessel vasculitis (giant cell arteritis and Takayasu arteritis).
- [^{18}F]FDG PET/CT can identify multi-vessel involvement of disease, grade intensity of vessel inflammation, monitor response to therapy, and patients with a greater risk of developing aneurysm or rupture.

14.4 Sarcoidosis

Sarcoidosis is a multisystem disease; lung involvement is present in about two thirds of the patients, but any organ can be affected. The severity of clinical manifestations ranges from an asymptomatic state to a life-threatening condition, depending on the organs involved. Diagnosis is based on the histopathologic pattern of non-caseating granulomatous inflammation, associated with characteristic clinical and/or radiographic findings [46].

Radiographic staging is based on plain chest X-ray and/or chest CT [47]. Lung sarcoidosis on a plain chest X-ray film presents with bilateral hilar and paratracheal enlarged lymph nodes, with or without parenchymal lung opacities [48]. Bilateral hilar adenopathy (especially in asymptomatic cases) and disease along the bronchovascular bundle are the "classical" findings supporting diagnosis of lung sarcoidosis on high-resolution CT [49]. *High-resolution CT* performs better than MRI in the assessment of interstitial lung diseases [50].

MRI is sensitive for detecting muscular, soft tissue, and bone involvement, revealing findings that are occult on radiographs [51, 52]. Additionally, MRI is very useful to evaluate cardiac sarcoidosis [53]. Gadolinium-enhanced MRI is the imaging technique of choice for the assessment of neurosarcoidosis. The most common abnormalities of neurosarcoidosis on MRI are non-enhancing periventricular white matter lesions and meningeal enhancement [54].

Several radiopharmaceuticals have been employed for the evaluation of sarcoidosis. ^{67}Ga-citrate scintigraphy makes the diagnosis of sarcoidosis highly probable when it shows the typical "lambda" sign (bilateral hilar and right paratracheal lymphadenopathy uptake) and the "panda" sign (uptake in bilateral lacrimal and parotid glands) (Figs. 14.4, 14.5 and 14.6) [55]. The presence of both the lambda and panda patterns is highly specific for sarcoidosis. However, the panda pattern by itself is not specific for sarcoidosis (as it can also be observed in, i.e., RA, and lymphoma) [56, 57]. ^{67}Ga-citrate uptake within the lung parenchyma per se is also nonspecific [58]. Among all methods described to estimate ^{67}Ga-citrate uptake in the sarcoid-involved lung parenchyma, the most common and the easiest to use is to visually compare lung uptake to that of soft tissue, bone marrow, and liver [59]. However, ^{67}Ga-citrate scintigraphy can also yield false-negative results [60]. ^{67}Ga-scanning has been evaluated also for monitoring therapeutic response and for prognostic purposes, resulting exquisitely sensitive in identifying patients with active sarcoidosis [57]. Despite its lack of specificity, ^{67}Ga-citrate scintigraphy can be useful in some clinical scenarios: (1) assisting in the diagnosis and staging of difficult cases, especially those with isolated extra-thoracic disease; (2) helping to identify active sites for biopsy; (3) detecting or excluding recurrent disease after steroid therapy; and (4) differentiating active disease from fibrosis in a lung transplant candidate [57].

In cardiac sarcoidosis, the ^{99m}Tc-sestamibi resting scan [61] typically reveals segmental areas of decreased uptake in the ventricular myocardium that often disappear or decrease in size during stress imaging or after the intravenous administration of dipyridamole [62]. The combined use of ^{201}Tl-chloride and ^{67}Ga-citrate imaging of the heart, particularly with SPECT, increases the identification of cardiac sarcoidosis [55]. ^{123}I-MIBG can also be employed in sarcoidosis patients [63].

Sarcoidosis is another area where [^{18}F]FDG PET has been successfully used. [^{18}F]FDG PET is an ideal technique to investigate patients with sarcoidosis, because in 25–50% of

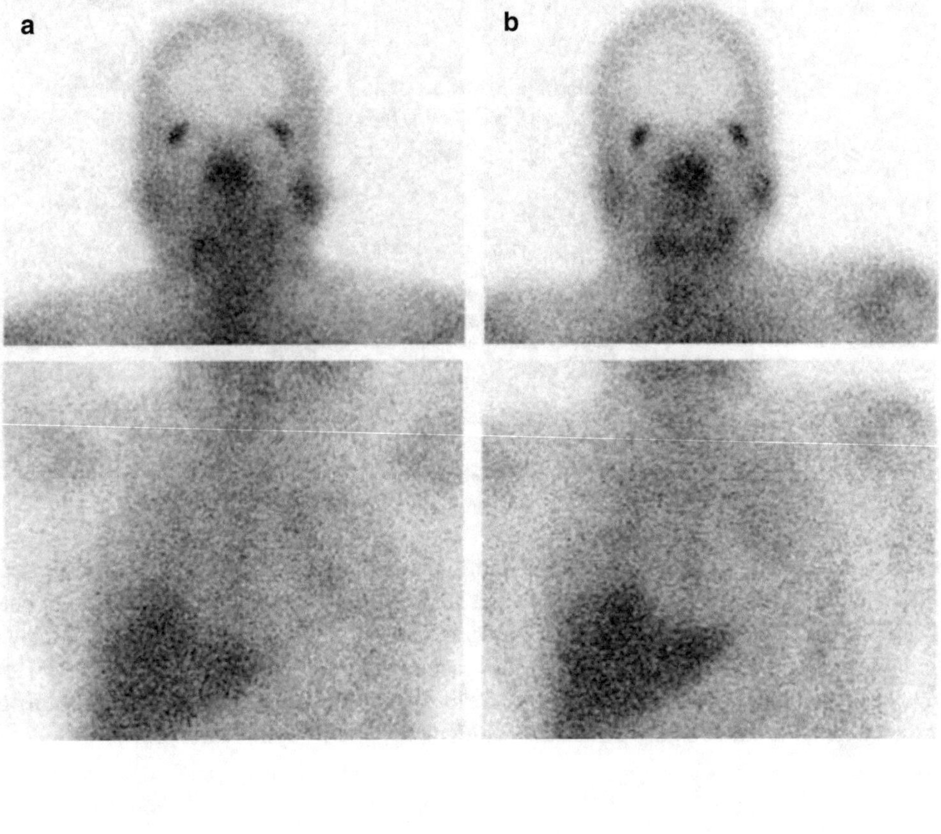

Fig. 14.4 ^{67}Ga-citrate scintigraphy in a patient with grade 4 sarcoidosis treated with steroids. Planar anterior images of the head (upper) and chest (lower) obtained 48 h (**a**) and 72 h (**b**) after tracer injection show the "panda" sign (uptake in bilateral lacrimal and left parotid gland) associated with diffuse lung uptake

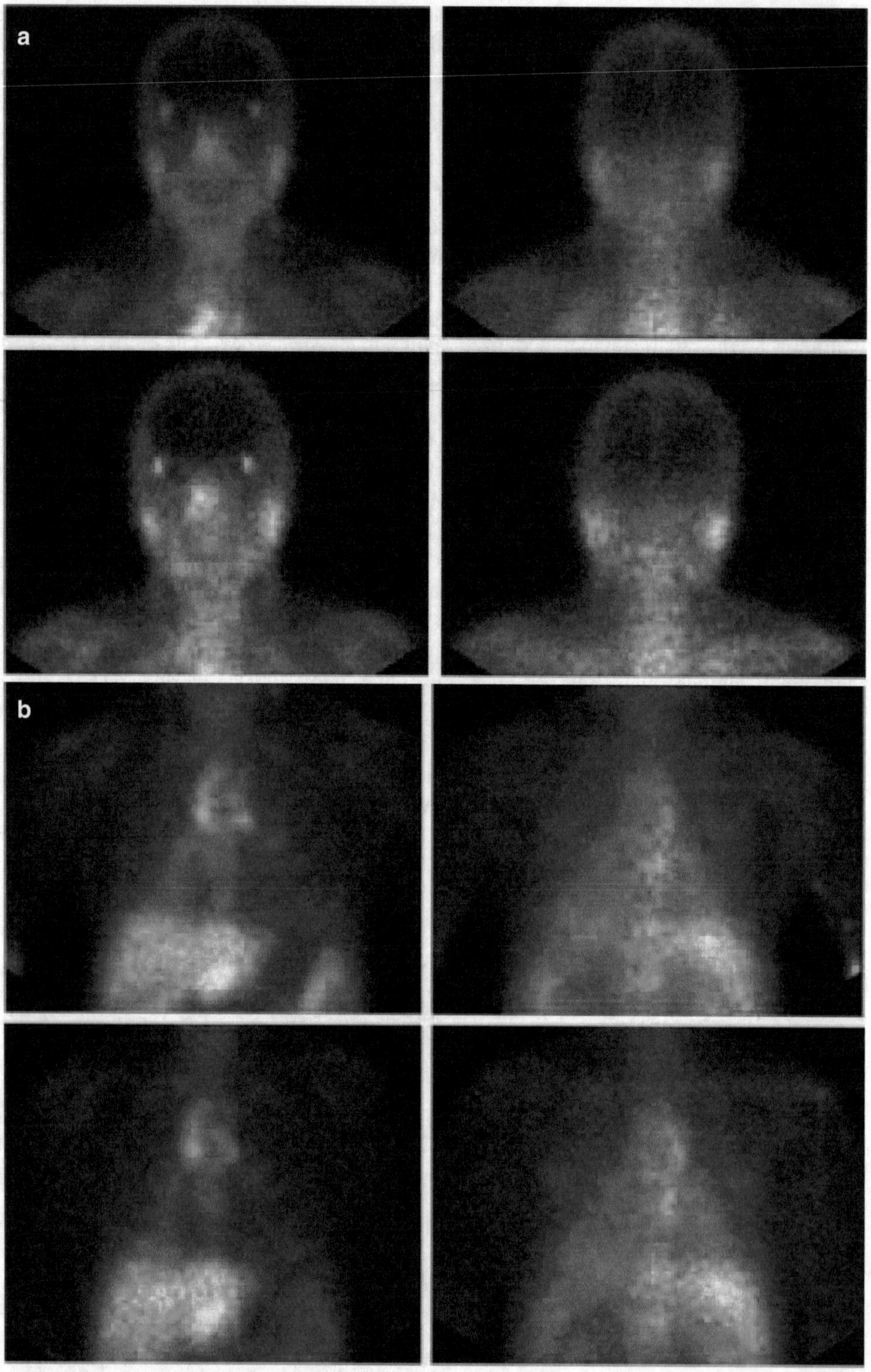

Fig. 14.5 ^{67}Ga-citrate scintigraphy in a patient with suspected sarcoidosis. Planar spots of the head (**a**) and chest (**b**) in anterior and posterior views obtained 48 h (upper) and 72 h (lower) after tracer injection. The images show the classical scintigraphic "panda" and "lambda" signs

cases the disease spreads beyond the lungs, potentially affecting multiple sites [64]. Although not per se diagnostic, [^{18}F]FDG PET can reveal with high-sensitivity active foci of inflammation (Figs. 14.7 and 14.8) [65], thus facilitating the choice of lesions that can be biopsied to secure the diagnosis. Compared with traditional ^{67}Ga-citrate scintigraphy, [^{18}F]FDG PET has a greater sensitivity [66], and has also been shown to be sensitive to change during treatment [67], thus helping to fine-tune therapy in the individual patient. A limitation of [^{18}F]FDG PET is its inability to reliably discriminate between inflammatory and neoplastic lesions, including lymphoma [68].

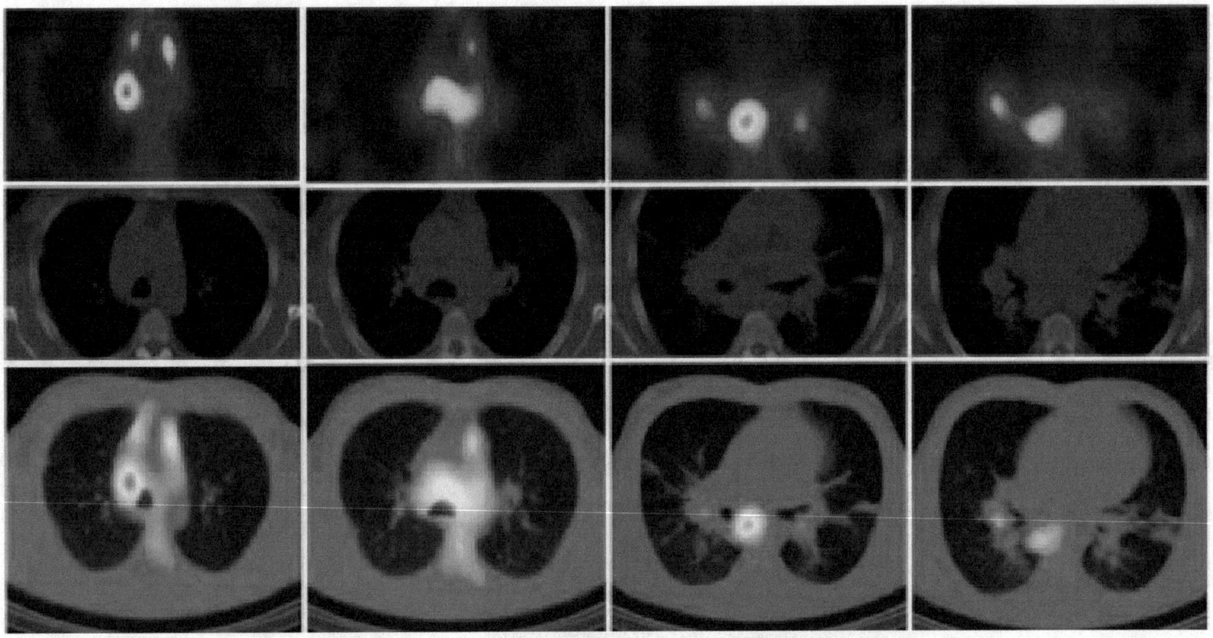

Fig. 14.6 ^{67}Ga-citrate scintigraphy in a patient with sarcoidosis and suspected myocardial involvement. SPECT/CT images (SPECT, upper; CT, middle; fused SPECT/CT, lower) obtained 72 h after tracer injection show increased uptake at multiple mediastinal lymph nodes, without however significant myocardial disease localization

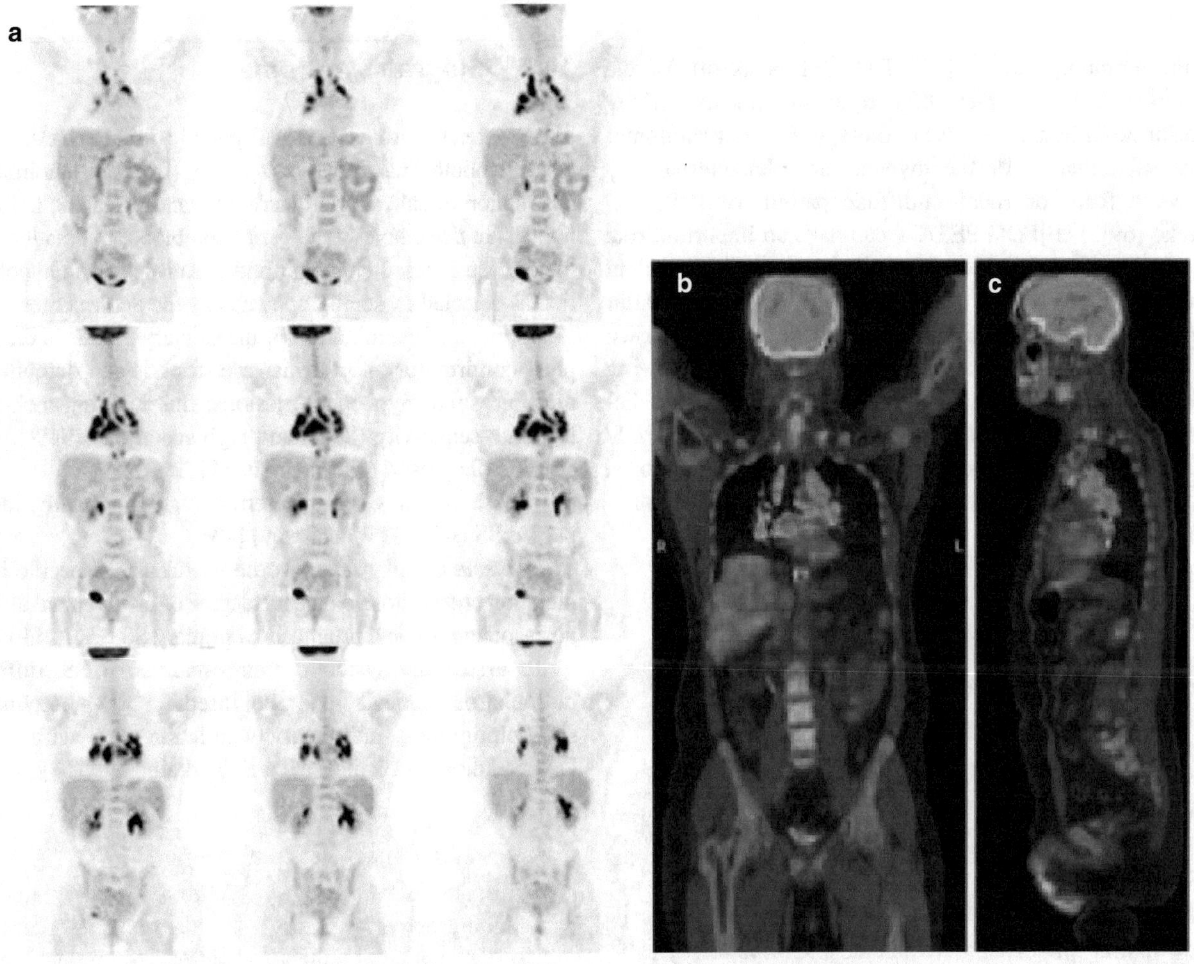

Fig. 14.7 [^{18}F]FDG PET/CT in a young woman with suspected lung sarcoidosis. Coronal PET (**a**) and fused PET/CT images in coronal (**b**) and sagittal (**c**) views demonstrate intense [^{18}F]FDG uptake in mediastinal lymph nodes, indicating active disease

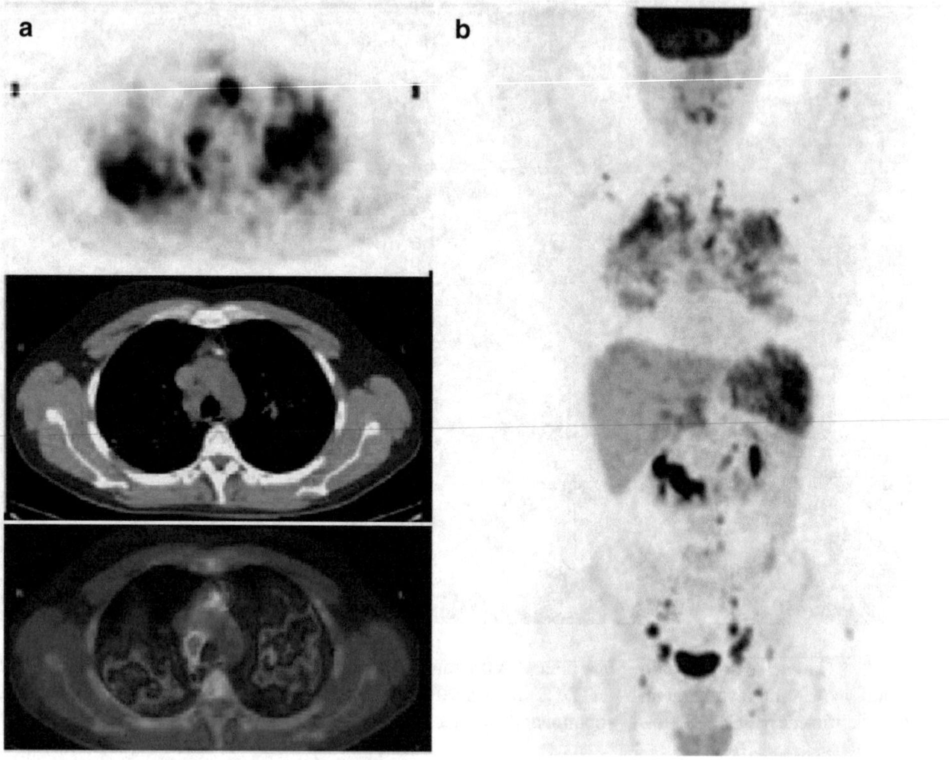

Fig. 14.8 [18F]FDG PET/CT in a patient with lung sarcoidosis. Transaxial images (PET, upper; CT, middle; fused PET/CT, lower) (**a**) show intense [18F]FDG uptake in mediastinal lymph nodes and in the parenchyma of both lungs, indicating stage 3 sarcoidosis. The MIP image (**b**) reveals multiple spots of tracer uptake also in left arm, supraclavicular regions, abdomen, pelvis, and groins. Moreover, inhomogeneous [18F]FDG uptake is present in the spleen

Furthermore, cardiac [18F]FDG PET is useful for the diagnosis and assessment of cardiac sarcoidosis activity and for monitoring response to therapy. Active granulomatous inflammation of the myocardium characteristically shows a focal or focal-on-diffuse pattern of [18F]FDG uptake [69]. [18F]FDG PET/CT can have an important role by enabling the detection of unexpected, clinically silent lesions. The decreased [18F]FDG acidity of a lesion after the initiation or modification of treatment has been shown to correlate with clinical signs of improvement, showing [18F]FDG PET to represent a good tool for monitoring disease activity [70]. In conclusion, although [18F]FDG PET/CT is not included in the standard work-up for sarcoidosis, it is valuable in the initial diagnosis and for disease management [70].

Key Learning Points

- Sarcoidosis can spread from lungs to multiple organs.
- Different radionuclide imaging techniques have been employed to evaluate patients with sarcoidosis: ^{67}Ga-citrate scintigraphy, ^{99m}Tc-sestamibi for cardiac sarcoidosis, [18F]FDG PET/CT.
- [18F]FDG PET/CT in an ideal and sensitive technique (better than ^{67}Ga-citrate scintigraphy) to identify the inflamed areas, to grade intensity/activity of the disease, and to monitor response to therapy.

14.5 Sjögren Syndrome

The Sjögren syndrome (SS) is a systemic disease characterized by dry mouth and dry eyes, resulting from an autoimmune destruction of salivary and lacrimal glands. Specific autoantibodies are detectable in the peripheral blood, but diagnosis of the disease is based on biopsy and/or salivary gland hypofunction as detected by scintigraphy and by the Schirmer test [71].

Ultrasound examination of the salivary glands is the simplest confirmatory non-invasive test, as it can demonstrate multiple small hypoechoic lesions; this imaging technique has high sensitivity (87%) and high specificity (91%) when specific diagnostic criteria are used [72].

MRI sialography is the preferred imaging modality in suspected SS (with 83% accuracy) [73].

Sialoscintigraphy may also be useful using specific interpretation criteria, to evaluate the degree of involvement at diagnosis, outcomes, and prognosis of primary SS (Fig. 14.9) [74].

To assess the systemic manifestations of SS, different radiopharmaceuticals can be used: ^{99m}Tc-pertechnetate sialoscintigraphy, pulmonary ventilation scan with ^{99m}Tc-DTPA radioaerosol, and ^{99m}Tc-ECD brain SPECT [75–77].

Key Learning Point

- In patients with Sjögren syndrome, salivary gland scintigraphy is used to evaluate the degree of involvement at diagnosis, during follow-up, and provides useful prognostic information.

a

b

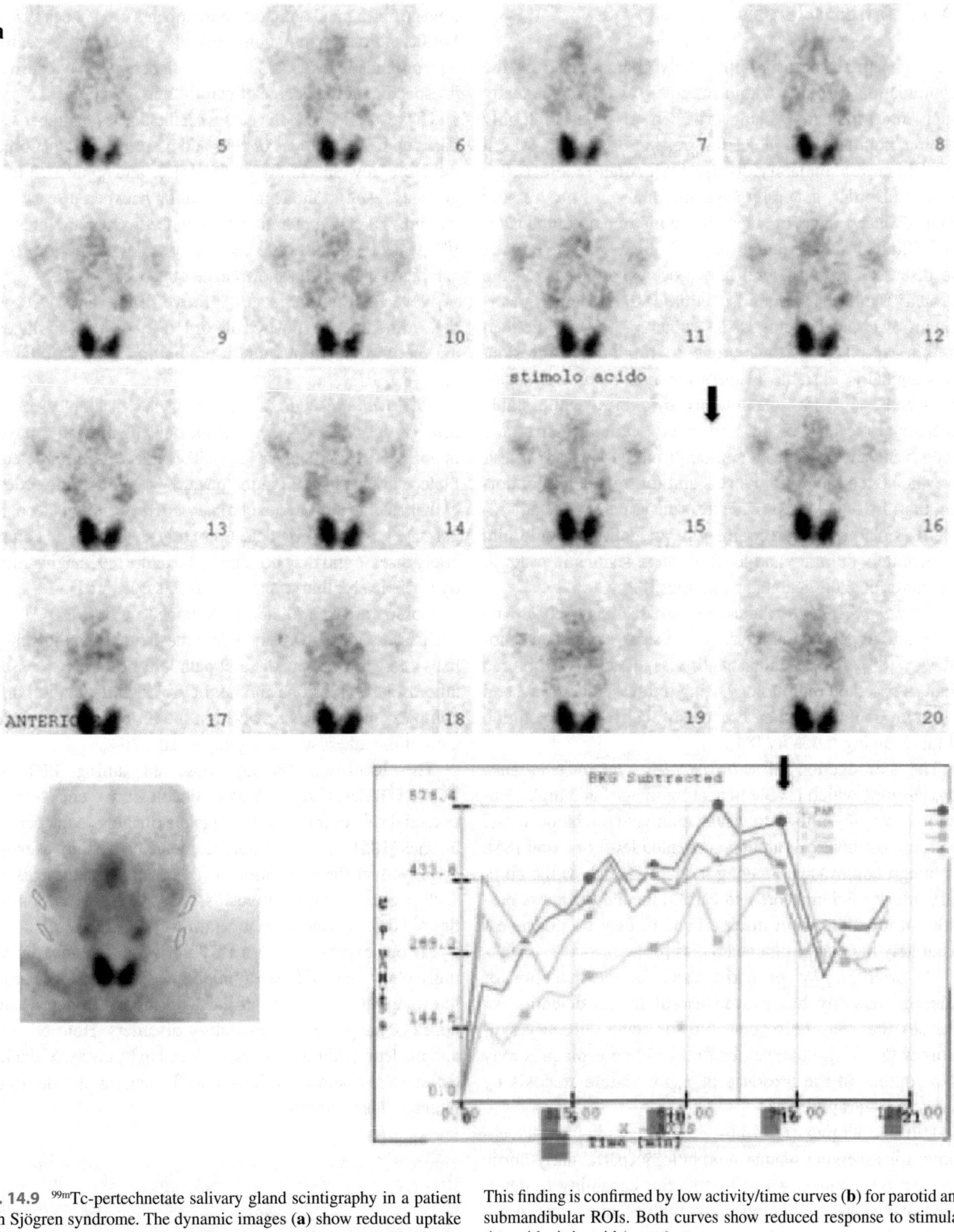

Fig. 14.9 ^{99m}Tc-pertechnetate salivary gland scintigraphy in a patient with Sjögren syndrome. The dynamic images (**a**) show reduced uptake of ^{99m}Tc-pertechnetate in the parotid and submandibular salivary glands. This finding is confirmed by low activity/time curves (**b**) for parotid and submandibular ROIs. Both curves show reduced response to stimulation with citric acid (arrow)

14.6 Atherosclerosis

Although atherosclerosis is primarily characterized by the accumulation of lipids within the artery wall, it is actually much more than that, being driven by a series of highly specific cellular and molecular responses which overall result in an inflammatory disease [78]. Atherosclerosis is a chronic disorder, generally systemic, that until progressing to an advanced stage, may remain asymptomatic for decades [79]. Clinical manifestations depend on site and severity of the disease (i.e., peripheral artery occlusive disease, acute coronary syndromes, brain ischemia) [80]. The main determinant of clinical events is the vulnerable plaque, defined as thin-cap fibroatheroma prone to rupture and erosion. Histologically, unstable plaques are rich in macrophages, foam cells, and pro-inflammatory cytokines, while stable atherosclerotic plaques are rich in extracellular matrix and smooth muscle cells [81]. Although biomarkers are useful to evaluate the blood lipid levels and for treatment monitoring, they are unable to provide information about the atherosclerosis plaque; therefore, imaging modalities should aim at accurately defining and locating these lesions in order to prevent critical clinical manifestations [82].

Ultrasonography of the carotid arteries has been proven successful to predict the future risk of stroke, based on echolucency [83]. On the other hand, visualization of ruptured plaques based on morphology using intravascular ultrasound results in doubtful finding because of the limited resolution of this imaging modality [84].

The introduction of *intravascular optical coherence tomography*, which is able to acquire images at a high resolution (~10 μm), allows to visualize in vivo the blood vessel wall microstructure at an unprecedented level of detail [85]. Although noninvasive imaging modalities such as the coronary artery calcium score and carotid medial thickness provide information about disease burden, they do not assess accurately the plaque characteristics [86].

CT angiography, primarily used for the detection of calcium, recently has proven useful in the detection of plaques that may be responsible for acute coronary syndromes [80, 87]; however, central lipid core plaques may also rupture in the presence of a not visible stenosis by X-ray angiography [88].

MRI is emerging as the most promising radiological technique for assessing plaque morphology (particularly aortic and carotid plaques), since its superior capability to determine plaque size and composition with accuracy and reproducibility provides the opportunity to evaluate the relationships between plaque morphology/composition and subsequent cardiovascular events [82, 88].

[^{18}F]FDG PET has been used to evaluate the degree of inflammation in documented atherosclerosis and metabolic syndrome [89–94] and to successfully monitor the effect of lipid-lowering and antioxidant treatments on plaques [95–99]. Furthermore, inflammation-related [^{18}F]FDG uptake seems to be a prognostic factor associated with early stroke recurrence, irrespective of the degree of carotid stenosis [100].

However, [^{18}F]FDG is a nonspecific metabolic tracer and is taken up by many types of cells and tissues in different organs; therefore, low specificity of this tracer and small size of target sites result in moderate correlation between disease activity and PET-based quantification. Indeed, association between [^{18}F]FDG PET and more conventional diagnostic tool of CT calcification has been shown to be quite weak [101].

Nevertheless, large prospective trials are needed to determine the prognostic role of [^{18}F]FDG PET in the evaluation of inflamed plaque for predicting cardiovascular disease [89, 101].

PET with ^{18}F-NaF (a marker of calcification/osteoblastic activity) can be used to evaluate the ongoing mineral deposition in atherosclerotic plaques [102]. This tracer used for detecting molecular calcification in the plaques has allowed detection of global calcification in the coronary arteries, and this technique has great promise for detecting early evidence for coronary artery disease and may become in the future the imaging modality of choice for this severe vascular disorder [101].

Comparative evaluations obtained with PET/CT with [^{18}F]FDG and ^{18}F-NaF show that these functional techniques may allow to evaluate distinct pathophysiologic processes in atherosclerotic lesions and might provide information on the complex interactions involved in the formation and progression of the atherosclerotic plaque [103, 104].

The incidental findings observed during PET with ^{68}Ga-DOTATATE in a series of oncologic patients suggest a potential role of this tracer for plaque imaging in the coronary arteries [105]. Moreover, nuclear medicine techniques may be employed in the evaluation of other inflammatory diseases such as coeliac disease, myositis, type 1 diabetes, autoimmune thyroid disease, and psoriatic arthritis [106–110].

As our experience with PET grows, it becomes increasingly clear that PET has a unique, well-defined role among the imaging procedures in the work-up of numerous diagnosed or suspected inflammatory disorders. Both clinicians and nuclear medicine specialists need to be aware of the indications and potential pitfalls of PET imaging in order to best manage their patients.

Key Learning Point

- In patients with atherosclerosis, PET/CT with [^{18}F]FDG and ^{18}F-NaF can evaluate distinct pathophysiologic processes in atherosclerotic lesions, providing information on the complex interactions involved in the formation and progression of the atherosclerotic plaque.

Acknowledgments All editors have contributed to the preparation of this chapter. We are particularly grateful to Dr. Diego De Palma (Varese, Italy), Dr. Paola A. Erba (Pisa, Italy), and Dr. Elena Lazzeri (Pisa, Italy) for providing images that have been included in this chapter.

Clinical Cases

Case 14.1

Paola A. Erba

Woman, 71 years old (50 kg; 158 cm). Atypical rheumatic polymyalgia treated with corticosteroid (4 mg of Medrol/daily), blood hypertension, anemia, bilateral scapula-humeral periarthrytis, erosive gastritis, deficit of vitamin D treated with Cacit and Dibase. October 21, 2009: thyroidectomy because of goiter. December 7, 2009: urinary culture positive for *E. coli*. Serotine fever responsive to corticosteroid treatment (from March 2009) associated with asthenia and articular pain. Infectious screening (anti-Toxo IgM, HCV, HIV, Coxackie virus, adenovirus, CMV, EBV, HSV-1 and -2, *Cryptococcus neoformans*, *Aspergillus*, and *Candida*) negative. Increased Ca 15.3 (=39.77 U/mL) and beta-2 microglobulin (=2.3 mg/L). Chest X-ray and mammography negatives. Anti-core and anticardiolipin antibodies were positive. Increased ESR (=50 mm/h), CRP (=27.16 mg/L), and fibrinogen (=503 mg/dL).

Suspected Site of Infection

Unknown.

Radiopharmaceutical Activity

Injection of 666 MBq of ^{99m}Tc-HMPAO-WBC.

Imaging

Whole-body, spot, and SPECT/CT images of the chest (Figs. 14.10, 14.11, and 14.12).

Conclusion/Teaching Point

Labeled leukocyte scintigraphy findings, suggestive for vasculitis, were confirmed by temporal artery biopsy. Labeled leukocyte scintigraphy may be performed in suspected vasculitis when [^{18}F]FDG PET/CT is not available.

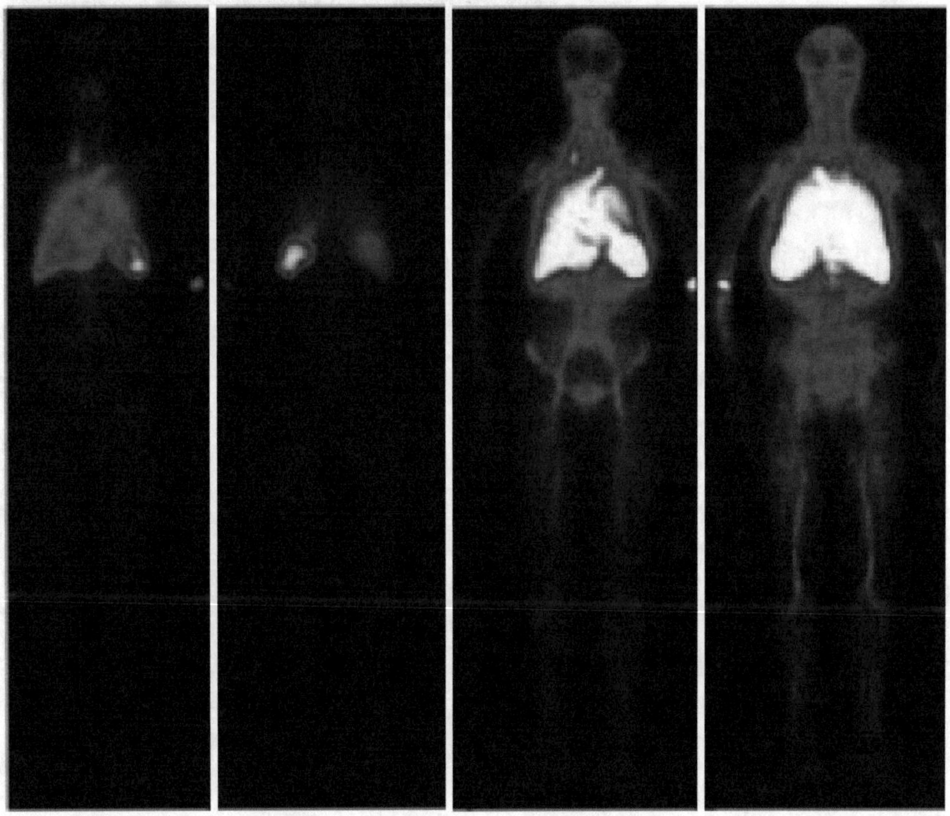

Fig. 14.10 ^{99m}Tc-HMPAO-WBC scintigraphy: whole-body images (anterior and posterior views) obtained at 30 min

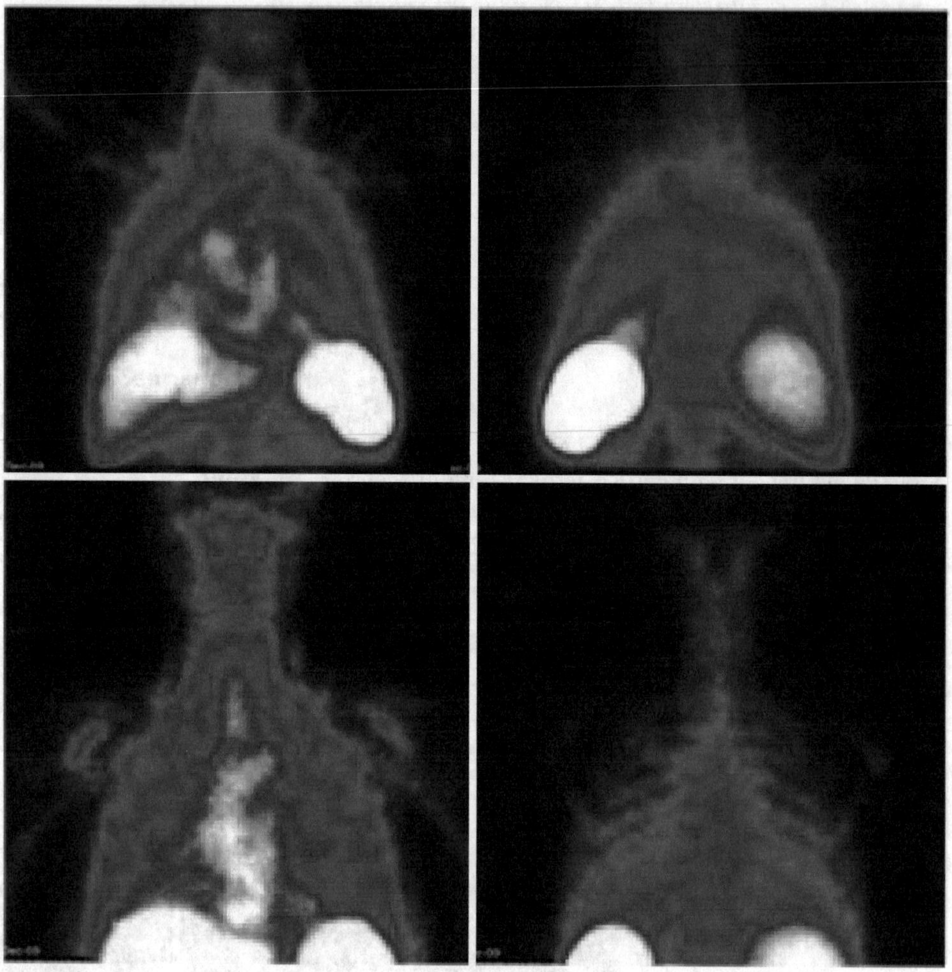

Fig. 14.11 ^{99m}Tc-HMPAO-WBC scintigraphy: spot images of the chest (anterior view, left; posterior view, right) at 4 h (upper images) and at 24 h (lower images) demonstrating accumulation of labeled leukocytes in the aortic root region

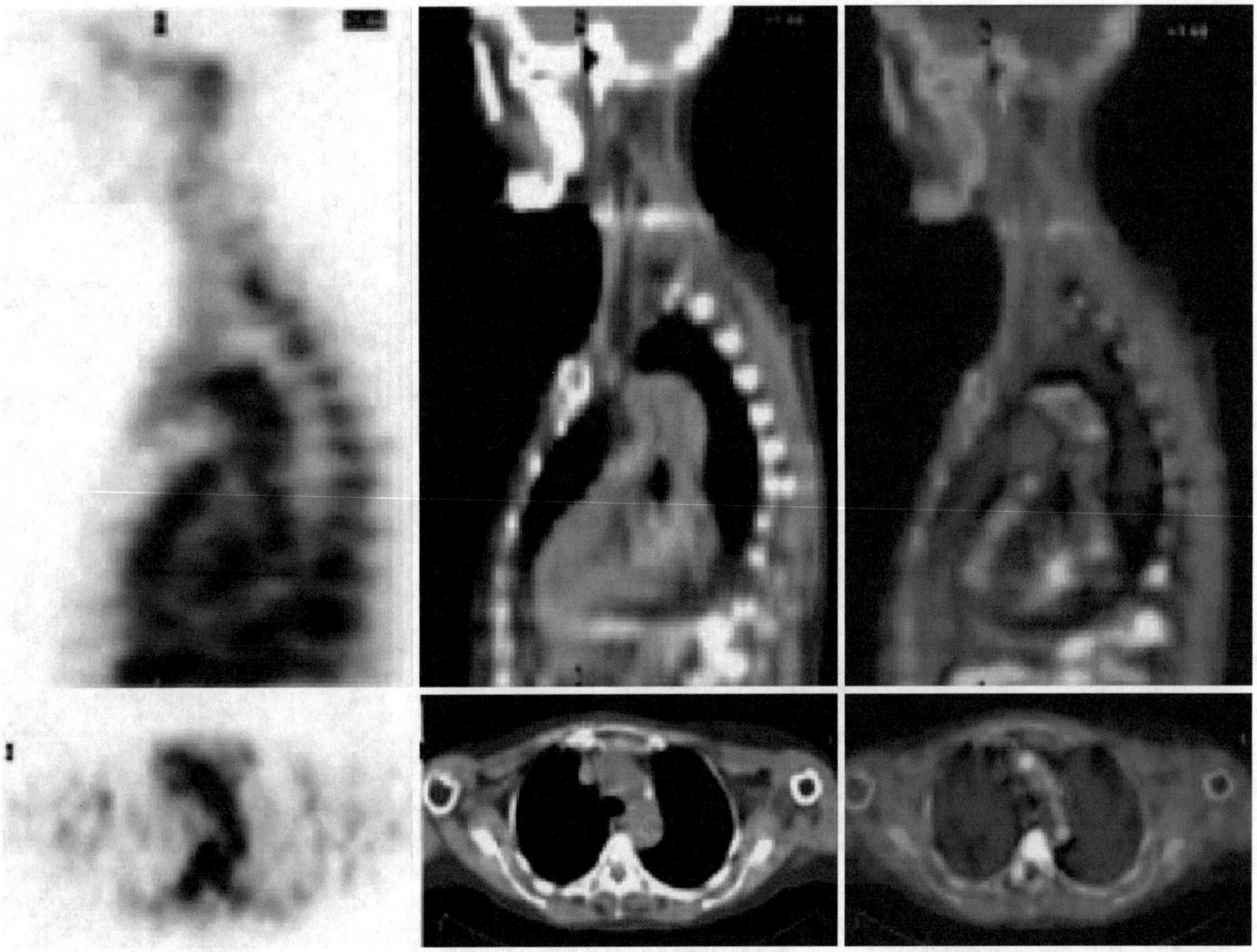

Fig. 14.12 SPECT/CT images showing abnormal accumulation of labeled leukocytes uptake at the epi-aortic vessels and aortic root

Case 14.2

Elena Lazzeri

Woman, 61 years old (weight, 62 kg; height, 162 cm). Suspected vasculitis in patient with mild increase of CRP, ESR, and hypertension. Medical treatment: February 4, 2011: [^{18}F]FDG PET/CT; February 17, 2011: CT scan of chest and abdomen; February 20, 2011: temporal artery biopsy, "giant cell arteritis."

Suspected Site of Inflammation

Large vessels.

Radiopharmaceutical Activity

February 2, 2011: Injection of 333 MGq of [^{18}F]FDG at 10.04 a.m., scan acquisition started at 11.20 a.m.

Imaging

[^{18}F]FDG PET/CT: 2D-mode acquisition (Figs. 14.13, 14.14, and 14.15).

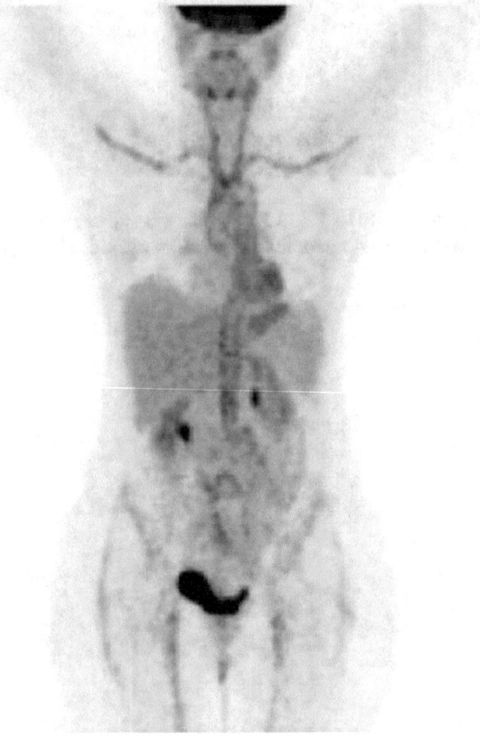

Fig. 14.13 MIP image of [^{18}F]FDG PET/CT

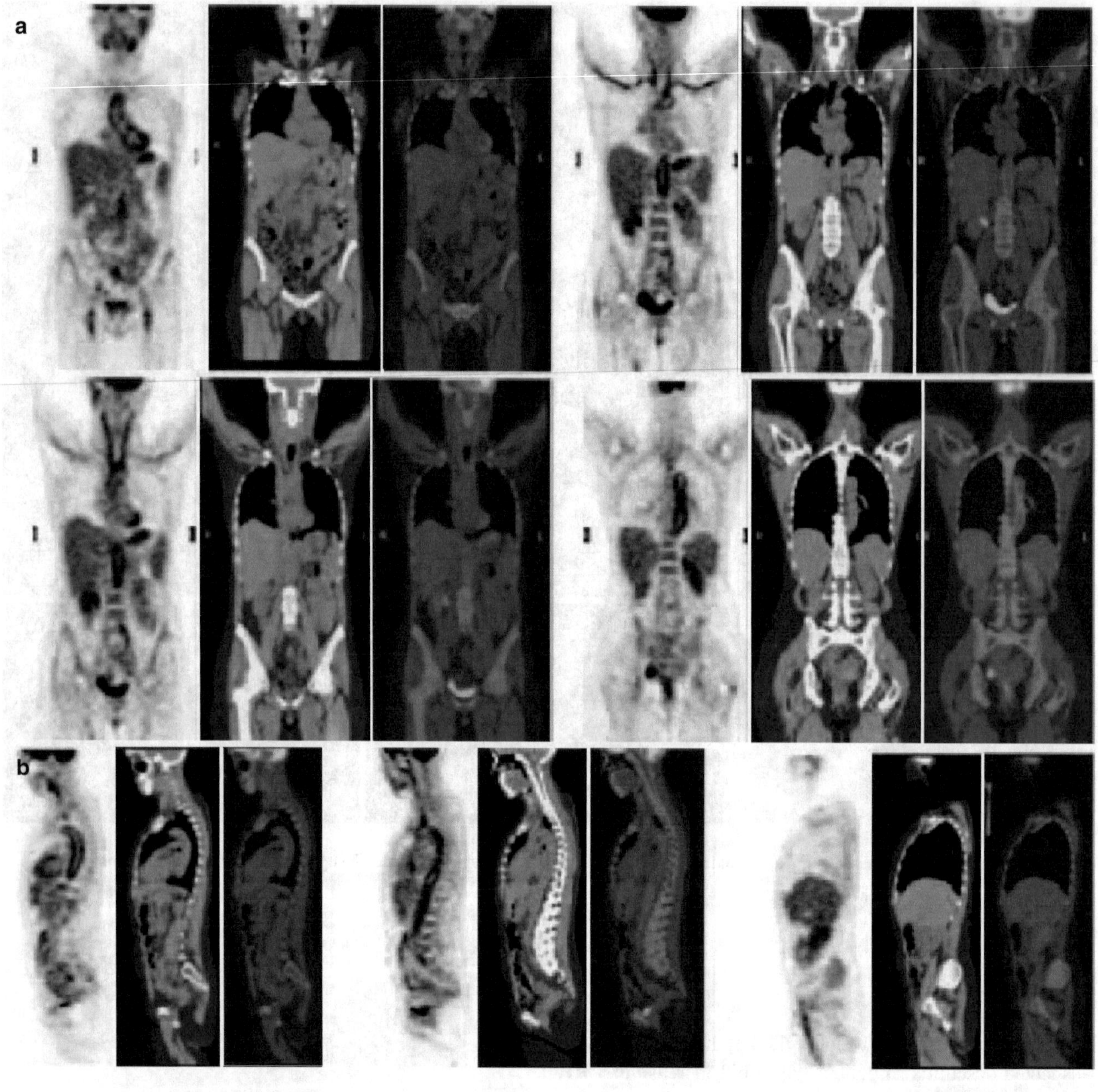

Fig. 14.14 [^{18}F]FDG PET/CT: coronal (a) and sagittal (b) sections showing diffuse [18F]FDG uptake along the vessels course (SUV_{max} = 5.4 aorta; SUV_{max} = 3.4 femoral; SUV_{max} = 4.4 carotid; SUV_{max} = 4.1 succlavia). These findings suggest large vessels vasculitis

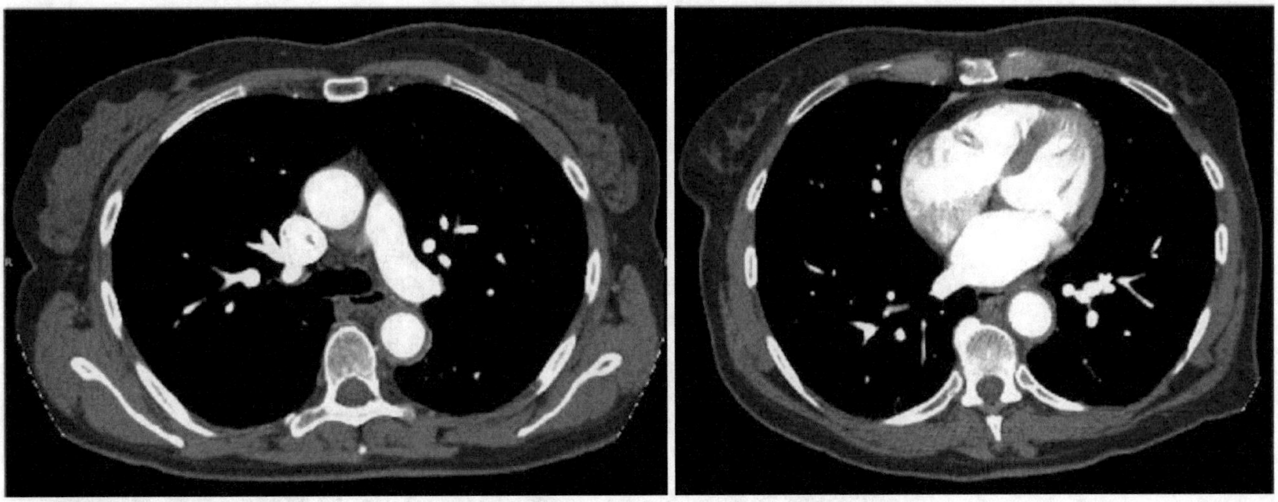

Fig. 14.15 CT slices show mild and diffuse concentric thickening of the aortic root, epiaortic vessels and descending aorta (which is thickened until the carrefour; maximum thickness 5 mm), consistent with vasculitis

Conclusion/Teaching Point

[^{18}F]FDG PET/CT allows the identification of the vessels involved in the inflammatory disease, often before the morphological changes can be detected on CT or MRI.

Case 14.3

Annibale Versari and Nicolò Pipitone

Woman, 60 years old. Patient with anxiety. Fever (temperature <38 °C) from June 2010. Treatment with nonsteroidal anti-inflammatory agents does not induce any improvement in contrast to what happens with steroids. ESR = 99 mm/h; CRP = 10.3. Other therapies: ranitidine, escitalopram, and lexotanil.

Suspected Site of Infection

Unknown.

Radiopharmaceutical Activity

August 6, 2011: injection of 204 MBq of [^{18}F]FDG. Glucose level of 81 mg/dL before radiopharmaceutical injection.

January 21, 2011: injection of 210 MBq of [^{18}F]FDG. Glucose level of 78 mg/dL before radiopharmaceutical injection.

April 16, 2012: injection of 227 MBq of [^{18}F]FDG. Glucose level of 87 mg/dL before radiopharmaceutical injection.

Imaging

PET/CT total body acquisitions were performed 1 h after radiopharmaceutical i.v. administration (Figs. 14.16, 14.17, 14.18, 14.19, and 14.20).

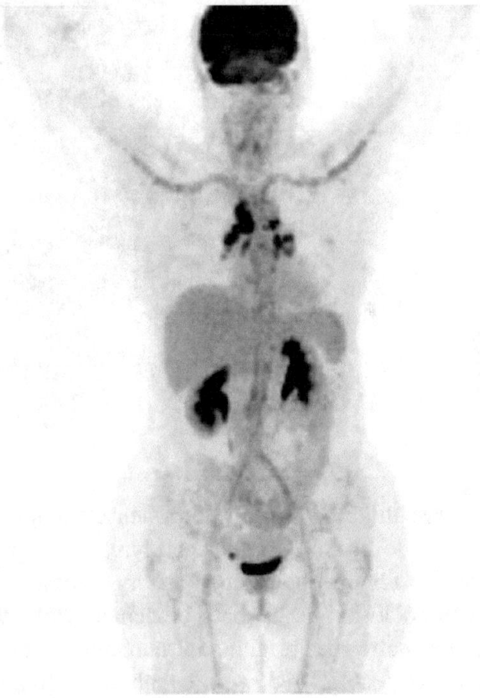

Fig. 14.16 [^{18}F]FDG PET/CT: the MIP image shows intense tracer uptake in the hilar and peri-hilar regions bilaterally, associated with uptake in large vessels, particularly the thoracic and abdominal aorta, subclavian, axillary, and iliac arteries

Conclusion/Teaching Point

In this case, baseline [^{18}F]FDG PET/CT has been useful to identify the cause of fever. On the basis of [^{18}F]FDG PET/CT findings, vasculitis has been diagnosed. An ultrasound study of the epiaortic vessels showed wall thickening with a positive "halo sign" in the common carotid arteries consistent

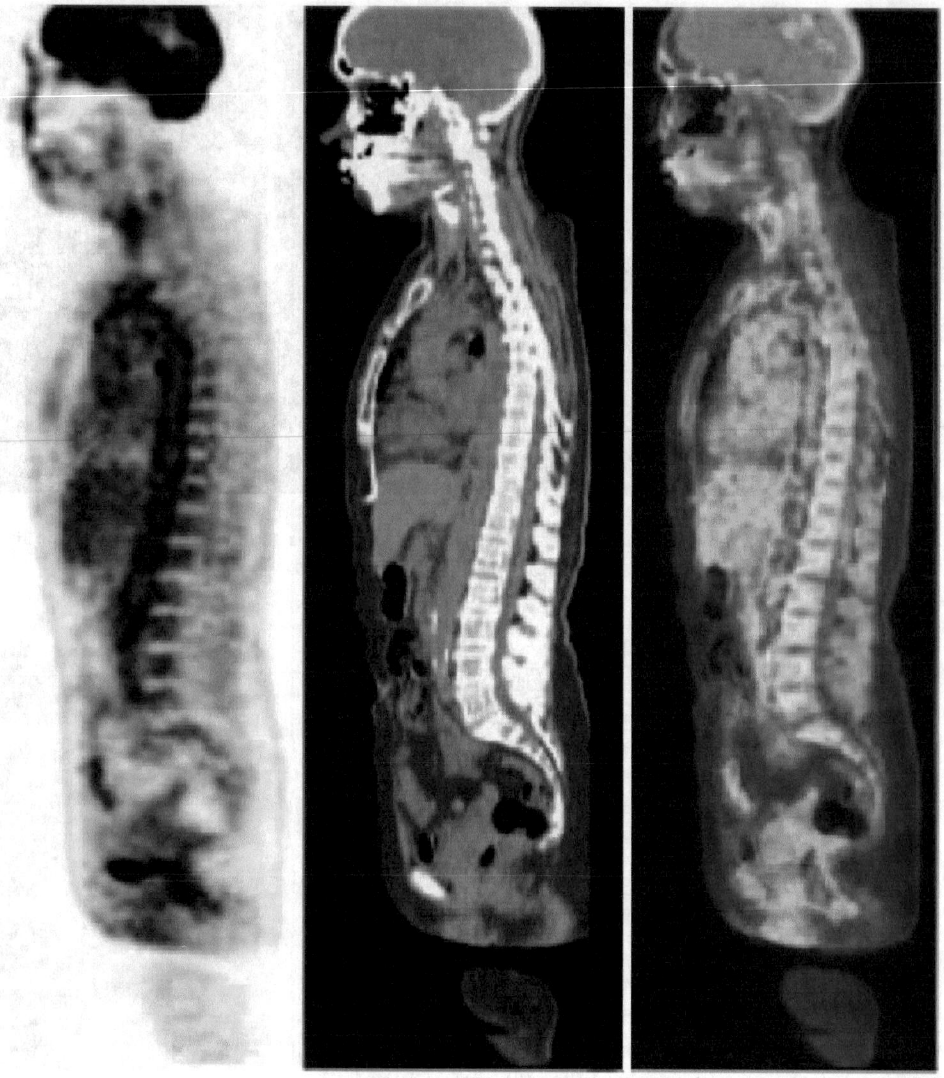

Fig. 14.17 [^{18}F]FDG PET/CT: sagittal views show intense tracer uptake (Grade 3) in the whole aorta wall

with active vasculitis. Additionally, the intense radiopharmaceutical uptake localized at mediastinal lymphadenopathies was suggestive for infectious/inflammatory disease (tubercolosis or sarcoidosis); hence, both bronchial cytology and histology were performed resulting in "numerous histiocytes and granulocytes associated with lymph node fragments with anthracosis" and "aspecific inflammation," respectively. Large-vessel vasculitis associated with probable sarcoidosis was the diagnosis and prednisone 50 mg/daily commenced with a tapering scheme. Treatment with steroids determines a significant improvement of clinical conditions and after 5 months of therapy, the patient presented with only occasional episodes of fever, which were completely resolved 15 months later. Therapy was continued with only a "maintaining" dosage.

Case 14.4

Annibale Versari and Carlo Salvarani

A 72-year-old lady was referred in February 2011 to the Hematology Department because of low-grade fever (37.5 °C), weight loss (>5 kg), neck and shoulder pain, and carotidodynia. She suffered from diabetes and glaucoma and also reported a previous episode of headache that had spontaneously resolved within a couple of weeks. Laboratory tests showed ESR 112 mm/h and CRP 8 mg/dL. Malignancy was suspected and further investigations organized. Coombs test, Bence Jones protein, and a bone marrow biopsy were normal or negative. The patient reported aches and pain in the scapular and pelvic girdles with morning stiffness lasting

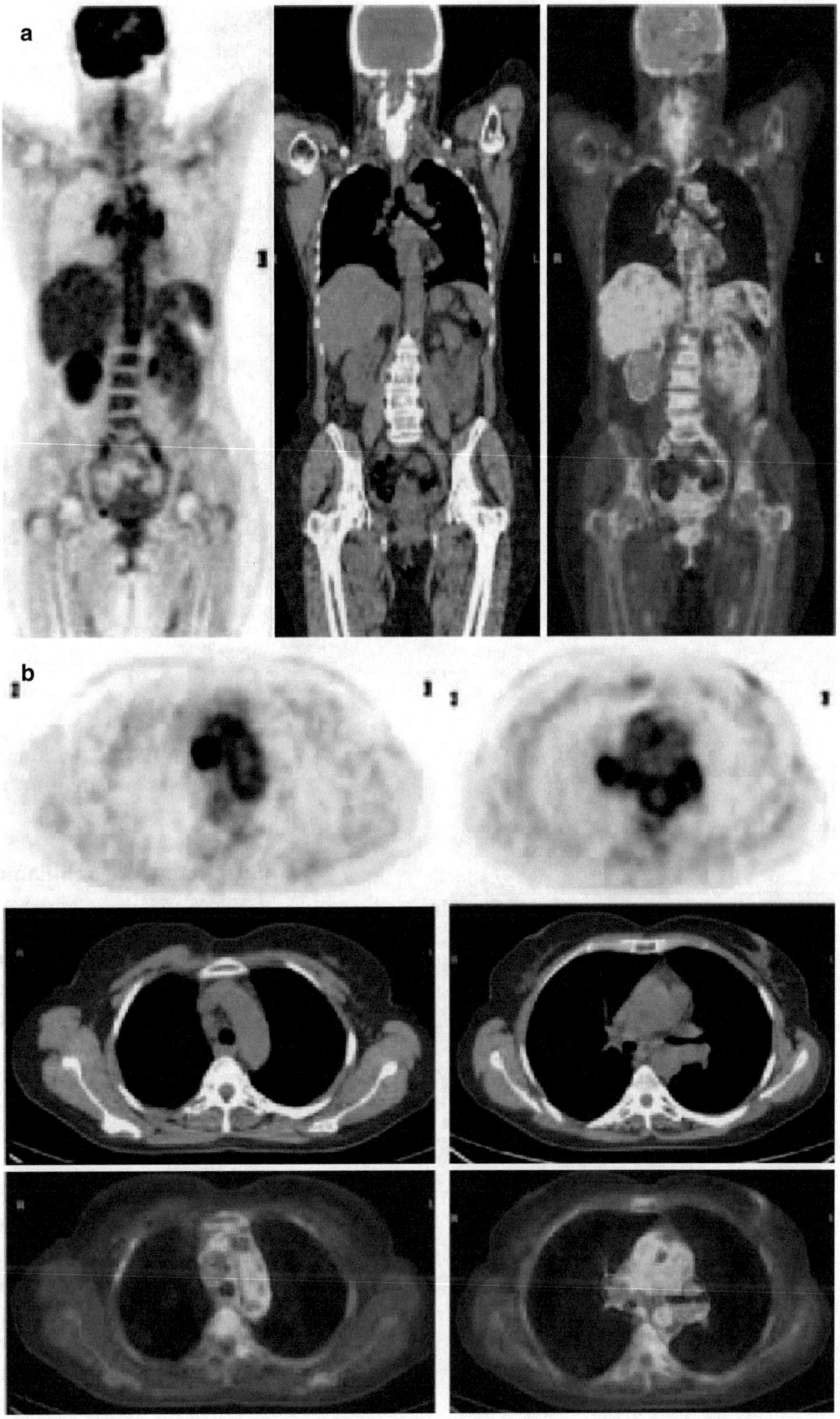

Fig. 14.18 [^{18}F]FDG PET/CT: the coronal (**a**) and transaxial (**b**) sections demonstrate intense [^{18}F]FDG uptake at both mediastinal lymphadenopathies and aorta

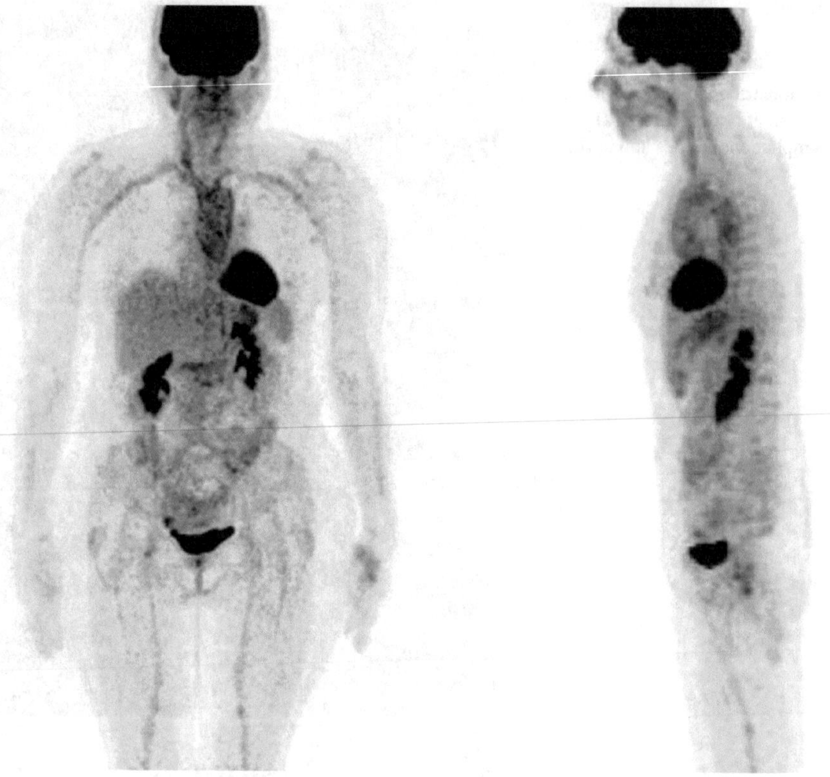

Fig. 14.19 MIP images of [18F]FDG PET/CT performed after 5 months of therapy show the persistence of intense vascular [18F]FDG uptake (Grade 2–3). Uptake in mediastinal lymph nodes is no longer detectable

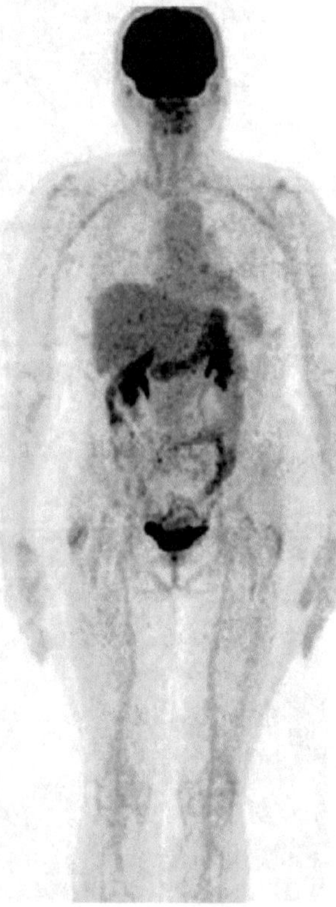

Fig. 14.20 MIP image of [18F]FDG PET/CT performed after 20 months of therapy shows residual mild (Grade 1) [18F]FDG uptake at carotids, subclavian, axillary arteries, and thoracic aorta

about 1 h. ESR was 120 mm/h and CRP 8.93 mg/dL. The patient was referred to us for suspected large-vessel vasculitis.

Suspected Site of Inflammation

Large vessels.

Radiopharmaceutical Activity

June 1, 2011: injection of 222 MBq of [18F]FDG.

February 15, 2012: injection of 227 MBq of [18F]FDG.

Imaging

PET/CT total body acquisition was performed 1 h after radiopharmaceutical i.v. administration (Figs. 14.21, 14.22, and 14.23).

Conclusion/Teaching Point

Giant cell arteritis with large-vessel involvement and polymyalgia rheumatica were diagnosed on the basis of the clinical, laboratory, and imaging findings. Four weeks after the onset of tocilizumab therapy, the patient reported feeling much better in herself. The clinical improvement was paralleled by a drop in ESR (28 mm/h) and CRP (0.11 mg/dL) levels. In December 2011, at the end of the tocilizumab course, the patient was in complete clinical remission, while ESR was 4 mm/h and CRP 0.02 mg/dL. In this case [18F]

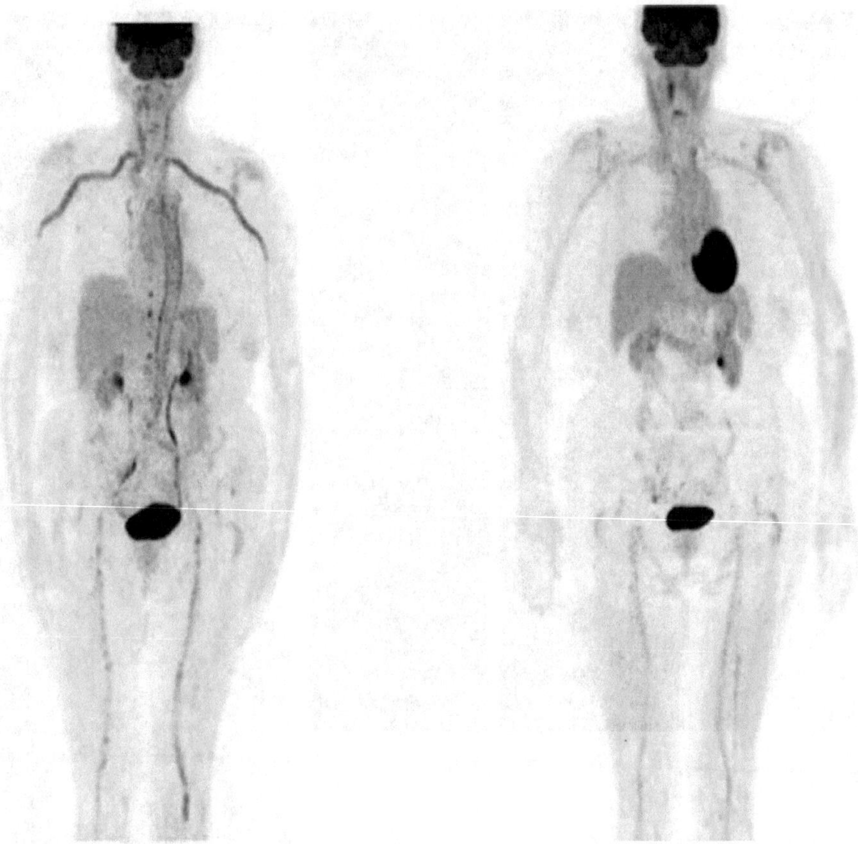

Fig. 14.21 MIP image of baseline [^{18}F]FDG PET/CT (left) and PET/CT scan performed after treatment (right). Images show initial diffuse large vessel vasculitis with good response to treatment

FDG PET/CT has been useful in also monitoring the treatment response.

Case 14.5

Annibale Versari and Giulia Pazzola

A 25-year-old woman was referred to the rheumatology department because of low-grade fever, joint aches and pains, cough, and carotidynia. Past medical history revealed quiescent ulcerative colitis. Laboratory tests showed ESR, 41 mm/h; CRP, 12.8 mg/dL; and positive antineutrophil cytoplasmic antibodies directed against cathepsin G. Chest X-ray was unremarkable. Vascular US disclosed vessel wall thickening of the common carotid arteries, more evident on the left, and possible stenosis of the right renal artery, which was subsequently confirmed by abdominal CT angiography. Takayasu arteritis was diagnosed and a [^{18}F] FDG PET/CT scan requested to assess the extent and activity of the vasculitis.

Suspected Site of Inflammation

Colon/large vessels.

Radiopharmaceutical Activity

March 5, 2008: injection of 239 MBq of [^{18}F]FDG.

January 13, 2010: injection of 240 MBq of [^{18}F]FDG.

Imaging

PET/CT total body acquisitions were performed 1 h after radiopharmaceutical administration (Figs. 14.24 and 14.25).

Conclusion/Teaching Point

This is an example of the usefulness of [^{18}F]FDG PET/CT in vasculitis to assess extent, disease activity, and treatment response. Radiopharmaceutical uptake in vessels reflects the disease course, also the decrease of [^{18}F]FDG uptake at the post-therapy scan coincides with clinical and laboratory results improvement.

Case 14.6

Annibale Versari and Giulia Pazzola

A 57-year-old man was referred to the rheumatology department because of fatigue, mild abdominal pain, and claudication in the lower limbs. Physical examination was noncontributory. In particular, no vascular bruits were heard, and arterial pulses

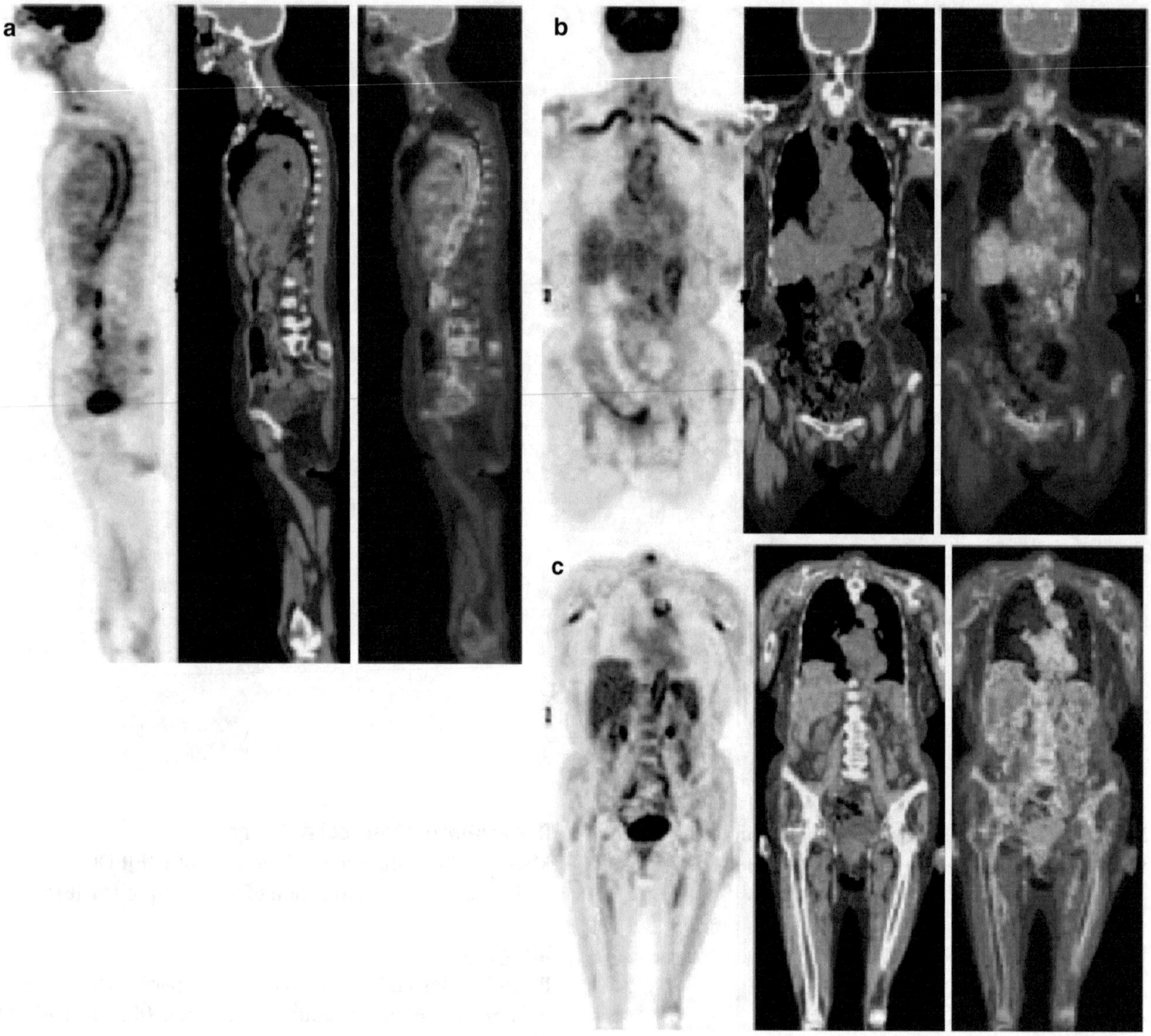

Fig. 14.22 Baseline [^{18}F]FDG PET/CT sagittal (**a**) and coronal (**b**, **c**) sections show increased (Grade 3) [^{18}F]FDG uptake in the common carotid, subclavian, and axillary arteries bilaterally, as well as in the thoracic and abdominal aorta up to the iliac arteries

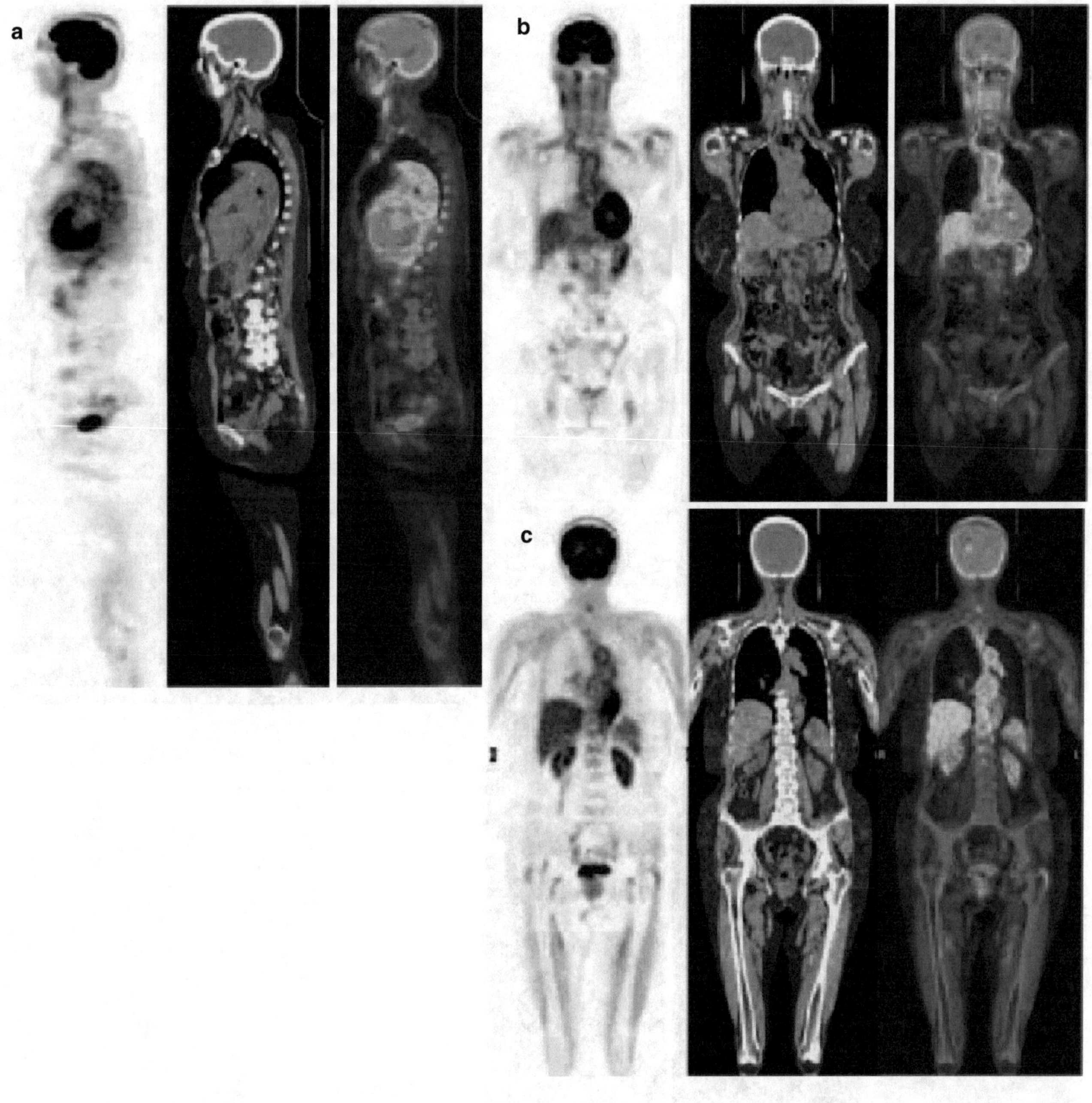

Fig. 14.23 [18F]FDG PET/CT: sagittal (**a**) and coronal (**b**, **c**) sections of scan acquired after 6 months of monotherapy (tocilizumab 8 mg/kg per month) show CT markedly decreased (Grade 1) vascular [18F]FDG uptake in the common carotid and subclavian arteries bilaterally, as well as in the thoracic and abdominal aorta up to the iliac arteries

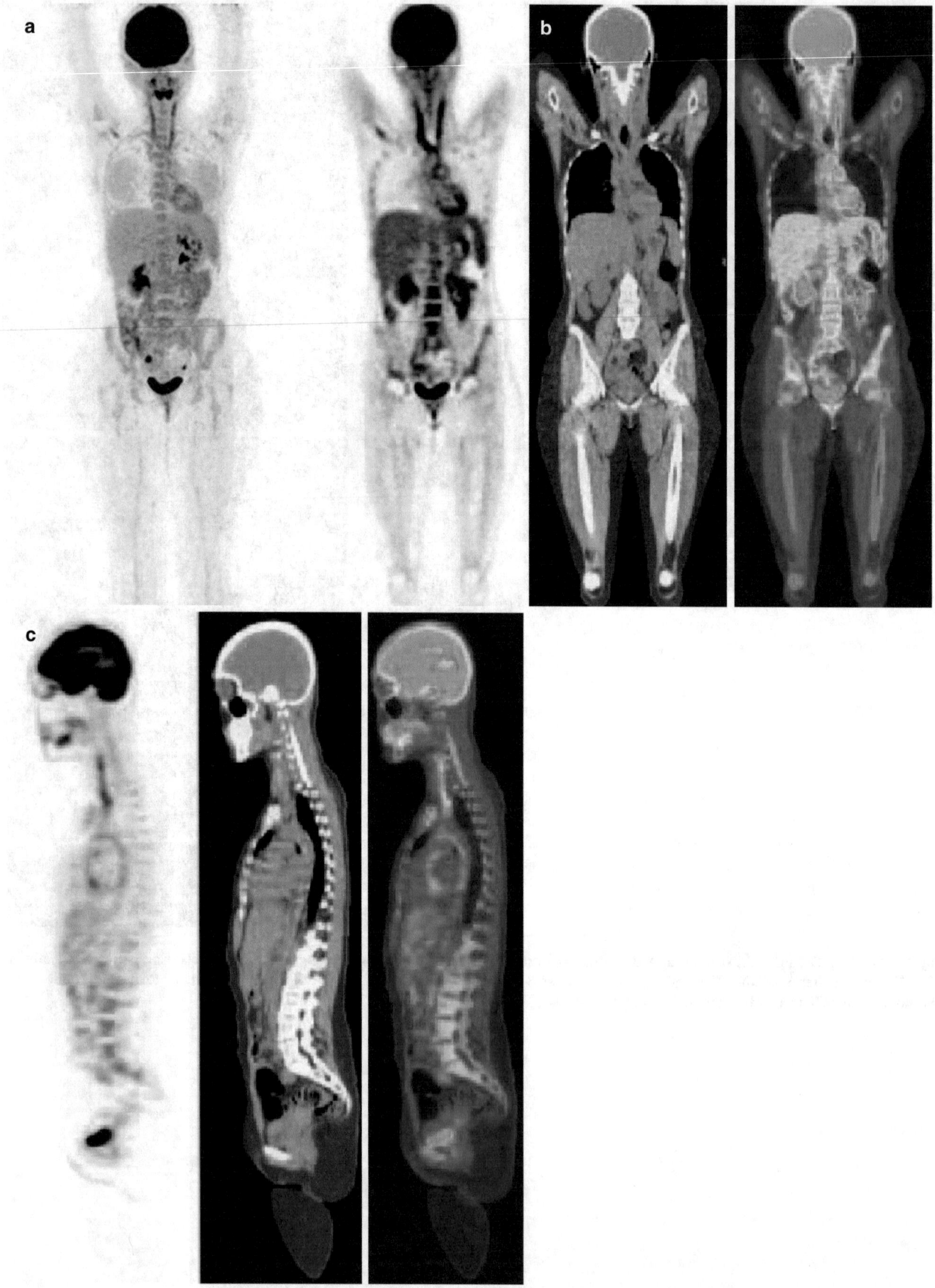

Fig. 14.24 MIP image from the baseline [^{18}F]FDG PET/CT MIP (**a**) shows tracer uptake in the common carotid arteries bilaterally and in the brachiocephalic trunk. Particularly, coronal (**b**) and sagittal (**c**) views demonstrate intense (Grade 3) [^{18}F]FDG uptake in the common carotid arteries bilaterally and in the brachiocephalic trunk

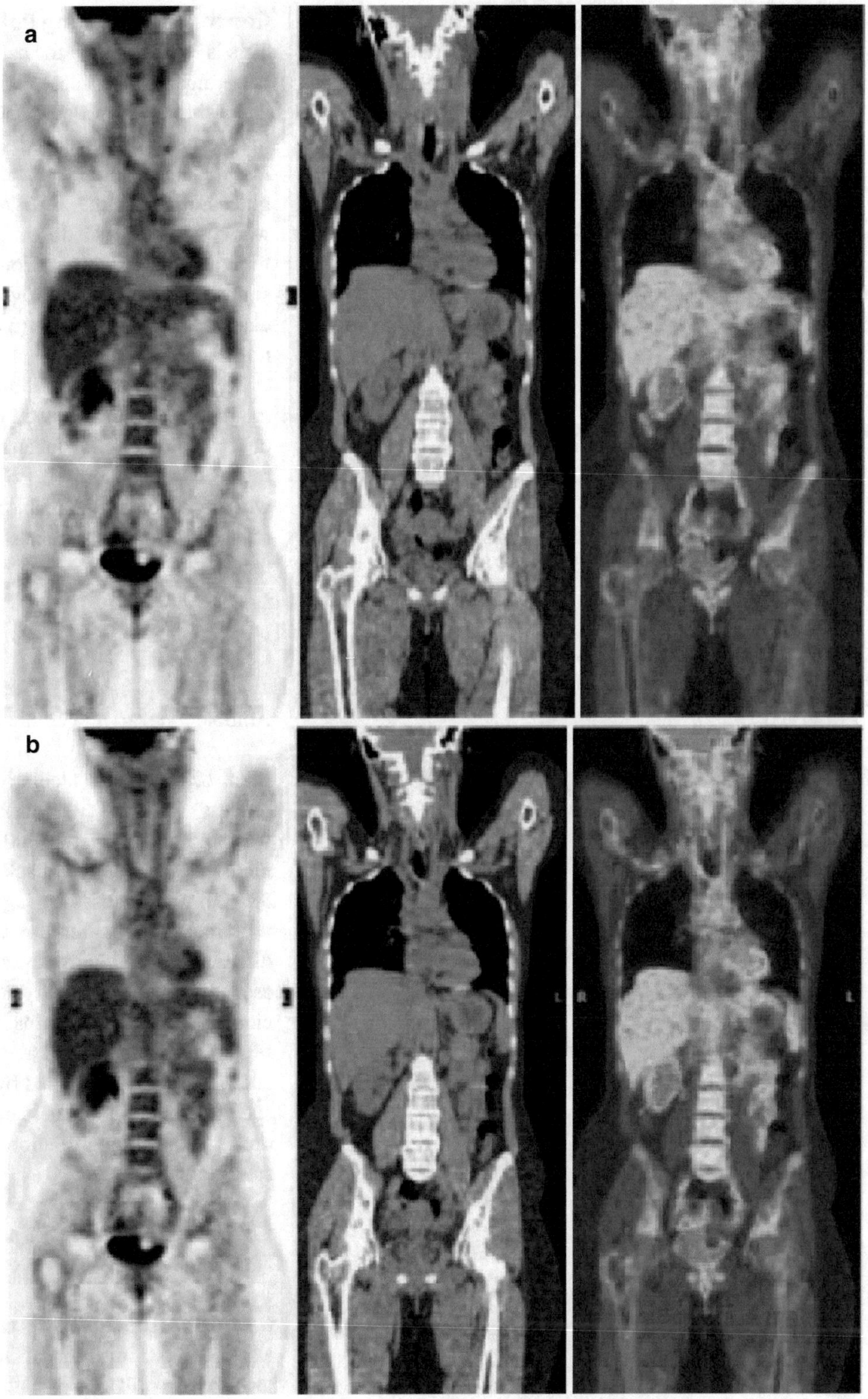

Fig. 14.25 [^{18}F]FDG PET/CT: coronal sections from the scan acquired after treatment with prednisone 1 mg/kg per day show a mild (Grade 1) tracer uptake in the carotid arteries (**a**), ascending aorta and left axillary artery (**b**)

were all normal. ESR was elevated at 89 mm/h (reference values <47), while CRP was 5.04 mg/dL (normal values <0.5 mg/dL). Infectious screening for common pathogens including HCV, HBV, *Mycobacterium tuberculosis*, and *Treponema pallidum* was entirely negative. Chest X-rays were unremarkable. An abdominal US revealed wall thickening of the abdominal aorta, while CT angiography of the abdomen showed diffuse concentric subintimal thickening of the abdominal aorta from the origin of left renal artery to the bifurcation of the common iliac arteries. Vasculitis was suspected.

Suspected Site of Inflammation

Large vessels.

Radiopharmaceutical Activity

July 15, 2011: injection of 255 MBq of [^{18}F]FDG. Glucose level = 89 mg/dL

January 26, 2012: injection of 278 MBq of [^{18}F] FDG. Glucose level = 87 mg/dL

Imaging

PET/CT total body acquisitions were performed 1 h after radiopharmaceutical administration (Figs. 14.26, 14.27, 14.28, and 14.29).

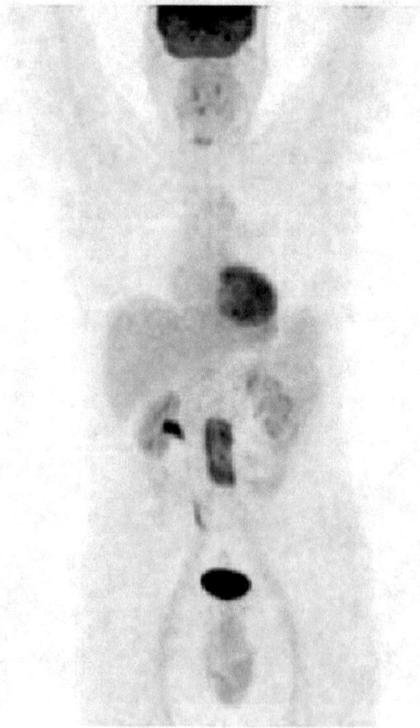

Fig. 14.26 MIP image from baseline [^{18}F]FDG PET/CT shows intense tracer uptake in a well-defined portion of abdominal aorta

Conclusion/Teaching Point

This is an example of the usefulness of [^{18}F]FDG PET/CT in the evaluation of disease activity and treatment response. On the basis of baseline [^{18}F]FDG PET/CT examination, abdominal aortitis was diagnosed. Because the patient had diabetes mellitus and arterial hypertension and was reluctant to take glucocorticoids, the IL-6 receptor antagonist tocilizumab was commenced at a dose of 8 mg/kg/month as monotherapy for 6 months. After the second infusion the patient reported a significant clinical improvement with only mild residual claudication, while ESR (6 mm/h) and CRP (0.03 mg/dL) normalized.

Repeat abdominal CT angiography performed after the tocilizumab course showed persistent wall thickening without pathological enhancement, while a repeated PET/CT revealed no abnormal [^{18}F]FDG vascular uptake. After withdrawal of tocilizumab, the patient has successfully been managed with methotrexate 10 mg/kg/week as maintenance therapy.

Case 14.7

Annibale Versari and Giulia Pazzola

Man, 67 years old; ulcerative gastritis; previous right lung abscess (40 years before); currently no drugs. Patient was referred in March 2008 to the rheumatology department because of low back pain, low-grade fever (up to 38 °C), weight loss of 8 kg, and shortness of breath. ESR was raised at 71 mm/h, while creatinine was 1.15 mg/dL. Echocardiography revealed a dilated aortic root in the ascending segment with moderate valvular aortic insufficiency, while an abdominal CT scan showed an aneurysm >6 cm of the abdominal aorta, below the renal arteries. The aneurysm was surrounded by hypodense, nonenhancing tissue of maximum thickness of 2.5 cm, which encased the left ureter with ensuing dilation of the excretory system on the same side.

Suspected Site of Inflammation

Abdominal aorta.

Radiopharmaceutical Activity

May 5, 2008: injection of 300 MBq of [^{18}F]FDG. Glucose level = 89 mg/dL.

March 18, 2009: injection of 295 MBq of [^{18}F] FDG. Glucose level = 87 mg/dL.

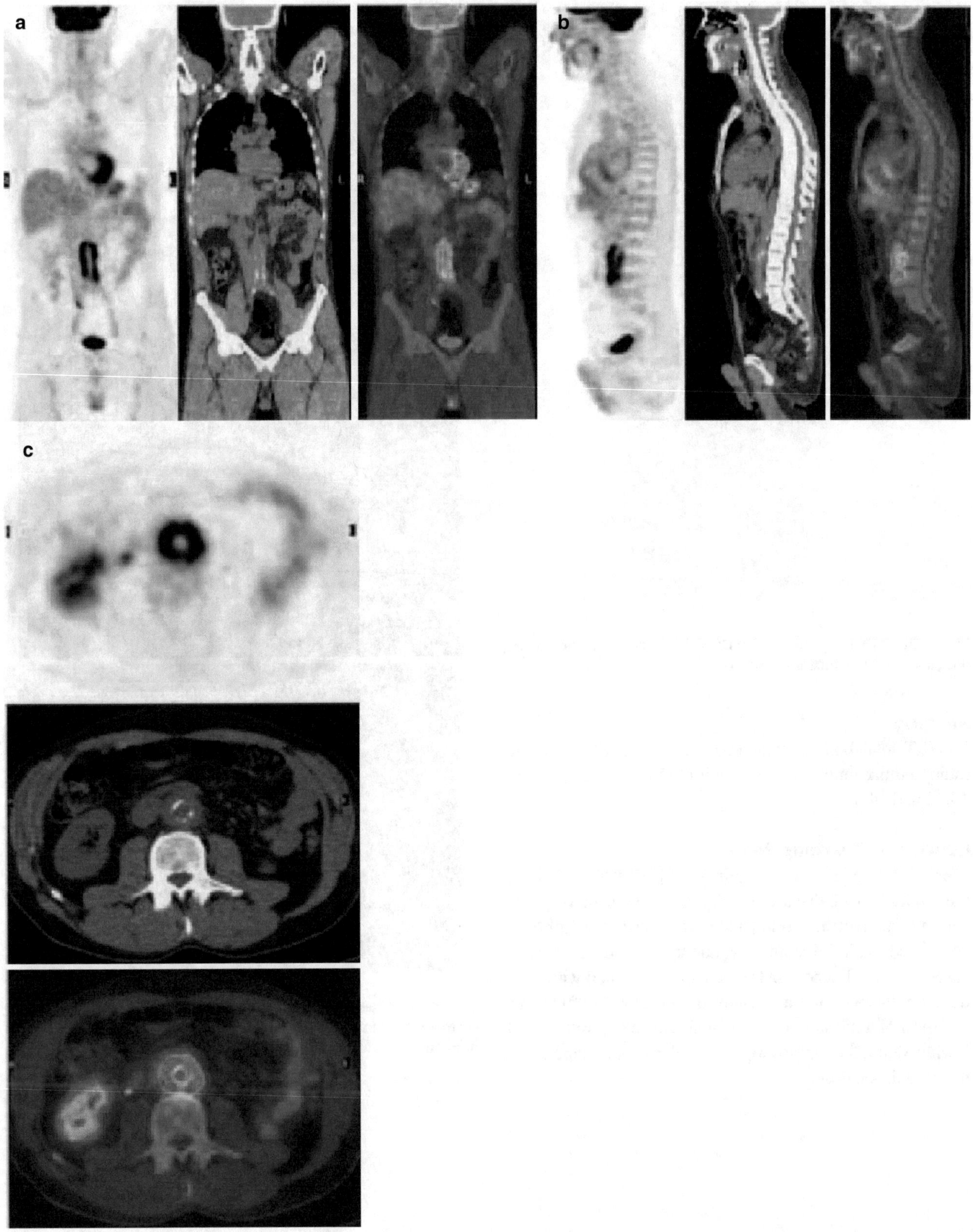

Fig. 14.27 [18F]FDG PET/CT coronal (**a**), sagittal (**b**), and transaxial (**c**) sections demonstrate increased (Grade 3) tracer uptake in the infrarenal abdominal aorta, with $SUV_{max} = 8.8$

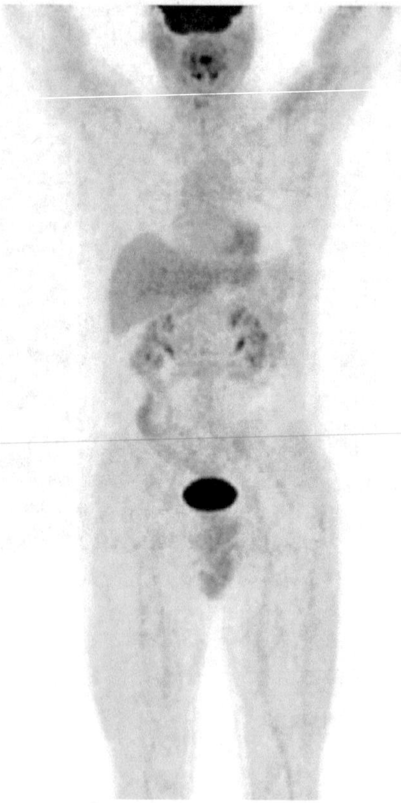

Fig. 14.28 MIP image from [^{18}F]FDG PET/CT acquired after therapy does not show abnormal tracer uptake

Imaging

PET/CT total body acquisitions were performed 1 h after radiopharmaceutical administration (Figs. 14.30, 14.31, 14.32 and 14.33).

Conclusion/Teaching Point

This is an example of the usefulness of [^{18}F]FDG PET/CT in the evaluation of disease activity and treatment response. Chronic periaortitis (idiopathic retroperitoneal fibrosis) associated with inflammatory aneurysm and large-vessel vasculitis was diagnosed. The patient was treated with high-dose prednisone tapering, endovascular stent-grafting, and insertion of a left ureter pigtail stent. However, over the following years, the disease repeatedly flared upon tapering of the prednisone dose.

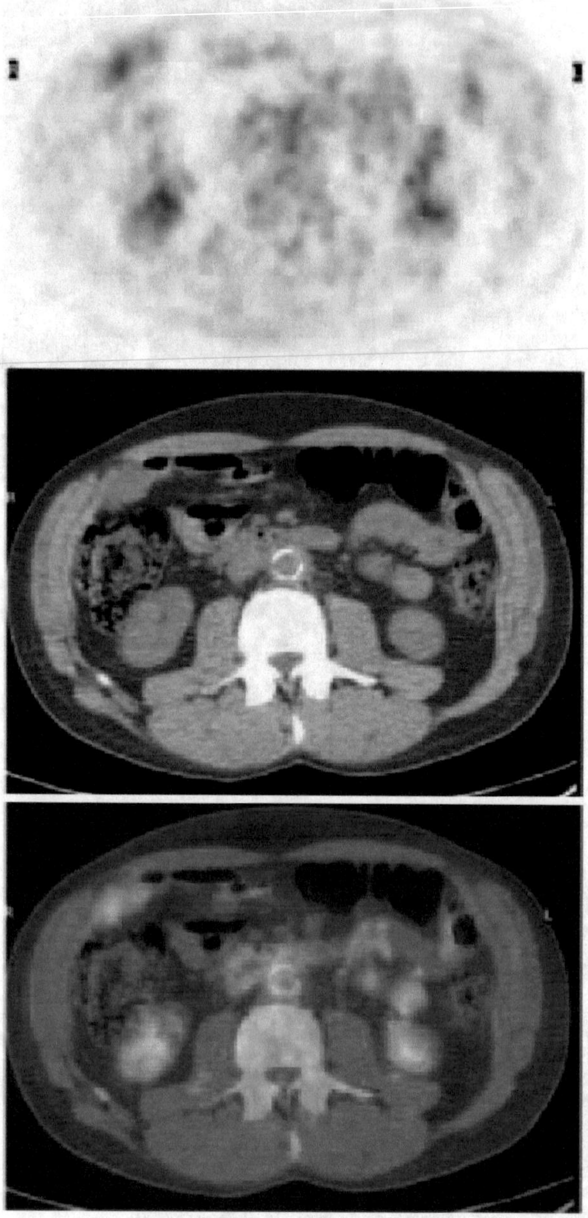

Fig. 14.29 Transaxial [^{18}F]FDG PET/CT sections acquired after medical treatment demonstrate the disappearance of significant uptake in the infrarenal abdominal aorta

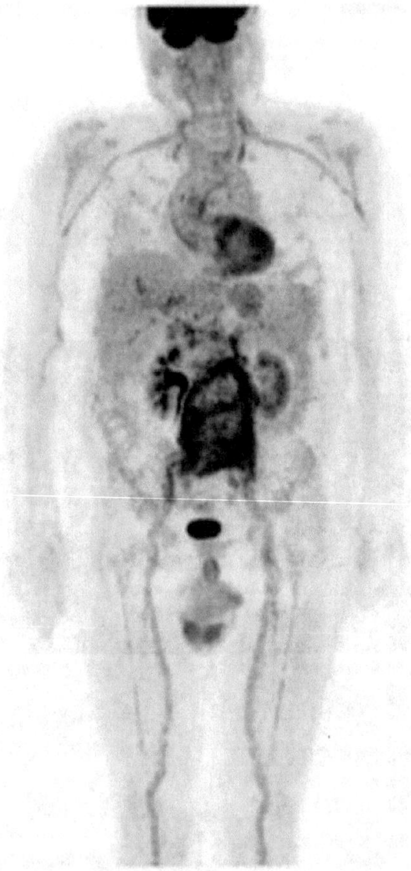

Fig. 14.30 MIP image from baseline [^{18}F]FDG PET/CT shows intense tracer uptake in the abdomen associated with diffuse uptake at thoracic aorta and subclavian, axillary, carotid, iliac, and femoral arteries bilaterally

Case 14.8

Annibale Versari and Nicolò Pipitone

Woman, 83 years old; anxiety therapy. Patient was referred in August 2010 to the rheumatologists because of the recent onset of muscle weakness affecting all four limbs. On examination, she had marked proximal muscle weakness (grade 3 of the Medical Research Council scale). Physical examination also disclosed erythema over the periorbital area and upper chest as well as Gottron papules. Antinuclear antibody (ANA) test was positive (1/160) with a homogeneous pattern, while ESR, extractable nuclear antigens, and creatine kinase were negative or normal. A muscle biopsy was noncontributory and resulted in lichenoid dermatitis (August 26, 2010). Dermatomyositis was diagnosed and treatment with combined prednisone and ciclosporin commenced. Approximately 1 month later, the patient developed a dry cough and shortness of breath. Auscultation of the lung revealed diffuse rales so chest X-ray was performed (September 15, 2010) (Fig. 14.34).

Suspected Site of Infection

Suspected paraneoplastic syndrome.

Radiopharmaceutical Activity

September 15, 2010: Injection of 210 MBq of [^{18}F]FDG. Glucose level of 87 mg/dL before radiopharmaceutical injection.

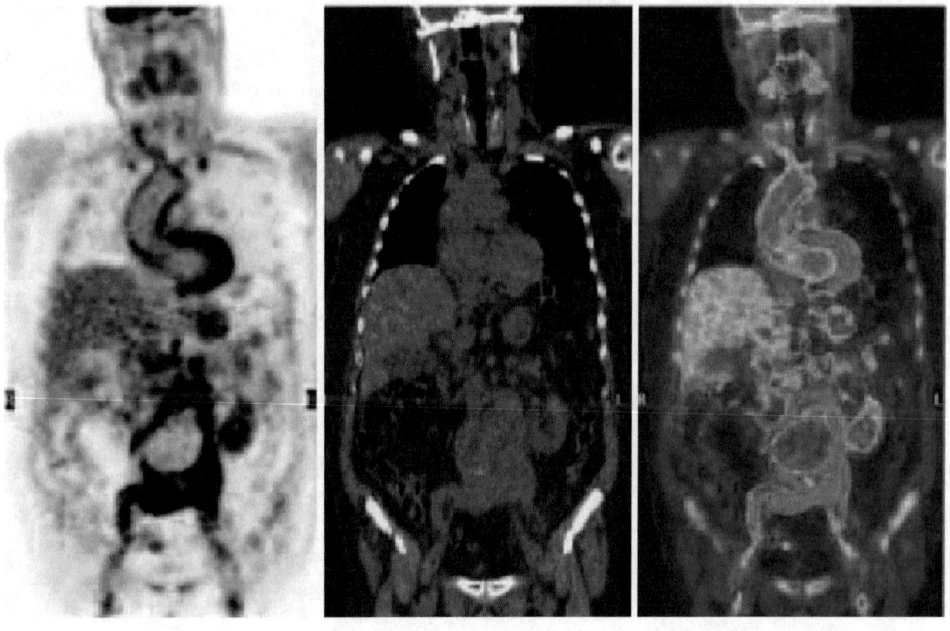

Fig. 14.31 [^{18}F]FDG PET/CT: coronal sections demonstrate intense tracer uptake in the abdominal aorta aneurysm wall and periaortic mass, ascendant aorta and iliac arteries

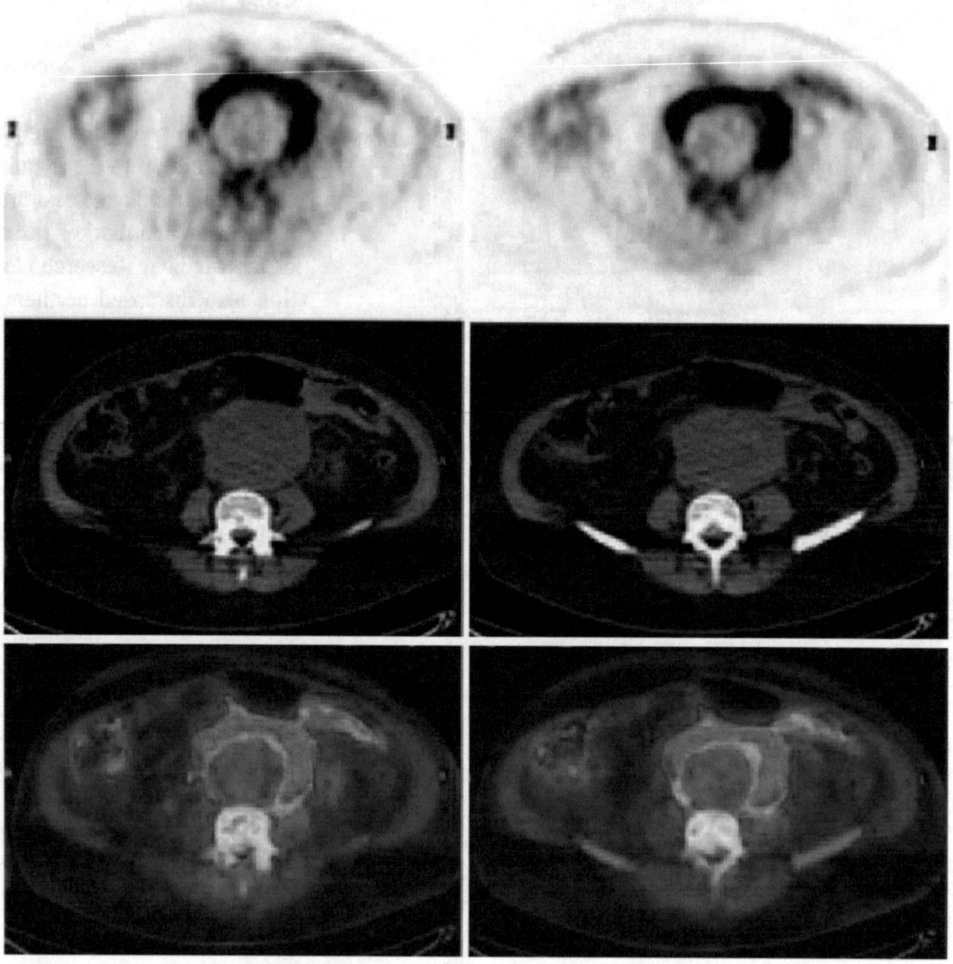

Fig. 14.32 The transaxial [^{18}F]FDG PET/CT sections show intense tracer uptake in the aneurysm wall and periaortic tissue

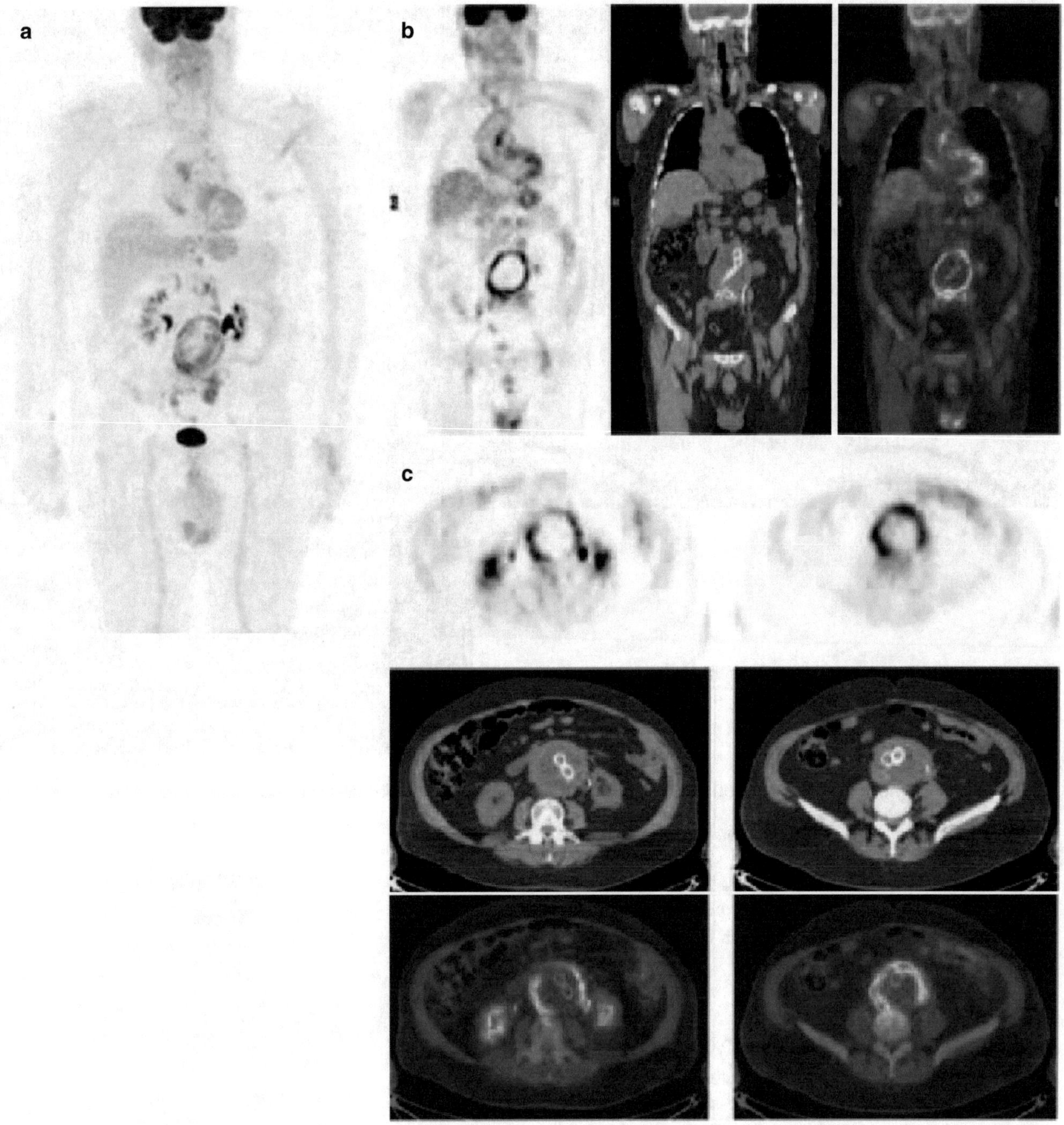

Fig. 14.33 MIP image of [^{18}F]FDG-PET/CT performed after 22 months of medical treatment show a reduction of extension and intensity of tracer uptake in the abdomen and vessels (**a**). The reduction of uptake is associated with a size reduction of the periaortic mass, as demonstrated by coronal (**b**) and transaxial (**c**) sections

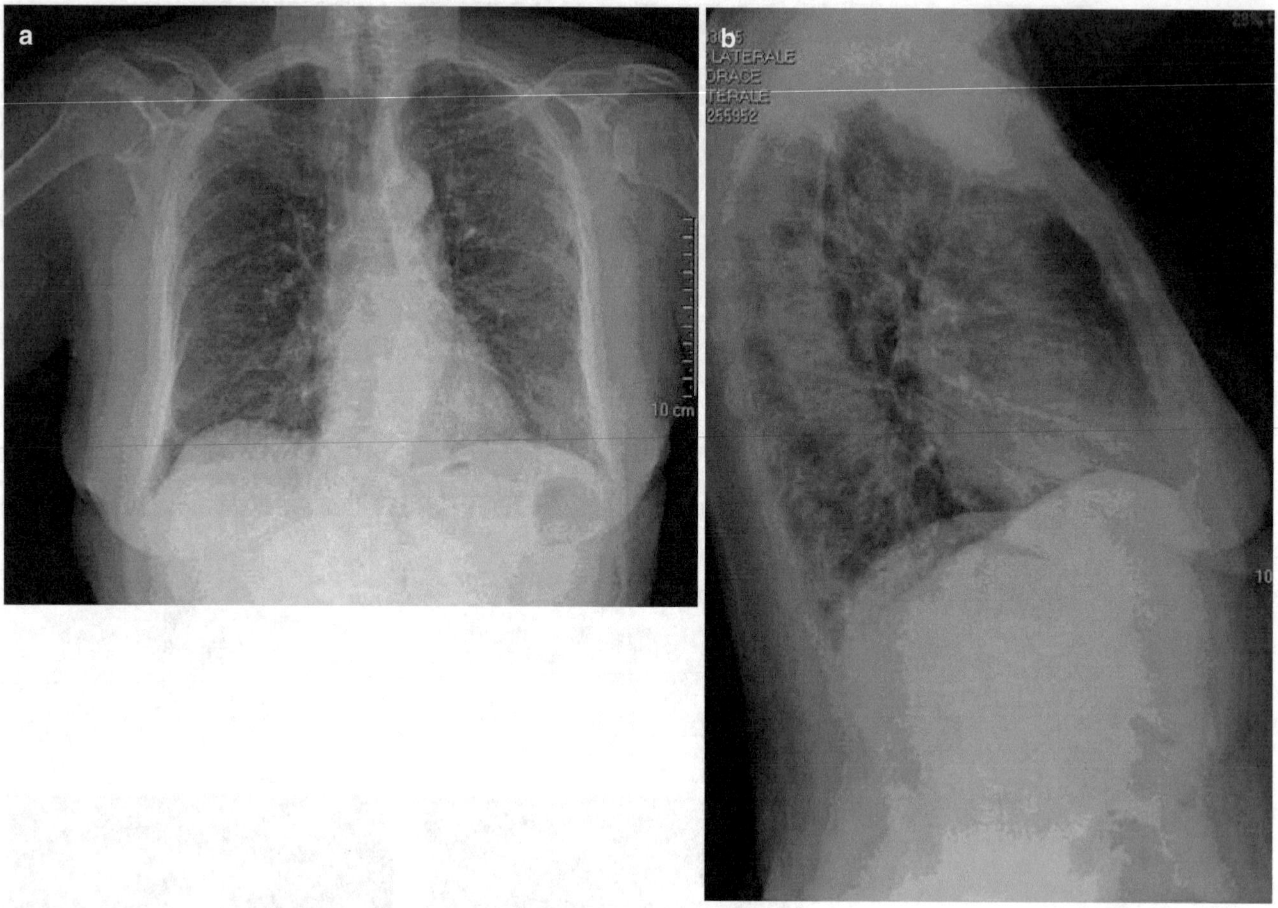

Fig. 14.34 Chest X-ray in posteroanterior (**a**) and lateral (**b**) projections revealed increased interstitial pattern associated with basal left lung parenchyma thickening

Imaging

PET/CT total body acquisition was performed 1 h after radiopharmaceutical i.v. administration (Figs. 14.35, 14.36, and 14.37).

Conclusion/Teaching Point

[^{18}F]FDG PET/CT was useful to identify interstitial pneumonia. The patient went on to develop pneumothorax related to vasculitis associated with her muscle disease and died a few weeks later despite aggressive medical therapy and endotracheal intubation with assisted respiration.

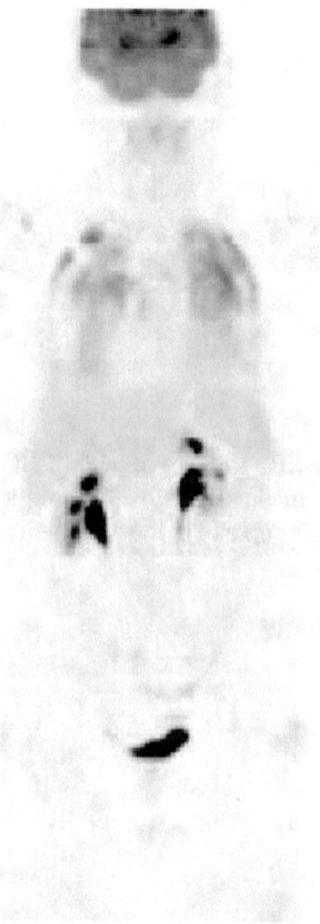

Fig. 14.35 MIP image of [^{18}F]FDG PET/CT shows diffusely increased, symmetrical, prevalently posterior [^{18}F]FDG uptake in the lung fields

Case 14.9

Paola A. Erba

Woman, 45 years old. 2001: diagnosis of psoriatic arthritis treated with methotrexate and ciclosporin until May 2009. June 2009: preventative antibiotic treatment (Augmentin, 10 days) because of dental surgery.

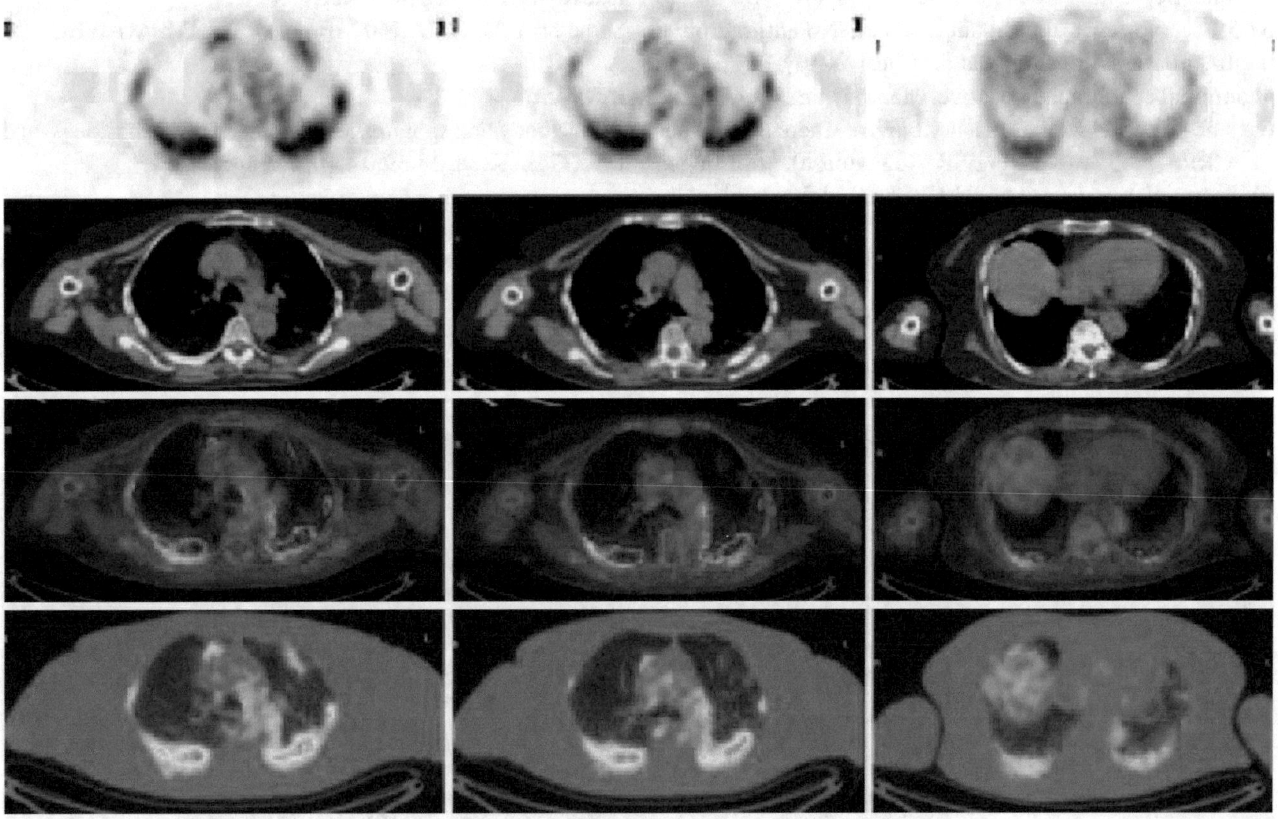

Fig. 14.36 Transaxial [^{18}F]FDG PET/CT sections demonstrate diffusely increased, symmetrical, prevalently posterior tracer uptake in the lung fields, considered to be consistent with interstitial lung disease secondary to dermatomyositis

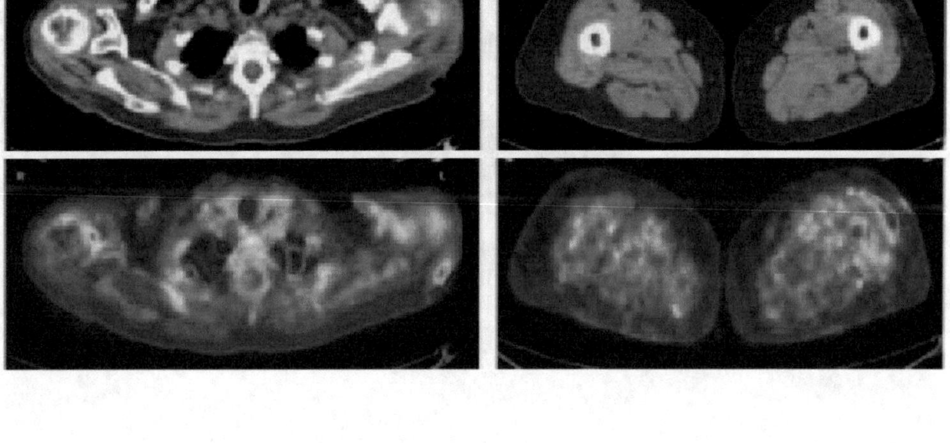

Fig. 14.37 [^{18}F]FDG PET/CT: transaxial sections demonstrate radiopharmaceutical uptake in posterior soft tissues, in deltoid muscle of left arm (**a**) and in proximal left thigh (**b**)

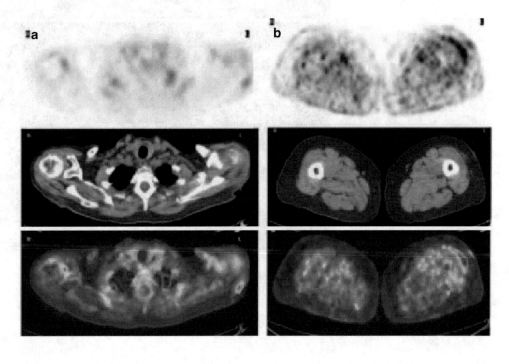

June–September 2009: fever (temperature up to 37.5 °C). No fever after about 2 weeks. No antimicrobial treatment. Pain to right hand. Chest X-ray, TTE, and abdominal echography negative. Mantoux and Leishmania tests negative, as well as urinary culture. Increased values of CRP (5.43 mg/dL), ESR (63 mm/h), fibrinogen (668 mg/dL), ALP (142 U/L), and alpha-2 globulin (14.9%).

Suspected Site of Infection

Joints.

Radiopharmaceutical Activity

September 23, 2009: 740 MBq of ^{99m}Tc-HMPAO-WBC.

Imaging

Whole body and spot images of chest, arms, hands, legs, and feet (Figs. 14.38, 14.39, 14.40, and 14.41).

Conclusion/Teaching Point

Labeled leukocyte scintigraphy allows the evaluation of the presence of the inflammatory infection process in all joints with high accuracy leading to adequate therapy.

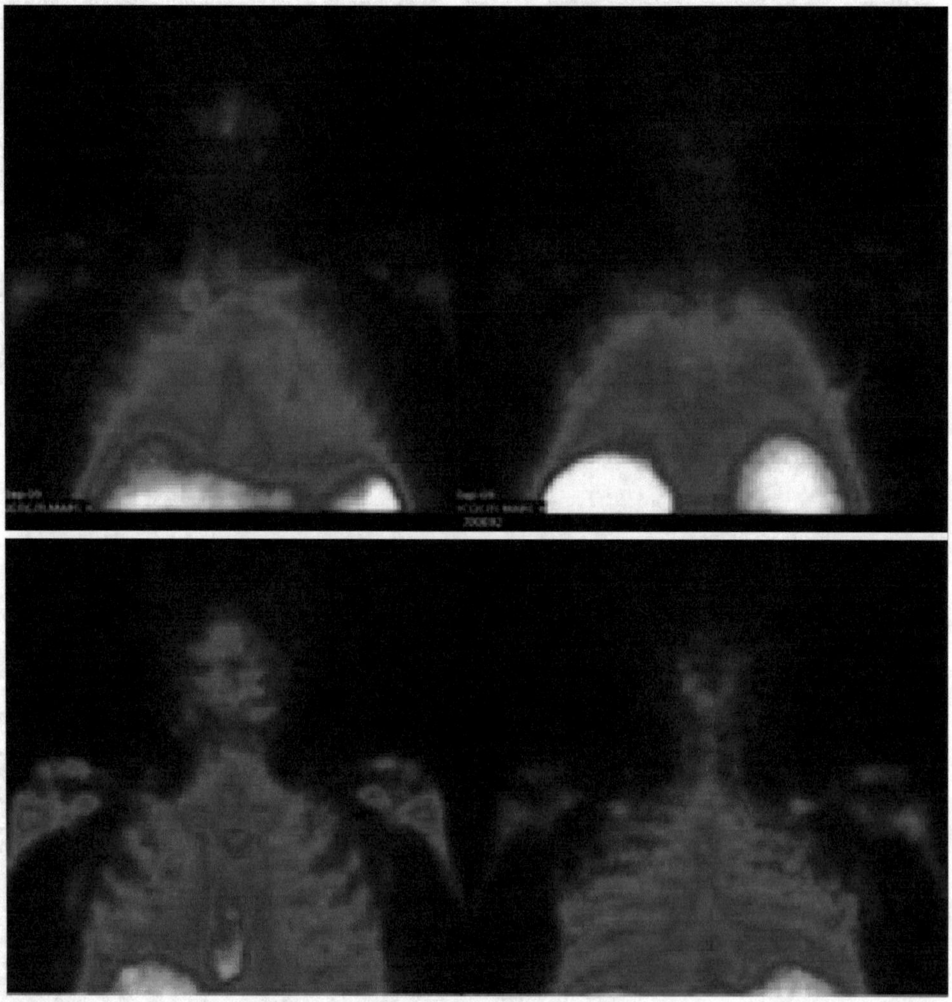

Fig. 14.38 ^{99m}Tc-HMPAO-WBC scintigraphy: spot planar images of the chest in anterior (left column) and posterior views (right column) obtained at 45 min (upper panels) and 6 h (lower panels)

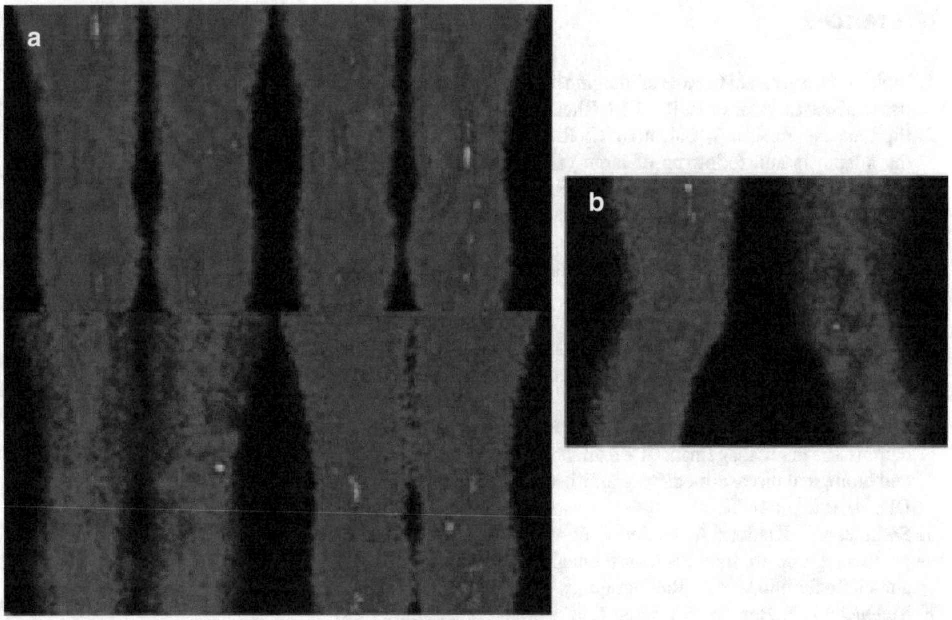

Fig. 14.39 (a) Spot planar images of the legs in anterior (left column) and posterior (right column) and lateral views (left column, only delayed images) obtained at 45 min (upper panels) and 6 h (lower panels). (b) Spot lateral view of the legs acquired at 6 h. Semi-quantitative analysis of radioactivity accumulation in left knee showed target/background ratio of 1.5 in the early acquisition, and 1.9 in the delayed acquisition

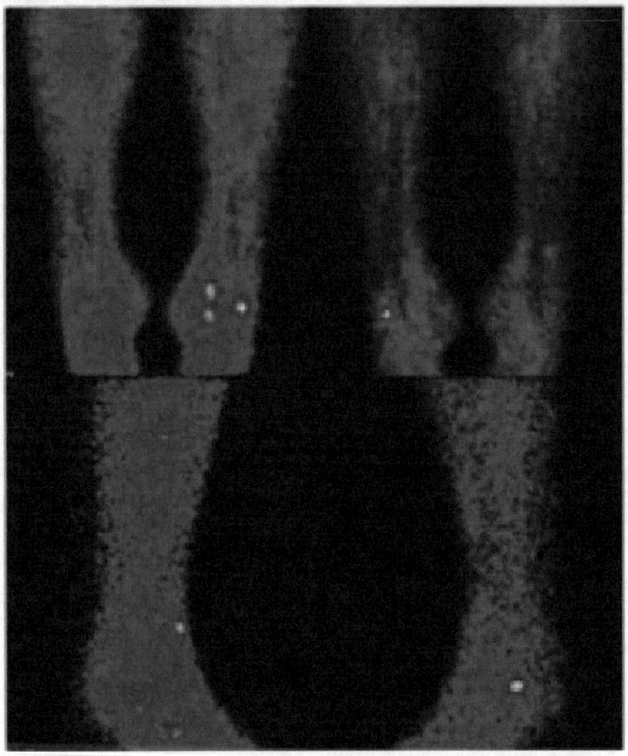

Fig. 14.40 Spot images of the legs and feet in anterior and posterior views (upper panels) and lateral view (lower panel) obtained at 6 h

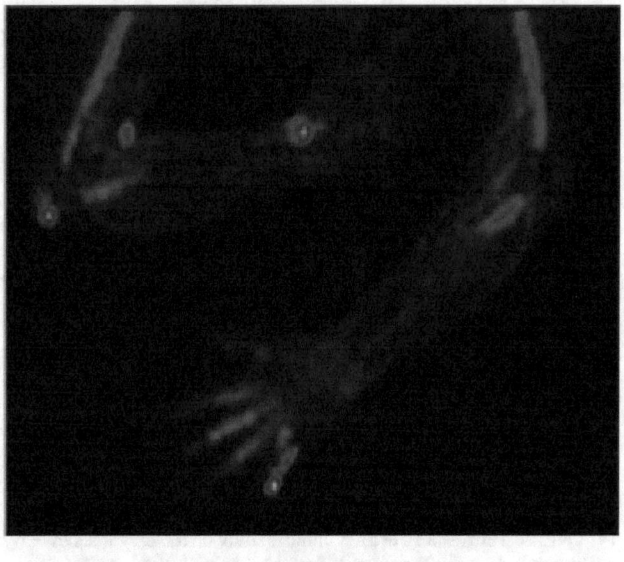

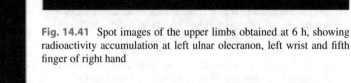

Fig. 14.41 Spot images of the upper limbs obtained at 6 h, showing radioactivity accumulation at left ulnar olecranon, left wrist and fifth finger of right hand

References

1. Pipitone N, Salvarani C. Role of imaging in vasculitis and connective tissue diseases. Best Pract Res Clin Rheumatol. 2008;22:1075–91.
2. Pipitone N, Versari A, Salvarani C. Role of imaging studies in the diagnosis and follow-up of large-vessel vasculitis: an update. Rheumatology (Oxford). 2008;47:403–8.
3. Gabriel SE. The epidemiology of rheumathoid arthritis. Rheum Dis Clin N Am. 2001;27:269–82.
4. Hurd ER. Extraarticular manifestations of rheumatoid arthritis. Semin Arthritis Rheum. 1979;8:151–76.
5. Aletaha D, Neogi T, Silman AJ, et al. 2010 rheumatoid arthritis classification criteria: an American College of Rheumatology/European League Against Rheumatism collaborative initiative. Ann Rheum Dis. 2010;69:1580–8.
6. Smolen JS, Landewé R, Breedveld FC, et al. EULAR recommendations for the management of rheumatoid arthritis with synthetic and biological disease-modifying antirheumatic drugs. Ann Rheum Dis. 2010;69:964–75.
7. Sommer OJ, Kladosk A, Weiler V, et al. Rheumatoid arthritis: a practical guide to state-of-the-art imaging, image interpretation, and clinical implications. Radiographics. 2005;25:381–98.
8. McQueen FM, Benton N, Crabbe J, et al. What is the fate of erosions in early rheumatoid arthritis? Tracking individual lesions using—rays and magnetic resonance imaging over the first two years of disease. Ann Rheum Dis. 2001;60:859–68.
9. Szkudlarek M, Klarlund M, Narvestad E, et al. Ultrasonography of the metacarpophalangeal and proximal interphalangeal joints in rheumatoid arthritis: a comparison with magnetic resonance imaging, conventional radiography and clinical examination. Arthritis Res Ther. 2006;8:R52.
10. Tan YK, Conaghan PG. Imaging in rheumatoid arthritis. Best Pract Res Clin Rheum. 2011;25:569–84.
11. McQueen FM, Benton N, Perry D, et al. Bone edema scored on magnetic resonance imaging scans of the dominant carpus at presentation predicts radiographic joint damage of the hands and feet six years later in patients with rheumatoid arthritis. Arthritis Rheum. 2003;48:1814–27.
12. Bøyesen P, Haavardsholm EA, Ostergaard M, et al. MRI in early rheumatoid arthritis: synovitis and bone marrow oedema are independent predictors of subsequent radiographic progression. Ann Rheum Dis. 2011;70:428–33.
13. Schwarz A, Elbracht T, Jeschke A, et al. Bone scintigraphy and clinical outcome in rheumatoid gonarthritis. Nuklearmedizin. 2003;42:94–8.
14. Qing C, Lei Y, Ma L, et al. A clinical study on the diagnosis of early rheumatoid arthritis using bone imaging with ^{99m}Tc-MDP. Sheng Wu Yi Xue Gong Cheng Xue Za Zhi. 2008;25:1193–6.
15. Ozgul A, Yasar E, Arslan N, et al. The comparison of ultrasonographics and scintigraphic findings of early arthritis in revealing rheumatoid arthritis according to criteria of American College of Rheumatology. Rheumatol Int. 2009;29:765–8.
16. Ostendorf B, Mattes-György K, Reichelt DC, et al. Early detection of bony alterations in rheumatoid and erosive arthritis of finger joints with high-resolution single photon emission computed tomography, and differentiation between them. Skelet Radiol. 2010;39:55–61.
17. Scherer A, Wirrwar A, Mattes-György K, et al. Bony pathologies of the metacarpophalangeal joints in early rheumatoid arthritis: comparison of MRI and high-resolution SPECT. RöFo. 2009;181:875–80.
18. Diot P, Le Pape A, Nolibe D, et al. Scintigraphy with J001X, a Klebsiella membrane glycolipid, for the early diagnosis of chronic berilliosis: results from an experimental model. Br J Int Med. 1992;49:359–64.
19. Tishler M, Lysyy O, Levy O, et al. ^{99m}Tc-albumin nanocolloid joint scintigraphy in rheumatoid arthritis patients who are in clinical remission—is remission real? Clin Exp Rheumatol. 2010;28:360–4.
20. Dos Anjos DA, do Vale GF, Campos CM, et al. Extra-articular inflammatory sites detected by F-18 FDG PET/CT in a patient with rheumatoid arthritis. Clin Nucl Med. 2010;35:540–1.
21. Goerres GW, Forster A, Uebelhart D, et al. F-18 FDG whole-body PET for the assessment of disease activity in patients with rheumatoid arthritis. Clin Nucl Med. 2006;31:386–90.
22. Vijayant V, Sarma M, Aurangabadkar H, et al. Potential of ^{18}F-FDG-PET as a valuable adjunct to clinical and response assessment in rheumatoid arthritis and seronegative spondyloarthropathies. World J Radiol. 2012;4:462–8.
23. Dhawan R, Lokitz K, Lokitz S, et al. FDG PET imaging of extremities in rheumatoid arthritis. J La State Med Soc. 2016;168:156–61.
24. Beckers C, Ribbens C, André B, et al. Assessment of disease activity in rheumatoid arthritis with ^{18}F-FDG PET. J Nucl Med. 2004;45:956–64.
25. Okamura K, Yonemoto Y, Arisaka Y, et al. The assessment of biologic treatment inpatient with rheumatoid arthritis using FDG-PET/CT. Rheumatology (Oxford). 2012;51:1484–91.
26. Elzinga EH, van der Laken CJ, Comans EF, et al. ^{18}F-FDG PET as a tool to predict the clinical outcome of infliximab treatment of rheumatoid arthritis: an exploratory study. J Nucl Med. 2011;52:77–80.
27. Roivainen A, Parkkola R, Yli-Kerttula T, et al. Use of positron emission tomography with methyl-^{11}C-choline and 2-^{18}F-fluoro-2-deoxy-*d*-glucose in comparison with magnetic resonance imaging for the assessment of inflammatory proliferation of synovium. Arthritis Rheum. 2003;48:3077–84.
28. Virtanen H, Autio A, Siitonen R, et al. ^{68}Ga-DOTA-Siglec-9: a new imaging tool to detect synovitis. Arthritis Res Ther. 2015;17:308.
29. Li XG, Autio A, Ahtinen H, et al. Translating the concept of peptide labeling with 5-deoxy-5-[^{18}F]fluororibose into preclinical practice: ^{18}F-labeling of Siglec-9 peptide for PET imaging of inflammation. Chem Commun (Camb). 2013;49:3682–4.
30. Bruijnen S, Tsang-A-Sjoe M, Raterman H, et al. B-cell imaging with zirconium-89 labelled rituximab PET-CT at baseline is associated with therapeutic response 24 weeks after initiation of rituximab treatment in rheumatoid arthritis patients. Arthritis Res Ther. 2016;18:266.
31. Johnston SL, Lock RJ, Gomples NM. Takayasu arteritis: a review. J Cin Pathol. 2002;55:481–6.
32. Jiemy WF, Heeringa P, Kamps JAAM, et al. Positron emission tomography (PET) and single photon emission computed tomography (SPECT) imaging of macrophages in large vessel vasculitis: current status and future prospects. Autoimmun Rev. 2018;17:715–26.
33. Bloch DA, Michel BA, Hunder GG, et al. The American College of Rheumatology 1990 criteria for the classification of vasculitis. Patients and methods. Arthritis Rheum. 1990;33:1068–73.
34. Blockmans D, Bley T, Schmidt W. Imaging for large-vessel vasculitis. Curr Opin Rheumat. 2009;21:19–28.
35. Blockmans D, De Ceuninck L, Vanderschueren S, et al. Repetitive 18-fluorodeoxyglucose positron emission tomography in isolated polymyalgia rheumatic: a prospective study in 35 patients. Rheumatology (Oxford). 2007;46:672–7.
36. Meller J, Strutz F, Siefker U, et al. Early diagnosis and follow-up of aortitis with [^{18}F]FDG PET and MRI. Eur J Nucl Med Mol Imaging. 2003;30:730–6.
37. Blockmans D. ^{18}F-fluoro-deoxyglucose positron emission tomography in patients with fever of unknown origin. Acta Clin Belg. 2004;59:134–7.
38. Walter MA, Melzer RA, Graf M, et al. [^{18}F]FDG-PET of giant-cell aortitis. Rheumatology (Oxford). 2005;44:690–1.

39. Salvarani C, Magnani L, Catanoso M, et al. Tocilizumab: a novel therapy for patients with large-vessel vasculitis. Rheumatology (Oxford). 2012;51:151–6.
40. de Leeuw K, Bijl M, Jager PL. Additional value of positron emission tomography in diagnosis and follow-up of patients with large vessel vasculitis. Clin Exp Rheumatol. 2004;22:S21–6.
41. Blockmans D. PET in vasculitis. Ann N Y Acad Sci. 2011;1228:64–70.
42. Glaudemans AWJM, de Vries EFJ, Galli F, et al. The use of ^{18}F-FDG-PET/CT for diagnosis and treatment monitoring of inflammatory and infectious disease. Clin Dev Immunol. 2013;2013:623036. Hindawi Publishing Corporation
43. Huang WS, Chiu PY, Kao A, et al. Decreased cerebral blood flow in neuro-Behcet's syndrome patients with neuropsychiatric manifestations and normal magnetic resonance imaging —a preliminary report. Neuroimaging. 2002;12:355–9.
44. Kaya E, Saglam H, Ciftci I, et al. Evaluation of myocardial perfusion and function by gated SPECT in patients with Behcet disease. Ann Nucl Med. 2008;22:287–95.
45. Kashyap R, Mittal BR, Bhattacharya A, et al. Exercise myocardial perfusion imaging to evaluate inducible ischaemia in children with Kawasaki disease. Nucl Med Commun. 2011;32:137–41.
46. Haimovic A, Sanchez M, Judson MA, et al. Sarcoidosis: a comprehensive review and update for the dermatologist. Part II. Extracutaneous disease. J Am Acad Dermatol. 2012;66:719.e1–10.
47. Lynch JP, Kazerooni EA, Gay SE. Pulmonary sarcoidosis. Clin Chest Med. 1997;18:755–85.
48. Puryear DW, Fowler AA. Sarcoidosis: a clinical overview. Compr Ther. 1996;22:649–53.
49. Judson MA. The diagnosis of sarcoidosis. Clin Chest Med. 2008;29:415–27.
50. Mañá J. Magnetic resonance imaging and nuclear imaging in sarcoidosis. Curr Opin Pulm Med. 2002;8:457–63.
51. Moore SL, Teirstein A, Golimbu C. MRI of sarcoidosis patients with musculoskeletal symptoms. AJR Am J Roentgenol. 2005;185:154–9.
52. Mortele KJ, Ros PR. Imaging of diffuse liver disease. Semin Liver Dis. 2001;21:195–212.
53. Sharma S. Cardiac imaging in myocardial sarcoidosis and other cardiomyopathies. Curr Opin Pulm Med. 2009;15:507–12.
54. Smith JK, Matheus MG, Castillo M. Imaging manifestations of neurosarcoidosis. AJR Am J Roentgenol. 2004;182:289–95.
55. Sulavik SB, Spencer RP, Weed DA, et al. Recognition of distinctive patterns of gallium-67 distribution in sarcoidosis. J Nucl Med. 1990;31:1909–14.
56. Sulavik SB, Spencer RP, Palestro CJ, et al. Specificity and sensitivity of distinctive chest radiographic and/or ^{67}gallium images in the noninvasive diagnosis of sarcoidosis. Chest. 1993;103:403–9.
57. Schuster DM, Alazraki N. Gallium and other agents in diseases of the lung. Semin Nucl Med. 2002;32:193–211.
58. Kramer EL, Divgi CR. Pulmonary applications of nuclear medicine. Clin Chest Med. 1991;12:55–75.
59. van der Wall H, McLanghlin AF, Southee AE. Gallium scintigraphy in tumor diagnosis and management. In: Murray IPC, Ell PJ, editors. Nuclear medicine in clinical diagnosis and treatment. 2nd ed. New York: Churchill Livingstone; 1998. p. 813–5.
60. Mañá J. Nuclear imaging. ^{67}Gallium, ^{201}Tallium, ^{18}F-labelled fluoro-2-deoxy-D-glucose positron emission tomography. Clin Chest Med. 1997;18:781–99.
61. Nakazara A, Ikeda K, Ito Y, et al. Usefulness of dual ^{67}Ga and ^{99m}Tc-sestamibi single-photon-emission CT scanning in the diagnosis of cardiac sarcoidosis. Chest. 2004;126:1372–6.
62. Mañá J, Gamez C. Molecular imaging in sarcoidosis. Curr Opin Pulm Med. 2011;17:325–31.
63. Van Kroonenburgh M, Mostard R, Vöö S. Metaiodobenzylguanidine scintigraphy in pulmonary and cardiac disease. Curr Opin Pulm Med. 2010;16:511–5.
64. Balan A, Hoey ET, Sheerin F, et al. Multi-technique imaging of sarcoidosis. Clin Radiol. 2010;65:750–60.
65. Teirstein AS, Machac J, Almeida O, et al. Results of 188 whole-body fluorodeoxyglucose positron emission scans in 137 patients with sarcoidosis. Chest. 2007;132:1949–53.
66. Nishiyama Y, Yamamoto Y, Fukunaga K, et al. Comparative evaluation of ^{18}F-FDG PET and ^{67}Gallium-scintigraphy in patients with sarcoidosis. J Nucl Med. 2006;47:1571–6.
67. Braun JJ, Kessler R, Constantinesco A, et al. ^{18}F-FDG PET/CT in sarcoidosis management: review and report of 20 cases. Eur J Nucl Med Mol Imaging. 2008;35:1537–43.
68. Kruger S, Buch AK, Mottaghy FM, et al. Use of integrated FDG PET/CT in sarcoidosis. Clin Imaging. 2008;32:269–73.
69. Tahara N, Tahara A, Nitta Y, et al. Heterogeneous myocardial FDG uptake and the disease activity in cardiac sarcoidosis. J Am Coll Cardiol. 2010;3:1219–28.
70. Gensuke A, Malak I, Shah H, et al. PET/CT in the diagnosis and workup of sarcoidosis: focus on atypical manifestations. Radiographics. 2018;38:1536–49.
71. Krusza P, O'Brian RJ. Diagnosis and management of Sjogren syndrome. Am Fam Physician. 2009;79:465–70.
72. Milic VD, Petrovic RR, Boricic IV, et al. Diagnostic value of salivary gland ultrasonographic scoring system in primary Sjogren's syndrome: a comparison with scintigraphy and biopsy. J Rheumatol. 2009;36:1495–500.
73. Tonami H, Higashi K, Matoba M, et al. A comparative study between MR sialography and salivary gland scintigraphy in the diagnosis of Sjögren syndrome. J Comput Assist Tomogr. 2001;25:262–8.
74. Ramos-Casals M, Brito-Zerón P, Perez-DE-Lis M, et al. Clinical and prognostic significance of parotid scintigraphy in 405 patients with primary Sjogren's syndrome. J Rheumatol. 2010;37:585–90.
75. Taura S, Murata Y, Aung W, et al. Decreased thyroid uptake of Tc-99m pertechnetate in patients with advanced-stage Sjögren syndrome: evaluation using salivary gland scintigraphy. Clin Nucl Med. 2002;27:265–9.
76. Le Guern V, Belin C, Henegar C, et al. Cognitive function and ^{99m}Tc-ECD brain SPECT are significantly correlated in patients with primary Sjogren syndrome: a case-control study. Ann Rheum Dis. 2010;69:132–7.
77. Pirildar T, Gumuser G, Ruksen E, et al. Assessment of alveolar epithelial permeability with Tc-99m DTPA aerosol scintigraphy in patients with Sjogren syndrome. Rheumatol Int. 2010;30:599–604.
78. Ross R. Atherosclerosis—an inflammatory disease. N Engl J Med. 1999;340:115–26.
79. Ross R. The pathogenesis of atherosclerosis: a perspective for the 1990s. Nature. 1993;362:801–9.
80. Maseri A, Fuster V. Is there a vulnerable plaque? Circulation. 2003;107:2068–71.
81. Finn AV, Nakano M, Narula J, et al. Concept of vulnerable/unstable plaque. Arterioscler Thromb Vasc Biol. 2010;30:1282–92.
82. Prati F, Di Vito L. Imaging of intraplaque haemorrhage. J Cardiovasc Med (Hagerstown). 2012;13:640–4.
83. Gronholdt ML, Nordestgaard BG, Nielsen TG, et al. Echolucent carotid artery plaques are associated with elevated levels of fasting and postprandial triglyceride-rich lipoproteins. Stroke. 1996;27:2166–72.
84. Rioufol G, Gilard M, Finet G, et al. Evolution of spontaneous atherosclerotic plaque rupture with medical therapy: long-term follow-up with intravascular ultrasound. Circulation. 2004;110:2875–80.

85. Tearney GJ, et al. Consensus standards for acquisition, measurement, and reporting of intravascular optical coherence tomography studies: a report from the International Working Group for Intravascular Optical Coherence Tomography Standardization and Validation. J Am Coll Cardiol. 2012;59:1058–72.
86. Doherty TM, Detrano RC, Mautner SL, et al. Coronary calcium: the good, the bad, and the uncertain. Am Heart J. 1999;137:806–14.
87. Kereiakes DJ. The Emperor's clothes: in search of the vulnerable plaque. Circulation. 2003;107:2076–7.
88. Bourque JM, Schietinger BJ, Kennedy JL, et al. Usefulness of cardiovascular magnetic resonance imaging of the superficial femoral artery for screening patients with diabetes mellitus for atherosclerosis. Am J Cardiol. 2012;110:50–6.
89. Tahara H, Kai H, Nakaura H, et al. The prevalence of inflammation in carotid atherosclerosis: analysis with fluorodeoxyglucose positron emission tomography. Eur Heart J. 2007;28:2243–8.
90. Tahara H, Kai H, Yamagishi S, et al. Vascular inflammation evaluated by [^{18}F]-fluorodeoxyglucose positron emission tomography is associated with the metabolic syndrome. J Am Coll Cardiol. 2007;49:1533–9.
91. Meirelles GS, Gonen M, Strauss HW. ^{18}F-FDG uptake and calcifications in the thoracic aorta on positron emission tomography/ computed tomography examinations: frequency and stability on serial scans. J Thorac Imaging. 2011;26:54–62.
92. Menezes LJ, Kayani I, Ben-Haim S, et al. What is the natural history of ^{18}F-FDG uptake in arterial atheroma on PET/CT? Implications for imaging the vulnerable plaque. Atherosclerosis. 2010;211:136–40.
93. Wassélius J, Larsson S, Jacobsson H. Time-to-time correlation of high-risk atherosclerotic lesions identified with [^{18}F]-FDG-PET/ CT. Ann Nucl Med. 2009;23:59–64.
94. Mehta NN, Torigian DA, Gelfand JM, et al. Quantification of atherosclerotic plaque activity and vascular inflammation using [^{18}F] fluorodeoxyglucose positron emission tomography/computed tomography (FDG-PET/CT). J Vis Exp. 2012;(63):e3777. https://doi.org/10.3791/3777.
95. Patel R, Janoudi A, Vedre A, et al. Plaque rupture and thrombosis are reduced by lowering cholesterol levels and crystallization with ezetimibe and are correlated with fluorodeoxyglucose positron emission tomography. Arterioscler Thromb Vasc Biol. 2011;31:2007–14.
96. Gaeta C, Fernández Y, Pavía J, et al. Reduced myocardial ^{18}F-FDG uptake after calcium channel blocker administration. Initial observation for a potential new method to improve plaque detection. Eur J Nucl Med Mol Imaging. 2011;38:2018–24.
97. Tahara N, Kai H, Ishibashi M, et al. Simvastatin attenuates plaque inflammation: evaluation by fluorodeoxyglucose positron emission tomography. J Am Coll Cardiol. 2006;48:1825–31.
98. Silvera SS, Aidi HE, Rudd JH, et al. Multimodality imaging of atherosclerotic plaque activity and composition using FDG-PET/ CT and MRI in carotid and femoral arteries. Atherosclerosis. 2009;207:39–143.
99. Ogawa M, Magata Y, Kato T, et al. Application of ^{18}F-FDG-PET for monitoring the therapeutic effect of antiinflammatory drugs on stabilization of vulnerable atherosclerotic plaques. J Nucl Med. 2006;47:1845–50.
100. Marnane M, Merwick A, Sheehan OC, et al. Carotid plaque inflammation on ^{18}F-fluorodeoxyglucose positron emission tomography predicts early stroke recurrence. Ann Neurol. 2012;71:709–18.
101. Moghbel M, Al-Zaghl A, Werner TJ, et al. The role of PET in evaluating atherosclerosis: a critical review. Semin Nucl Med. 2018;48:488–97.
102. Rudd JH, Myers KS, Bansilal S, et al. Relationships among regional arterial inflammation, calcification, risk factors, and biomarkers: a prospective fluorodeoxyglucose positron-emission tomography/ computed tomography imaging study. Circ Cardiovasc Imaging. 2009;2:107–15.
103. Derlin T, Wisotzki C, Richter U, et al. In vivo imaging of mineral deposition in carotid plaque using ^{18}F-sodium fluoride PET/CT: correlation with atherogenic risk factors. J Nucl Med. 2011;52:362–8.
104. Derlin T, Tóth Z, Papp L, et al. Correlation of inflammation assessed by ^{18}F-FDG PET, active mineral deposition assessed by ^{18}F-fluoride PET, and vascular calcification in atherosclerotic plaque: a dual-tracer PET/CT study. J Nucl Med. 2011;52:1020–7.
105. Rominger A, Saam T, Vogl E, et al. In vivo imaging of macrophage activity in the coronary arteries using ^{68}Ga-DOTATATE PET/CT: correlation with coronary calcium burden and risk factors. J Nucl Med. 2010;51:193–7.
106. Takata T, Taniguchi Y, Ohnishi T, et al. ^{18}FDG PET/CT is a powerful tool for detecting subclinical arthritis in patients with psoriatic arthritis and/or psoriasis vulgaris. J Dermatol Sci. 2011;64:144–7.
107. Pipitone N, Versari A, Zuccoli G, et al. ^{18}F-fluorodeoxyglucose positron emission tomography for the assessment of myositis. Clin Exp Rheumatol. 2012;30:570–3.
108. Holzmann H, Krause BJ, Kaltwasser JP, et al. Psoriatic osteoarthropathy and bone scintigraphy. Hautarzt. 1996;47:427–31.
109. Rydgren L, Wollmer P, Hultquist R, et al. ^{111}Indium-labelled leukocytes for measurement of inflammatory activity in arthritis. Scand J Rheumatol. 1991;20:319–25.
110. Usai P, Serra A, Marini B, et al. Frontal cortical perfusion abormalities related to gluten intake and associate autoimmune disease in adult coeliac disease: ^{99m}Tc-ECD brain SPECT study. Dig Liver Dis. 2004;36:513–8.

Radionuclide Imaging of Inflammatory Vascular Diseases: Vasculitis and Atherosclerosis

15

Riemer H. J. A. Slart, Florent L. Besson, and Jan Bucerius

Contents

R. H. J. A. Slart (✉)
Medical Imaging Center, Department of Nuclear Medicine and Molecular Imaging, University of Groningen, University Medical Center Groningen, Groningen, The Netherlands

Department of Biomedical Photonic Imaging, Faculty of Science and Technology, University of Twente, Enschede, The Netherlands
e-mail: r.h.j.a.slart@umcg.nl

F. L. Besson
Department of Biophysics and Nuclear Medicine-Molecular Imaging, Hôpitaux Universitaires Paris-Saclay, Assistance Publique-Hôpitaux de Paris, CHU Bicêtre, Le Kremlin Bicêtre, France

Université Paris Saclay, CEA, CNRS, Inserm, BioMaps, Orsay, France

J. Bucerius
Department of Nuclear Medicine, University Medicine Göttingen, Georg-August-University Göttingen, Göttingen, Germany

Learning Objectives

- To learn more about acquisition, reconstruction, and quantification of [^{18}F]FDG PET/CT imaging in large vessel vasculitis and atherosclerosis
- To update the value of [^{18}F]FDG PET/CT imaging in large vessel vasculitis and atherosclerosis, including treatment monitoring and prognosis
- To learn possible pitfalls [^{18}F]FDG PET/CT imaging in large vessel vasculitis and atherosclerosis
- To share the perspectives in large vessel vasculitis and atherosclerosis imaging, including novel radiopharmaceuticals

E. Lazzeri et al. (eds.), *Radionuclide Imaging of Infection and Inflammation*, https://doi.org/10.1007/978-3-030-62175-9_15

15.1 Introductory Background

The spectrum of vascular inflammatory disease ranges from atherosclerosis and hypertension (widespread conditions affecting large proportions of the population) to the vasculitis spectrum. In both conditions, inflammatory cells such as macrophages and T lymphocytes play a major role in initiating the disease and in its progression. Large vessel vasculitis (LVV) is defined as a disease mainly affecting the large arteries, with two major variants, Takayasu arteritis (TA) and giant cell arteritis (GCA) [1]. Vasculitis can be distributed locally in the branches of the internal and external carotid artery or the aorta and its main branches more centrally in the thorax. TA and GCA are different diseases with different age of onset, ethnic distribution, immunogenic background [2], anatomic distribution, and responsiveness to therapy [3, 4] of the affected arteries. In vasculitis, mural thickening usually involves the complete circumference of the vessel wall, whereas in atherosclerosis (vulnerable) plaque formation starts from a focal point rather than circumferentially. Atherosclerosis progresses over decades, causing major complications when the vessel wall lesion ruptures, giving rise to lumen-occlusive atherothrombosis which can result in cardiovascular events such as myocardial infarction, cerebrovascular accidents (CVA), and peripheral critical limb ischemia.

2-[^{18}F]-fluorodeoxyglucose ([^{18}F]FDG) positron emission tomography/computed tomography (PET/CT) is a functional imaging technique which is an established tool in oncology and has also demonstrated a role in the field of inflammatory diseases. [^{18}F]FDG PET is based on the ability to detect enhanced glucose uptake from high glycolytic activity of inflammatory cells in inflamed arterial walls and synovia/bursa [5]. This chapter describes the procedures and current status of [^{18}F]FDG PET/CT imaging in large vessel vasculitis and atherosclerosis. General background information on LVV and atherosclerosis, and procedural information such as patients' preparation, imaging protocols, scoring methodology, diagnostic and prognostic performance, and response monitoring are also given.

15.2 Large Vessel Vasculitis

15.2.1 Background

Large vessel vasculitis (LVV) are chronic idiopathic inflammatory diseases affecting the large- to medium-sized arteries [1]. Granulomatous infiltration of the vascular wall leads to segmental stenoses and aneurysm formations.

Two major variants with different clinical features and outcome are identified: giant cell arteritis (GCA) and Takayasu arteritis (TA). GCA is the most common primary vasculitis in western countries and typically concerns women older than 50 years [6], whereas TA is a rare vasculitis that typically concerns far-eastern and Asian women younger than 50 years [7]. In both the cases, aorta and its main branches may be involved, with several specificities: GCA may predominantly involve either cranial arteries (temporal and vertebral arteries mainly), and is named "*cGCA*," or large thoracic arteries (aorta, subclavian, and carotid arteries), which is named "*lvvGCA*." Overlapping between those two sub-entities is not systematic [8]. GCA is frequently associated with polymyalgia rheumatica (PMR) [9], and clinical symptoms depend on the GCA subtype. Headache, ocular symptoms, or claudication of the jaw are observed in *cGCA*, whereas *lvvGCA* frequently presents with nonspecific systemic inflammation. PMR-associated symptoms are characterized by inflammatory pain and stiffness of the scapular and pelvic girdles. Although *lvvGCA* is more prone to cause aortic aneurysms [10], overall disease-related morbidity is dominated by the *cGCA* complications. On the other hand, TA mainly involves thoracic arteries, with a particular tropism for pulmonary arteries. TA disease generally evolves in two phases: the former one being characterized by nonspecific systemic symptoms and the second one being characterized by vascular wall inflammation with vascular stenoses that may ultimately lead to severe hypertension and organ deficiencies [11].

Glucocorticoids (GC) are the first-line therapy for both the diseases. Frequent relapses and long-term GC side effects motivate the use of GC-sparing agents, such as disease-modifying anti-rheumatic drugs (methotrexate, leflunomide) or biological targeted treatments (tumor necrosis factor antagonist and monoclonal IL-6 receptor blockers) [12, 13].

15.2.2 Diagnostic Approach

Diagnostic tests of LVV are currently not well established. The traditional American College of Rheumatology criteria for LVV [14] are not systematically adopted in the clinical routine: first, they were initially designed for LVV classification; second, a majority of patients does not fulfill all the required criteria; and third, invasive procedures are currently avoided (biopsy of the temporal artery is frequently negative both in *cGCA* and in *lvvGCA*) [15–17]. Arteriography in TA is not relevant for early stage disease and involves a high radiation dose.

Thus, the diagnosis of LVV is rather based on a set of nonspecific clinical-biological features with suggestive imaging findings, and histopathological features for *cGCA*, when available. International efforts have recently been undertaken to promote the use of noninvasive whole-body imaging procedure such as [^{18}F]FDG PET/CT for the early diagnosis of LVV.

15.2.3 [^{18}F]FDG PET/CT

Positron emission tomography/computed tomography (PET/CT) is a nuclear hybrid imaging modality that combines emission-based functional imaging approach (PET) with a transmission-based morphological imaging approach (CT). [^{18}F]FDG is an analog of glucose capitalizing on the Warburg effect [18], which has been and still is being widely used in oncology. As inflammatory processes also demonstrate avidity for [^{18}F]FDG [19], the vascular wall inflammation of large vessels is observable on PET/CT. Current hybrid PET/CT devices have an intrinsic spatial resolution of 3–4 mm, thus making possible the visualization of large but also medium size arteries, such as the cranial ones (Fig. 15.1).

15.2.4 Patient Preparation and Imaging Protocol

Efforts have recently been made to standardize patient preparation and image acquisition in LVV [20]. A typical fasting of 6 h before the [^{18}F]FDG administration is required, and intense physical activities should be avoided within the 24 h (level II, grade B). Particularly for GCA patients, [^{18}F]FDG PET/CT should be performed ideally within the 3–7 days after the start of glucocorticoids, and serum glucose level should not exceed 7 mmol/L (126 mg/dL) for optimal image quality (level III, grade B) [20]. After [^{18}F]FDG injection into a venous branch of the arm, a minimum of 1-h relaxation time is recommended in a temperature-controlled room before image acquisition. If necessary, beta-blocking drugs may be orally administered to prevent [^{18}F]FDG uptake in brown fat. Whole-body [^{18}F]FDG PET/CT acquisition from the vertex of the skull to the knee in supine position is then performed, with the arms next to the body. For that purpose, a low-dose non-contrast CT scan is systematically performed for unbiased attenuation correction and anatomical localization, followed by PET acquisition. Optionally, arterial contrast-enhanced CT scan may complete the acquisition procedure, especially for the assessment of vascular wall thickening or stenosis.

15.2.5 Scoring [^{18}F]FDG PET/CT

For clinical routine, interpretation criteria should be based on a standardized 0–3 visual grading scale as illustrated in the Fig. 15.2 and Table 15.1, as follows: grade 0 = no uptake;

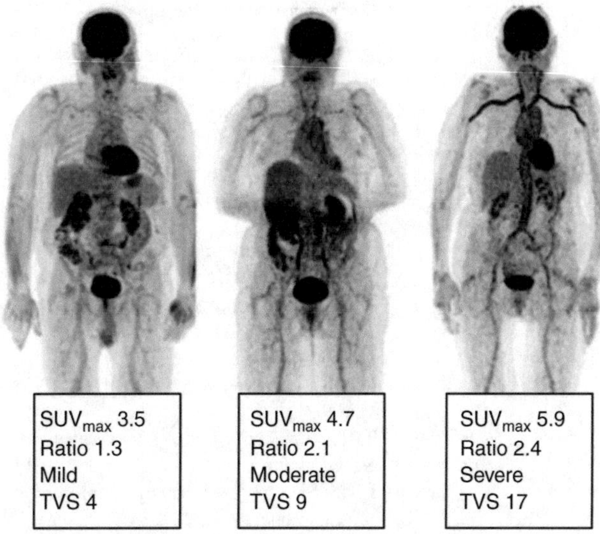

Fig. 15.2 [^{18}F]FDG-PET whole-body MIP images of patients with increasing severity *lvvGCA*. From left to right: low (grade 1), intermediate (grade 2), and high (grade 3) [^{18}F]FDG uptake patterns. SUV_{max} values refer to the thoracic aorta. Ratio is defined as the average SUV_{max} of the thoracic aorta divided by the liver region. The total vascular score (TVS) is also shown (highest for the rightmost patient). (*Reproduced with permission from* [20])

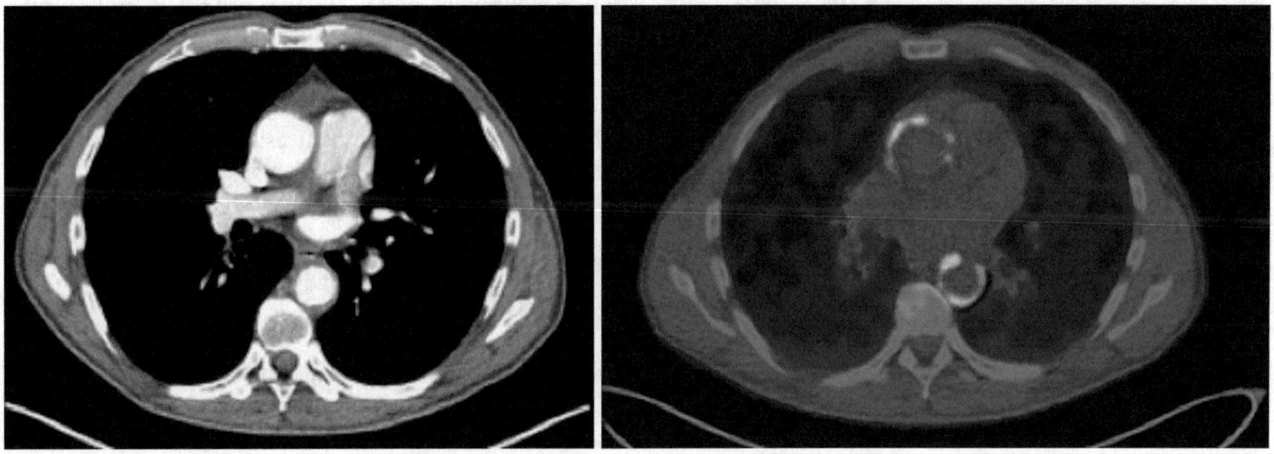

Fig. 15.1 [^{18}F]FDG PET/CTA of a 67-year-old man with CGA. On the left: transaxial view of the contrast chest CT, showing severely increased wall thickness (4.7 mm) of the descending aorta (30 × 31 mm in diameter); the ascending aorta (not shown) was enlarged (41 × 41 mm in diameter) and had moderately increased wall thickness (3.1 mm). On the right: fused transaxial image of the contrast chest CT and [^{18}F]FDG PET, showing markedly increased [^{18}F]FDG uptake (average SUV_{max} 5.5) in the ascending and descending aorta. (*Reproduced with permission from* [20])

Table 15.1 Proposed standardized [18F]FDG-PET/CT(A) interpretation criteria in large vessel vasculitis

Recommended PET interpretation criteria	
For clinical use	*LVV visual grading (GCA and TA)* Grade 0: No vascular uptake (≤mediastinum) Grade 1: Vascular uptake < liver uptake Grade 2: Vascular uptake = liver uptake, may be PET-positive Grade 3: Vascular uptake > liver uptake, considered PET-positive PMR associated visual assessment (only GCA) Grade 0: No uptake Grade 1: Uptake < liver uptake Grade 2: Uptake = liver uptake Grade 3: Uptake > liver uptake Increased metabolic activity of the scapular and pelvic girdles Increased metabolic activity of the knee bursae and capsule Increased metabolic activity at the site of the cervical and lumbar interspinous bursae Increased metabolic activity of the trochanteric and ischial bursae
In general for research only	*PET semiquantitative analysis* [a] Target: Average SUV_{max} artery of the vascular ROIs Blood pool: Average SUV_{max} of several vein ROIs TBR = (average SUV_{max} artery)/(average SUV_{max} vein) Liver: SUV_{max} of a liver region, preferably the right lobe TBR = (average SUV_{max} artery/(SUV_{max} of a liver region) Vascular targets: – Carotid arteries – Subclavia arteries – Axillary arteries – Vertebral arteries – Ascending aorta – Aortic arch – Pulmonary arteries – Abdominal aorta Joints: Scapulae and pelvic girdles, knees, cervical and lumbar Interspinous bursae, trochanteric and ischial bursae
For clinical use	*Contrast-enhanced (PET/)CTA* Regular vascular wall thickness (mm) Contrast enhancement Presence of stenosis and/or aneurysm

TBR target-to-background ratio, *SUV* standardized uptake value, *ROI* region of interest, *TA* Takayasu arteritis, *PMR* polymyalgia rheumatica, *CGA* giant cell arteritis

[a]SUV using EARL criteria (Boellaard R, Delgado-Bolton R, Oyen WJ, Giammarile F, Tatsch K, Eschner W, et al. FDG-PET/CT: EANM procedure guidelines for tumour imaging: version 2.0. Eur J Nucl Med Mol Imaging. 2015;42:328–54). (*Reproduced with permission from* [20], *slightly modified*)

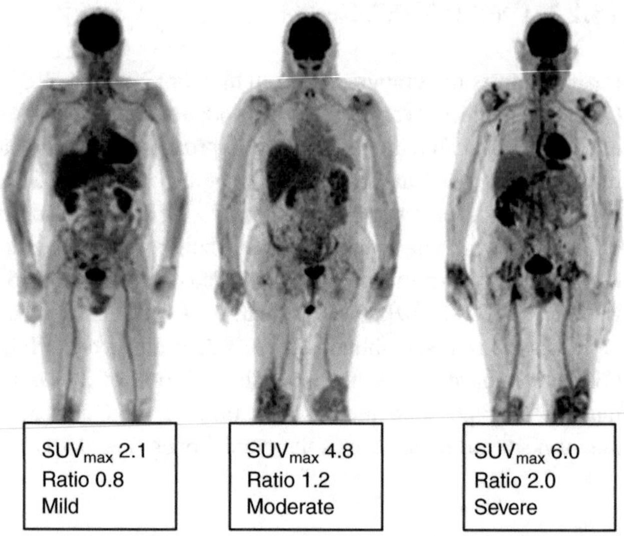

Fig. 15.3 [18F]FDG-PET whole-body MIP images of patients by PMR, with increasing severity of [18F]FDG uptake in the large joint regions (from left to right). SUV_{max} values refer to the shoulders. Ratio is defined as the average SUV_{max} in the shoulders divided by the liver region. The total number and intensity of affected joints are highest for the rightmost patient. (*Reproduced with permission from* [20])

grade 1 = vascular uptake inferior to liver; grade 2 = vascular uptake equal to liver; grade 3 = vascular uptake superior to liver uptake [20]. In active large vessel vasculitis, a smooth linear and segmental pattern of grade 3 visual [18F]FDG uptake in the wall of aorta (thoracic mainly) or its main branches (subclavian, carotid or vertebral arteries) is considered a positive [18F]FDG PET. Under treatment, a grade 2 may be possibly considered as positive [20].

Possible [18F]FDG uptake in the temporal arteries should also be carefully evaluated, a feature that can be better assessed on recent time-of-flight PET/CT systems [21, 22]. In GCA patients, PMR is frequently associated and should be searched for, and visually scored using the same grading system (Fig. 15.3 and Table 15.1). Peri-articular [18F]FDG uptake is typically seen in scapular and pelvic girdles, associated with less specific interspinous vertebral or trochanteric/ischial bursa uptakes. Semi-quantitative interpretation criteria based on vascular to background ratios (liver or vascular blood pool) are used for investigational purpose and are currently not validated in the clinical setting [20].

15.2.6 Diagnostic Performance of [18F]FDG PET/CT

The diagnostic performance parameters of [18F]FDG PET/CT are overall good in LVV. Meta-analyses mainly based on retrospective data provided sensitivities of 80–83.3% for *lvvGCA* [23, 24] and 70.1–87% for TA [25, 26], whereas specificities were 89% for *lvvGCA* and 73–93% for

TA. Pooling GCA and TA provided 76% of sensitivity and 93% specificity for the diagnosis of LVV [27]. An interesting European retrospective case–control study showed that considering [^{18}F]FDG PET/CT in the diagnostic workflow of GCA patients impacted the patient management in one third of the cases [28]. However, a systematic review specifically performed for the European League Against Rheumatism (EULAR) recently highlighted the lack of prospective studies using [^{18}F]FDG PET for the diagnosis of LVV [29], and the related recommendations published by the EULAR for the use of [^{18}F]FDG PET in LVV are thus mainly based on consensus of experts [30]. Based on those recommendation, [^{18}F]FDG PET/CT may be used as an early imaging test to support the diagnosis of *lvvGCA* and should be considered as an alternative to MRI for the diagnosis of TA [30].

Although ultrasound or MRI should be preferred for the diagnosis of *cGCA*, two very recent works highlighted the good diagnostic performance of time-of-flight PET/CT for the detection of *cGCA* specifically, with sensitivities of 71–82% and specificities of 91–100% [21, 22]. Finally, comparison with other imaging modalities remains scarce. Ultrasound has a high level of evidence for the diagnosis of *cGCA* and is currently considered as the modality of choice in this setting [30]. For *lvvGCA,* there is currently no evidence of superiority of one modality to the others. The few comparative studies between PET and CTA or MRI showed weak concordance between vascular thickness or contrast-enhancement and [^{18}F]FDG uptake at the vascular regional level [31–34]. One explanation would be the typical dyssynchrony between morphological changes (thickening reduction), which can be very delayed, and early metabolic changes observed on [^{18}F]FDG PET/CT. In TA, due to the age of onset and the need of long-term follow-up, [^{18}F]FDG PET/CT should be considered as an alternative to MRI [30].

15.2.7 Prognostic Value of [^{18}F]FDG PET/CT and Assessment of Response to Treatments (Conventional and New Therapies)

Currently, [^{18}F]FDG PET/CT is not recommended for monitoring treatment response in LVV. Typically, vascular [^{18}F]FDG uptake rapidly decreases after several days of GC therapy [35]. However, long-term residual vascular [^{18}F]FDG uptake has been frequently observed in many GCA patients despite clinical and biological remission [32, 36]. The pathophysiological meaning of this residual uptake under GC remains unknown, possibly due to physiological vascular remodeling or subclinical residual disease. The frequently observed weak correlation between clinical-biological features and [^{18}F]FDG PET/CT findings adds interpretation difficulties (for review see [24, 37]). Dose of GC treatment influenced the signal on [^{18}F]FDG PET/CT. When treatment is increased, there is significant reduction in disease activity by imaging, clinical, and inflammatory markers ($P \leq 0.01$ for each) [38]. When treatment is unchanged, disease activity remained similarly unchanged over 6-month intervals. When treatment is reduced, PET activity significantly worsens ($P = 0.02$) but clinical and serologic activity will not significantly change [38].

Treatment of GCA and TA with tocilizumab and tumor necrosis factor inhibitors resulted in significant improvement in imaging and clinical assessments of disease activity, but only rarely did the assessments both become normal [38]. Furthermore, it has been shown that an alternative strategy using a short-term treatment with tocilizumab can be proposed to spare GC for the treatment of GCA [39]. Very few studies focused on the risk of relapse based on [^{18}F]FDG PET/CT, and the results are discrepant: in their prospective study including 35 *lvvGCA* patients, Blockmans et al. did not find significant relationship between baseline PET and the risk of relapse at 3 months [36]; in their study including 17 confirmed LVV patients, Dellavedova et al. showed changes in [^{18}F]FDG PET findings to predict the clinical course of the disease [40]; in TA, Tezuka et al. retrospectively found [^{18}F]FDG PET/CT to outperform biological features for the assessment of disease activity in TA relapsing patients [41]. Finally, [^{18}F]FDG aortic uptake has been shown to be associated with late aortic complications [42, 43].

Key Learning Points

- [^{18}F]FDG PET/CT is of value for diagnostic purposes in LVV patients and demonstrated high accuracy.
- Prognostic value of [^{18}F]FDG PET/CT and assessment of response to treatments (conventional and new therapies) is valuable, but needs additional evaluation.
- Standardized patient preparation, image acquisition, and scoring methodology in LVV is up-most important.
- Be aware of pitfalls, such as the long-standing use of glucocorticoids that may result in false-negative findings.

15.3 Atherosclerosis

15.3.1 Background

Atherosclerosis is a disease of the arterial wall with endothelial dysfunction, expression of adhesion molecules, and binding of circulating inflammatory cells to the endothelium. Progression of these vessel wall changes over the time leads to the development of atherosclerotic plaques. When looking more specifically at those arterial plaques, the so-called high-risk plaques are more vulnerable (prone) to rupture and are characterized by larger invasion of inflammatory cells, necrotic lipid core, microcalcifications, neovascularization, and a thinning fibrous cap compared to low-risk plaques [44, 45]. It is currently well accepted that inflammation plays a crucial role in the different stages of atherosclerotic plaque development and especially in the evolution from a stable plaque to an instable plaque. The latter might, by rupturing and, consecutively, releasing embolic material, lead to clinical manifestations such as myocardial infarction and stroke [46, 47].

15.3.2 Diagnostic Approach

In current clinical routine, diagnosis of atherosclerosis still relies mainly on the assessment of the degree of intraluminal arterial stenosis using invasive angiography or CT angiography. However, angiography in general suffers from substantial limitations, as it does not image the vessel wall including information on the plaque vulnerability. Therefore, there is a recognized need for noninvasive, highly sensitive, measures to identify those high-risk plaques, which might be, at least partly, undetected by all "conventional" imaging methods such as CT or MRI. Therefore, since more than two decades, a scientific focus was set on in vivo molecular imaging of signature pathological mechanisms in atherosclerosis by using PET. Numerous studies were published on all different aspects of PET imaging in atherosclerosis, providing insights into the biological processes within an arterial wall lesion, improving risk stratification, and enabling the evaluation of novel therapies and interventions.

15.3.3 [^{18}F]FDG PET/CT

[^{18}F]FDG is currently the most commonly used and evaluated tracer for PET imaging of atherosclerosis (Fig. 15.4). The use of [^{18}F]FDG in atherosclerosis imaging is based on the high glucose metabolism of activated macrophages, which are part of the inflammatory changes in more advanced arterial plaques [48, 49]. Arterial wall [^{18}F]FDG uptake was indeed shown to be related to the macrophage content of atherosclerotic plaques, to well-known clinical risk factors for atherosclerosis, and to emerging cardiovascular events [50–52], and it is well established as an endpoint surrogate marker in several interventional studies [47, 53]. However, despite its proven value in atherosclerosis imaging, the clinical use of [^{18}F]FDG is limited in atherosclerosis due to its accumula-

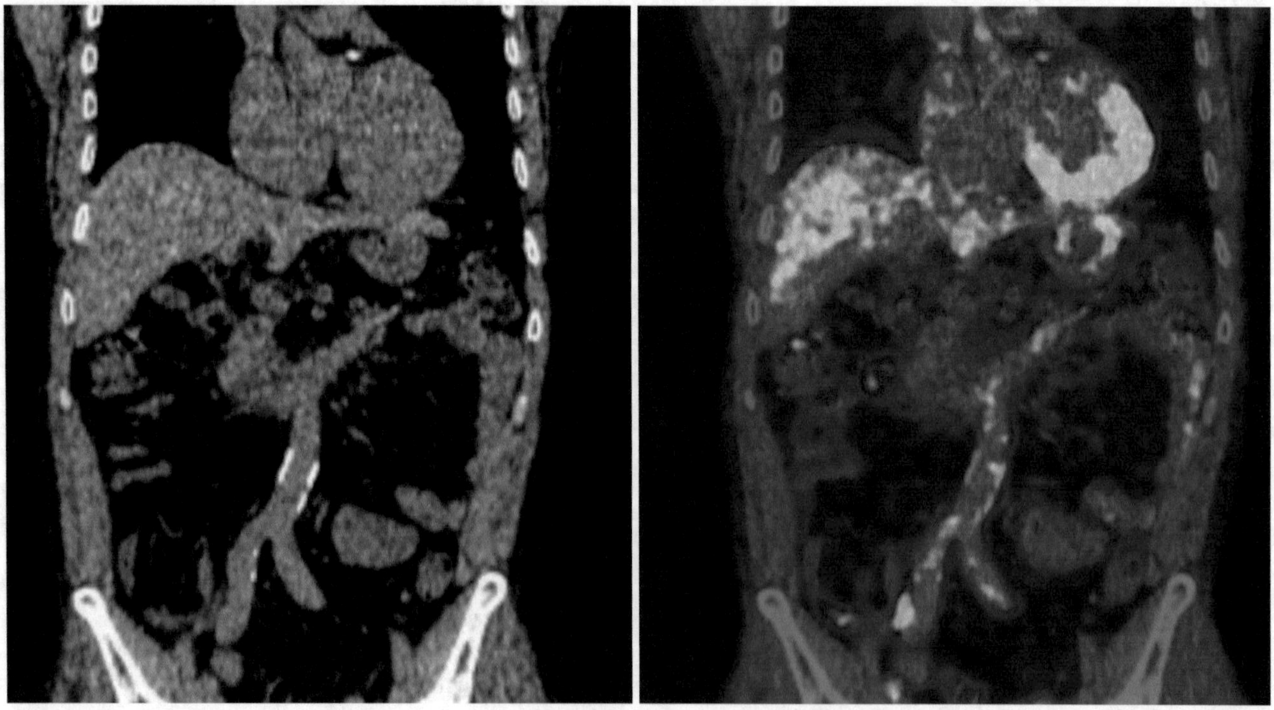

Fig. 15.4 Coronal views from a [^{18}F]FDG PET/CT scan in a 63-year-old man with medical history of prior cardiovascular disease history (previously submitted to coronary-artery bypass graft), now presenting with active atherosclerosis of the abdominal aorta. The low-dose CT component of the scan (left panel) shows macrocalcifications affecting different portions of the abdominal aorta, some of them with increased [^{18}F]FDG uptake indicating inflammatory atherosclerotic process (right panel)

tion in any active tissue like muscles, inflammatory lymph nodes, cancer tissue, etc. For example, uptake in lymph nodes or the myocardium may cause spillover of activity into the target tissue (atherosclerotic changes of the arterial wall) and may therefore hamper accurate quantification. Furthermore, up to now clearly defined and well-evaluated cut-off values for arterial [^{18}F]FDG uptake to accurately discriminate plaques at risk for rupture from more stable plaques are still lacking. For this reason, investigations continue to explore other PET tracers to visualize plaque inflammation or other plaque characteristics that might have a close correlation to plaque rupture.

15.3.4 Patient Preparation and Imaging Protocol

Over the last years, several efforts have been made to overcome at least some of the well-known limitations of [^{18}F]FDG PET in atherosclerosis imaging. In this scenario, it was also attempted to standardize the practice of arterial PET imaging in nuclear medicine centers and thereby to facilitate (multicenter) clinical studies on the imaging of atherosclerosis with PET. A position paper on atherosclerosis imaging with [^{18}F]FDG PET published in 2016 by the Cardiovascular Committee of the European Association of Nuclear Medicine (EANM) stated and addressed the limitations of [^{18}F]FDG PET in atherosclerosis [54], as summarized here below.

The acquisition of PET images should not to be started earlier than 2 h (circulation time) after injection of the tracer, to assure an adequate compromise between a low background (blood) and a high target (plaque) signal. Consequently, this would allow a reliable quantification of [^{18}F]FDG uptake in the arterial vessel wall and/or plaques. Furthermore, a circulation time of approximately 2 h is considered as an acceptable duration of the PET study for patients [54]. Considering a desired circulation time of 2 h for arterial imaging, the EANM Cardiovascular Committee recommends an injected activity of [^{18}F]FDG between 3 and 4 MBq/kg body weight for atherosclerotic plaque imaging, to allow sufficient image quality. In settings of patient screening and/or repeated PET studies, lower [^{18}F]FDG activities are required to further limit the patient's total radiation exposure. From a technical point of view, new PET technologies like digital PET might facilitate that approach [54]. Pre-scan glucose levels lower than approximately 130 mg/dL (approximately 7.0–7.2 mmol/L) are recommended for [^{18}F]FDG PET imaging in atherosclerosis. If these blood glucose levels cannot be achieved by other approaches (fasting protocol, pre-scan diet, etc.), correction of the vascular [^{18}F]FDG uptake according to the EANM recommendations for oncological PET imaging may be considered [54]. However, this "mathematical" correction clearly needs to be more extensively evaluated and, finally, validated in the setting of arterial wall imaging with [^{18}F]FDG PET (for more detailed information see [54]).

15.3.5 Parameters for Quantification of Radiotracer Uptake in Atherosclerotic Plaques

For the quantification of [^{18}F]FDG uptake in atherosclerotic plaques, application of target-to-background (TBR) analysis rather than SUV is recommended. The use of a ratio between two measurements limits the effects on signal quantification of errors in patient weight, in the activity of the injected radiotracer and of the imaging time point. Furthermore, comparison of the arterial [^{18}F]FDG uptake between sequential PET studies requires any effort to compare the same arterial territories. This is due to the intrinsically variable [^{18}F]FDG uptake patterns in different arterial regions, which may significantly bias the results of the studies—mainly those investigating the effect of interventions on arterial [^{18}F]FDG uptake. Different uptake parameters were previously evaluated and applied in several studies on atherosclerotic PET imaging [TBR_{max}, TBR_{mean}, most diseased segment (MDS), active segment (AS)]. The choice of one or more of these parameters depends mainly on the aim of the study (for more detailed information see [54], Fig. 15.5).

Reconstruction parameters for PET images may influence SUV and TBR quantification. The implementation of dedi-

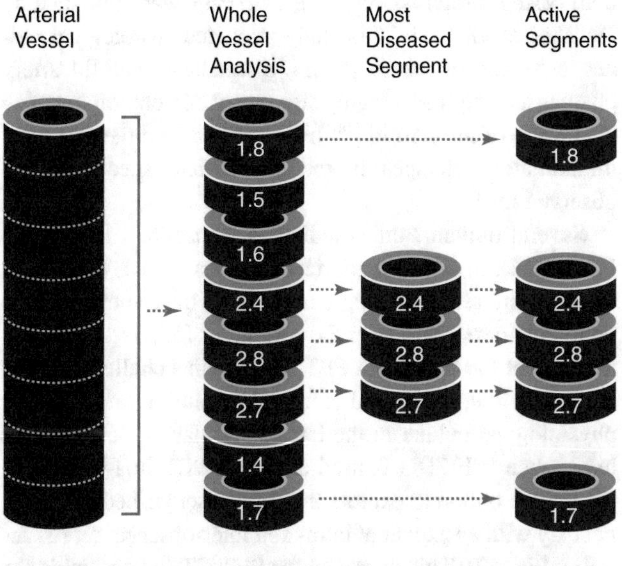

Fig. 15.5 Current most frequently used approaches to quantifying arterial [^{18}F]FDG uptake for clinical studies. All values given are maximal target to background ratios (TBR_{max}). A TBR threshold of >1.6 was considered significant for the active segment analysis. The mean TBR_{max} of the whole vessel would be 1.99, and the mean TBR_{max} of the most diseased segment would be 2.63. (*Reproduced with permission from* [54])

cated PET acquisition, processing, and reconstruction protocols for arterial imaging is therefore recommended (for more detailed information see [54]).

15.3.6 [^{18}F]FDG PET as Surrogate Endpoint in Interventional Studies

Measurement of [^{18}F]FDG uptake in atherosclerotic plaques is highly reproducible between PET studies and provides robust information on beneficial or deleterious effects of the drug under evaluation. Changes in [^{18}F]FDG uptake are detectable as early as 3–4 months after the initiation of drug treatment. In contrast, morphological changes (for instance in plaque volume, as detected by CT and/or MRI) may be visualized significantly later within the disease process (12–24 months). For recommendations regarding the arterial territories to be analyzed depending on the different study settings, see [54].

15.3.7 Diagnostic Performance

One of the very first studies evaluating the diagnostic performance of [^{18}F]FDG PET in atherosclerosis was published by Rudd et al. in 2002 [55]. Patients with symptomatic carotid atherosclerosis were imaged with [^{18}F]FDG PET/CT and showed a 27% higher [^{18}F]FDG uptake in the symptomatic plaque compared to the asymptomatic contralateral lesions [55]. Four years later, the second milestone publication in the field of atherosclerosis imaging with PET was published by Tawakol et al. [51]. This study provided histological evidence for the increased [^{18}F]FDG uptake in carotid artery plaques as a high and highly significant correlation between the degree of the carotid [^{18}F]FDG uptake, and the degree of inflammatory changes in the histological specimen was observed [51].

Several human studies indicated a specific arterial [^{18}F]FDG uptake in different arterial territories such as the carotid arteries, different aortic regions, the iliac, the femoral and the popliteal arteries and even the coronaries [56, 57]. However, imaging of the latter with PET still remains challenging due the rather low spatial and temporal resolution and the high physiological uptake in the left ventricular myocardium, at least when [^{18}F]FDG is used as tracer. PET imaging offers the unique option to explore multiple vascular beds simultaneously with an excellent intra- and inter-observer reproducibility [56, 57]. This is crucial for PET/CT to be reliable for studying atherosclerotic plaques, especially when using this technique in interventional trials as well as for tracking changes occurring within the plaque over time.

With regard to clinical cardiovascular risk factors, arterial [^{18}F]FDG uptake was shown to be increased in patients with an increased number of cardiovascular risk factors and with preexisting distinct diseases, such as diabetes mellitus and the metabolic syndrome [58, 59]. Tahara et al. showed that carotid inflammation was associated with waist circumference, hypertension, glucose intolerance, and the metabolic syndrome [59]. Furthermore, in patients with type 2 diabetes or impaired glucose tolerance, Kim et al. reported higher arterial [^{18}F]FDG uptake values in both the study groups compared to controls [58]. Furthermore, an increasing prevalence of diabetes with increments of maximum [^{18}F]FDG uptake values as depicted by tertiles was observed in this study [58]. Two prospective trials published by Bucerius et al. confirmed these findings by showing a significant correlation between the carotid [^{18}F]FDG uptake and hypertension, obesity, higher patients age, smoking, and male gender [52]. Strikingly, it was also observed that, with an increasing number of components of the metabolic syndrome, [^{18}F]FDG uptake in the carotid arteries increased significantly [52]. A highly significant association between [^{18}F]FDG uptake in the carotid arteries and type 2 diabetes mellitus was also reported by this group [60]. In addition, a significant relation between the arterial [^{18}F]FDG uptake and increasing patient's fasting blood glucose values was also observed, a fact which emphasizes the importance of an appropriate treatment regimen in patients suffering from diabetes [60].

Only few studies have been published so far regarding defined [^{18}F]FDG uptake threshold values for identifying patients at risk for emerging cardiovascular events. This is to some degree due to the fact that those studies need to follow a well-designed and, above all, a well-powered study protocol. In an effort to at least partly overcome this shortcoming, van der Valk et al. analyzed the arterial [^{18}F]FDG uptake in the carotid arteries and the ascending aorta of 83 subjects, which were classified into three groups: healthy controls, patients at increased for cardiovascular disease (CVD), and patients with known CVD [20]. They reported [^{18}F]FDG uptake thresholds for healthy subjects, which are exceeded by >52% of risk factor patients and >67% of CVD patients. This remained true, regardless of readout vessel (carotid artery or aorta), signal quantification method, or the use of background correction. However, due to overlap between subject categories and the relatively small population studied, the results of this study are only limited generalizable and larger, well-designed studies regarding this topic are still lacking [61].

15.3.8 Prognostic Value and Clinical Relevance

Several efforts have been made over the last years to evaluate the predictive value of arterial [^{18}F]FDG uptake and emerging cardiovascular events. In a study by Rominger et al. published in 2009 on arterial [^{18}F]FDG PET for the identification of patients at risk for subsequent cardiovascular events, a cohort of 932 cancer patients who underwent a whole-body [^{18}F]FDG PET/CT were retrospectively analyzed [62]. Based on the results of the study, an increased arterial TBR ≥1.7 was identified to predict the cardiovascular risk in those patients after a median follow-up time of 29 months. Arterial [^{18}F]FDG uptake had a greater prognostic value than did arterial calcified plaque burden [62]. In 2012, Marnane et al. included 60 patients (25 stroke, 29 TIA, 6 retinal embolism) in their study, aiming to investigate the relation between the [^{18}F]FDG uptake in the carotids and stroke recurrence [63]; 13 (22%) of their patients suffered from stroke recurrence within the follow-up period of 90 days [63]. The ipsilateral carotid plaque was significantly higher in patients suffering from recurrent stroke compared to asymptomatic patients. Furthermore, corrected for several other variables, the mean plaque [^{18}F]FDG uptake was the only independent predictor of stroke recurrence [63].

A more recent article by Kelly et al. reported a multicenter prospective cohort study [BIOVASC (Biomarkers/Imaging Vulnerable Atherosclerosis in Symptomatic Carotid disease)] of patients with carotid stenosis and recent stroke/transient ischemic attack with 90-day follow-up [64]. They analyzed the association of SUV_{max} with all recurrent nonprocedural stroke (before and after PET) and with recurrent stroke after PET only. In the pooled cohort (n = 196), 37 recurrent strokes occurred (29 before and 8 after PET). Plaque SUV_{max} was higher in patients with all recurrence ($P < 0.0001$) and post-PET recurrence ($P = 0.009$). The fully adjusted hazard ratio of any recurrent stroke was 2.19 (CI, 1.41–3.39; $P < 0.001$) and for post-PET recurrent stroke it was 4.57 (CI, 1.5–13.96; $P = 0.008$). Recurrent stroke risk increased across SUV_{max} quartiles (log-rank $P = 0.003$). The area under receiver operating curve for all recurrence was 0.70 (CI, 0.59–0.78) and for post-PET recurrence was 0.80 (CI, 0.64–0.96). They concluded that plaque inflammation-related [^{18}F]FDG uptake independently predicted future recurrent stroke post-PET, and [^{18}F]FDG PET may improve patient selection for carotid revascularization, and the study suggested that anti-inflammatory agents may have benefit for poststroke vascular prevention [64]. The group of Tawakol and colleagues in Boston evaluated the incremental value of arterial [^{18}F]FDG PET in predicting CVD beyond traditional cardiovascular risk factors [65]. They included 53 individuals who underwent an [^{18}F]FDG PET/CT and defined CVD events as stroke, transient ischemic attack, acute coronary syndrome, revascularization, new-onset angina, peripheral arterial disease, heart failure, or CVD death. The TBR, as measured in the ascending aorta, strongly predicted subsequent CVD independent of traditional risk factors (hazard ratio: 4.71; $P < 0.001$) and (hazard ratio: 4.13; $P = 0.004$) after further adjustment for the coronary calcium score. Furthermore, arterial TBR was also inversely associated with the onset of CVD events (β −0.096; $P < 0.0001$), with as higher the aortic TBR as earlier the CVD event emerged [65].

For investigating the performance of arterial [^{18}F]FDG uptake as an independent prognostic indicator of cardiovascular events and to evaluate its incremental predictive value in addition to the Framingham risk score (FRS) and carotid intima-media thickness (CIMT), Moon et al. analyzed 1089 asymptomatic adults who underwent [^{18}F]FDG PET/CT [66]. High carotid [^{18}F]FDG uptake and high CIMT were identified as independent predictors of events. By adding carotid [^{18}F]FDG uptake, but not CIMT, to the FRS, the time-dependent area under the receiver-operating characteristic curve could be significantly increased from 0.60 to 0.73 ($P = 0.04$). Therefore, high carotid [^{18}F]FDG uptake not only predicts cardiovascular events independent of traditional risk factors and CIMT in asymptomatic adults, but may also add to risk stratification beyond the FRS and CIMT [66].

One of the latest studies on the prognostic value of arterial [^{18}F]FDG PET was published by Cho et al. in 2017 [67]. In this study the predictive value of [^{18}F]FDG uptake in the large arteries (carotid arteries, ascending and abdominal aorta) for coronary artery calcium (CAC) progression in asymptomatic individuals (n = 96) was evaluated. In 31 subjects (32.3%) with CAC progression, significantly higher TBR values in all of the three arteries analyzed compared to patients without CAC progression were observed. Besides the peak TBR in the abdominal aorta, age ≥58 years and a positive baseline CAC were significantly associated with CAC progression as revealed by multivariate regression analysis. However, a higher TBR peak of the abdominal aorta (≥2.11) was only associated with CAC progression in patients with a negative baseline CAC. In those with a positive baseline CAC, only the amount of baseline CAC showed a significant association with CAC progression [67].

15.3.9 Response Monitoring (Conventional and New Drugs)

Up to now, arterial [^{18}F]FDG PET has been used as a surrogate endpoint marker to monitor changes in arterial inflammation in several trials, of which some will be described hereinafter. One of the very first studies in this regard was published in 2006, when patients were randomly assigned to a diet-only or to a statin group and monitored by [^{18}F]FDG PET at baseline and at the 3 months follow-up. Low-dose simvastatin led to a significant decline of the arterial [^{18}F]FDG uptake, whereas in the diet-only group, no significant change at all could be observed [47]. In another study evaluating the effects of statins on arterial inflammation, the effect of 5 mg per day atorvastatin versus 20 mg per day was compared. As evaluated by [^{18}F]FDG PET imaging, treatment with 20 mg atorvastatin per day yielded a significant reduction of [^{18}F]FDG uptake in the ascending aorta and the femoral artery after 6 months of treatment. On the contrary, changes of the arterial [^{18}F]FDG PET signal in patients receiving 5 mg atorvastatin per day led to not statistically significant changes [53]. This dose-dependent effect of atorvastatin on arterial inflammation was confirmed in a consecutive well-designed prospective multicenter trial; 77 patients without high-dose statin treatment but with a cardiovascular risk profile or known atherosclerosis randomly received either 10 mg or 80 mg of atorvastatin per day and underwent arterial [^{18}F]FDG PET/CT at baseline as well as at 4 and 12 weeks [68]. A significant reduction in the index vessel [^{18}F]FDG uptake compared with baseline was observed at 4 weeks in both groups with an additional relative reduction at 12 weeks. However, this decrease was only observed in the high-dose group receiving 80 mg of atorvastatin per day. It has to be pointed out that changes in TBR did not correlate with lipid profile changes indicating an independent effect of statins on vascular inflammation [68].

Over the last decade, the effects of several other drugs besides statins on arterial inflammation have been evaluated with [^{18}F]FDG PET. In 2011, the results of a large double-blind multicenter trial on the effect of dalcetrapib, a modulator of the cholesteryl ester transfer protein (CETP), to raise high-density lipoprotein cholesterol (HDL-C) were published by Fayad et al. [69]. Patients with or without high risk of coronary heart disease were randomly assigned to dalcetrapib 600 mg per day or placebo for 24 months. Co-primary endpoint besides the MRI-assessed indices was the assessment of arterial inflammation with [^{18}F]FDG PET/CT within an index vessel (right carotid, left carotid, or ascending thoracic aorta) after 6 months. After 24 months, MRI revealed a reduction in total vessel enlargement in patients receiving dalcetrapib compared with those receiving placebo, with an absolute change from baseline relative to placebo of −4.01 mm^2 (nominal $P = 0.04$). Regarding the PET data, the index vessel most-diseased-segment TBR was not different between groups. In addition, the carotid artery analysis revealed a 7% reduction in most-diseased-segment TBR in the dalcetrapib group; however, this decline in arterial inflammation did not reach statistical significance ($P = 0.07$) [69].

The systemic anti-inflammatory properties of losmapimod (a p38 mitogen-activated protein kinase inhibitor) were demonstrated in 2012 with [^{18}F]FDG PET. Losmapimod reduced vascular inflammation in the most inflamed regions, concurrent with a reduction in inflammatory biomarkers and [^{18}F]FDG uptake in visceral fat in patients with atherosclerosis [70]. The results of a randomized, placebo-controlled trial on a p38 mitogen-activated protein kinase (p38MAPK, an important element of inflammatory pathways in atherothrombosis) inhibitor, failed to show a significant reduction of atherosclerotic plaque inflammation as assessed by [^{18}F]FDG PET imaging [71]. In contrast, further stressing the beneficial effects of statins on arterial inflammation, statin intensification was associated with significant reduction of hs-CRP and arterial inflammation in active slices as compared to placebo [71]. The results of a randomized controlled trial on the anti-inflammatory effects of dipeptidyl peptidase (DPP)-4 inhibitors were published by a Dutch group were published in 2017. DPP-4 inhibitors are a class of oral anti-diabetic agents with potentially beneficial cardiovascular effects [72, 73]. After 26 weeks of treatment with the DPP-4 inhibitor linagliptin in 45 patients with early type 2 diabetes but without CVD and naive to anti-diabetic treatment, linagliptin led to a significant decrease ($P = 0.015$) in arterial [^{18}F]FDG uptake compared to placebo [73].

Key Learning Points

- [^{18}F]FDG is currently the most commonly used and evaluated tracer for PET imaging of atherosclerosis, but still is in the clinical investigation phase.
- Standardized patient preparation, image acquisition, and scoring methodology in atherosclerosis imaging with [^{18}F]FDG PET/CT are up-most important.
- [^{18}F]FDG uptake independently predicted cardiovascular events and is highly related to risk factors.
- Arterial [^{18}F]FDG PET has been used as a surrogate endpoint marker to monitor changes in arterial inflammation.

15.4 Perspectives in Large Vessel Vasculitis and Atherosclerosis Imaging

The present chapter provides background information and recommendations to assist imaging specialists and clinicians of [^{18}F]FDG PET procedurals in patients with suspected LVV and PMR. Based on the present clinical data, [^{18}F]FDG PET/CT(A) has an important role in the diagnosis of extracranial vascular involvement in patients with LVV/PMR, but additional randomized studies are needed to support this conclusion. Visual methods are most commonly used, but semiquantitative methods such as the vascular/blood ratio and vascular/liver ratio using SUVs are increasingly being used. The role of [^{18}F]FDG PET/CT in patient management and in treatment monitoring must be further established. When to use [^{18}F]FDG PET/CT in the diagnosis, in the follow-up, and how often, and what time point after [^{18}F]FDG injection (1 or 2 h)? The use of vasculitis-specific tracers, directed against cells/proteins involved in and unique for the pathophysiology of LVV and PMR, should be investigated.

The addition of CTA to PET provides high-resolution imaging of vascular morphology that can potentially improve diagnostic accuracy, but more importantly provides information on the presence of possible complications such as stenosis, organ ischemia, aneurysm formation, and dissection. New developments in camera systems, such as PET/MRI, enable us to combine metabolism or other molecular targets (PET) with vascular tissue layer characterization (MRI), including a reduction in radiation dose. New digital camera techniques or novel reconstruction of the skull that enable visualization of the superficial cranial arteries, which will result in better comparison of local LVV with TABLE [21]. These were important recommendation to tackle in previous consensus papers [20, 30].

[^{18}F]FDG PET imaging in atherosclerosis revealed promising results, but several limitations still prevent its application in clinical routine. Besides limitations of the PET technique per se, like the rather low spatial and temporal resolution that are obviously "tracer-independent," [^{18}F]FDG might not be the most optimal tracer for assessing arterial inflammation due to its rather low specificity. In this regard, other PET tracers might be superior to [^{18}F]FDG, and, in addition, they might also be more suitable for imaging of coronary artery disease as they are not physiologically taken up by the myocardium as is [^{18}F]FDG.

Two of the most intensively evaluated tracers beyond [^{18}F]FDG are ^{68}Ga-DOTATATE and ^{18}F-sodium fluoride (^{18}F-NaF). ^{68}Ga-labeled somatostatin receptor tracers like ^{68}Ga-DOTATATE were introduced into clinical routine for imaging of neuroendocrine tumors (NET). Similarly as observed in NET, certain somatostatin receptors are also overexpressed in activated macrophages and damaged endothelial cells, in which they facilitate modulating inflammation and angiogenesis [74–76]. One of the most important studies on arterial ^{68}Ga-DOTATATE imaging was published by Tarkin et al. in 2017 [76]. They not only confirmed ^{68}Ga-DOTATATE binding in macrophages and excised carotid plaques but also compared ^{68}Ga-DOTATATE with [^{18}F]FDG PET imaging in patients with atherosclerosis [76]. ^{68}Ga-DOTATATE showed a specific ligand binding to somatostatin receptors in CD68-positive macrophage-rich carotid plaque regions, and, most strikingly, ^{68}Ga-DOTATATE uptake not only identified culprit versus non-culprit arteries in patients with acute coronary syndrome as well as in transient ischemic attack/stroke but also predicted high-risk features in coronary computed tomography. On the other hand, also [^{18}F]FDG correctly differentiates culprit from non-culprit carotid lesions and high-risk from low-risk coronary arteries, but due to the well-known physiological myocardial [^{18}F]FDG uptake, there was uninterpretable coronary [^{18}F]FDG information in up to 64% of the patients [76].

The second PET tracer gaining more and more interest over the past years in imaging of atherosclerosis is ^{18}F-NaF. ^{18}F-NaF is primarily used in clinical routine for imaging of benign and malignant osseous lesions and has nowadays been reported as a useful marker of valvular and vascular calcification activity in patients with aortic stenosis [77–80]. One of the milestone studies regarding ^{18}F-NaF imaging in atherosclerosis was published in 2014 by Joshi et al. [80]. Patients with myocardial infarction and stable angina underwent both ^{18}F-NaF and [^{18}F]FDG PET/CT, as well as invasive coronary angiography. In the majority of patients with myocardial infarction (93%), the highest ^{18}F-NaF uptake was observed in the culprit plaque (Fig. 15.6). Not unexpectedly, [^{18}F]FDG uptake in the coronary arteries was frequently masked due to overspill from the myocardial [^{18}F]FDG uptake. Furthermore, if well analyzable, no significant difference between culprit and non-culprit plaques was seen with [^{18}F]FDG [80]. Several other promising PET tracers are currently evaluated for the identification of different targets within the atherosclerotic disease process—in both the preclinical and the clinical setting. It has to be seen whether one or more of those tracers will further facilitate noninvasive imaging of atherosclerosis including high-risk (vulnerable) arterial plaques.

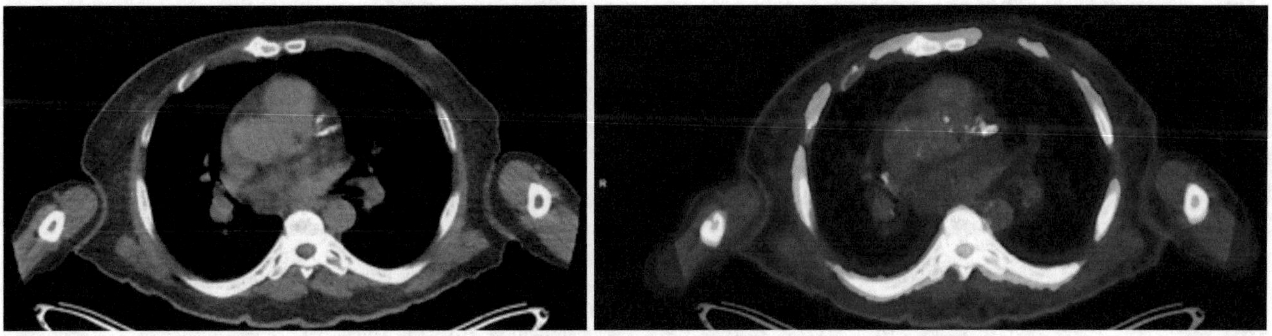

Fig. 15.6 Midthoracic transaxial sections from a PET/CT scan with ^{18}F-NaF in a 60-year-old man with type 2 diabetes and active atherosclerosis in the coronary left anterior descending coronary. The low-dose CT component (left panel) shows coronary artery calcifications, with increased ^{18}F-NaF uptake in the PET component (right panel)

In conclusion, PET imaging has shown its unique capability to further characterize the pathophysiological processes of inflammatory vascular diseases. Substantial efforts have been made to standardize the PET imaging procedures at the international level, highlighting the interest of the worldwide nuclear medicine community for this topic. Multimodal hybrid imaging and new PET radiotracers are two key research topics for the coming few years that could significantly improve the patient's management and prognosis capabilities in this field.

Key Learning Points

- Based on the clinical data currently available, [^{18}F]FDG PET/CT(A) has an important role in the diagnosis of extracranial vascular involvement in patients with LVV/PMR.
- Visual methods are most commonly used, but semi-quantitative methods such as the vascular/blood ratio and vascular/liver ratio using SUVs are increasingly being used for [^{18}F]FDG PET/CT.
- The role of [^{18}F]FDG PET/CT in patient management and in treatment monitoring in LVV/PMR and atherosclerosis must be further validated.
- New developments, such as new digital cameras, advantageous reconstruction, and novel, more specific PET radiotracers will overcome the current limitations of [^{18}F]FDG PET/CT for the diagnosis and monitoring of LVV/PMR and atherosclerotic disease.

Glossary

AS	Active segment
CAC	Coronary artery calcium
CETP	Cholesteryl ester transfer protein
cGCA	Cranial giant cell arteritis
CIMT	Carotid intima-media thickness
CT	Computed tomography
CTA	CT angiography
CVA	Cerebrovascular accidents
CVD	Cardiovascular disease
DPP	Dipeptidyl peptidase
[^{18}F]FDG	2-[^{18}F]fluorodeoxyglucose
^{18}F-NaF	Sodium [^{18}F]fluoride
FRS	Framingham risk score
^{68}Ga-DOTATATE	^{68}Ga-DOTA-octreotide
GC	Glucocorticoids
GCA	Giant cell arteritis
HDL-C	High-density lipoprotein cholesterol
LVV	Large vessel vasculitis
lvvGCA	Large vessel vasculitis-giant cell arteritis
MDS	Most diseased segment
MRI	Magnetic resonance imaging
NET	Neuroendocrine tumors
PET	Positron emission tomography
PET/CT	Positron emission tomography/computed tomography
PMR	Polymyalgia rheumatica
SUV	Standardized uptake value
TA	Takayasu arteritis
TBR	Target-to-background ratio
TVS	Total vascular score

References

1. Jennette JC, Falk RJ, Bacon PA, Basu N, Cid MC, Ferrario F, et al. 2012 Revised International Chapel Hill Consensus Conference nomenclature of vasculitides. Arthritis Rheum. 2013;65:1–11.
2. Spanish GCA Study Group, Italian GCA Study Group, Turkish Takayasu Study Group, Vasculitis Clinical Research Consortium, Carmona FD, Coit P, et al. Analysis of the common genetic component of large-vessel vasculitides through a meta-immunochip strategy. Sci Rep. 2017;7:43953.
3. Langford CA, Cuthbertson D, Ytterberg SR, Khalidi N, Monach PA, Carette S, et al. A randomized, double-blind trial of abatacept (CTLA-4Ig) for the treatment of giant cell arteritis. Arthritis Rheumatol. 2017;69:837–45.
4. Langford CA, Cuthbertson D, Ytterberg SR, Khalidi N, Monach PA, Carette S, et al. A randomized, double-blind trial of abatacept (CTLA-4Ig) for the treatment of Takayasu arteritis. Arthritis Rheumatol. 2017;69:846–53.
5. Kubota R, Yamada S, Kubota K, Ishiwata K, Tamahashi N, Ido T. Intratumoral distribution of fluorine-18-fluorodeoxyglucose in vivo: high accumulation in macrophages and granulation tissues studied by microautoradiography. J Nucl Med. 1992;33:1972–80.
6. Ninan J, Lester S, Hill C. Giant cell arteritis. Best Pract Res Clin Rheumatol. 2016;30:169–88.
7. de Souza AWS, de Carvalho JF. Diagnostic and classification criteria of Takayasu arteritis. J Autoimmun. 2014;48–49:79–83.
8. de Boysson H, Liozon E, Ly KH, Dumont A, Delmas C, Aouba A. The different clinical patterns of giant cell arteritis. Clin Exp Rheumatol. 2019;37(Suppl 117):57–60.
9. Weyand CM, Goronzy JJ. Giant-cell arteritis and polymyalgia rheumatica. Solomon CG, editor. N Engl J Med. 2014;371:50–7.
10. de Boysson H, Daumas A, Vautier M, Parienti J-J, Liozon E, Lambert M, et al. Large-vessel involvement and aortic dilation in giant-cell arteritis. A multicenter study of 549 patients. Autoimmun Rev. 2018;17:391–8.
11. Comarmond C, Biard L, Lambert M, Mekinian A, Ferfar Y, Kahn J-E, et al. Long-term outcomes and prognostic factors of complications in Takayasu arteritis: a multicenter study of 318 patients. Circulation. 2017;136:1114–22.
12. Salvarani C, Magnani L, Catanoso M, Pipitone N, Versari A, Dardani L, et al. Tocilizumab: a novel therapy for patients with large-vessel vasculitis. Rheumatology. 2012;51:151–6.
13. Mekinian A, Comarmond C, Resche-Rigon M, Mirault T, Kahn JE, Lambert M, et al. Efficacy of biological-targeted treatments in Takayasu arteritis: multicenter, retrospective study of 49 patients. Circulation. 2015;132:1693–700.
14. Bloch DA, Michel BA, Hunder GG, McShane DJ, Arend WP, Calabrese LH, et al. The American College of Rheumatology 1990 criteria for the classification of vasculitis: patients and methods. Arthritis Rheum. 2010;33:1068–73.

15. Breuer GS, Nesher R, Nesher G. Negative temporal artery biopsies: eventual diagnoses and features of patients with biopsy-negative giant cell arteritis compared to patients without arteritis. Clin Exp Rheumatol. 2008;26:1103–6.
16. Grossman C, Barshack I, Koren-Morag N, Ben-Zvi I, Bornstein G. Baseline clinical predictors of an ultimate giant cell arteritis diagnosis in patients referred to temporal artery biopsy. Clin Rheumatol. 2016;35:1817–22.
17. Muratore F, Kermani TA, Crowson CS, Green AB, Salvarani C, Matteson EL, et al. Large-vessel giant cell arteritis: a cohort study. Rheumatology. 2015;54:463–70.
18. Vander Heiden MG, Cantley LC, Thompson CB. Understanding the Warburg effect: the metabolic requirements of cell proliferation. Science. 2009;324:1029–33.
19. Vaidyanathan S, Patel CN, Scarsbrook AF, Chowdhury FU. FDG PET/CT in infection and inflammation—current and emerging clinical applications. Clin Radiol. 2015;70:787–800.
20. Slart RHJA, Writing Group, Reviewer Group, Members of EANM Cardiovascular, Members of EANM Infection & Inflammation, Members of Committees, SNMMI Cardiovascular, et al. FDG-PET/CT(A) imaging in large vessel vasculitis and polymyalgia rheumatica: joint procedural recommendation of the EANM, SNMMI, and the PET Interest Group (PIG), and endorsed by the ASNC. Eur J Nucl Med Mol Imaging. 2018;45:1250–69.
21. Nielsen BD, Hansen IT, Kramer S, Haraldsen A, Hjorthaug K, Bogsrud TV, et al. Simple dichotomous assessment of cranial artery inflammation by conventional ^{18}F-FDG PET/CT shows high accuracy for the diagnosis of giant cell arteritis: a case-control study. Eur J Nucl Med Mol Imaging. 2019;46:184–93.
22. Sammel AM, Hsiao E, Schembri G, Nguyen K, Brewer J, Schrieber L, et al. Diagnostic accuracy of positron emission tomography/computed tomography of the head, neck, and chest for giant cell arteritis: a prospective, double-blind, cross-sectional study. Arthritis Rheumatol. 2019;71:1319–28.
23. Lee YH, Choi SJ, Ji JD, Song GG. Diagnostic accuracy of ^{18}F-FDG PET or PET/CT for large vessel vasculitis: a meta-analysis. Z Rheumatol. 2016;75:924–31.
24. Besson FL, Parienti J-J, Bienvenu B, Prior JO, Costo S, Bouvard G, et al. Diagnostic performance of ^{18}F-fluorodeoxyglucose positron emission tomography in giant cell arteritis: a systematic review and meta-analysis. Eur J Nucl Med Mol Imaging. 2011;38:1764–72.
25. Soussan M, Nicolas P, Schramm C, Katsahian S, Pop G, Fain O, et al. Management of large-vessel vasculitis with FDG-PET: a systematic literature review and meta-analysis. Medicine. 2015;94:e622.
26. Cheng Y, Lv N, Wang Z, Chen B, Dang A. 18-FDG-PET in assessing disease activity in Takayasu arteritis: a meta-analysis. Clin Exp Rheumatol. 2013;31:S22–7.
27. Lee S-W, Kim S-J, Seo Y, Jeong SY, Ahn B-C, Lee J. F-18 FDG PET for assessment of disease activity of large vessel vasculitis: a systematic review and meta-analysis. J Nucl Cardiol. 2019;26:59–67.
28. Fuchs M, Briel M, Daikeler T, Walker UA, Rasch H, Berg S, et al. The impact of ^{18}F-FDG PET on the management of patients with suspected large vessel vasculitis. Eur J Nucl Med Mol Imaging. 2012;39:344–53.
29. Duftner C, Dejaco C, Sepriano A, Falzon L, Schmidt WA, Ramiro S. Imaging in diagnosis, outcome prediction and monitoring of large vessel vasculitis: a systematic literature review and meta-analysis informing the EULAR recommendations. RMD Open. 2018;4:e000612.
30. Dejaco C, Ramiro S, Duftner C, Besson FL, Bley TA, Blockmans D, et al. EULAR recommendations for the use of imaging in large vessel vasculitis in clinical practice. Ann Rheum Dis. 2018;77:636–43.
31. Daumas A, Rossi P, Bernard-Guervilly F, Francès Y, Berbis J, Durand J-M, et al. Clinical, laboratory, radiological features, and outcome in 26 patients with aortic involvement amongst a case series of 63 patients with giant cell arteritis. Rev Med Interne. 2014;35:4–15.
32. de Boysson H, Dumont A, Liozon E, Lambert M, Boutemy J, Maigné G, et al. Giant-cell arteritis: concordance study between aortic CT angiography and FDG-PET/CT in detection of large-vessel involvement. Eur J Nucl Med Mol Imaging. 2017;44:2274–9.
33. Meller J, Strutz F, Siefker U, Scheel A, Sahlmann CO, Lehmann K, et al. Early diagnosis and follow-up of aortitis with [^{18}F]FDG PET and MRI. Eur J Nucl Med Mol Imaging. 2003;30:730–6.
34. Einspieler I, Thürmel K, Pyka T, Eiber M, Wolfram S, Moog P, et al. Imaging large vessel vasculitis with fully integrated PET/MRI: a pilot study. Eur J Nucl Med Mol Imaging. 2015;42:1012–24.
35. Nielsen BD, Gormsen LC, Hansen IT, Keller KK, Therkildsen P, Hauge E-M. Three days of high-dose glucocorticoid treatment attenuates large-vessel ^{18}F-FDG uptake in large-vessel giant cell arteritis but with a limited impact on diagnostic accuracy. Eur J Nucl Med Mol Imaging. 2018;45:1119–28.
36. Blockmans D, de Ceuninck L, Vanderschueren S, Knockaert D, Mortelmans L, Bobbaers H. Repetitive^{18}F-fluorodeoxyglucose positron emission tomography in giant cell arteritis: a prospective study of 35 patients. Arthritis Rheum. 2006;55:131–7.
37. Gomez L, Chaumet-Riffaud P, Noel N, Lambotte O, Goujard C, Durand E, et al. Effect of CRP value on ^{18}F–FDG PET vascular positivity in Takayasu arteritis: a systematic review and per-patient based meta-analysis. Eur J Nucl Med Mol Imaging. 2018;45:575–81.
38. Banerjee S, Quinn KA, Gribbons KB, Rosenblum JS, Civelek AC, Novakovich E, et al. Effect of treatment on imaging, clinical, and serologic assessments of disease activity in large-vessel vasculitis. J Rheumatol. 2020;47:99–107.
39. Samson M, Devilliers H, Ly KH, Maurier F, Bienvenu B, Terrier B, et al. Tocilizumab as an add-on therapy to glucocorticoids during the first 3 months of treatment of Giant cell arteritis: a prospective study. Eur J Intern Med. 2018;57:96–104.
40. Dellavedova L, Carletto M, Faggioli P, Sciascera A, Del Sole A, Mazzone A, et al. The prognostic value of baseline ^{18}F-FDG PET/CT in steroid-naïve large-vessel vasculitis: introduction of volume-based parameters. Eur J Nucl Med Mol Imaging. 2016;43:340–8.
41. Tezuka D, Haraguchi G, Ishihara T, Ohigashi H, Inagaki H, Suzuki J, et al. Role of FDG PET-CT in Takayasu arteritis. JACC Cardiovasc Imaging. 2012;5:422–9.
42. Blockmans D, Coudyzer W, Vanderschueren S, Stroobants S, Loeckx D, Heye S, et al. Relationship between fluorodeoxyglucose uptake in the large vessels and late aortic diameter in giant cell arteritis. Rheumatology. 2008;47:1179–84.
43. de Boysson H, Liozon E, Lambert M, Parienti J-J, Artigues N, Geffray L, et al. ^{18}F-fluorodeoxyglucose positron emission tomography and the risk of subsequent aortic complications in giant-cell arteritis: a multicenter cohort of 130 patients. Medicine. 2016;95:e3851.
44. Bergheanu SC, Bodde MC, Jukema JW. Pathophysiology and treatment of atherosclerosis: current view and future perspective on lipoprotein modification treatment. Neth Heart J. 2017;25:231–42.
45. Falk E. Pathogenesis of atherosclerosis. J Am Coll Cardiol. 2006;47:C7–12.
46. Rafieian-Kopaei M, Setorki M, Doudi M, Baradaran A, Nasri H. Atherosclerosis: process, indicators, risk factors and new hopes. Int J Prev Med. 2014;5:927–46.
47. Tahara N, Kai H, Ishibashi M, Nakaura H, Kaida H, Baba K, et al. Simvastatin attenuates plaque inflammation. J Am Coll Cardiol. 2006;48:1825–31.
48. Marnane M, Prendeville S, McDonnell C, Noone I, Barry M, Crowe M, et al. Plaque inflammation and unstable morphology are associated with early stroke recurrence in symptomatic carotid stenosis. Stroke. 2014;45:801–6.

49. Carr S, Farb A, Pearce WH, Virmani R, Yao JST. Atherosclerotic plaque rupture in symptomatic carotid artery stenosis. J Vasc Surg. 1996;23:755–66.
50. Tarkin JM, Joshi FR, Rudd JHF. PET imaging of inflammation in atherosclerosis. Nat Rev Cardiol. 2014;11:443–57.
51. Tawakol A, Migrino RQ, Bashian GG, Bedri S, Vermylen D, Cury RC, et al. In vivo ^{18}F-fluorodeoxyglucose positron emission tomography imaging provides a noninvasive measure of carotid plaque inflammation in patients. J Am Coll Cardiol. 2006;48:1818–24.
52. Bucerius J, Duivenvoorden R, Mani V, Moncrieff C, Rudd JHF, Calcagno C, et al. Prevalence and risk factors of carotid vessel wall inflammation in coronary artery disease patients. JACC Cardiovasc Imaging. 2011;4:1195–205.
53. Ishii H, Nishio M, Takahashi H, Aoyama T, Tanaka M, Toriyama T, et al. Comparison of atorvastatin 5 and 20 mg/d for reducing F-18 fluorodeoxyglucose uptake in atherosclerotic plaques on positron emission tomography/computed tomography: a randomized, investigator-blinded, open-label, 6-month study in Japanese adults scheduled for percutaneous coronary intervention. Clin Ther. 2010;32:2337–47.
54. On behalf of the Cardiovascular Committee of the European Association of Nuclear Medicine (EANM), Bucerius J, Hyafil F, Verberne HJ, Slart RHJA, Lindner O, et al. Position paper of the Cardiovascular Committee of the European Association of Nuclear Medicine (EANM) on PET imaging of atherosclerosis. Eur J Nucl Med Mol Imaging. 2016;43:780–92.
55. Rudd JHF, Warburton EA, Fryer TD, Jones HA, Clark JC, Antoun N, et al. Imaging atherosclerotic plaque inflammation with [^{18}F]-fluorodeoxyglucose positron emission tomography. Circulation. 2002;105:2708–11.
56. Rudd JHF, Myers KS, Bansilal S, Machac J, Rafique A, Farkouh M, et al. ^{18}Fluorodeoxyglucose positron emission tomography imaging of atherosclerotic plaque inflammation is highly reproducible. J Am Coll Cardiol. 2007;50:892–6.
57. Rudd JHF, Myers KS, Bansilal S, Machac J, Pinto CA, Tong C, et al. Atherosclerosis inflammation imaging with ^{18}F-FDG PET: carotid, iliac, and femoral uptake reproducibility, quantification methods, and recommendations. J Nucl Med. 2008;49:871–8.
58. Kim TN, Kim S, Yang SJ, Yoo HJ, Seo JA, Kim SG, et al. Vascular inflammation in patients with impaired glucose tolerance and type 2 diabetes: analysis with ^{18}F-fluorodeoxyglucose positron emission tomography. Circ Cardiovasc Imaging. 2010;3:142–8.
59. Tahara N, Kai H, Yamagishi S, Mizoguchi M, Nakaura H, Ishibashi M, et al. Vascular inflammation evaluated by [^{18}F]-fluorodeoxyglucose positron emission tomography is associated with the metabolic syndrome. J Am Coll Cardiol. 2007;49:1533–9.
60. Bucerius J, Mani V, Moncrieff C, Rudd JHF, Machac J, Fuster V, et al. Impact of noninsulin-dependent type 2 diabetes on carotid wall ^{18}F-fluorodeoxyglucose positron emission tomography uptake. J Am Coll Cardiol. 2012;59:2080–8.
61. van der Valk FM, Verweij SL, Zwinderman KAH, Strang AC, Kaiser Y, Marquering HA, et al. Thresholds for arterial wall inflammation quantified by ^{18}F-FDG PET imaging. JACC Cardiovasc Imaging. 2016;9:1198–207.
62. Rominger A, Saam T, Wolpers S, Cyran CC, Schmidt M, Foerster S, et al. ^{18}F-FDG PET/CT identifies patients at risk for future vascular events in an otherwise asymptomatic cohort with neoplastic disease. J Nucl Med. 2009;50:1611–20.
63. Marnane M, Merwick A, Sheehan OC, Hannon N, Foran P, Grant T, et al. Carotid plaque inflammation on ^{18}F-fluorodeoxyglucose positron emission tomography predicts early stroke recurrence. Ann Neurol. 2012;71:709–18.
64. Kelly PJ, Camps-Renom P, Giannotti N, Martí-Fàbregas J, Murphy S, McNulty J, et al. Carotid plaque inflammation imaged by ^{18}F-fluorodeoxyglucose positron emission tomography and risk of early recurrent stroke. Stroke. 2019;50:1766–73.
65. Figueroa AL, Abdelbaky A, Truong QA, Corsini E, MacNabb MH, Lavender ZR, et al. Measurement of arterial activity on routine FDG PET/CT images improves prediction of risk of future CV events. JACC Cardiovasc Imaging. 2013;6:1250–9.
66. Moon SH, Cho YS, Noh TS, Choi JY, Kim B-T, Lee K-H. Carotid FDG uptake improves prediction of future cardiovascular events in asymptomatic individuals. JACC Cardiovasc Imaging. 2015;8:949–56.
67. Cho S-G, Park KS, Kim J, Kang S-R, Kwon SY, Seon HJ, et al. Prediction of coronary artery calcium progression by FDG uptake of large arteries in asymptomatic individuals. Eur J Nucl Med Mol Imaging. 2017;44:129–40.
68. Tawakol A, Fayad ZA, Mogg R, Alon A, Klimas MT, Dansky H, et al. Intensification of statin therapy results in a rapid reduction in atherosclerotic inflammation. J Am Coll Cardiol. 2013;62:909–17.
69. Fayad ZA, Mani V, Woodward M, Kallend D, Abt M, Burgess T, et al. Safety and efficacy of dalcetrapib on atherosclerotic disease using novel non-invasive multimodality imaging (dal-PLAQUE): a randomised clinical trial. Lancet. 2011;378:1547–59.
70. Elkhawad M, Rudd JHF, Sarov-Blat L, Cai G, Wells R, Davies LC, et al. Effects of p38 mitogen-activated protein kinase inhibition on vascular and systemic inflammation in patients with atherosclerosis. JACC Cardiovasc Imaging. 2012;5:911–22.
71. Emami H, Vucic E, Subramanian S, Abdelbaky A, Fayad ZA, Du S, et al. The effect of BMS-582949, a P38 mitogen-activated protein kinase (P38 MAPK) inhibitor on arterial inflammation: a multicenter FDG-PET trial. Atherosclerosis. 2015;240:490–6.
72. Scheen AJ. Cardiovascular effects of gliptins. Nat Rev Cardiol. 2013;10:73–84.
73. de Boer SA, Heerspink HJL, Lefrandt JD, Hovinga-de Boer MC, van Roon AM, Juárez Orozco LE, et al. Effect of linagliptin on arterial ^{18}F-fluorodeoxyglucose positron emission tomography uptake. J Am Coll Cardiol. 2017;69:1097–8.
74. Adams RL, Adams IP, Lindow SW, Zhong W, Atkin SL. Somatostatin receptors 2 and 5 are preferentially expressed in proliferating endothelium. Br J Cancer. 2005;92:1493–8.
75. Armani C, Catalani E, Balbarini A, Bagnoli P, Cervia D. Expression, pharmacology, and functional role of somatostatin receptor subtypes 1 and 2 in human macrophages. J Leukoc Biol. 2007;81:845–55.
76. Tarkin JM, Joshi FR, Evans NR, Chowdhury MM, Figg NL, Shah AV, et al. Detection of atherosclerotic inflammation by ^{68}Ga-DOTATATE PET compared to [^{18}F]FDG PET imaging. J Am Coll Cardiol. 2017;69:1774–91.
77. Dweck MR, Chow MWL, Joshi NV, Williams MC, Jones C, Fletcher AM, et al. Coronary arterial ^{18}F-sodium fluoride uptake. J Am Coll Cardiol. 2012;59:1539–48.
78. Dweck MR, Jones C, Joshi NV, Fletcher AM, Richardson H, White A, et al. Assessment of valvular calcification and inflammation by positron emission tomography in patients with aortic stenosis. Circulation. 2012;125:76–86.
79. Dweck MR, Khaw HJ, Sng GKZ, Luo ELC, Baird A, Williams MC, et al. Aortic stenosis, atherosclerosis, and skeletal bone: is there a common link with calcification and inflammation? Eur Heart J. 2013;34:1567–74.
80. Joshi NV, Vesey AT, Williams MC, Shah ASV, Calvert PA, Craighead FHM, et al. ^{18}F-fluoride positron emission tomography for identification of ruptured and high-risk coronary atherosclerotic plaques: a prospective clinical trial. Lancet. 2014;383:705–13.

Radionuclide Imaging of Infection and Inflammation in Pediatrics

16

Maria Carmen Garganese, Maria Felicia Villani, and Giovanni D'Errico

Contents

Learning Objectives

- To acquire basic knowledge of the most frequent indications for radiolabeled leukocyte scintigraphy in children
- To become familiar with typical features of radiolabeled leukocyte scintigraphy in children

Infections are a frequent occurrence in children, ranging from mild to severe diseases [1], and are often caused by bacteria [2]. The most common infections in childhood involve bones, lungs, kidneys, brain, and heart [2].

Nuclear medicine imaging tests are often necessary in the diagnostic work-up and when assessing response to therapy in pediatric infections. In particular:

- Three-phase bone scintigraphy with ^{99m}Tc-diphosphonates (most frequently ^{99m}Tc-MDP) helps in the diagnosis of acute and chronic osteomyelitis; this diagnostic procedure is characterized by high sensitivity, but low specificity.
- The role of PET/CT with the metabolic tracer [^{18}F]FDG is steadily growing in many conditions, such as osteomyelitis [3–5], inflammatory bowel disease [3, 6–8], and fever of unknown origin [3, 9–11]; despite some limitations (e.g., low specificity, high costs) [12], it has many advantages, such as high spatial resolution and high sensitivity [3].
- Scintigraphy with radiolabeled autologous leukocytes is used in several clinical conditions [13]; its limitations include a relatively high radiation burden and complexity of the labeling procedure.

Scintigraphy with radiolabeled leukocytes is a useful and often essential tool in the evaluation of many infectious conditions in children. The most common indications for this procedure include cardiovascular system infections (endocarditis, prosthetic vascular graft infections), orthopedic hardware infections (prosthetic joints, fixation devices), inflammatory bowel disease, and fever of unknown origin [13].

Performing the scan and interpreting the images so obtained in children require both full knowledge of the technical and clinical aspects and a coordinated teamwork of professionals experienced in pediatrics. For these reasons, in this chapter, we choose to discuss in particular scintigraphy with radiolabeled leukocytes in order to emphasize its complexity and to focus on image features, describing the procedure we apply and discussing some interesting cases we dealt with in our Nuclear Medicine Unit.

M. C. Garganese (✉) · M. F. Villani
Nuclear Medicine Unit, Department of Imaging, "Bambino Gesù" Pediatric Hospital, Rome, Italy
e-mail: mcarmen.garganese@opbg.net

G. D'Errico
Department of Nuclear Medicine, Private Hospital "Pio XI", Rome, Italy

E. Lazzeri et al. (eds.), *Radionuclide Imaging of Infection and Inflammation*, https://doi.org/10.1007/978-3-030-62175-9_16

For isolation and labeling of leukocytes, a closed disposable sterile system (Leukokit®, GE Healthcare) is currently used in our Nuclear Medicine Unit for labeling leukocytes with ^{99m}Tc-HMPAO, strictly following the manufacturer's instructions. Although the optimal volume of blood to be withdrawn is 50 mL in adults, it is difficult to achieve this volume in children; therefore, smaller volumes are usually drawn, according to body weight (but at least 20 mL) [13]. The appropriate activity of ^{99m}Tc-HMPAO-leukocytes, according to patient' weight [14], is injected.

Five minutes after the administration of radiolabeled leukocytes, two static images are acquired: one including the thorax and abdomen (necessary to evaluate biodistribution in lungs, liver and spleen), the other one over the region of interest. Two hours later, a whole-body acquisition and a static image of the region of interest are recorded; a SPECT (preferably SPECT/CT) acquisition is usually added at this time.

The final acquisitions at 24 h post-injection include a static vies and a SPECT acquisition of the region of interest. All the images are acquired without anesthesia and sedation.

Although manual fusion of the images is possible, the use of a hybrid SPECT/CT gamma camera facilitates image fusion and correction for attenuation.

Clinical Cases

Case 16.1

Background

A 4-year-old boy with severe dilative cardiomyopathy was hospitalized in cardiovascular intensive care unit, waiting to be listed for heart transplantation; a biventricular assist device (BIVAD)—Berlin heart—and a tracheostomy were placed in order to support blood circulation and mechanic ventilation, respectively. On the 95th day of hospitalization, the patient developed fever resistant to antibiotic treatment; swab tests on the skin surrounding BIVAD tubes revealed the presence of *Staphylococcus aureus*, *Escherichia coli*, and Klebsiella. The plain chest X-ray showed severe cardiomegaly, a retrocardiac consolidation in left lung, and diffuse interstitial involvement (Fig. 16.1). A radiolabeled leucocyte scintigraphy was performed in order to rule out infection of BIVAD and/or an endocarditis.

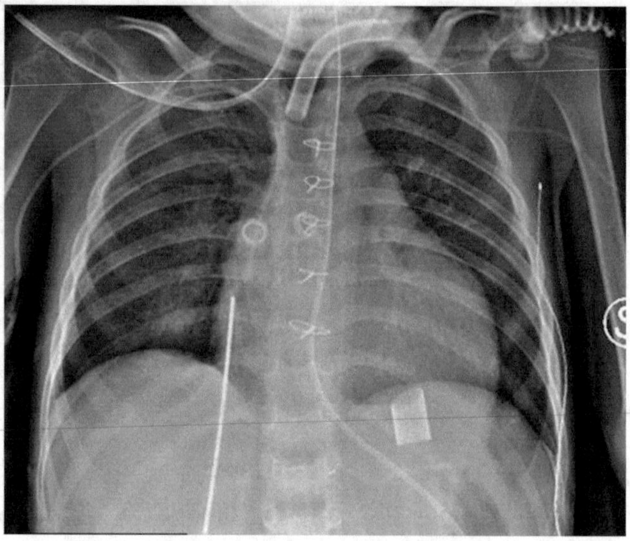

Fig. 16.1 Plain chest X-ray, showing severe cardiomegaly, retrocardiac opacity in left lung, and diffuse interstitial involvement

Findings

Planar imaging did not show any focus of abnormal accumulation of radiolabeled leukocytes (Fig. 16.2). The manually fused SPECT/CT images showed abnormally high accumulation of the radiolabeled leukocytes into multiple consolidations in both lungs (Fig. 16.3), but no other focal abnormalities were detected in the BIVAD or in the endocardium (Fig. 16.4). Antibiotic therapy was subsequently modified, with resolution of fever.

Conclusion/Teaching Points

SPECT/CT images are mandatory in order to improve diagnostic accuracy, to define the localization of uptake and to confirm the absence of abnormal uptake evident on static images.

Case 16.2

A 17-year-old boy, followed in our Cardiology Department for Laubry and Pezzi syndrome and aortic insufficiency surgically treated multiple times (last surgery: aortic valve replacement with bioprosthetic valve, 6 years earlier), was referred to the accident and emergency unit for vomit and fever and was hospitalized.

Chest CT showed a large fluid collection in the anterior mediastinum, close to the aortic conduit. Blood culture yielded *Staphylococcus aureus*, but there were no signs of endocarditis on echocardiography. Suspecting an involvement of the conduct, a radiolabeled leucocyte scintigraphy was scheduled, and appropriate antibiotic therapy was prescribed.

Findings

Planar imaging at 2 h showed a focal area of increased accumulation in the thorax, near the left side of the sternal manubrium, increasing in intensity at 24 h (Fig. 16.4). The manually fused SPECT/CT images showed radiolabeled

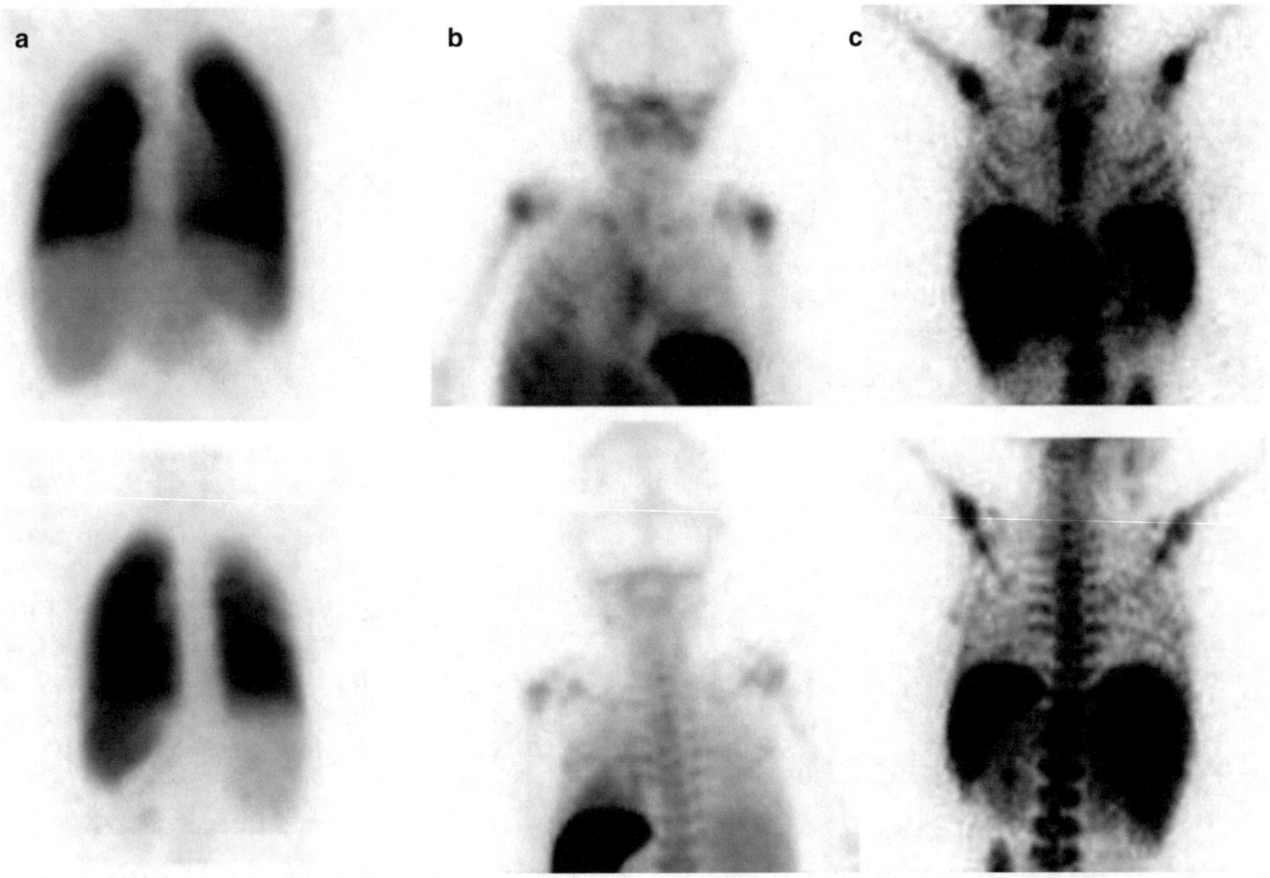

Fig. 16.2 Planar radiolabeled leukocyte anterior and posterior views, showing normal biodistribution in lungs, liver, and spleen at 5 min (**a**); a faint area of leukocyte accumulation in the base of left lung is detected at 2 h (**b**) and at 24 h (**c**)

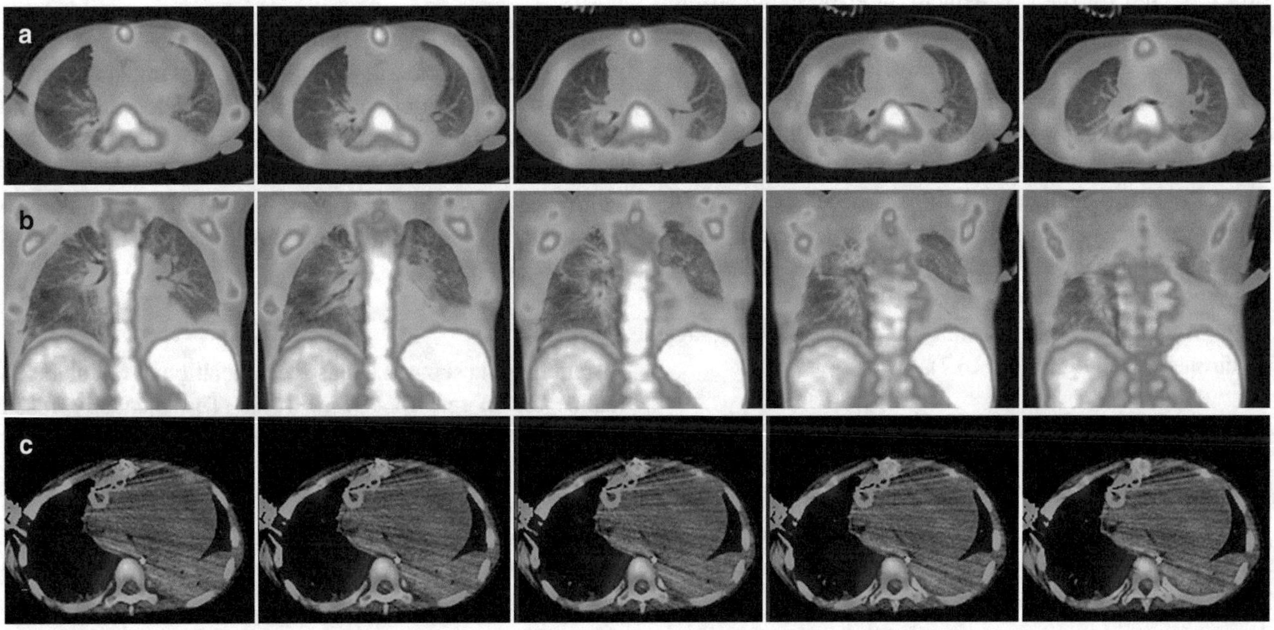

Fig. 16.3 Manually fused SPECT/CT images, demonstrating radiolabeled leukocyte accumulation into multiple consolidations in the apical posterior segment of right superior lobe, in the apical segment of the right inferior lobe and in the left inferior lobe, respectively (**a**, transaxial sections; **b**, coronal sections); no abnormal accumulation of labeled leukocytes can be detected on the endocardium (**c**)

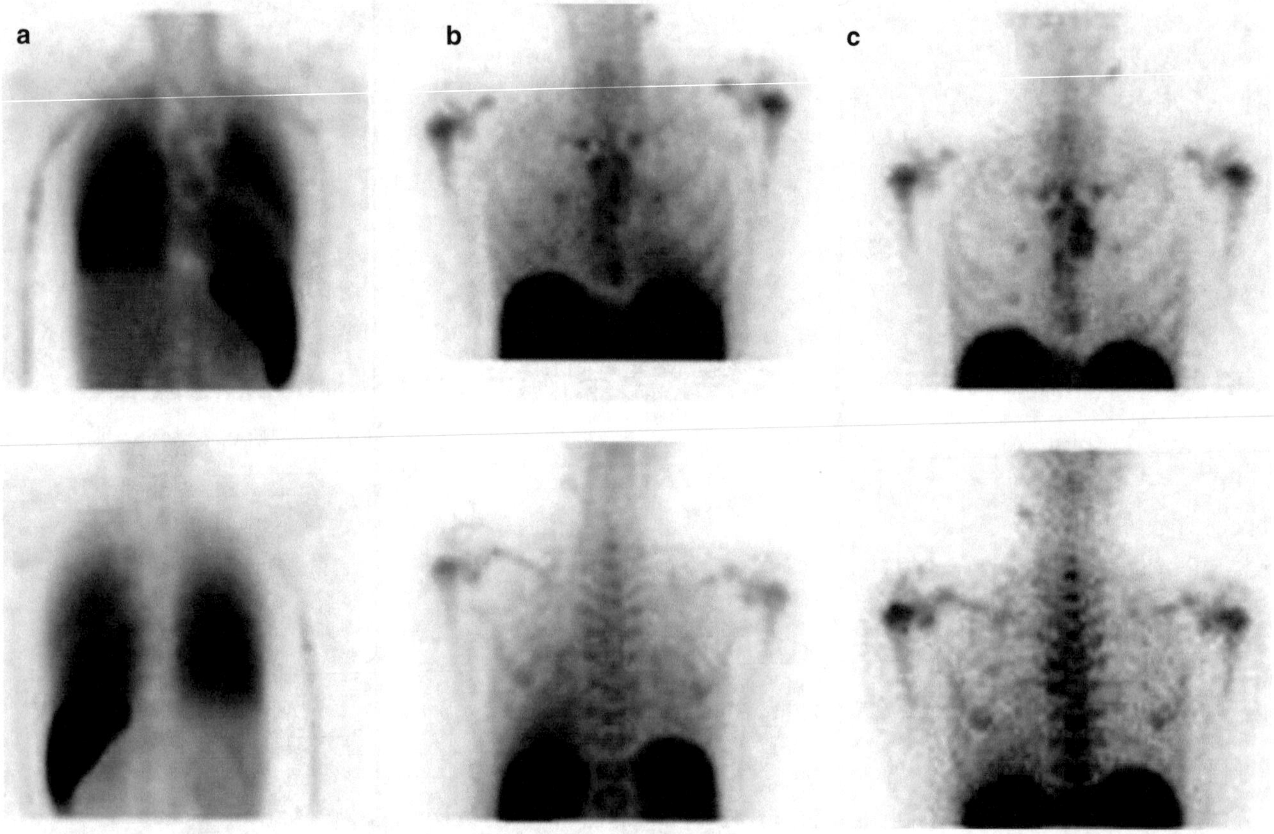

Fig. 16.4 Planar radiolabeled leukocyte anterior and posterior views, showing normal biodistribution in lungs, liver, and spleen at 5 min (**a**), abnormal accumulation in the thorax, near the left side of the sternal manubrium at 2 h (**b**), increasing in intensity at 24 h (**c**)

leukocytes accumulation into the known fluid collection detected on the CT scan in anterior mediastinum, but no foci of abnormal accumulation of radiolabeled leukocytes on the aortic conduit nor on the valve (Fig. 16.5).

Antibiotic therapy was subsequently modified, and the collection was surgically drained, with resolution of fever. At the end of antibiotic therapy, radiolabeled leucocyte scintigraphy was repeated in order to confirm resolution of the infection. Planar imaging images did not show any focus of abnormal accumulation of radiolabeled leukocytes (Fig. 16.6), and also the manually fused SPECT/CT images confirmed this finding (Fig. 16.7).

Conclusion/Teaching Points

Radiolabeled leukocyte scintigraphy helps in the differential diagnosis of fluid collections in post-surgical patients (abscess versus sterile collection), allowing better definition of therapeutic management. This procedure is also useful to verify the efficacy of antibiotic therapy.

Case 16.3

A 10-year-old boy with left tibial osteosarcoma, previously treated with chemotherapy, amputation, and implant of prosthesis, 4 months after surgery presented dehiscence of the wound, fever, and pain in the left foot. An ultrasound scan showed nonspecific thickening of soft tissue in left ankle. Left leg and foot showed no signs of osteomyelitis. A radiolabeled leukocyte scintigraphy was performed in order to rule out osteomyelitis.

Findings

Planar imaging showed intense accumulation of radiolabeled leukocytes in left foot (Fig. 16.8). The manually fused SPECT/CT images showed abnormally high accumulation of radiolabeled leukocytes in astragalus, around the prosthesis, and additional foci of accumulation in tarsus and metatarsus (Fig. 16.9).

Antibiotic therapy was started, with resolution of fever and pain relief within 7 days.

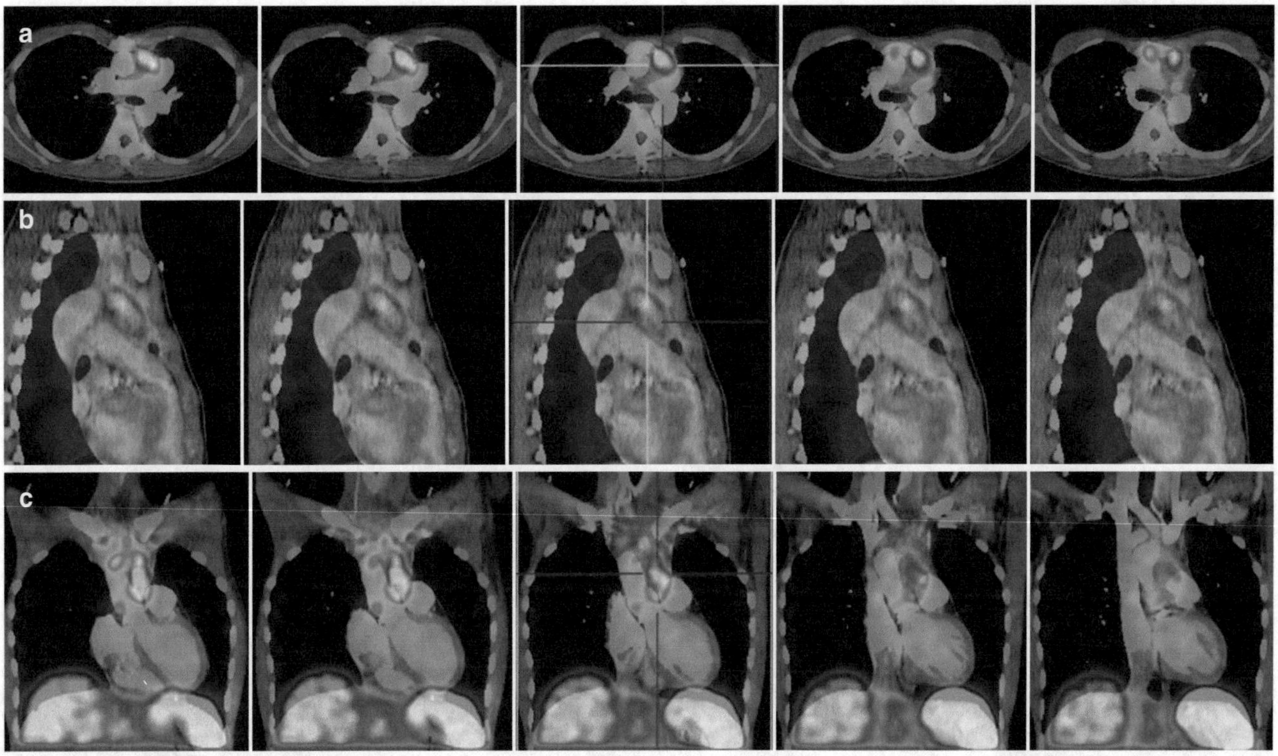

Fig. 16.5 Manually fused SPECT/CT images, showing accumulation of radiolabeled leukocytes into the fluid collection in anterior mediastinum; no focus of abnormal accumulation of radiolabeled leukocytes is detected on the aortic conduit nor on the valve (**a**, transaxial sections; **b**, sagittal section; **c**, coronal section)

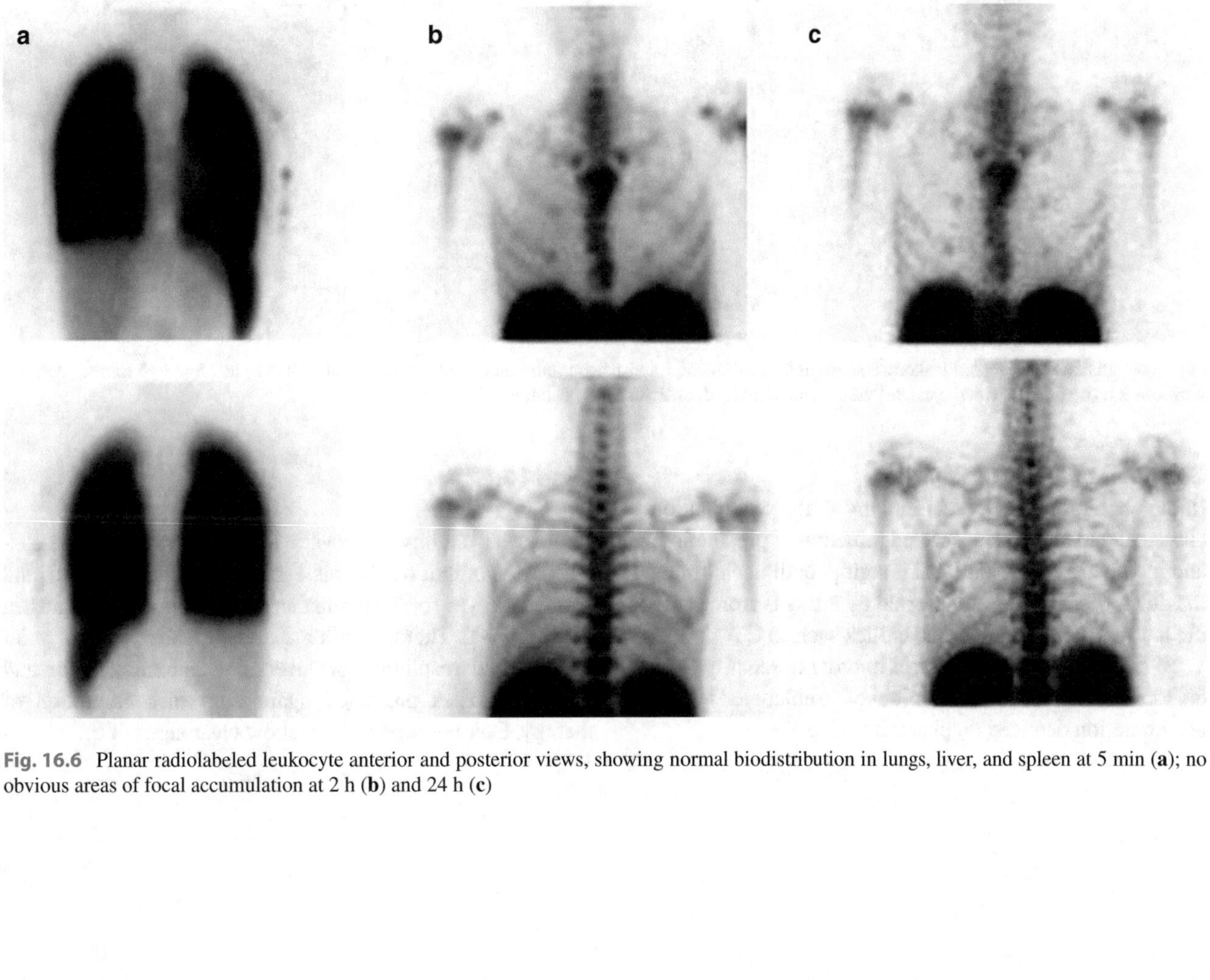

Fig. 16.6 Planar radiolabeled leukocyte anterior and posterior views, showing normal biodistribution in lungs, liver, and spleen at 5 min (**a**); no obvious areas of focal accumulation at 2 h (**b**) and 24 h (**c**)

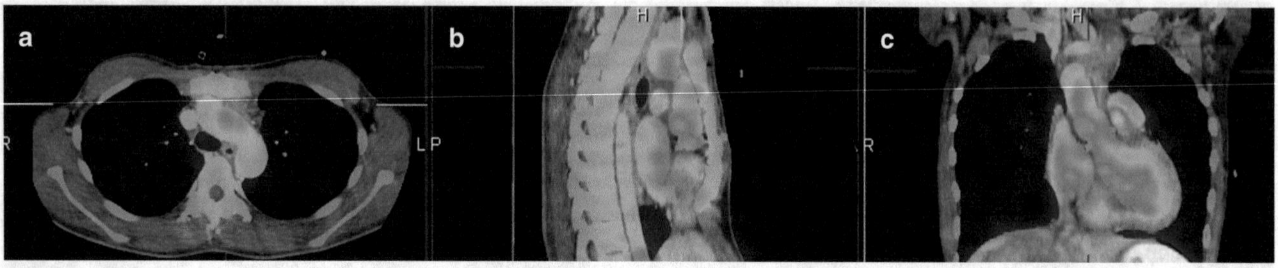

Fig. 16.7 Manually fused SPECT/CT images, showing no evidence of abnormal accumulation in the mediastinum (**a**, transaxial section; **b**, sagittal section; **c**, coronal section)

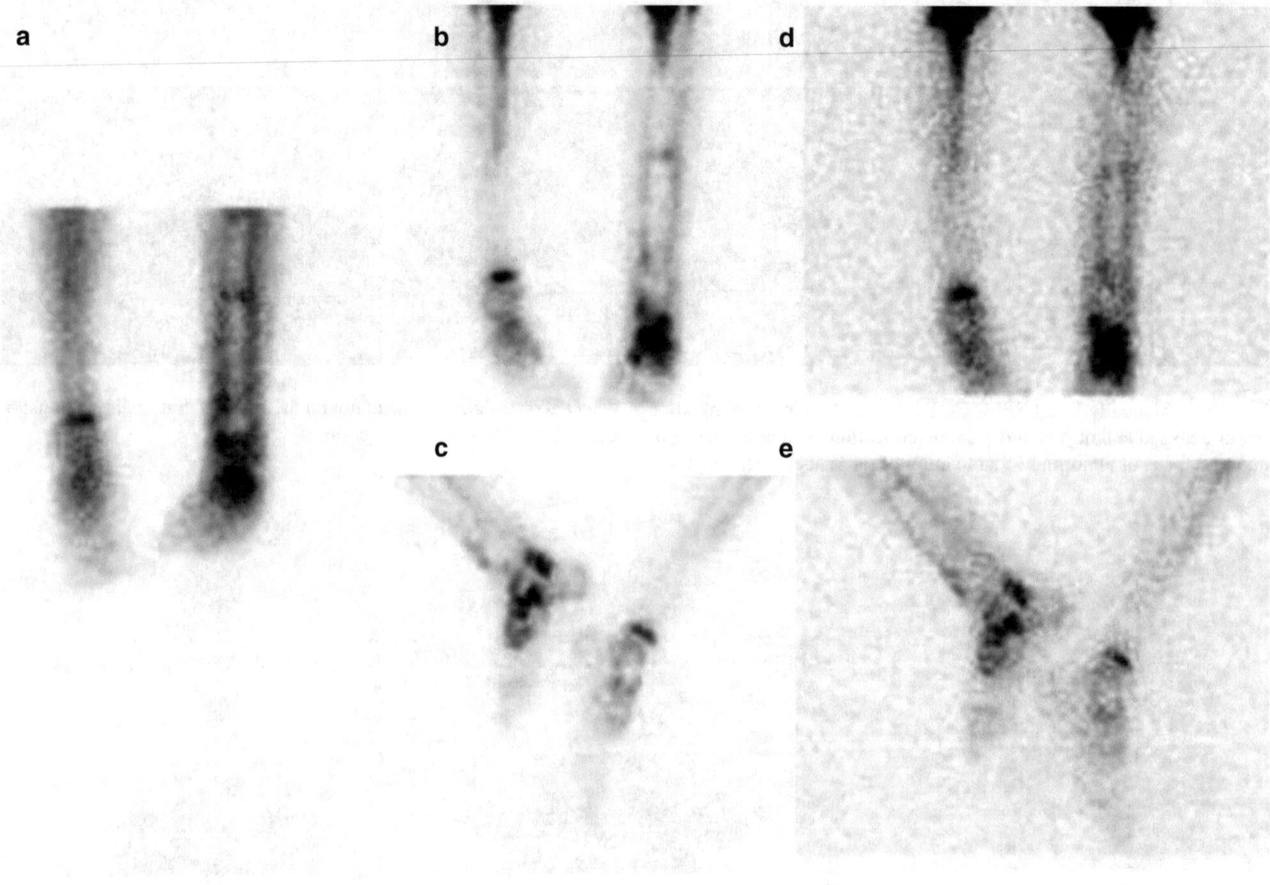

Fig. 16.8 Planar radiolabeled leukocyte static images, showing intense accumulation of radiolabeled leukocytes in left foot at 5 min (**a**, anterior view), at 2 h (**b**, anterior view; **c**, lateral view), and at 24 h (**d**, anterior view; **e**, lateral view)

Conclusion/Teaching Points

Radiolabeled leukocyte scintigraphy is the examination of choice in patients with suspected infection of prosthetic joint and inconclusive conventional imaging, both in children and in adults, because it is not affected by artifacts from orthopedic hardware, unlike other modalities such as CT.

SPECT/CT images are useful in order to identify the precise anatomical localization of foci of radiolabeled leukocyte accumulation detected on planar imaging.

Case 16.4

An 18-year-old boy with cystic fibrosis followed by the cystic fibrosis unit of our hospital presented abdominal pain and recurring fever for 2 months; an episode of bloody diarrhea also occurred. Therapy with mesalazine lead to prompt relief of pain and resolution of fever, but abdominal pain and bloody diarrhea presented again after discontinuation of therapy. Colonoscopy did not show clear signs of inflamma-

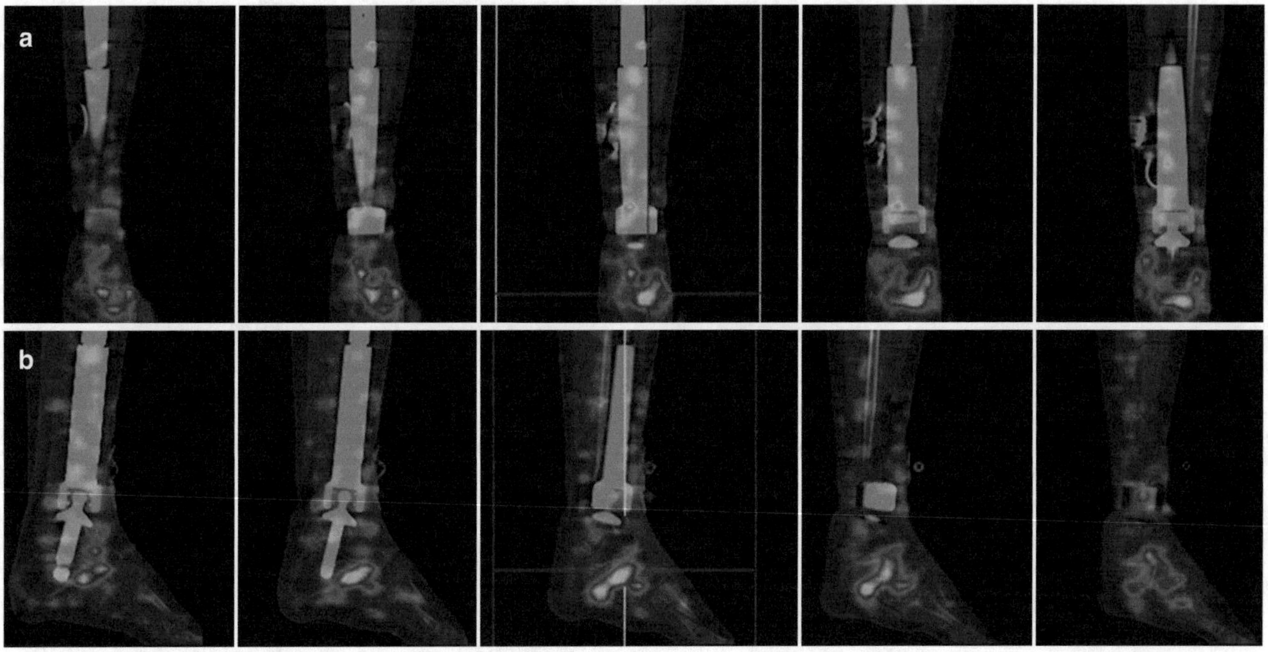

Fig. 16.9 Manually fused SPECT/CT images, showing diffuse radiolabeled leukocytes accumulation in astragalus, around the prosthesis (**a**, coronal sections), and additional foci of accumulation in tarsus and metatarsus (**b**, sagittal sections)

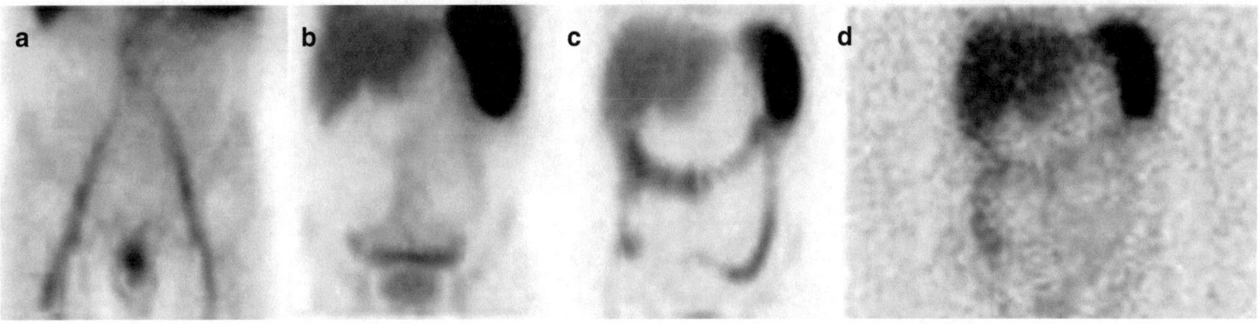

Fig. 16.10 Planar radiolabeled leukocytes anterior views, showing normal biodistribution in liver and spleen at 5 min (**a**), diffuse radiolabeled leukocyte accumulation in ascending, transverse, and descending colon at 2 h (**b**) and 24 h (**c**); abnormal accumulation persisted at 48 h (**d**)

tion, but histological examination revealed nonspecific inflammatory infiltration. A radiolabeled leukocytes scintigraphy was scheduled in order to confirm the clinical diagnosis of inflammatory bowel disease.

Findings

Planar imaging showed diffuse accumulation of radiolabeled leukocytes in the colon, persisting at 24 and 48 h (Fig. 16.10); this pattern suggested inflammatory bowel disease. Long-term therapy with mesalazine was therefore started again, with resolution of signs and symptoms.

Conclusion/Teaching Points

Radiolabeled leukocyte scintigraphy can help to confirm the diagnosis in patients with symptoms suggestive of inflammatory bowel disease (abdominal pain and/or fever and/or bloody diarrhea), but inconclusive endoscopy. Additional imaging at 48 h is useful to distinguish physiological excretion in the bowel from pathological accumulation of radiolabeled leukocytes.

References

1. Schuster JE, Newland JG. Old and new infections of childhood. Infect Dis Clin N Am. 2018;32:xiii–xiv.
2. Signore A, Glaudemans AWJM, Gheysens O, et al. Nuclear medicine imaging in pediatric infection or chronic inflammatory diseases. Semin Nucl Med. 2017;47:286–303.
3. Parisi MT, Otjen JP, Stanescu AL, Shulkin BL. Radionuclide imaging of infection and inflammation in children: a review. Semin Nucl Med. 2018;48:148–65.

Index

E. Lazzeri et al. (eds.), *Radionuclide Imaging of Infection and Inflammation*, https://doi.org/10.1007/978-3-030-62175-9

Printed in the United States
by Baker & Taylor Publisher Services